Viva and OSCE Exams in Ophthalmology

Timothy H. M. Fung
Winfried M. K. Amoaku
Editors

Viva and OSCE Exams in Ophthalmology

A Revision Study Guide

Second Edition

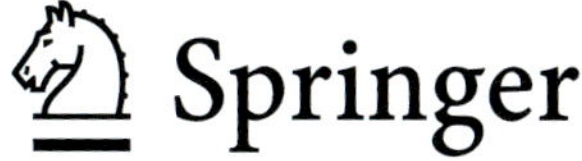

Editors
Timothy H. M. Fung
University Hospitals of Derby & Burton
NHS Foundation Trust,
Royal Derby Hospital
Derby, UK

Winfried M. K. Amoaku
Eye, Ear, Nose and Throat Centre,
Queens Medical Centre
Nottingham University
Hospitals NHS Trust
Nottingham, UK

ISBN 978-3-031-97400-7 ISBN 978-3-031-97401-4 (eBook)
https://doi.org/10.1007/978-3-031-97401-4

This Springer imprint is published by the registered company Springer Nature Switzerland AG
The registered company address is: Gewerbestrasse 11, 6330 Cham, Switzerland

Preface

Readers of the first edition will understand that this textbook aims to provide a comprehensive revision resource for ophthalmology examination candidates preparing for their Viva and OSCE exams. Since the publication of the first edition in 2020, there have been significant developments, including new clinical trials that have impacted practices, as well as updates to national clinical guidelines and technology appraisal guidance from the National Institute for Health and Care Excellence. This edition has been thoroughly revised and expanded to reflect the latest information and treatments across various subspecialties in ophthalmology, making it valuable for both new and returning users of the book.

The second edition continues to primarily target individuals preparing for the Part 2 FRCOphth Oral examination. Since the release of the first edition, this examination has expanded internationally to include locations such as Singapore, Egypt, Greece, Dubai, India, Pakistan, and Malaysia. We hope this book will also benefit candidates preparing for other ophthalmology membership or fellowship exams in different jurisdictions, as well as allied health professionals seeking to enhance their general knowledge of ophthalmology.

Given the visual nature of the subject matter and the importance of recognising signs in various ophthalmic pathologies, we are pleased to include an increased number of images in this edition. For the first time, all images published in this edition will be available online in an enlarged, higher-resolution format. Additionally, we have provided some ocular motility videos, which will also be accessible online, adding further value to the text. Our thanks to Shery Thomas and Emily Hogan for making these videos available.

Finally, we would like to express our gratitude to all candidates, trainers, and examiners who provided valuable feedback on the book, along with their compliments and support. To all prospective candidates, we wish you great success in your exams and future careers, and we hope this book contributes to your achievements in some way.

Derby, UK Timothy H. M. Fung
Nottingham, UK Winfried M. K. Amoaku

Contents

About the Editors

Timothy H. M. Fung is a practicing consultant ophthalmologist specialising in vitreoretinal surgery. He has published numerous peer-reviewed articles on a variety of clinical ophthalmic topics.

Winfried M. K. Amoaku is also a practicing consultant ophthalmologist, with a subspecialty interest in medical retina. He serves as an examiner for the FRCOphth Part 2 oral exam and has an extensive publication record, with over 120 peer-reviewed publications on clinical and other ophthalmic topics.

Glossary of Abbreviations

AAC	Acute angle closure
ABK	Aphakic bullous keratopathy
AC	Anterior chamber
ACE	Angiotensin converting enzyme
ACG	Angle closure glaucoma
ACIOL	Anterior chamber intraocular lens
AD	Autosomal dominant
AF	Atrial fibrillation
AIM	Acute idiopathic maculopathy
AION	Anterior ischaemic optic neuropathy
AKC	Atopic keratoconjunctivitis
AL	Axial length
AMD	Age-related macular degeneration
ANA	Anti-nuclear antibodies
ANCA	Anti-neutrophil cytoplasmic antibodies
APMPPE	Acute posterior multifocal placoid pigment epitheliopathy
AR	Autosomal recessive
ARN	Acute retinal necrosis
AS-OCT	Anterior segment optical coherence tomography
AZT	Azathioprine
BALAD	Bacillary layer detachment
BCC	Basal cell carcinoma
BCL	Bandage contact lens
BCVA	Best corrected visual acuity
BD	Twice a day
BK	Band keratopathy
BMD	Best's macular dystrophy
BMO	Bruch's membrane opening
BMO-MRW	Bruch's membrane opening-minimum rim width
BP	Blood pressure
BPES	Blepharophimosis epicanthus syndrome
BRAO	Branch retinal artery occlusion
BRVO	Branch retinal vein occlusion
BSV	Binocular single vision
CAR	Cancer associated retinopathy
CAS	Clinical activity score
CCT	Central corneal thickness

CDR	Cup-to-disc ratio
CHED	Congenital hereditary endothelial dystrophy
CJD	Creutzfeldt-Jakob disease
CKD	Chronic kidney disease
CL	Contact lens
CLRAO	Cilioretinal artery occlusion
CME	Continuing medical education
CMO	Cystoid macular oedema
CMV	Cytomegalovirus
CN	Cranial nerve
CNLDO	Congenital nasolacrimal duct obstruction
CNS	Central nervous system
CNV	Choroidal neovascularisation
CRA	Central retinal artery
CRV	Central retinal vein
COAG	Chronic open angle glaucoma
CPD	Continuing professional development
CPEO	Chronic progressive external ophthalmoplegia
CPSD	Corrected pattern standard deviation
CRA	Central retinal artery
CRAO	Central retinal artery occlusion
CRP	C-reactive protein
CRVO	Central retinal vein occlusion
CSF	Cerebrospinal fluid
CSMO	Clinically significant macular oedema
CSNB	Congenital stationary night blindness
CSR	Central serous chorioretinopathy
CT	Computed tomography
CTA	Computed tomography angiography
CTR	Capsular tension ring
CVA	Cerebrovascular accident
CWS	Cotton wool spot
CXR	Chest X-ray
DALK	Deep anterior lamellar keratoplasty
DCG	Dacryocystography
DCR	Dacryocystorhinostomy
DESP	Diabetic eye screening programme
DIC	Disseminated intravascular coagulation
DM	Diabetes mellitus
DME	Diabetic macular oedema
DMEK	Descemet's membrane endothelial keratoplasty
DMO	Diabetic macular oedema
DR	Diabetic retinopathy
DSAEK	Descemet's stripping automated endothelial keratoplasty
DSEK	Descemet's stripping endothelial keratoplasty
DSG	Dacryoscintigraphy
EBMD	Epithelial basement membrane dystrophy
EBV	Epstein-Barr virus

ECG	Electrocardiogram
ECLO	Eye clinic liaison officer
ED	Epithelial defect
EDT	Electrodiagnostic tests
ETDA	Ethylenediaminetetraacetic acid
EMG	Electromyography
EMGT	Early manifest glaucoma trial
EOG	Electrooculogram
EOM	Extraocular muscle
EPP	Exposure prone procedures
ERG	Electroretinogram
ERM	Epiretinal membrane
ESR	Erythrocyte sedimentation rate
ET	Esotropia
FAF	Fundus autofluorescence
FB	Foreign body
FBC	Full blood count
FED	Fuchs endothelial dystrophy
FFA	Fundus fluorescein angiogram
FHx	Family history
GA	Geographic atrophy/general anaesthetic
GCA	Giant cell arteritis
GC-IPL	Ganglion cell-inner plexiform layer
GDI	Glaucoma drainage implant
GHT	Glaucoma hemifield test
GI	Gastrointestinal
GMC	General medical council
GP	General practitioner
GPA	Granulomatosis with polyangiitis
GPC	Giant papillary conjunctivitis
GRT	Giant retinal tear
HES	Hospital eye service
HM	Hand motions
HTN	Hypertension
HRT	Heidelberg retinal tomography
HSV	Herpes simplex virus
HTLV-1	Human T-lymphotropic virus-1
HVF	Humphrey visual field
Hx	History
HZV	Herpes zoster virus
ICA	Internal carotid artery
ICE	Iridocorneal endothelial
ICK	Infectious crystalline keratopathy
ICP	Intracranial pressure
IFIS	Intraoperative floppy iris syndrome
IIH	Idiopathic intracranial hypertension
IK	Interstitial keratitis
ILM	Inner limiting membrane

IM	Intramuscular
IOFB	Intraocular foreign body
IOL	Intraocular lens
IOP	Intraocular pressure
INO	Internuclear ophthalmoplegia
IO	Inferior oblique
IR	Inferior rectus
IRF	Intraretinal fluid
IRMA	Intraretinal microvascular abnormalities
ITC	Iridotrabecular contact
IV	Intravenous
IVCM	In vivo confocal microscopy
JIA	Juvenile idiopathic arthritis
KC	Keratoconus
KP	Keratic precipitates
LASIK	Laser-assisted in situ keratomileusis
LCA	Lebers congenital amaurosis
LCAT	Lecithin-cholesterolacyltransferase
LESC	Limbal epithelial stem cell
LF	Levator function
LFT	Liver function test
LHON	Leber hereditary optic neuropathy
LP	Lumbar puncture
LR	Lateral rectus
LRI	Limbal relaxing incision
LTS	Lateral tarsal strip
Ma	Microaneurysm
MacTel	Macular telangiectasia
MAR	Melanoma-associated retinopathy
MALT	Mucosa-associated lymphoid tissue
MD	Mean defect
MFC	Multifocal choroiditis and panuveitis
mfERG	Multifocal electroretinogram
MH	Macular hole
MG	Myasthenia gravis
MGD	Meibomian gland dysfunction
MI	Myocardial infarction
MIGS	Minimally invasive glaucoma surgery
MR	Medial rectus
MRA	Magnetic resonance angiography
MRD1	Marginal reflex distance 1
MRI	Magnetic resonance imaging
MS	Multiple sclerosis
MTMT	Maximum tolerated medical therapy
MTX	Methotrexate
MVZ	Macular vulnerability zone
NAI	Non-accidental injury
NF	Neurofibromatosis

NFL	Nerve fibre layer
NLD	Nasolacrimal duct
NLDO	Nasolacrimal duct obstruction
NPDR	Non-proliferative diabetic retinopathy
NSAIDS	Non-steroidal anti-inflammatory drugs
NTG	Normal tension glaucoma
NVA	Neovascularisation of the angle
NVD	Neovascularisation of the disc
NVE	Neovascularisation elsewhere
NVG	Neovascular glaucoma
NVI	Neovascularisation of the iris
OCP	Oral contraceptive pill/ocular cicatricial pemphigoid
OCT	Optical coherence tomography
OCT-A	Optical coherence tomography angiography
OD	Once a day
ODD	Optic disc drusen
ODDS	Optic disc drusen studies
OIS	Ocular ischaemic syndrome
ORT	Outer retinal tubulations
OSA	Obstructive sleep apnoea
OVD	Ophthalmic viscosurgical devices
PA	Palpebral aperture
PAC	Primary angle closure
PACG	Primary angle closure glaucoma
PACS	Primary angle closure suspect
PAN	Polyarteritis nodosa
PAS	Peripheral anterior synechiae
PBK	Pseudophakic bullous keratopathy
PC	Posterior capsule
PCG	Primary congenital glaucoma
PCIOL	Posterior chamber intraocular lens
PCR	Polymerase chain reaction
PCV	Polypoidal choroidal vasculopathy
PDP	Personal development plan
PDR	Proliferative diabetic retinopathy
PDS	Pigment dispersion syndrome
PDT	Photodynamic therapy
PED	Pigment epithelial detachment
PERG	Pattern electroretinogram
PESS	Post enucleation socket syndrome
PGAs	Prostaglandin analogues
PHOMS	Peripapillary hyperreflective ovoid mass-like structures
PI	Peripheral iridotomy
PL	Perception of light
PK	Penetrating keratoplasty
PMD	Pellucid marginal degeneration
POHS	Presumed ocular histoplasmosis syndrome
PPA	Peripapillary atrophy

PPCD	Posterior polymorphous corneal dystrophy
PPV	Pars plana vitrectomy
PRP	Panretinal photocoagulation
PSD	Pattern standard deviation
Pt	Patient
PTK	Phototherapeutic keratectomy
PVD	Posterior vitreous detachment
PVR	Proliferative vitreoretinopathy
PXF	Pseudoexfoliation
RA	Rheumatoid arthritis
RAP	Retinal angiomatous proliferation
RAPD	Relative afferent pupillary defect
RCOphth	Royal college of ophthalmologists
RCT	Randomised controlled trial
RD	Retinal detachment
RK	Radial keratotomy
RNFL	Retinal nerve fibre layer
RNIB	Royal national institute of blind people
ROP	Retinopathy of prematurity
RRD	Rhegmatogenous retinal detachment
RP	Retinitis pigmentosa
RPE	Retinal pigment epithelium
RVO	Retinal vein occlusion
SAC	Seasonal allergic conjunctivitis
SCD	Schnyder's crystalline dystrophy
SCR	Sickle cell retinopathy
SD-OCT	Spectral domain optical coherence tomography
SF	Short term fluctuations
SJS	Stevens-Johnson syndrome
SLD	Superluminescent diode
SLE	Systemic lupus erythematosus
SLO	Scanning laser ophthalmoscopy
SLT	Selective laser trabeculoplasty
SO	Superior oblique
SPA	Subperiosteal abscess
SR	Superior rectus
SRF	Subretinal fluid
STI	Sexually transmitted infection
TA	Triamcinolone
TAB	Temporal artery biopsy
TASS	Toxic anterior segment syndrome
TB	Tuberculosis
TBUT	Tear film break up time
TED	Thyroid eye disease
TEN	Toxic epidermal necrolysis
TIA	Transient ischaemic attack
TM	Trabecular meshwork
TPD	Training programme director

TTP	Thrombotic thrombocytopenic purpura
UES	Uveal effusion syndrome
URTI	Upper respiratory tract infection
US	Ultrasound
VA	Visual acuity
VDRL	Venereal disease research laboratory
VEGF	Vascular endothelial growth factor
VEP	Visual evoked potential
VF	Visual field
VFI	Visual field index
VHL	Von Hippel Lindau
VKC	Vernal keratoconjunctivitis
VKH	Vogt-Koyanagi-Harada
VMT	Vitreomacular traction
VR	Vitreoretinal
XR	X-linked recessive
XT	Exotropia

Part I

Structured VIVA

1 VIVA Technique: Do's and Don'ts

Timothy H. M. Fung and Winfried M. K. Amoaku

Abstract

A viva is an oral examination that allows examiners to assess a candidate's knowledge and understanding of a specific subject. To succeed in the viva, candidates need to have a thorough grasp of a topic and be able to communicate their knowledge effectively to the examiners. This chapter offers guidance on enhancing candidates' communication skills and provides strategies for answering examiners' questions effectively.

1.1 Formalities

- It is expected that you have prepared yourself for the examination (and not there for a rehearsal)
- Ensure that you have adequate amounts of sleep and rest in the lead up to the exam
- Dress professionally on the day of the exam
- Arrive at the exam venue in good time

1.2 Answering Examiners Questions

- Listen to the questions
- Answer the question that you have been asked
- Take a moment or two to gather your thoughts before answering the questions
- Maintain eye contact with the examiner when talking (and not at the floor, or elsewhere!)
- Speak clearly and succinctly. Do not speak too quietly or too quickly
- Try to give a well-structured answer to the questions
- Be confident in your answer if you think you are right, but do not argue with the examiner!
- The examiner may ask "*are you sure?*" in response to your answer. Have a think about your answer and do not feel afraid to stick to your answer (if you believe it to be correct), or afraid to retract statements (if you feel you were wrong)
- If you do not know the answer to a question, be honest and say so
- Really important that you avoid saying anything that would pose a danger to patients

T. H. M. Fung (✉)
University Hospitals of Derby & Burton NHS Foundation Trust, Royal Derby Hospital, Derby, UK
e-mail: timothy.fung@nhs.net

W. M. K. Amoaku
Eye, Ear, Nose and Throat Centre, Queens Medical Centre, Nottingham University Hospitals NHS Trust, Nottingham, UK

T. H. M. Fung, W. M. K. Amoaku (eds.), *Viva and OSCE Exams in Ophthalmology*,
https://doi.org/10.1007/978-3-031-97401-4_1

1.3 Communications Skills (for the Communication Skills Station)

- Practice with your colleagues and fellow candidates before your real VIVA examination. Watch good communicators at work to see how they would handle different scenarios
- Try to imagine yourself with a real-life patient in your communication skills scenario
- Always maintain good eye-contact, show good body language and show empathy
- Do not forget to introduce yourself and to check the patient's identity before proceeding
- Remember to keep the delivery of information to the patient (actor) simple with the avoidance of medical jargon
- Remember to identify and address any patient concerns

1.4 When You Think Things are Going Badly

- Remember that difficult stations are likely to be difficult to all candidates
- Each VIVA station is marked separately. Try to stay positive (easier said than done) if you feel you have performed badly in a particular station. A poor performance in a station does not necessarily mean that you will fail the exam overall.

2 Patient Investigation & Interpretation

Timothy H. M. Fung, Jacob S. Heng, and Winfried M. K. Amoaku

Abstract

Candidates preparing for ophthalmology examinations must grasp the principles and indications of various eye investigations to ensure accurate diagnoses while minimising the inconvenience to patients. This chapter provides essential knowledge on the fundamental principles, indications, and interpretation of common ophthalmic investigations that are vital in eye care.

2.1 Optical Coherence Tomography (OCT)

2.1.1 Principles

- OCT of the retina and choroid is a non-invasive diagnostic technique that renders in-vivo cross-sectional view of the retina and choroid (see Fig. 2.1).
- OCT is based on the principle of low-coherence interferometry, in which the signal carrying light returning from the eye is allowed to interfere with light that has travelled a known path length. This is achieved in a Michelson interferometer.
- Infrared (830 nm) incident beam created by a superluminescent diode (SLD) source is divided into 2 beams by a beam splitter. One beam axially project to the patient's retina whist the second beam (internal reference beam) is projected to a reference mirror at a known distance.
- When the 2 light beams (internal reference beam and the back-scattered and back-reflected light from the retina) attempt to recombine at a detector, the reference beam must be altered in order to combine with the diagnostic beam.
- The amount the reference beam is altered compared to its baseline to match the probe signal (optical path length difference) results in a signal generation.
- Anterior segment OCT (AS-OCT) provides both quantitative and qualitative information on the cornea, anterior chamber angle, iris and crystalline lens (see Figs. 2.2 and 2.3). Modern spectral-domain AS-OCT imaging devices employs an SLD of 1310 nm, which enables good penetration through scattering tissue such as the sclera.

T. H. M. Fung (✉)
University Hospitals of Derby & Burton NHS Foundation Trust, Royal Derby Hospital, Derby, UK
e-mail: timothy.fung@nhs.net

J. S. Heng
The John Hopkins Hospital, Baltimore, Maryland, USA

W. M. K. Amoaku
Eye, Ear, Nose and Throat Centre, Queens Medical Centre, Nottingham University Hospitals NHS Trust, Nottingham, UK

T. H. M. Fung, W. M. K. Amoaku (eds.), *Viva and OSCE Exams in Ophthalmology*,
https://doi.org/10.1007/978-3-031-97401-4_2

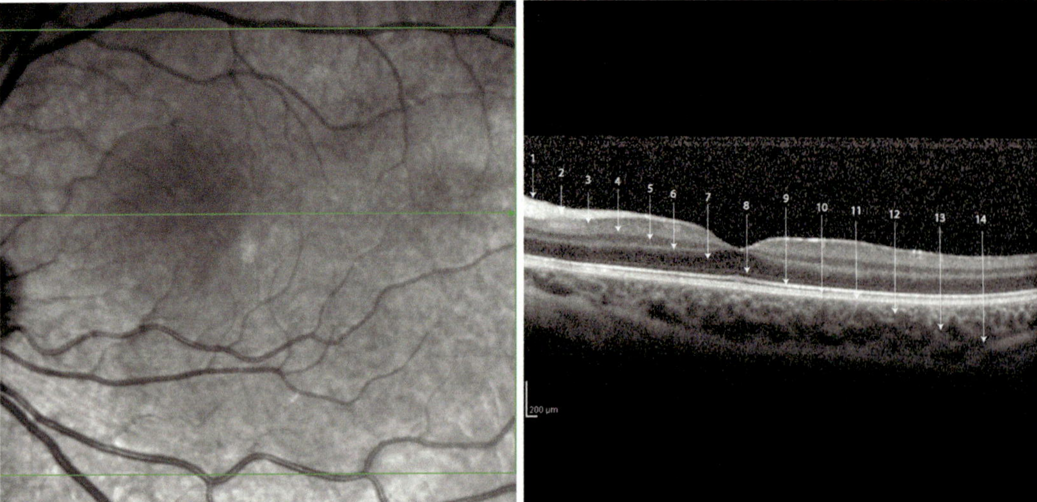

Fig. 2.1 OCT image of a patient with a normal macula. 1: Inner Limiting Membrane; 2: Nerve Fiber Layer; 3: Ganglion Cell Layer; 4: Inner Plexiform Layer; 5: Inner Nuclear Layer; 6: Outer Plexiform Layer; 7: Outer Nuclear Layer; 8: External Limiting Membrane; 9: Ellipsoid Zone; 10: Interdigitation Zone; 11: RPE / Bruch's Complex; 12: Choriocapillaris; 13: Sattler's Layer; 14: Haller's Layer

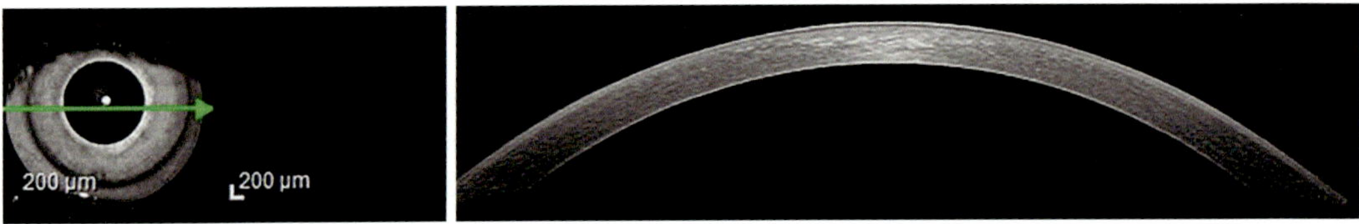

Fig. 2.2 Heidelberg AS-OCT image of the cornea

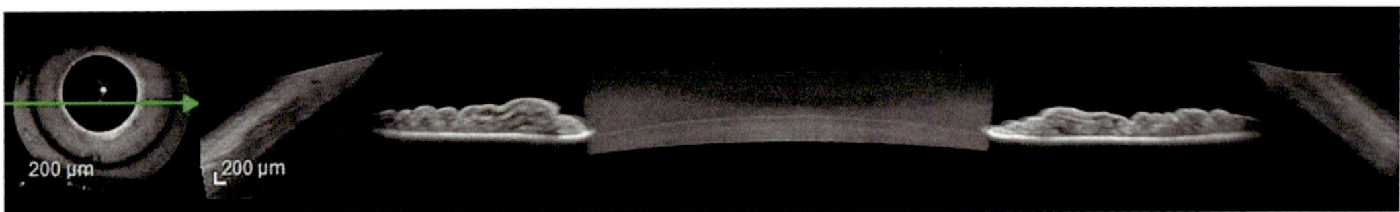

Fig. 2.3 Heidelberg AS-OCT image of the anterior chamber angle

2.1.2 Indications

- Anterior segment surgery (see Sect. 2.1.3)
- Macular pathology (see Sect. 2.1.4)
- Optic nerve pathology (see Sect. 2.1.5)

2.1.3 Application of AS-OCT

2.1.3.1 Corneal Transplantation

- AS-OCT is useful for visualisation of the complications of lamellar keratoplasty such as graft detachment (see Fig. 2.4), which is often difficult to detect with slit-lamp examination

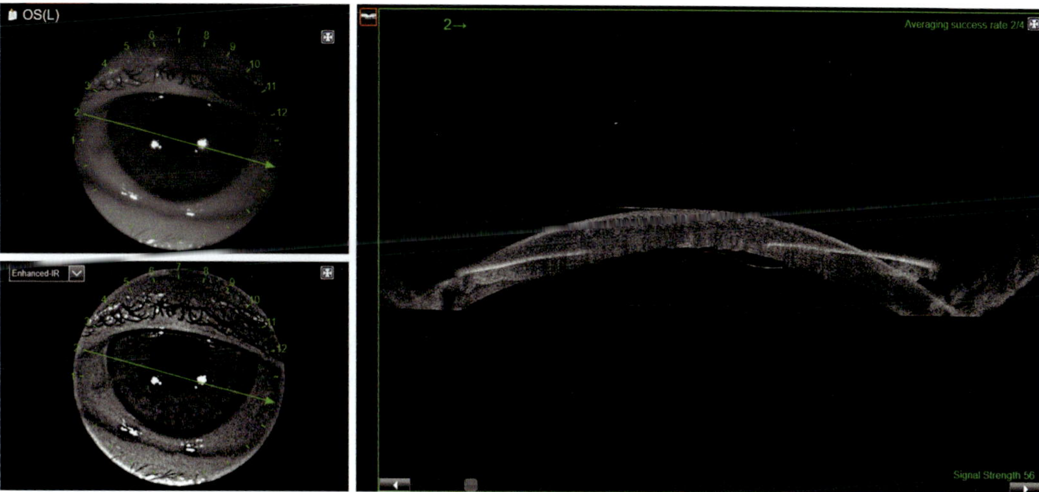

Fig. 2.4 AS-OCT image demonstrating a Descemet's membrane detachment after DMEK

2.1.4 OCT Images of Common Macular Pathologies

2.1.4.1 Macular Oedema

Causes of Macular Oedema

- Inflammatory disorders: post-operative (cataract, VR, corneal), post-laser (PI, PRP), post-cryotherapy, uveitis (anterior/intermediate/posterior)
- Retinal vascular diseases: DR, RVO, OIS, hypertensive retinopathy, radiation retinopathy, MacTel
- Choroidal vascular disease: CNV
- Drugs: latanoprost, topical adrenaline, glitazones, niacin, chemotherapy agents (e.g paclitaxel)
- Inherited retinal dystrophies: RP, autosomal dominantly inherited CMO
- Disorders of vitreoretinal interface: VMT, ERM
- Optic nerve head abnormalities: optic disc pit, optic disc coloboma
- Tumours of the choroid/retina

Mechanisms of Macular Oedema

- Increased vascular permeability: PGAs, VEGF, loss of vascular structure or vascular wall dysfunction—DR, RVO, uveitis, posterior scleritis
- Increased blood flow—post-op
- Dysfunction of RPE barrier/pump: retinal dystrophies
- Tractional stress—VMT, ERM (may not be true oedema, but tractional disruption of macula architecture)
- Drug reactions
- Fluid migration from optic nerve head abnormalities—optic disc pit

History

- Past medical history: diabetes, hypertension, hypercholesterolaemia, coagulopathies (e.g myeloma) or autoimmune conditions, any previous radiation exposure of orbit, globe, sinuses or nasopharynx,
- Past ocular history: any previous operations or laser procedures
- Social history: smoker
- Drug history: prostaglandin analogues, glitazones, topical epinephrine, nicotinic acid, OCP
- Family history: retinal dystrophies, autosomal dominantly inherited CMO

Examination

- Visual acuity
- Blood pressure: hypertension in RVO and hypertensive retinopathy

- RAPD: Ischaemic CRVO
- Prominent collateral vessels on forehead (connect external carotid artery on one side of head to the other): OIS
- IOP: may be low in OIS from ciliary body hypoperfusion, may be high in patients with NVA
- AC for flare/cells: OIS—flare out of proportion to cells, post-op, post-laser, post-cryotherapy, uveitis
- Gonioscopy for NVA: DR, OIS, RVO, radiation retinopathy
- Examine undilated iris for rubeosis: DR, OIS, RVO, radiation retinopathy
- Anterior vitreous for cells: uveitis
- Fundus examination: snowballs/snowbanking (intermediate uveitis), chorioretinal lesions (posterior uveitis), optic disc pits and colobomas, optic disc swelling (CRVO, hypertensive retinopathy), retinal haemorrhages (DR—bilateral, RVO—unilateral, OIS—unilateral, hypertensive retinopathy—bilateral, radiation retinopathy—bilateral), tortuosity and dilatation of retinal veins (RVO, OIS only has dilated veins with no tortuosity, DR—dilated and beaded), venous beading and IRMA (DR), attenuation of retinal arteries (OIS, RP), NVD/NVE (DR, OIS, RVO), bone spicules and waxy pale optic disc (RP), hard exudates at posterior pole (DR), retinal/choroidal masses

Investigations

- Fasting glucose and lipids: DR, OIS
- FBC, BP, Glucose, ESR: RVO [15]
- B-scan (choroidal mass)
- OCT: ERM, VMT, RVO (CMO respects horizontal raphe), DMO (see Fig. 2.5)
- OCT-A: detect macular ischaemia
- FFA:
  - Delayed arm-to-choroid & arm-to-retina (normally 8–12 s) circulation times (depend whether dye injected in ACF or hand): OIS
  - Patchy &/or delayed choroidal filling [choroidal filling normally complete within 5 s after the first appearance of dye]: OIS, *not* present in CRVO or DR
  - Prolongation of the retinal AV transit time (major retinal veins in the temporal vascular arcade are completely filled normally within 10–11 s after the first appearance of dye within the corresponding retinal arteries): OIS, RVO, CRAO
  - Petaloid pattern of leakage: CMO

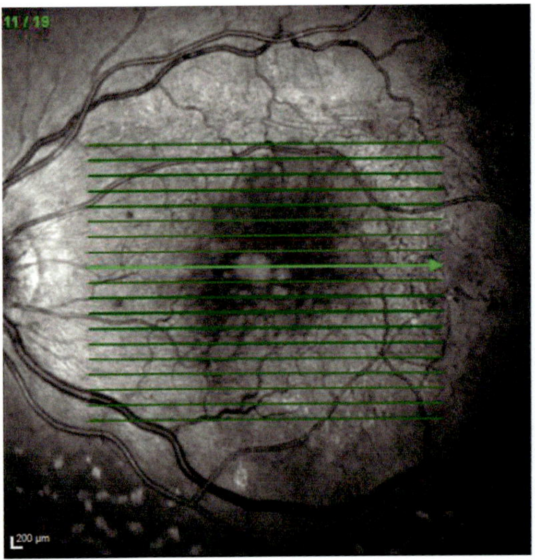

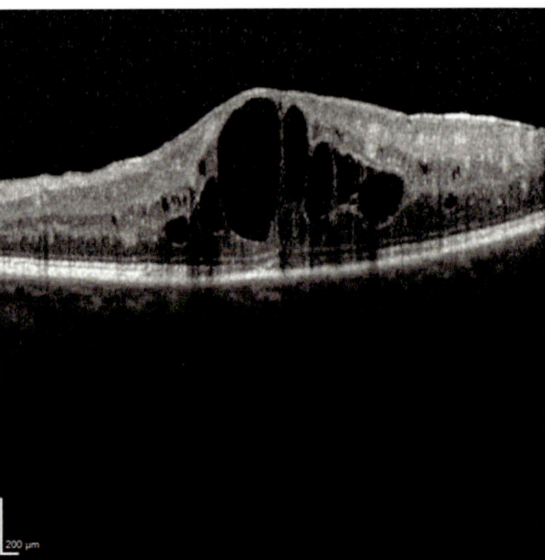

Fig. 2.5 OCT image of a patient with diabetic macular oedema. There are large intraretinal hyporeflective spaces with an intact RPE/Bruch's membrane complex and ILM

- Capillary non-perfusion: RVO, OIS, DR
- Staining of retinal vessel walls: OIS—arteries stain more than veins, RVO—only veins stain
- Hyperfluorescence of optic disc: OIS, RVO, absent in DR
- Early hyperfluorescence and late leakage suggestive of NVD or NVE: OIS, RVO, DR

- Carotid artery imaging (e.g. carotid artery duplex scan to look for 90% or more internal or common carotid artery stenosis: OIS

Management

- Co-manage with GP/physicians for systemic vascular risk factors (DR, RVO, OIS).
- Stop predisposing drugs if possible
- Carotid endarterectomy (OIS)
- PRP if NVI, NVD or NVE present (DR, RVO, OIS, Radiation retinopathy)
- Macular oedema—laser (RVO, DMO, optic disc pit), intravitreal anti-VEGF (DMO, RVO), topical steroids/NSAIDS (Post-op, Post-Cryo, Post-laser), peri-ocular steroid (post-op, post-cryo, post-laser, non-infectious uveitis), intravitreal TA (post-op), Ozurdex (DMO, non-infectious uveitis), Iluvien (DMO), topical/oral CAIs (RP), oral prednisolone (post-op, non-infectious uveitis)
- CNV—intravitreal anti-VEGF therapies (aflibercept, ranibizumab, faricimab, brolucizumab, bevacizumab)
- PPV (VMT) /PPV + ERM peel (ERM)

2.1.4.2 Subretinal Fluid (SRF) at the Fovea

Causes of SRF at the Fovea

- AMD
- Pachychoroid spectrum (group of clinical entities with a common characteristic of a thickened choroid): CSR (see Fig. 2.6), PCV, pachychoroid pigment epitheliopathy, pachychoroid neovasculopathy
- Infections and inflammatory disorders—POHS, VKH/SO, posterior scleritis, UES
- Optic disc pit with serous macular detachment

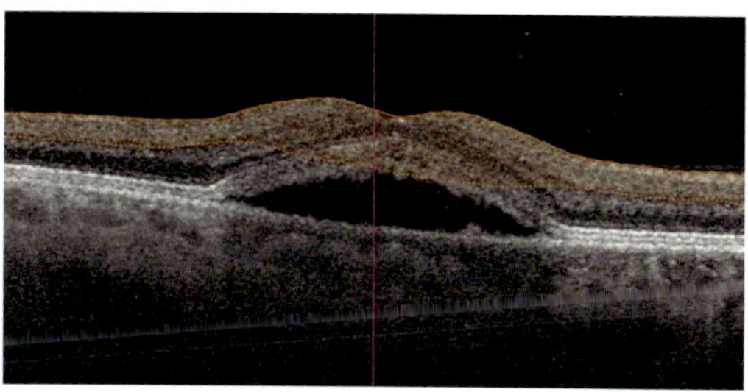

Fig. 2.6 OCT scan showing subretinal fluid at the fovea secondary to CSR

- Tumours—choroidal melanoma, choroidal haemangioma, choroidal metastases, choroidal osteoma, leukaemic infiltrates
- Vascular disorders—SLE, PAN, scleroderma, dermatomyositis, relapsing polychondritis, DIC/TTP, toxaemia of pregnancy, malignant HTN
- Dome shaped maculopathy (High myopia without CNV)—cap of hyporeflective subretinal space ('SRF') in absence of CNV, associated with inward bowing of the sclera-choroid complex in the central area (see Fig. 2.7)

History

- Ask about risk factors for CSR—steroid use (all forms), pregnancy, Hx of cushings disease
- Ask about risk factors for AMD—smoking, diet, spectacle prescription (hypermetropia), HTN, hypercholesterolaemia
- Ask about risk factors for PCV—HTN
- Ask about Hx of known primary tumour—choroidal metastases
- Ask about symptoms of vascular disorders—SLE (rashes, photosensitivity, chest pain, arthritis, oral ulcers, seizures), scleroderma (raynaud's phenomenon), dermatomyositis (pains and weakness in the shoulders or hips, rash affecting eyelids—heliotrope, cheeks, nose, chest, and extensor surfaces), relapsing polychondritis (ear and nose pain)

Examination

- Look for signs of Cushings disease (moon shaped face, buffalo neck hump, purple abdominal striae), well-demarcated oval shaped area of neurosensory RD in posterior pole—CSR

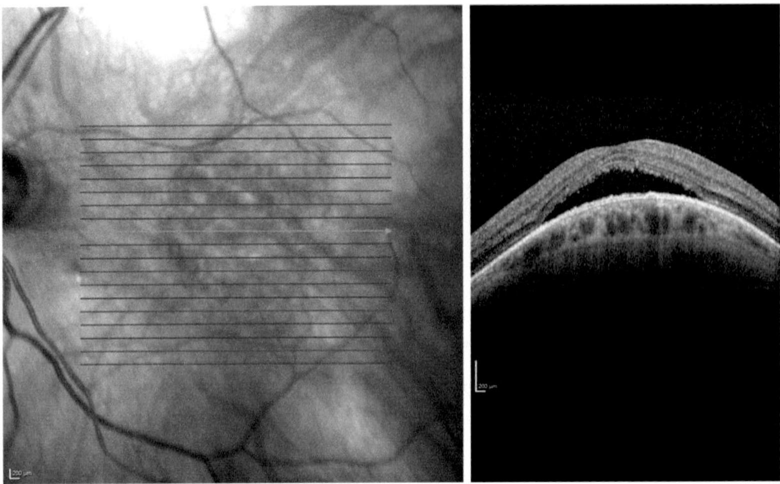

Fig. 2.7 OCT scan showing subretinal fluid at the fovea secondary to dome shaped maculopathy

- Look for drusen, RPE focal hyperpigmentation, GA—AMD
- Look for protruding orange red elevated subretinal lesions, subretinal haemorrhage, subretinal lipid exudation—PCV
- Look for presence of peripheral "punched out" chorioretinal lesions, PPA, and arcuate striae in the mid-periphery—POHS
- Look for presence of vitritis, optic disc hyperaemia, dalen fuch nodules (peripheral yellow white choroidal granulomas), sugiura sign (perilimbal vitiligo), associated systemic manifestations (vitiligo, poliosis, alopecia)—VKH/SO
- Look for ciliochoroidal detachments (brown-orange, solid-appearing elevations with smooth, convex surfaces. Choroidal detachments do not undulate appreciably with ocular movements, and this helps to distinguish them from RRD), visible ora serrata without scleral indentation, leopard spots in the fundus (diffuse depigmentation and multifocal hyperplasia of RPE)—UES
- Look for optic disc pit
- Look for creamy yellow mass in posterior pole—choroidal metastases, choroidal osteoma
- Look for circumscribed orange-red elevated mass posterior to equator—choroidal haemangioma
- Look for signs of vascular disorders—SLE (malar rash, discoid rash, oral ulcers, arthritis, pericarditis, pleuritis), scleroderma (thickening and tightening of skin especially in hands and fingers), dermatomyositis (rash affecting eyelids—heliotrope, cheeks, nose, chest, and extensor surfaces, plaques over knuckles of fingers—Gottron's papules), relapsing polychondritis (auricular nasal chondritis)
- Check BP and look for signs of malignant HTN (optic disc swelling, retinal haemorrhages, CWS, focal arteriolar narrowing, choroidal infarcts that are focal (elschnig's spots—grey-yellow spots) or linear along choroidal arteries (siegrist's streaks—linear hyperpigmented streaks)

Investigations

- Liaise with GP/medics to rule out suspected Cushings disease if signs are present—24 h urine collection for cortisol
- Liaise with GP/medics to rule out suspected SLE (urine dip for proteinuria, thrombocytopenia, lymphopenia, ANA, anti-dsDNA), PAN, scleroderma (CXR—pulmonary fibrosis), dermatomyositis (raised ESR, muscle biopsy, elevated skeletal muscle enzymes, abnormal EMG), or relapsing polychondritis if suspected.
- B scan—T sign (scleral thickening with a echolucent area at the posterior pole behind the echo of the sclera) for posterior scleritis, smooth thick dome-shaped membrane with little aftermovement in UES, low internal reflectivity (choroidal melanoma), high internal reflectivity (choroidal metastases, choroidal osteoma, choroidal haemangioma)

- FFA—ink blot/expansile dot pattern (CSR), smoke stake (dye rises within the neurosensory detachment and expands laterally in a mushroom-like or umbrella-like fashion at the upper limit of the detachment—only present in 10% of cases of CSR)
- OCT-A—detect CNV membrane (see Figs. 2.34, 2.35 and 2.36)
- ICG (choroidal lesions less obscured than FFA as ICG absorbs and emits near-infrared light, which readily penetrates the RPE and binding affinity of ICG to plasma proteins means that it does not leak from the choriocapillaris in the same was as fluorescein)—look for branching network of inner choroidal vessels (PCV), nodular polypoidal aneurysms or dilatation at the edge of these abnormal vessel networks (PCV), look for mutifocal hyperpermeable choroidal patches that are best seen as areas of hyperfluorescence in the mid-phase (CSR)

Management

- Intravitreal anti-VEGF (aflibercept, ranibizumab, faricimab, brolucizumab, bevacizumab; know regulatory status): AMD, PCV
- Conservative: CSR has high rate of spontaneous remission (80% spontaneously recover to 6/12 VA or better within 1–6 months). Pregnancy related CSR usually resolves 1–2 months post-delivery. Lifestyle modification and avoidance of glucocorticoid medication
- Indications for intervention in CSR: persistence more than 6 months, multiple recurrences, occupational needs, contralateral persistent visual impairment from CSR
- Laser photocoagulation: extrafoveal CSR; (caution with potential visual loss)
- Half-fluence PDT: subfoveal CSR

2.1.4.3 Pigment Epithelial Detachment (PED)

Causes of a PED

- AMD (see Sect. 10.7)
- PCV (see Sect. 10.7.8)
- Idiopathic CSR
- Ocular inflammation—VKH (see Sect. 3.11)/ Sympathetic ophthalmia
- Multifocal idiopathic PEDs

Classification of PED

- Drusenoid PED: represents large areas of confluent soft drusen)
- Serous PED
- Fibrovascular PED: growth of a CNV membrane in the sub-RPE space—type 1 CNV membrane
- Haemorrhagic PED: blood from CNV lesion is noted beneath or exterior to the RPE

Natural History of PED

- The spontaneous rate of RPE tear in the natural history of serous/fibrovascular PED associated with AMD has been reported to be 10% [1].
- At 5 years, 19% and 23% of patients with drusenoid PED associated with AMD progress to geographic atrophy and neovascular AMD, respectively [4].
- Most recognised risk factor for RPE tear is a large PED height (more than 400 μm). Additional risk factors include larger PED diameters and small ratio of CNV size to PED size.

Examination

- Drusenoid PED: appear as well-circumscribed yellow or yellow-white elevations of the RPE that are usually found within the macula. They may have scalloped borders and a slightly irregular surface.
- Serous PED: appear as a distinct circular or oval-like detachment of the RPE. Clear or yellowish-orange in colour, this dome shaped elevation of the RPE has a sharply demarcated border
- Fibrovascular PED: seen as an irregularly elevated lesion on clinical examination; flattened or notched border of the PED is a frequent and important sign of hidden associated CNV. Yellow subretinal or intraretinal exudates that occur typically at the PED margins, subretinal haemorrhages at PED

margins, sub-RPE blood which appears darker than subretinal blood with a fluid level sign, irregular elevation of the PED, radial chorioretinal folds surrounding the PED are caused by the contraction of Bruch membrane and the CNV.

Investigations

- OCT:
  - Elevation of highly reflective external band, which usually conforms to a concave smooth elevation with an optically quiet zone within the dome-shaped elevation. The highly reflective band should be continuous on both sides of the PED; a discontinuity may raise suspicion for an RPE tear or could be the result of blocking of the incident OCT beam by overlying exudate, blood, or fibrosis.
  - Drusenoid PED (see Fig. 2.8)—smooth contour of detached hyperreflective RPE band that may demonstrate an undulating appearance with moderate or high hyperreflectivity
  - Serous PED (see Fig. 2.9)—appear as dome shaped elevation of the RPE seen overlying a homogenously hyporeflective space, with Bruch's membrane often visible as a thin hyper-reflective line at the outer aspect of the PED
  - Fibrovascular PED (see Fig. 2.10)—appear as broad elevations of the RPE band relative to Bruch's membrane that are filled with solid layers of medium reflectivity separated by hyporeflective clefts
- FFA (see also Sect. 2.3):
  - Serous PED—uniform bright intense hyperfluorescence in the early phase, with a smooth contour to the RPE by the middle phase, and little, if any, leakage at the borders of the PED by the late phase. Brisk progressive pooling within the serous PED in a homogenous and well-demarcated manner. Late staining of serous PED is typical.
  - Fibrovascular PED—stippled hyperfluorescence along the surface of the RPE by the middle phase and may show pooling of dye in the overlying subsensory retinal space in the late phase.
  - Drusenoid PED—hyperfluoresce faintly during the transit and do not progress to bright hyperfluorescence in the late phase. No late leakage will be present.
  - Look for ink blot/smoke stake pattern: CSR
- ICG:
  - Look for branching vascular network (BVN)—PCV
  - Look for hyperfluorescent hot spot—RAP

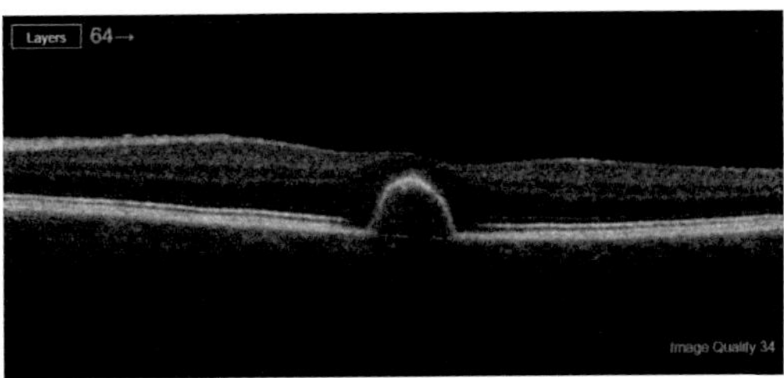

Fig. 2.8 OCT image of a patient with a drusenoid PED

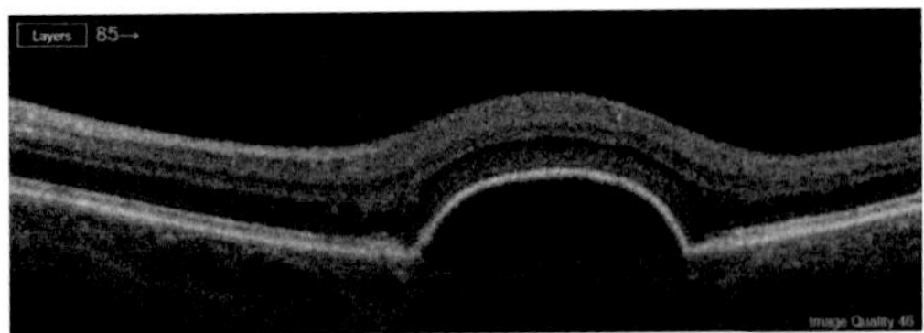

Fig. 2.9 OCT image of a patient with a serous PED

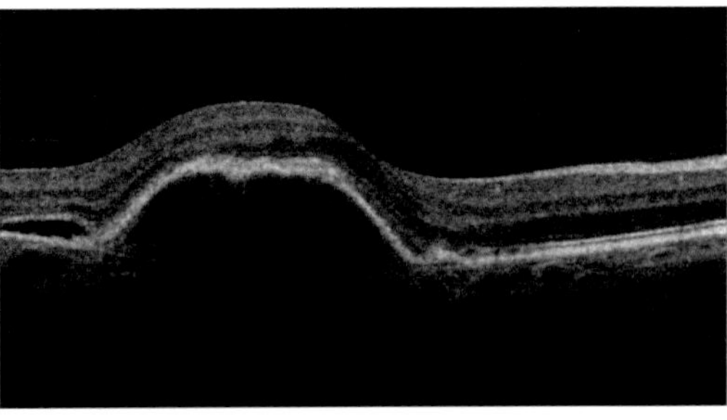

Fig. 2.10 OCT image showing a fibrovascular PED with adjacent SRF

2.1.4.4 Retinal Pigment Epithelium (RPE) Tears

Causes of RPE Tears

- Long standing substantial sub-RPE fluid collection due to active CNV (spontaneous RPE tear).
- Following verteporfin PDT or laser photocoagulation of lesions overlying a serous PED
- Following intravitreal injections of anti-VEGF agents

Mechanisms of RPE Tears

- RPE is put on stretch as a result of increasing or considerable SRF accumulation, and contraction of fibrovascular element of CNV; this stress leads to a tear in the RPE. Tear occurs at junction of detached and attached RPE.
- Sheet of RPE cells then contracts and scrolls up upon itself in a radial fashion, leaving an area of retina without underlying RPE
- Traction from CNV contraction and adhesion form the RPE that is still attached.

Examination

- Subretinal haemorrhages frequently accompanies an RPE tear, which appears ophthalmoscopically as an area of well-demarcated hyperpigmentation immediately adjacent to an area of relative hypopigmentation (see Fig. 2.11). Size is variable depending on extent of fibrovascular tissue and size of tear

Investigations

- OCT (directly through RPE tear)—irregular highly reflective outer band that appears thicker than the normal band due to scrolling of the RPE. This is immediately adjacent to an area where there is increased reflectivity from the choroid (posterior thickening of the external band) from the absence of the RPE (absence of RPE in region of tear allows for deeper penetration of the OCT signal, creating the characteristic reverse shadowing or hypertransmission sign). A sharply demarcated vertical discontinuity can also be seen in some instances (see Fig. 2.12)

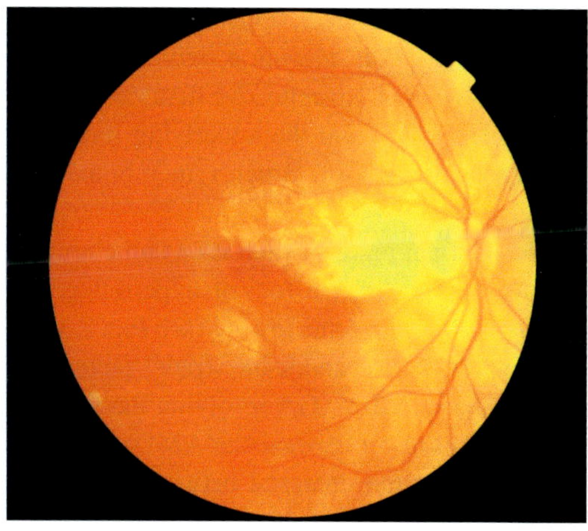

Fig. 2.11 Colour fundus image of a patient with an RPE tear following an intravitreal injection of an anti-VEGF agent

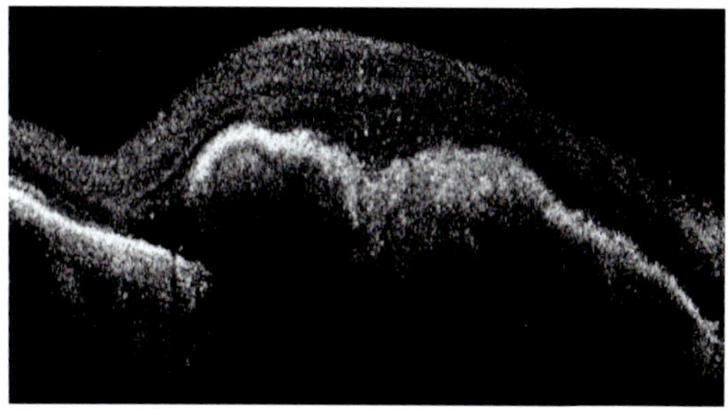

Fig. 2.12 OCT image of the same eye of the patient in Fig. 2.11 confirming an RPE tear

- FFA—absolute window defect, with well-circumscribed hyperfluorescence that does not increase in intensity or leak as the angiogram progresses, with an area of adjacent relative hypofluorescence corresponding to the scrolled RPE. Lack of fluorescein leakage distinguishes an RPE tear from a totally (100%) classic CNV membrane

2.1.4.5 Age-Related Macular Degeneration (AMD)

OCT Features of Non-neovascular AMD

(a) Small and intermediate typical drusen appear as discrete areas of RPE elevation with variable reflectivity

(b) Large typical drusen appear as dome-shaped areas of RPE elevation with underlying hypo- or medium-reflective material separating the RPE from the underlying inner collagenous zone of Bruch's membrane (see Fig. 2.13)
(c) Intraretinal pigment migration and clumping appears as discrete foci of hyperreflectivity with underlying shadowing (see Fig. 2.14)
(d) Reticular pseudodrusen (risk factor for advanced AMD—GA involving the fovea or any features of neovascular AMD) appear as hyperreflective material between the IS/OS junction and the RPE i.e. subretinal space (see Fig. 2.15)
(e) Vitelliform lesions appear as hyperreflective material in the subretinal space (see Fig. 2.16)
(f) GA appears as areas of sharply demarcated choroidal hyper-reflectivity from loss of the overlying RPE (see Fig. 2.17)

OCT Features of Neovascular AMD

(a) Intraretinal fluid (IRF), subretinal fluid (SRF), outer retinal tubulations (ORTs): IRF and SRF appear as hyporeflective spaces, ORTs (see Fig. 2.18) are branching tubular structures that appear as round or ovoid hyporeflective spaces with hyperreflective

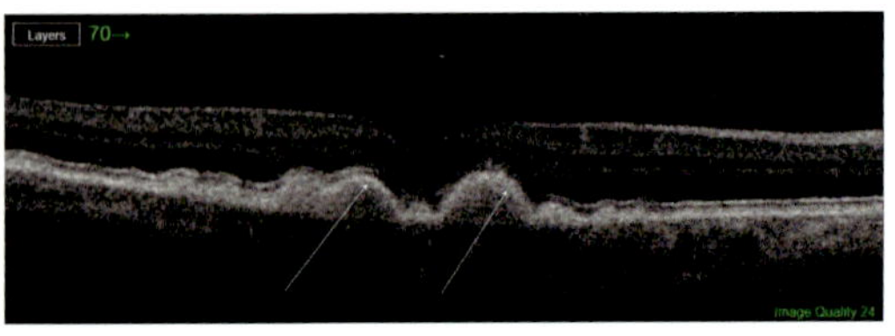

Fig. 2.13 OCT image showing large drusen. Discrete mounds (see white arrows), exhibiting medium reflectivity below the RPE, and above the choroid are obvious. The ellipsoid zone is present over some of the elevations, and less obvious over others

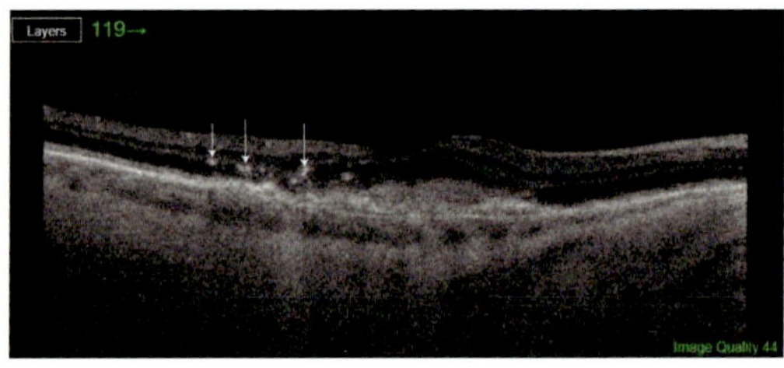

Fig. 2.14 OCT image showing multiple hyperreflective foci (white arrows) representing RPE clumping and migration and an adjacent subretinal CNV membrane

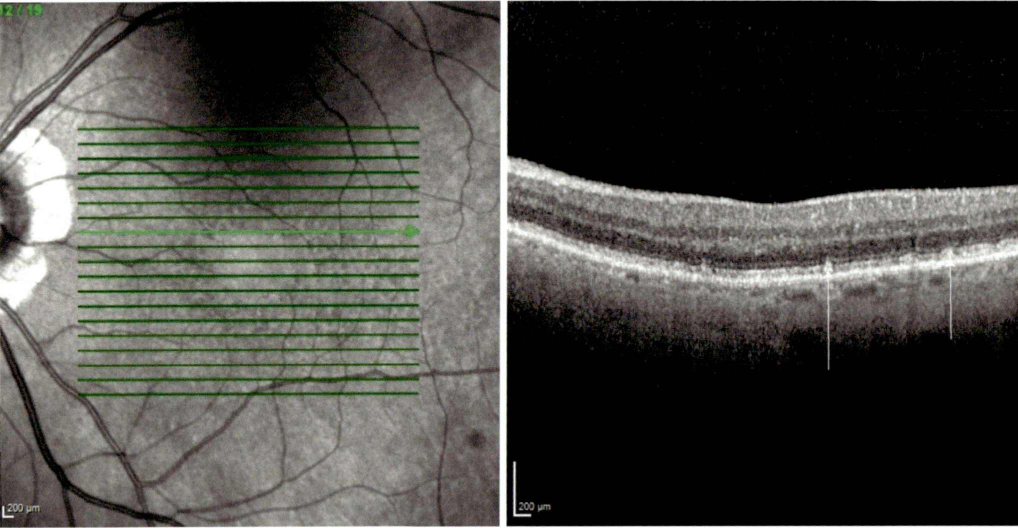

Fig. 2.15 OCT image of reticular pseudodrusen (RPD) showing accumulation of material (represented by focal subretinal hyper-reflective foci) in the subretinal space (see white arrows)

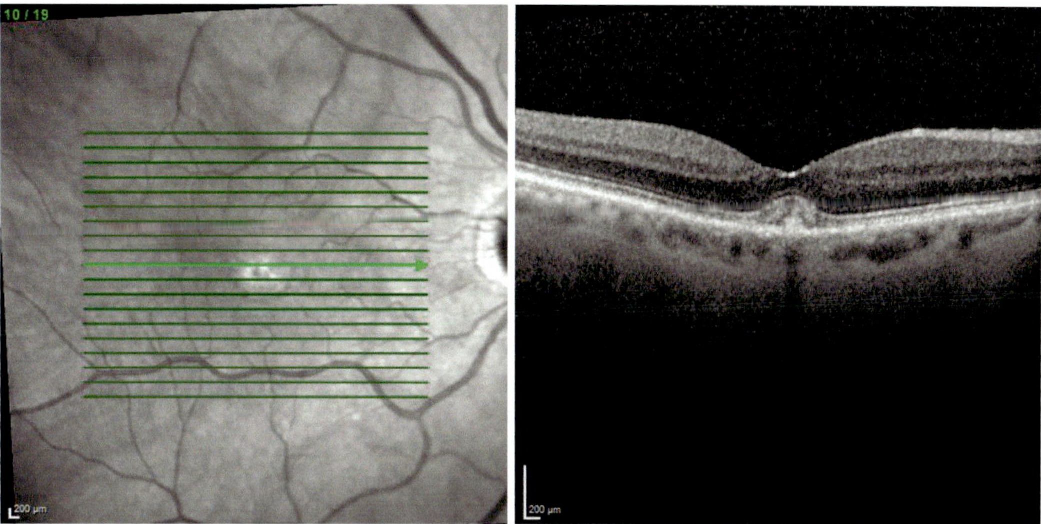

Fig. 2.16 OCT image of a patient with a vitelliform lesion showing a well-defined hyperreflective material in the subretinal space and splitting the RPE, without disruption of the overlying tissue

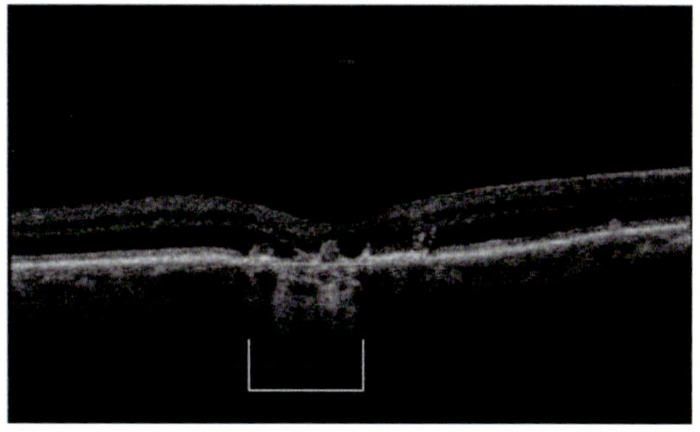

Fig. 2.17 OCT image showing areas of increased choroidal hyper-reflectivity from overlying RPE atrophy. There are associated localised hypo-reflective spaces overlying the RPE atrophy

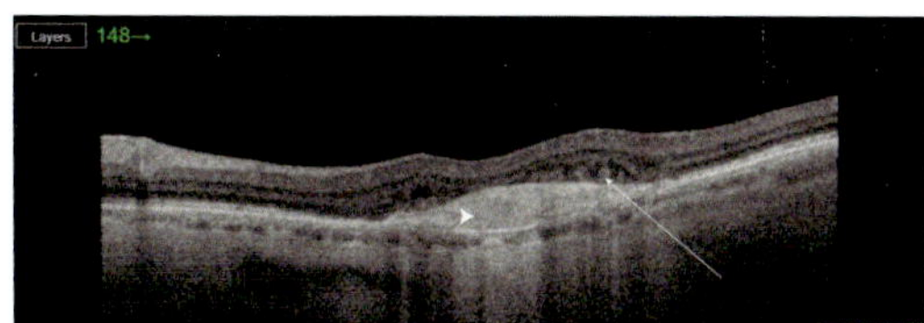

Fig. 2.18 OCT image showing a disciform scar (highly hyperreflective subretinal material—white arrowhead) and the presence of overlying ORTs (at the right edge of scar—white arrow)

borders in the ONL overlying areas of subretinal fibrosis or PED. ORTs represent a rearrangement of photoreceptors in response to injury and RPE loss.

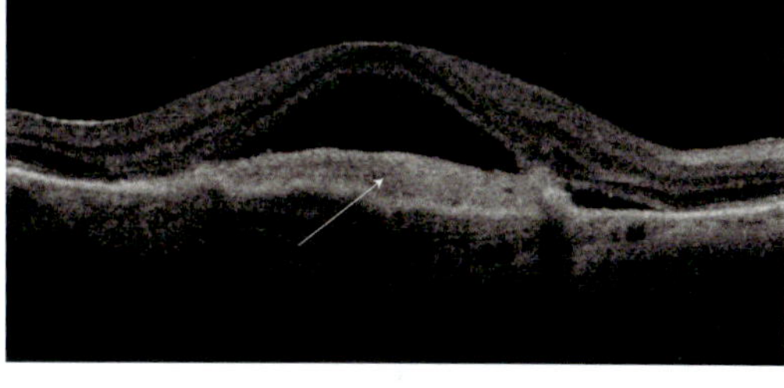

Fig. 2.19 OCT image showing an active CNV membrane (hyperreflective 'sausage-shaped' material overlying RPE/Bruch's membrane complex—white arrow) in the subretinal space with adjacent SRF

(b) Subretinal hyper-reflective material/ Disciform scar: CNV membranes in the subretinal space (type 2 CNV membrane—see Fig. 2.19) appear as an amorphous lesion of medium- to high-reflectivity above the RPE, disciform scar formation (see Fig. 2.18) appears as a well demarcated highly hyper-reflective lesion
(c) Serous PED (see Fig. 2.9)
(d) Fibrovascular PED (see Fig. 2.10)
(e) Haemorrhagic PED (frank haemorrhage from proliferating blood vessels in the sub-RPE space)
(f) Polypoidal choroidal vasculopathy (PCV)—black and asian populations, reddish-orange

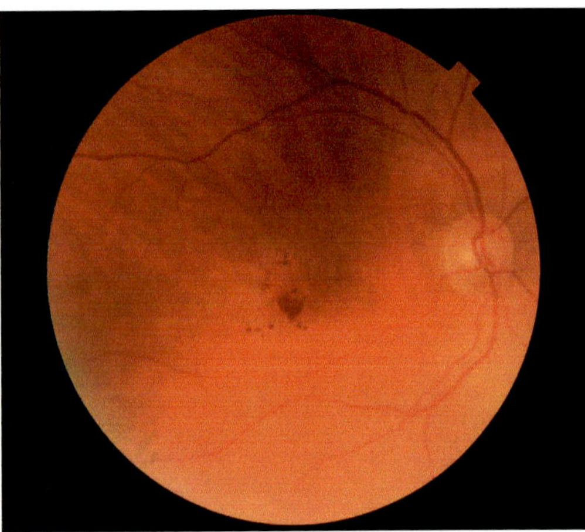

Fig. 2.20 Colour fundus image of a patient with RAP showing focal areas of intraretinal haemorrhage and right-angled venules

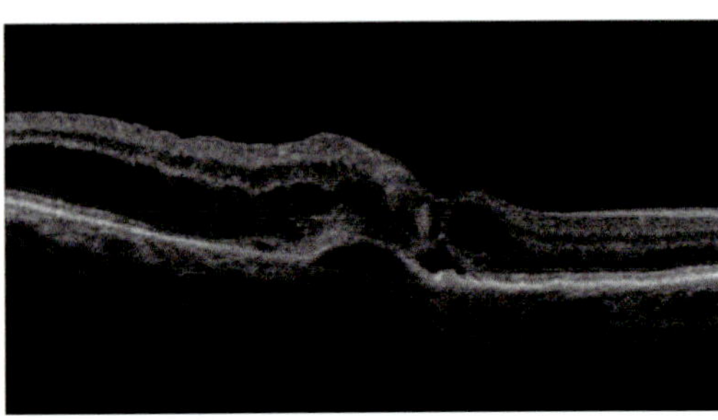

Fig. 2.21 OCT image of the same eye of the patient in Fig. 2.20 showing frank CMO (IRF) overlying a fibrovascular PED and accompanied by SRF

polypoidal lesions and is often associated with serosanguineous PEDs, branching vascular network (BVN) appear as a shallow elevation of the RPE, while the polypoidal lesions appear as sharper protuberances (see Sect. 10.7.8)

(g) RAP (intraretinal neovascularisation with retino-choroidal anastomosis—seen clinically as focal areas of intraretinal haemorrhage, right-angled venules and circinate collection of hard exudates—see Fig. 2.20): active RAP lesions have a characteristic OCT appearance typified by frank CMO overlying a fibrovascular PED and accompanied by SRF (see Fig. 2.21), "kissing sign"—a focal funnel shaped defect in the RPE associated with an intraretinal hyper-reflective lesion

2.1.4.6 Epiretinal Membrane (ERM)

Causes of ERM

- Idiopathic
- Postsurgical—RD surgery, cryotherapy, photocoagulation
- Trauma—penetrating or blunt accompanied by persistent vitreous haemorrhage
- Ocular inflammatory diseases—posterior uveitis, sarcoidosis, pars planitis
- Retinal vascular diseases—RVO, telangiectasias, arteriolar macroaneurysms, DR, SCR
- Intraocular tumours—retinal angiomas or hamartomas
- Inherited retinal dystrophies—RP

Mechanisms of ERM

- Glial cells (fibrous astrocytes and muller cells) of retinal origin proliferate through defects in the ILM. Defects in ILM usually associated with vitreous separation.
- In cases of membrane formation before vitreous detachment, glial cells may grow into the vitreous cavity. As the membrane extends over the surrounding retina, a layer of vitreous is trapped against the ILM.

Examination

- Look for complications of ERM including retinal striae (contraction of ILM), tortuosity of retinal vessels, pseudohole (negative watzke-allen test), fovea ectopia (diplopia), intra−/pre-retinal haemorrhages and tractional macular detachment
- Look for signs of DR including retinal haemorrhages, venous beading, IRMA, previous PRP scars, NVD/NVE, macular exudates and CSMO
- Look for signs of RVO including retinal haemorrhages, optic disc collaterals, telangiectatic vessels, venous dilatation and tortuosity

Investigations

- OCT: ERM (see Fig. 2.22) +/− CMO
- FFA: macular ischaemia (RVO, DR), delayed arteriovenous transit time (RVO), capillary

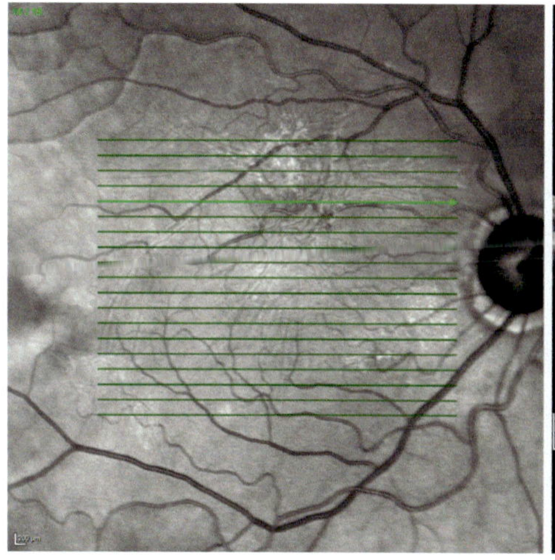
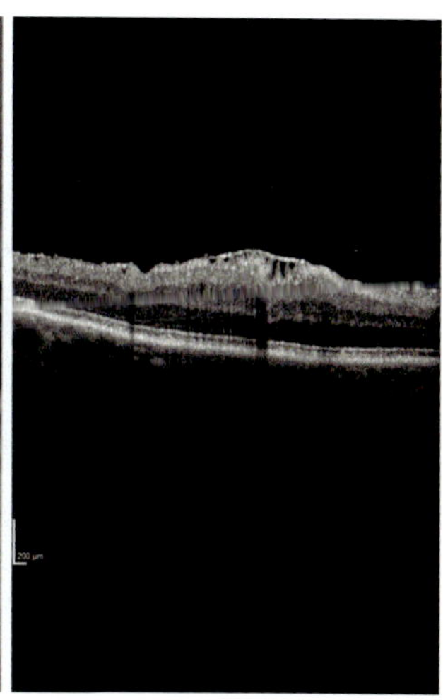

Fig. 2.22 OCT image of a patient with an idiopathic ERM. The inner retinal is distorted and irregular, with a hyper-reflective membrane with inner retinal hyporeflective spaces. Note RPE and outer retinal layers are intact in this scan. Occasionally, the outer retinal disruption may be shown as outer retinal hyporeflective spaces

non-perfusion (DR, RVO, SCR), optic disc hyperfluorescence (RVO), staining of retinal vessel walls (RVO)

Management

- Ensure that macular function is not limited by an additional underlying pathology (e.g. ischaemia due to RVO)
- PPV + ERM peel indicated for severely symptomatic membranes
- Consenting for PPV + ERM peel: up to 80% develop nuclear sclerotic cataract within 2 years [3], retinal tears/detachment may occur in 2.5% [10], retinal toxicity from dyes, up to 15% worsened acuity, 5% symptomatic recurrence

Prognosis

- 75% show no deterioration in vision after diagnosis
- With surgery, 60–85% patients show 2 or more snellen lines of visual improvement [6]
- Poor prognostic features are longer duration of symptoms before surgery, underlying macular pathology, lower preoperative visual acuity, thinner membranes and no retinal elevation [5]

2.1.4.7 Bacillary Layer Detachment (BALAD)

OCT Features of BALAD

- BALAD is characterised by a split of the photoreceptors posterior to the ELM, within the myoid zone of the photoreceptors (see Figs. 2.23 and 2.24)

Causes of BALAD

- Inflammatory (infectious and non-infectious): toxoplasma chorioretinitis, VKH, sympathetic ophthalmia, posterior scleritis, APMPPE, AIM, tuberculous serpiginous choroiditis, tubercular choroidal granuloma
- Degenerative: AMD
- Pachychoroid spectrum: CSR
- Drug induced: checkpoint inhibitors
- Tumours: choroidal melanoma, choroidal osteoma, choroidal lymphoma
- Ocular trauma with choroidal rupture
- Rhegmatogenous retinal detachment

2.1.5 OCT Images of Common Optic Nerve Pathologies

2.1.5.1 Glaucoma

Topographic RNFL Thickness Report

Spectralis RNFL Single Exam Report (see Fig. 2.25):

1. **Near-infrared image** of the right eye showing the location of the peripapillary RNFL circular scan (green circle) centered on the optic disc (green cross)
2. **Peripapillary SD-OCT B-scan** of the right eye. The red segmentation line should correspond to the location of the ILM (anterior bor-

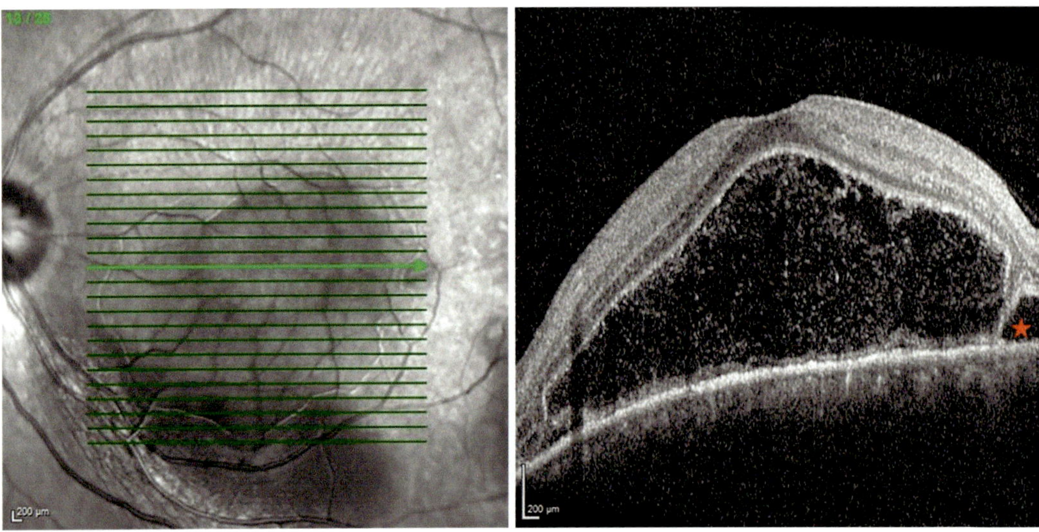

Fig. 2.23 OCT B-scan image of the left eye of a patient showing large fluid accumulation between the ELM and the ellipzoid zone, suggestive of bacillary layer detachment; and an area of neurosensory detachment (red star)

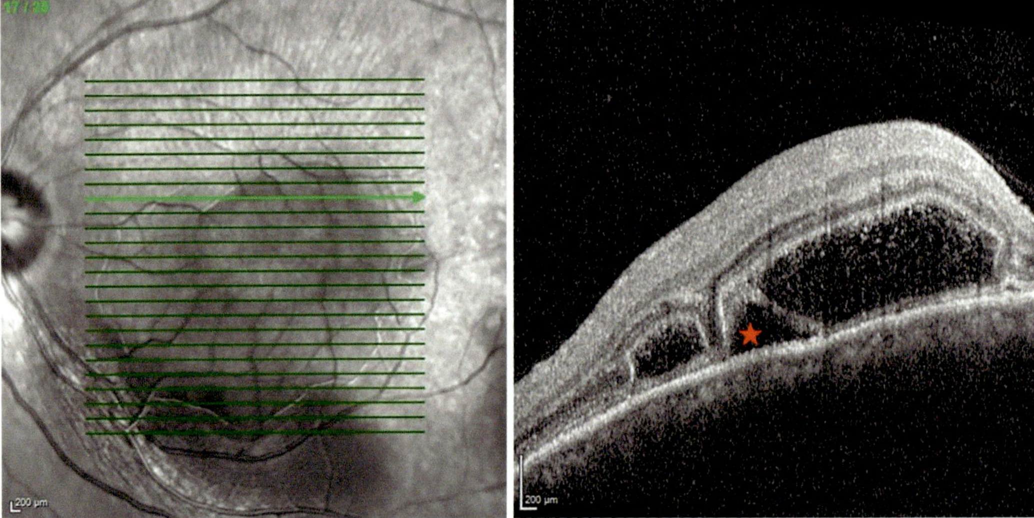

Fig. 2.24 Another OCT B-scan image of same eye as shown in Fig. 2.23 showing multiple pockets of fluid accumulated between the ELM and ellipsoid zone, suggestive of bacillary layer detachment; and an area of neurosensory detachment (red star)

der of the RNFL). The green segmentation line should correspond to the interface between the ganglion cell nerve fibers and ganglion cell bodies (posterior border of the RNFL).

3. **TSNIT RNFL thickness plot** of the right eye. The black line represents the thickness values of the patients scan around the optic disc from temporal, superior, nasal, inferior, superior to nasal (TSNIT). Colours indicate age-matched normative data ranges. The dark green line plots the average thickness values from the normative database.
4. **Classification bar**. Colours indicate age-matched normative data ranges. The colour yellow (borderline) indicates an anomaly that

RNFL Single Exam Report OU
SPECTRALIS® Tracking Laser Tomography

HEIDELBERG ENGINEERING

Patient: **DOB:** **Sex:**
Patient ID: **Exam.:**
Diagnosis: **Comment:**

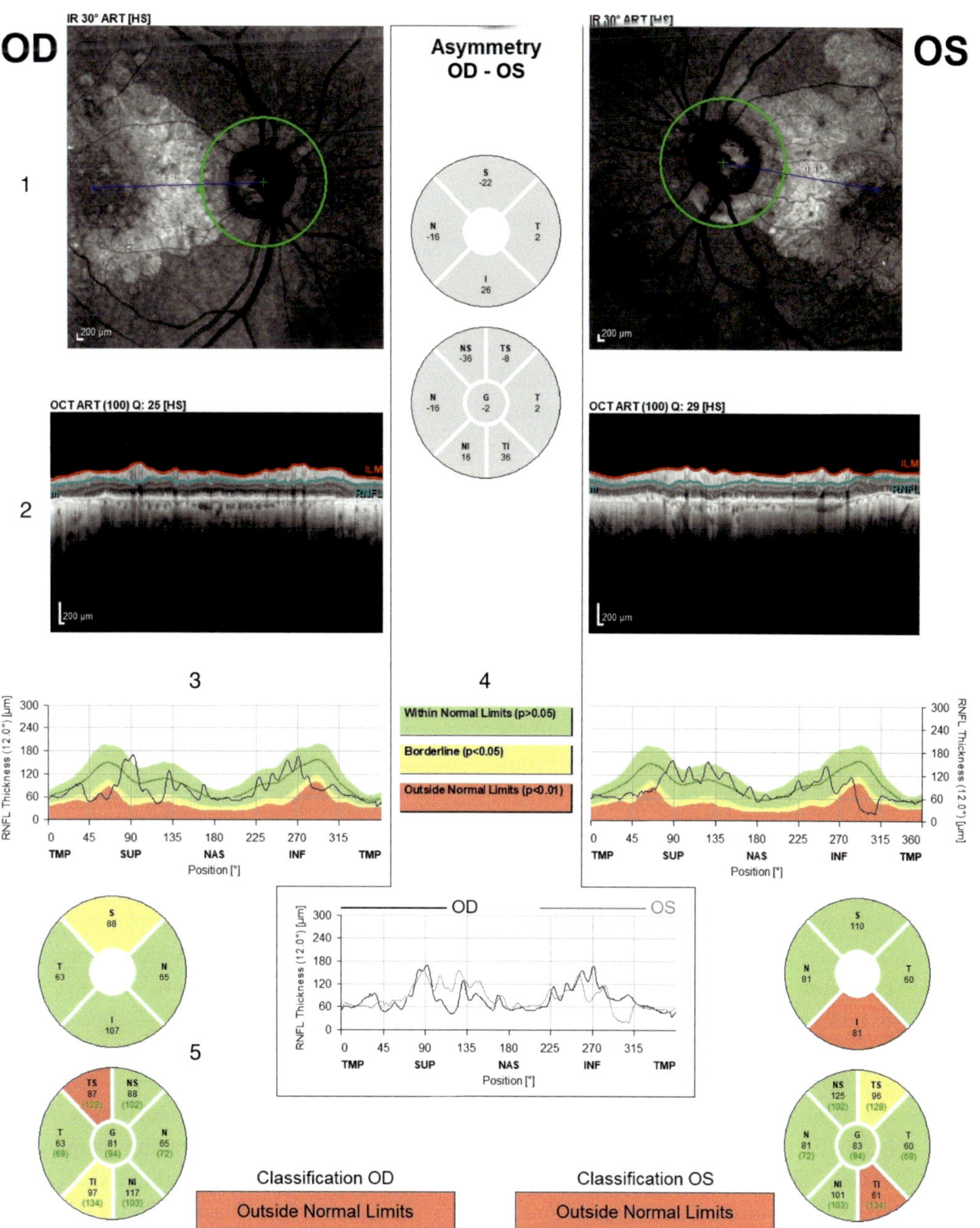

Fig. 2.25 Spectralis RNFL exam report showing thinning of the RNFL in both eyes

occurs in less than 5% of the population and red (outside normal limits) indicates an anomaly that occurs in less than 1% of the population.

5. **Classification pie chart** (four sector and seven sector) of the right eye showing the average RNFL thickness (in microns) for each sector. Global (G) average is shown in the center. Sector colour indicates classification versus normative database. The papillomacular bundle thickness is in the temporal sector, and the symmetry ratio of nasal compared to temporal (N/T) is in the nasal sector.

Topographic RNFL Thickness Interpretation

1. **Check correct patient details**
   - The thickness measurements obtained from OCT machines are compared against age-matched controls (normative database) in order to identify significant RNFL thinning or thickening. With ageing, there is a natural attrition of the RNFL. Therefore, not accounting for age effects can significantly affect the estimate of disease progression
   - Having the incorrect date of birth entered could cause abnormalities in the probability plots of the thickness measurements that could lead to erroneous interpretation
2. **Check scan quality, alignment, segmentation**
   - Quality:
     - Focal media opacities, such as corneal opacities, cataract or vitreous opacities, can cause loss of signal strength giving a false appearance of local areas of RNFL drop out that can lower the average RNFL thickness or artificially create segmental areas of thinning
     - In the Cirrus platform (Carl Zeiss), once signal strength drops below a value of 7 (10 being maximum), the segmentation algorithm can often fail and produce large regional errors in the derived RNFL thickness
   - Alignment:
     - Improper alignment of the scan could introduce variability in repeat scans and changes in sectoral RNFL thickness, mostly through horizontal shifts of the scan placement.
     - To detect changes over time, images from different visits must be accurately aligned by using technology such as eye tracking or by measuring relative to a stable landmark (e.g., BMO). Alignment of a RNFL peripapillary circle scan should be along a stable axis (e.g., fovea to BMO axis)
   - Segmentation:
     - All OCT algorithms attempt to identify the ILM as the upper boundary of the RNFL
     - In the Cirrus platform (Carl Zeiss), failed segmentation can often be identified as rectangular-shaped areas of absolute loss in the RNFL deviation map that does not follow the normal arcuate pathway of the RNFL.
     - In the Spectralis platform (Heidelberg), errors in segmentation of the RNFL can be seen by inspecting the red segmentation line in the SD-OCT B-scan. A prominent ERM (see Fig. 2.26) or vitreoretinal interface (see Fig. 2.27) can be incorrectly identified as the ILM, which will result in an artifactually thickened RNFL measurements
     - Errors in segmentation can also be seen by examining the TSNIT RNFL thickness plot. A RNFL thickness approaching 0 μm on the TSNIT RNFL thickness plot can only be due to segmentation error because prior studies have shown that the RNFL thickness can only drop to approximately 30–40 μm despite long-standing optic neuropathies with NPL vision because of residual glial cells, retinal blood vessels, gliosis, and non-functioning ganglion cell axons that contribute to the RNFL [2]
     - Errors in segmentation of the RNFL can also occur from decentration of the scan in the z-axis, which can cause truncation of the image, resulting in areas of absolute

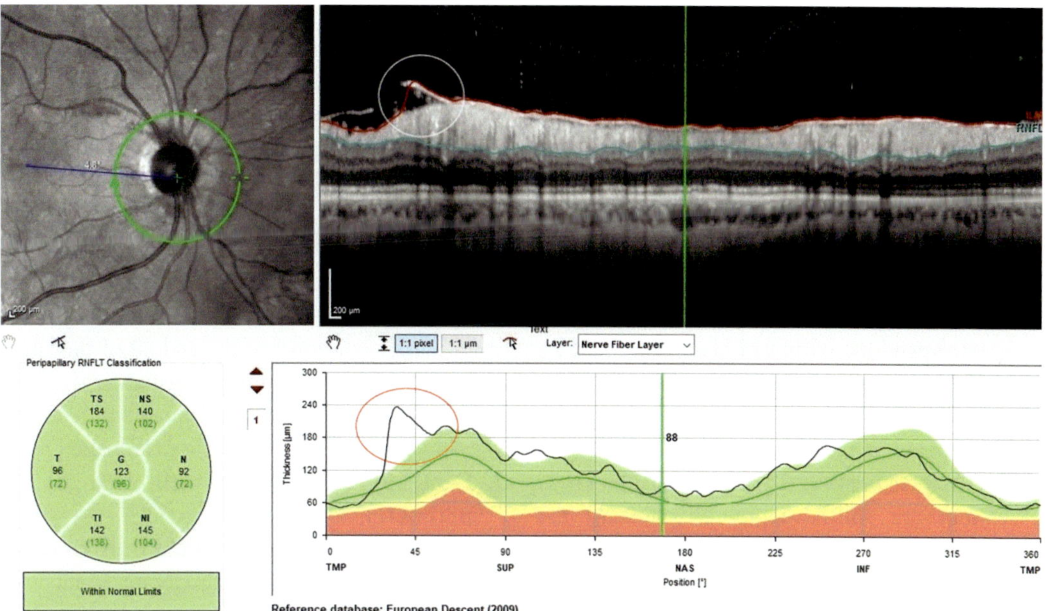

Fig. 2.26 Spectralis B-scan demonstrating an error in segmentation whereby an ERM is incorrectly identified as the ILM (see white circle), which has resulted in an artificially thickened sectoral RNFL measurement visible in the TSNIT thickness plot (see red circle)

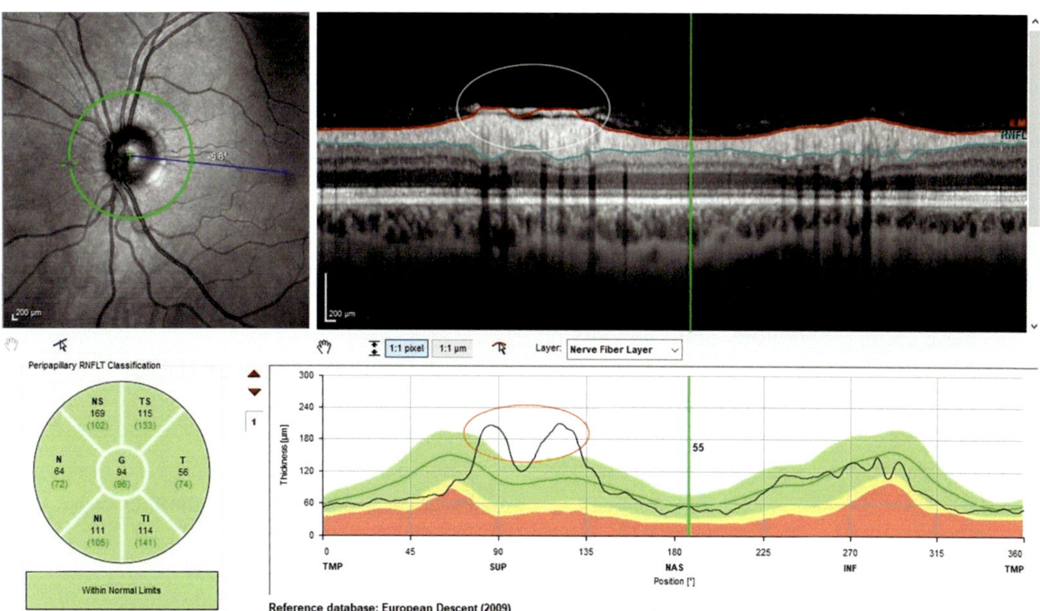

Fig. 2.27 Spectralis B-scan demonstrating an error in segmentation whereby the posterior vitreous interface is incorrectly identified as the ILM (see white circle), which has resulted in an artificially thickened sectoral RNFL measurement visible in the TSNIT thickness plot (see red circle)

loss on the RNFL thickness plot [2]. Examination of the B-scans will demonstrate an area of the scan that is truncated. This artifact can be reduced by ensuring that the data are well centered on the z-axis during acquisition

3. **Consider if the normative database is appropriate and applicable to the patient**
   - High myopia is associated with a thinner RNFL compared to the normal population However, the normative database excludes subjects with high myopia (−7.0 diopters in the Spectralis platform and −12 diopters in the Cirrus platform)
   - The peaks on the TSNIT RNFL thickness plot are shifted temporally toward the fovea in myopes compared to the normal population [2]. With increasing myopia, there is an increase in prevalence of a more temporal angle of the arcuate nerve bundles as they enter the optic nerve head. Due to the more temporal shift of the RNFL peaks in myopia, the temporal RNFL thickness may be elevated, while the superior and inferior RNFL thickness may be reported as decreased in myopic patients compared to the average arcuate bundle distribution of a normative database [2]
4. **Look at the whole scan**
   - Sectoral averaging of RNFL thickness, as shown in the classification pie chart, is helpful to highlight more localised loss but can still mask very focal defects within these sectors. Therefore, don't just rely on the classification pie chart alone. it is important to trace the whole TSNIT thickness plot.
5. **Compare RNFL thickness and macular GC-IPL OCT**
   - Compare and correlate the RNFL thickness with the macular GC-IPL thickness
6. **Look for changes in glaucoma hotspots**
   - Look for areas where glaucomatous damage is more likely to occur:
     - Inferotemporal and superotemporal RNFL
     - Macular vulnerability zone (MVZ): macular damage is typically arcuate in nature and often associated with local RNFL thinning in a narrow region of the disc, which is called the MVZ [7]. Most of the inferior region of the macula projects to the MVZ, which is located largely in the inferior quadrant of the disc (just adjacent to a major inferior temporal artery or vein), a region that is particularly susceptible to glaucomatous damage [7]. A small (cecocentral) region of the inferior macula, and all of the superior macula (inferior visual field), projects to the temporal quadrant, a region that is less susceptible to damage [7]
7. **Look for agreement with changes on perimetry**
   - The OCT is often consistent with the visual field in early and moderate glaucoma, except in young patients where the OCT impairment is greater than the impairment of the visual field (due to the redundancy of receptor fields in the ganglion cells)
8. **Don't rely on OCT alone and always consider other pathology**
   - Consider and exclude other pathologies including:
     - Non-glaucomatous optic neuropathies (congenital, compressive, inflammatory, toxic, trauma, AION)
     - Neurological diseases (stroke, MS, tumour)
     - Other ocular diseases (ERM, VMT, RVO, optic disc drusen)

2.1.5.2 Optic Disc Drusen (ODD)

Differential Diagnosis

- Papilloedema
- Pseudopapilloedema from another cause
- Pseudotumour cerebri
- Myelinated nerve fiber layer
- Crowded disc with associated hyperopia
- Tilted disc

Associations of ODD

- Retinitis pigmentosa
- Angioid streaks
- Usher syndrome

- Noonan syndrome
- Alagille syndrome

History

- Often asymptomatic. Rarely, patients can experience transient visual obscurations and gradual visual field loss

Examination

- Elevated optic disc with blurring of optic disc margins (pseudopapilloedema)
- Round yellow-white calcified deposits seen on the surface of the nerve (see Fig. 2.28) or buried beneath it
- Anomalous vascular branching pattern (tortuosity, optociliary shunt vessels)

Investigations

- B-scan ultrasonography: ODD is elevated and highly reflective
- Fundus autofluorescence (FAF): Superficial ODD will demonstrate autofluorescence (see Fig. 2.29)
- EDI-OCT: The ODDS Consortium [8] defined ODD as hyporeflective structures often seen with a full or partial hyperreflective margin (see Fig. 2.30). ODD are always located above

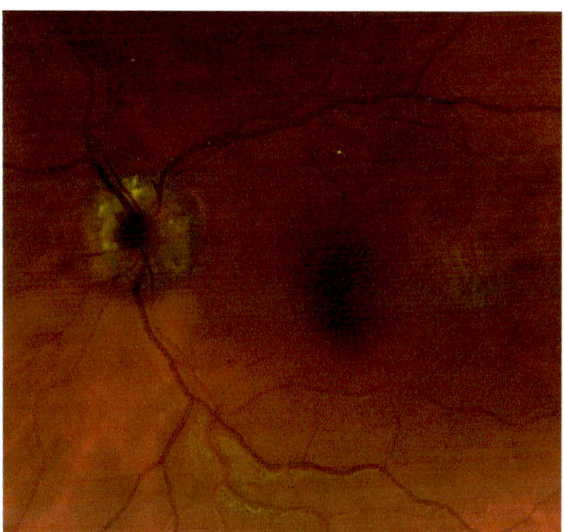

Fig. 2.28 Pseudocolour fundus image of the left eye of a patient with Pseudopapilloedema secondary to optic disc drusen

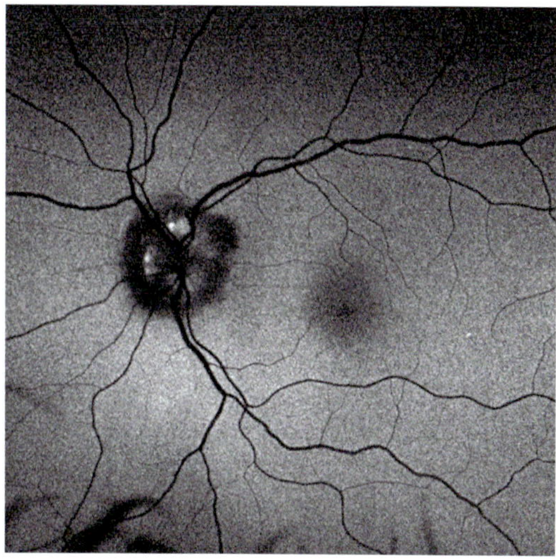

Fig. 2.29 Fundus autofluorescence image of the left eye of the same patient as shown in Fig. 2.28 showing autofluorescence of the optic disc drusen

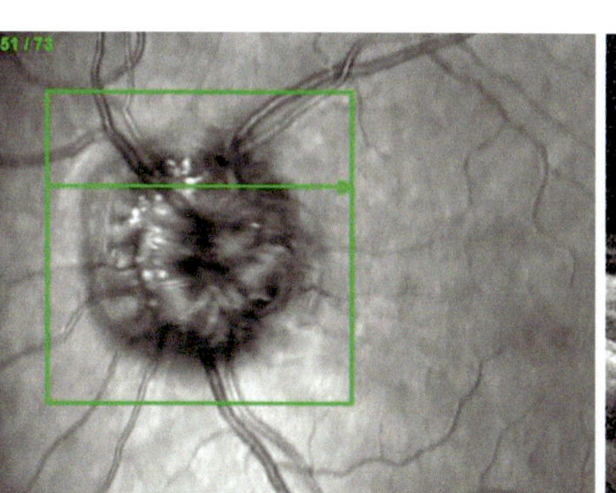

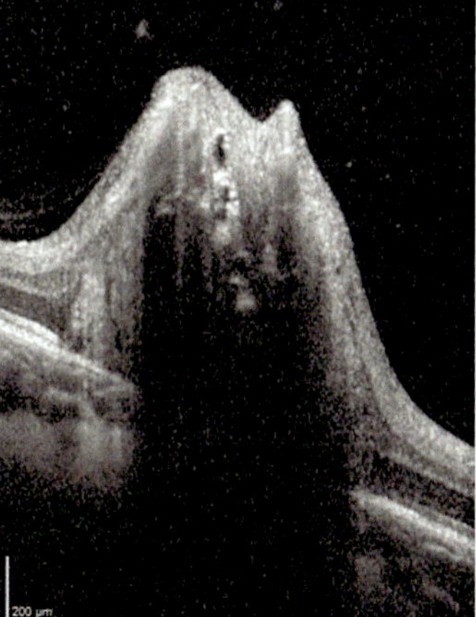

Fig. 2.30 OCT B-scan image of the left eye of the same patient as shown in Fig. 2.28 showing the presence of optic disc drusen (hyporeflective structure with a hyperreflective margin)

the lamina cribrosa and always have a signal-poor (hyporeflective) core. ODD are sometimes seen as conglomerates of smaller ODD with internal reflectivity within the signal-poor core
- FFA: Focal blockage of fluorescence in early frames with nodular staining without leakage in late frames

Complications
- Non-arteritic anterior ischaemic optic neuropathy
- Retinal vascular occlusions (CRAO)
- Peripapillary CNV membranes

Management
- ODD itself does not require treatment
- No effective treatment for patients who have gradual loss of visual fields from ODD
- Anti-VEGF therapies or focal laser treatment for CNV membranes

2.1.5.3 Peripapillary Hyperreflective Ovoid Mass-Like Structures (PHOMS)

- PHOMS are hyperreflective homogenous ovoid structures (see Fig. 2.31)
- PHOMS are situated in the peripapillary area encircling the optic nerve (see Fig. 2.32)
- PHOMS do not autofluoresce and are not visible on B-scan ultrasound despite their superficial location
- PHOMS might correspond to the lateral bulging or herniation of distended/swollen axons into the peripapillary retina as they exit the lamina cribrosa and enter the optic disc [8]
- PHOMS are a non-specific OCT finding present in various conditions, such as ODD, papilloedema, NA-AION, MS-related optic neuritis

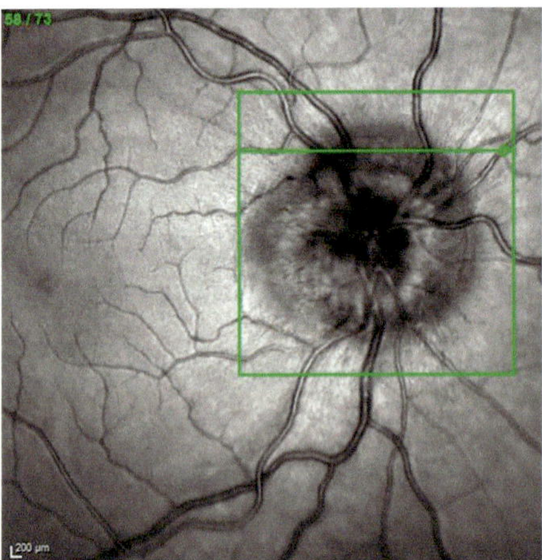

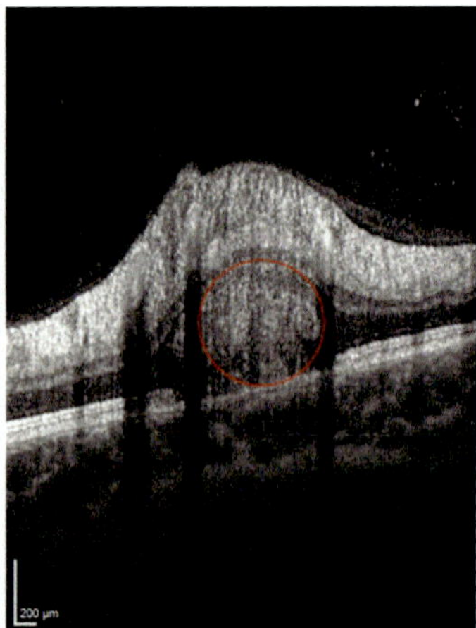

Fig. 2.31 OCT B-scan image of the right eye of a patient with pseudopapilloedema showing the presence of a PHOMS (red circle)

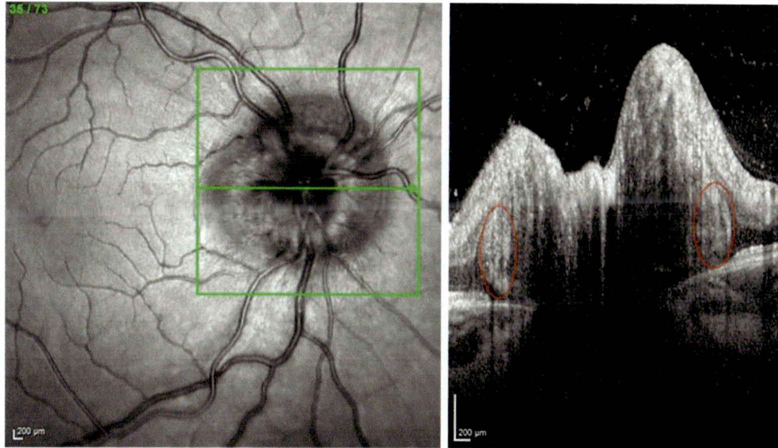

Fig. 2.32 OCT B-scan image of the right eye of the same patient in Fig. 2.31 showing the presence of PHOMS surrounding the optic disc (red circles)

2.2 OCT-Angiography (OCT-A)

2.2.1 Principles

- Non-invasive imaging method for high-resolution and cross-sectional visualisation of the vasculature of the retina and choroid without the injection of any intravenous dye
- OCT-A detects flow within blood vessels rather than imaging the blood vessels directly
- Since only the light reflectance off the surface of circulating red blood cells would differ between multiple time-lapse OCT images of the same tissue whereas all other tissue components would remain constant, the changing light reflectance between images is interpreted using software algorithm as intravascular flow
- OCT-A reconstructs the flow within the vasculature in separate layers in an en-face manner: namely the superficial capillary plexus, the deep capillary plexus and the choriocapillaris (See Fig. 2.33)

2.2.2 Indications

- Choroidal neovascularisation—conventionally OCT-A has been used to detect choroidal neovascularization in the macula e.g. in neovascular age-related macular degeneration (see Fig. 2.34), pathologic myopia (see Fig. 2.35), CSR (see Fig. 2.36)

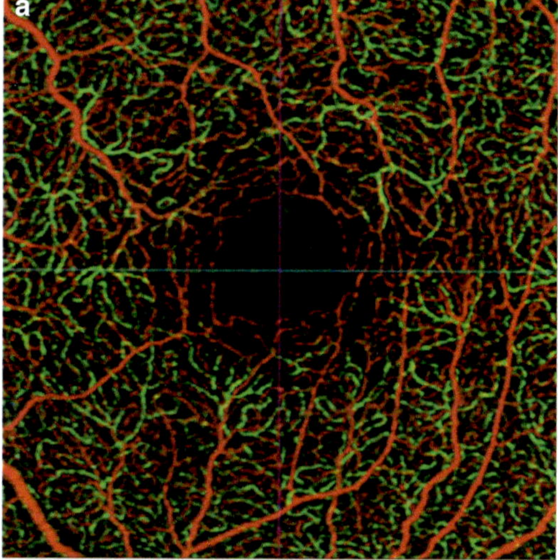

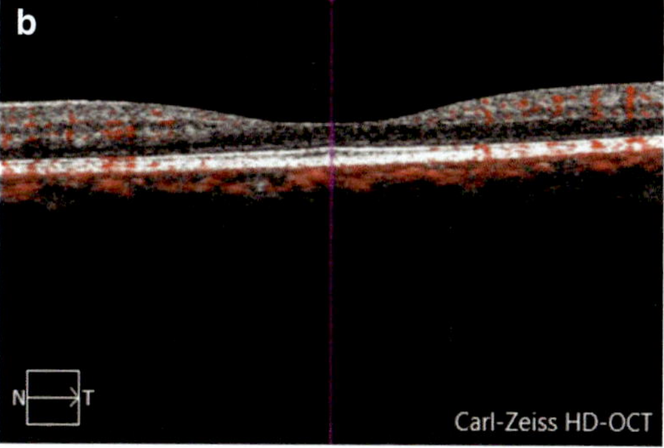

Fig. 2.33 (Top) depth encoded 3 mm × 3 mm OCT-A image of a normal macula centered on the fovea. The superficial capillary layer is coloured red while the deep capillary layer is coloured green. (Bottom) B-scan OCT image showing cross section through the fovea of the same retina

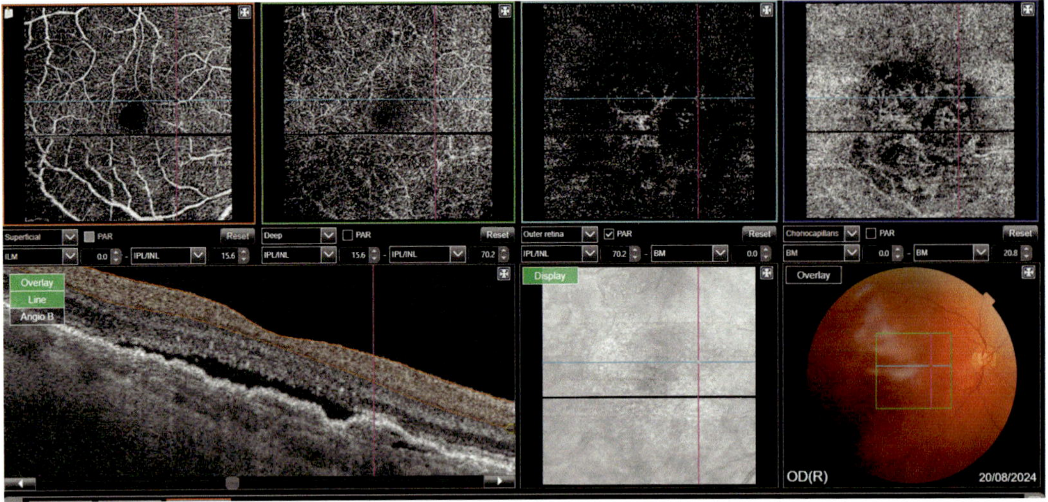

Fig. 2.34 OCT-A images of the right eye showing the presence of a CNV membrane in the setting of neovascular age-related macular degeneration

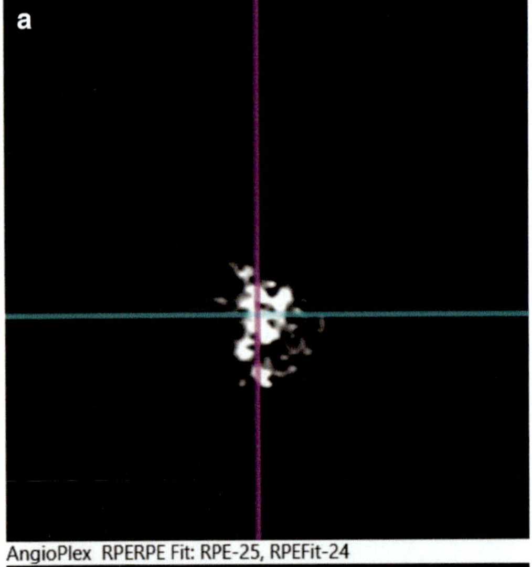

Fig. 2.35 (Top) OCT-A image showing a choroidal neovascular membrane (CNVM) in the setting of pathologic myopia. (Bottom) B-scan OCT image showing cross section through the fovea of the same retina

- Retinal neovascularisation—OCT-A can also be used to characterise retinal neovascularization e.g. in proliferative diabetic retinopathy. With wide-field and ultra-widefield OCT-A, this can be used to image the posterior pole for neovascularization elsewhere (NVE)
- Macular ischaemia (Figs. 2.37 and 2.38)—as OCT-A detects flow, it can be used to delineate the area of level at which ischaemia occurs in the retina or even in the choriocapillaris

2.2.3 Limitations

- Unable to detect leakage—OCT-A only detects intravascular flow and is unable to detect leakage unlike fluorescein angiography
- Need for stable fixation—OCT-A requires the patient to fixate stably for a longer period of time than conventional OCT; the inability to do so would preclude acquisition of useable OCT-A images or result in significant motion artifacts
- Flow outside of temporal window—flow that is too fast or too slow may not be detected
- Limited field of view—even widefield or ultra-widefield OCT-A has a limited field of view, which makes it less able to detect any flow abnormalities in the periphery compared to ultra-widefield fluorescein angiography

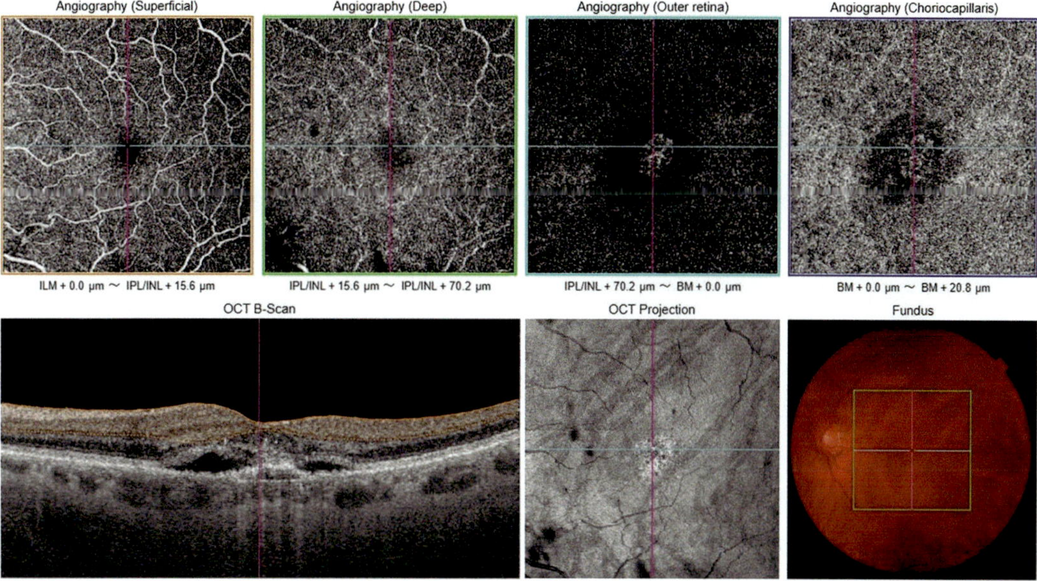

Fig. 2.36 OCT-A images of the left eye showing the presence of a secondary CNV membrane in the setting of CSR

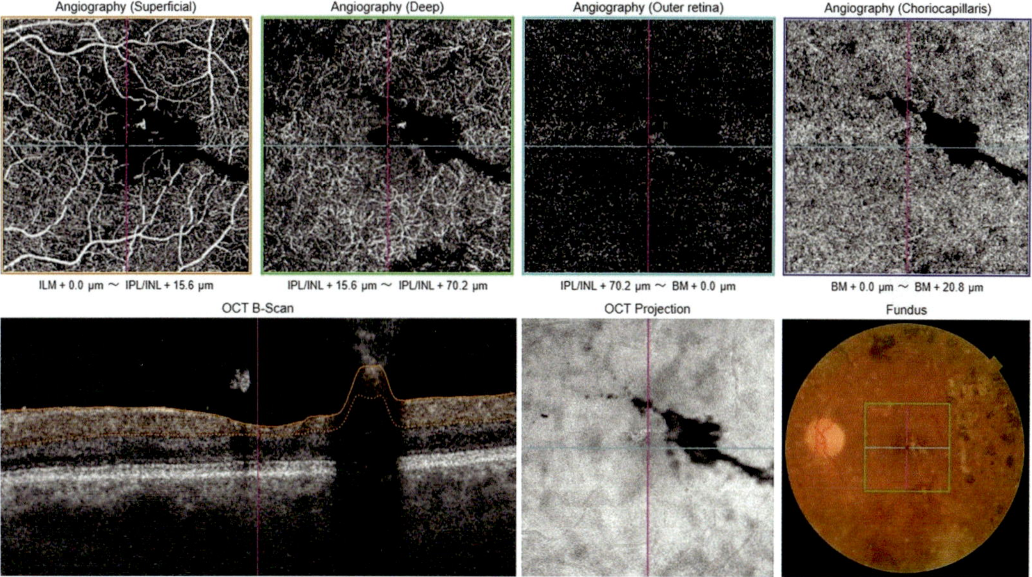

Fig. 2.37 OCT-A images of the left eye showing the presence of macular ischaemia in the setting of diabetic maculopathy

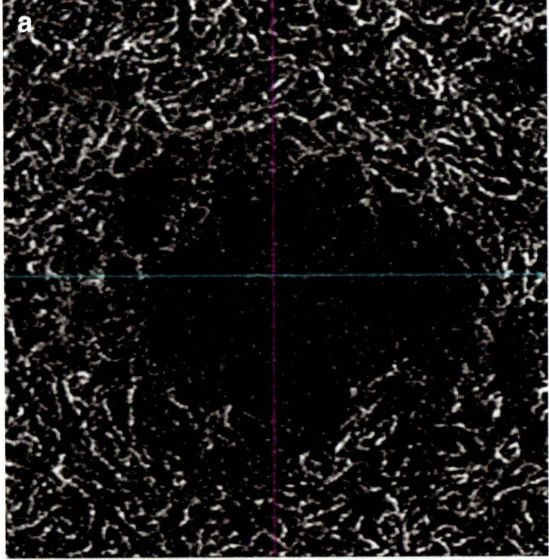

Fig. 2.38 (Top) OCT-A image showing multiple flow voids corresponding to multiple areas of non-perfusion in the deep capillary plexus in the setting of sickle cell retinopathy. (Bottom) B-scan OCT image showing cross section through the fovea of the same retina

- Need for clear medium—any significant media opacity can impede the acquisition of usable OCT-A images

2.3 Fundus Fluorescein Angiography (FFA)

2.3.1 Principles

- Based on the principle of fluorescence whereby excitation at one wavelength occurs and is emitted immediately through a longer wavelength.
- 5 ml of 10% Sodium fluorescein is injected intravenously into the patient's blood stream. 20% of sodium fluorescein remains unbound to protein and is available for fluorescence.
- Unbound sodium fluorescein molecules within the bloodstream or the sodium fluorescein molecules that have leaked out of blood vessels are excited with a blue flash (wavelength of 465–490 nm) of a camera. On cessation of the blue flash the excited fluorescein molecules will immediately emit a green-yellow light at a higher wavelength of 520–530 nm. The higher wavelength (green-yellow) light is then absorbed by the camera film to generate angiographic images.

2.3.2 Indications

- Look for vascular filling defects (e.g. areas of capillary non-perfusion)
- Look for neovascularisation (e.g. CNV membrane)

2.3.3 Contraindications

- Women who are pregnant, especially those in the first trimester
- Severe reactions to sodium fluorescein

2.3.4 Possible Side-Effects

- Extravasation of fluorescein under the skin +/− subsequent local-tissue necrosis
- Nausea and vomiting
- Transient skin and urine discolouration
- Vasovagal reaction (bradycardia, hypotension, sweating, patients sense of feeling cold)
- Allergic reaction (hives, itching) /anaphylaxis
- Death

2.3.5 Treatment of Anaphylaxis

- Crash call
- Oxygen

- Hydrocortisone 200 mg IV
- Adrenaline IM (1:1000 in 0.5 ml) or IV (1:10,000 in 0.5 ml)
- Chlorpheniramine 10 mg IV

2.3.6 Interpretation

Identify Phases of FFA

- These timings are only valid if the patient has been cannulated in the antecubital fossa and the patient's arm is fully stretched (i.e. the elbow joint is not flexed) when dye is injected intravenously.
- Choroidal phase:
  - Fluorescence begins to appear in the choroid approximately 10–12 s after dye injection in young patients and 12–15 s after injection in older patients. Appears as faint, patchy, and irregularly scattered throughout the posterior fundus
  - A cilioretinal artery, if present, will usually begin to fluoresce as the choroid fluoresces
- Arterial phase (see Fig. 2.39):
  - Starts 1–2 s after choroidal fluorescence is visible or approximately 10–15 s after dye injection
  - Extends from first appearance of dye in the arteries until whole arterial circulation is filled
- Arteriovenous phase (see Fig. 2.40):
  - Starts 1–2 s after the arterial phase

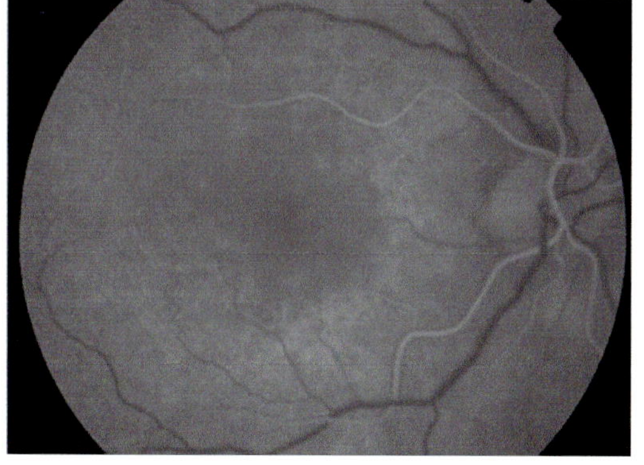

Fig. 2.39 Arterial phase of a fluorescein angiogram showing complete filling of arterial circulation with no filling of retinal veins

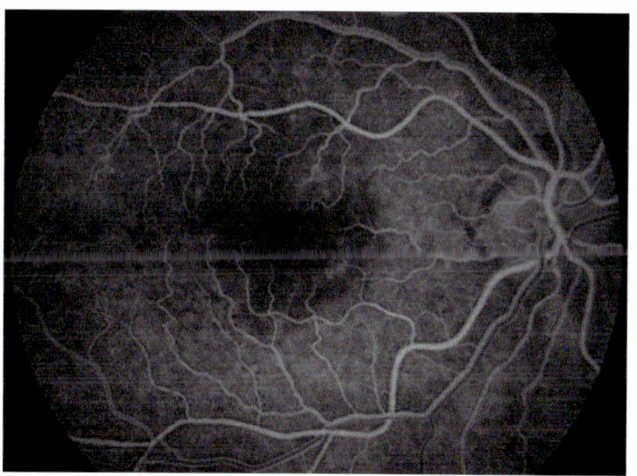

Fig. 2.40 Arteriovenous phase of a fluorescein angiogram showing laminar flow in the retinal veins

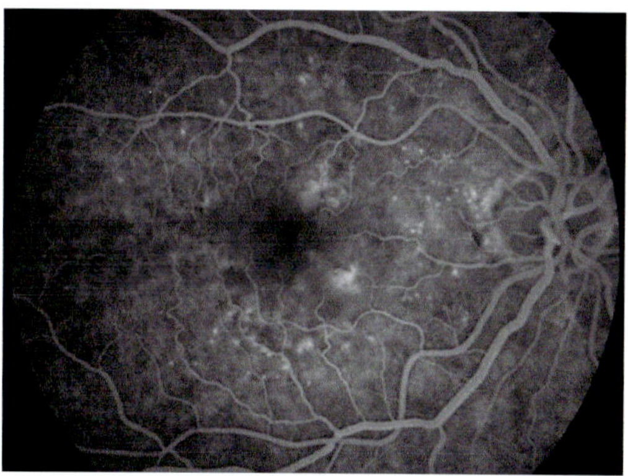

Fig. 2.41 Venous phase of a fluorescein angiogram showing complete filling of the retinal veins

  - Retinal veins begin to fill with a white line of fluorescence visible only along the margins of the retinal veins (laminar flow)
- Venous (see Fig. 2.41):
  - Occurs at approximately 30 s after dye injection
  - Complete fluorescence of retinal veins
- Recirculation phase (see Fig. 2.42):
  - Starts approximately 2–4 m after dye injection
  - Gradual elimination of dye from the choroidal and retinal vessels with a subsequent grey appearance to the vessels

Identify the Presence of Abnormal Hypofluorescence on FFA

- Hypofluorescence is a reduction or absence of normal fluorescence (abnormally dark area)
- Causes:

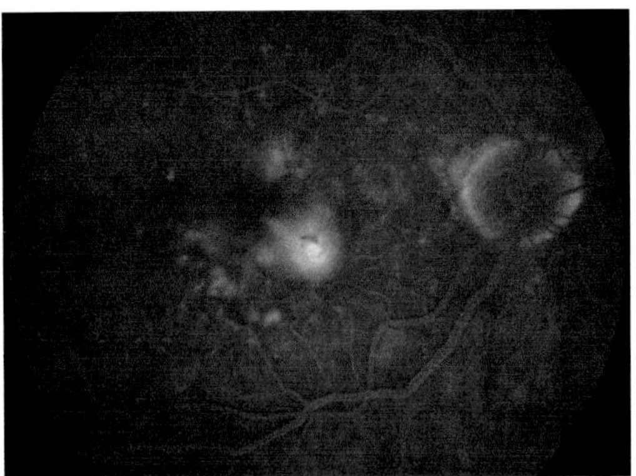

Fig. 2.42 Re-circulation phase of a fluorescein angiogram showing a grey appearance to the retinal vessels as fluorescein dye is eliminated from the retinal circulation

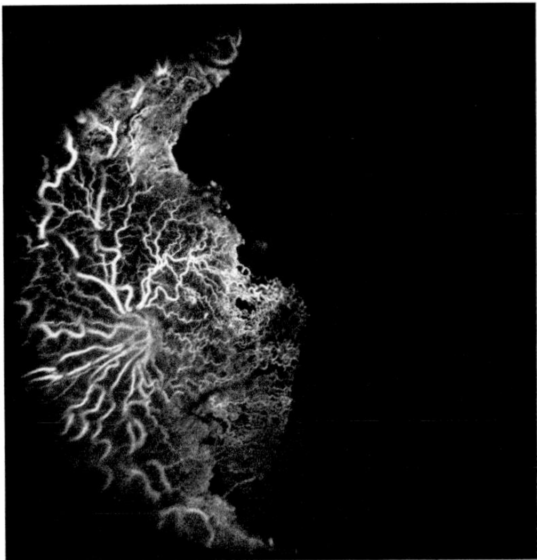

Fig. 2.43 Abnormal hypofluorescence in a fluorescein angiogram from a vascular filling defect due to an absence of retinal vasculature (extensive retinal capillary non-perfusion)

- Vascular filling defect:
  - Absence of vascular tissue (see Fig. 2.43) or complete/partial obstruction of retinal vessels (see Fig. 2.44)
- Blocked fluorescence (see Fig. 2.45):
  - Visualisation of fluorescence from the retinal or choroidal circulation prevented by material located anterior to the retinal or choroidal circulation
- To differentiate blocked fluorescence from a vascular filling defect, correlate the hypofluorescence on the FFA with the ophthalmoscopic view or with a colour fundus image. If there is visible material ophthalmoscopically or on the colour fundus image that corresponds to the area of the hypofluorescence then blocked fluorescence is present. If no correspondence exists, the hypofluorescence is a vascular filling defect.

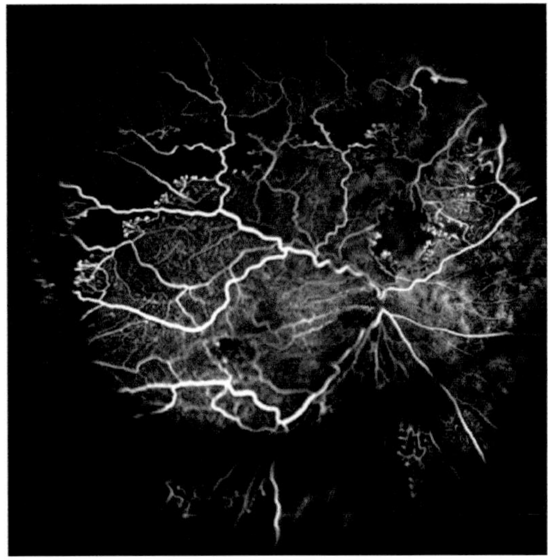

Fig. 2.44 Abnormal hypofluorescence in a fluorescein angiogram from a vascular filling defect due to scattered areas of retinal capillary non-perfusion

Identify the Presence of Abnormal Hyperfluorescence on FFA

- Hyperfluorescence is abnormally excessive hyperfluorescence (abnormally bright area)
- Causes:
  - Window defects (see Fig. 2.46):
    - Increased choroidal fluorescence due to the absence of RPE which normally forms a barrier to choroidal fluorescence
    - 4 characteristics:
      - Appears in the choroidal phase of the FFA
      - Fluorescence increases in intensity as dye concentration in the choroid increases as the FFA progresses

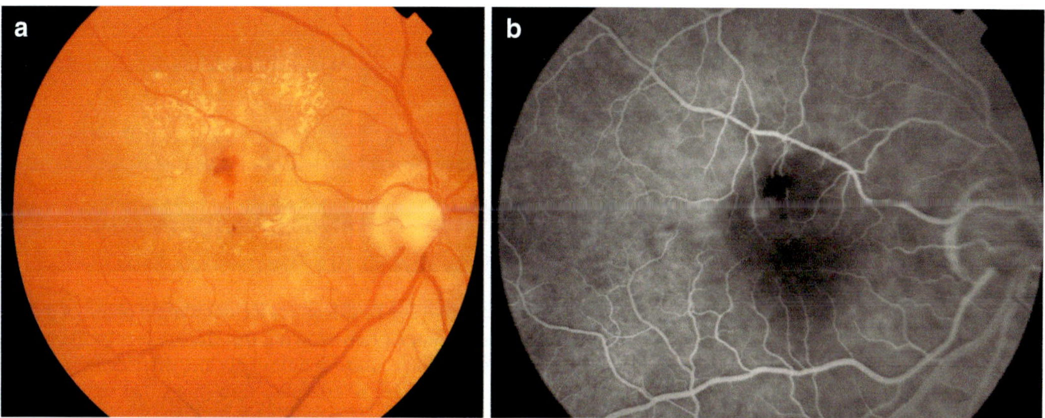

Fig. 2.45 (**a**) Colour fundus image showing an area of subretinal haemorrhage at the macula (**b**) Venous phase of a fluorescein angiogram showing the subretinal haemorrhage seen in image (**a**) as an area of hypofluorescence from blockage

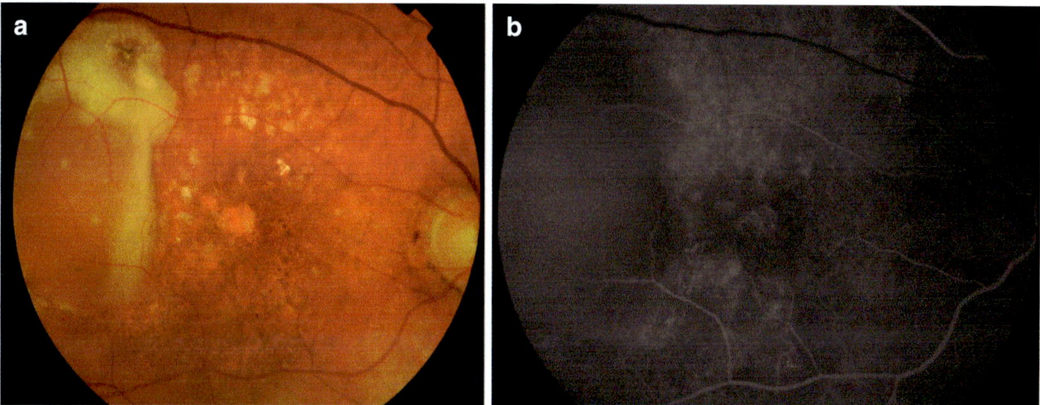

Fig. 2.46 (**a**) Colour fundus image showing areas of temporal subretinal scarring and chorioretinal atrophy at the macula (**b**) Arterial phase of a fluorescein angiogram showing the areas of macular chorioretinal atrophy seen in the colour fundus image in (**a**) as hyperfluorescence areas from window defects

    - Fluorescence does not increase in size or shape during the FFA later phases
    - Fluorescence fades or disappears as dye is eliminated from the choroid at the end of FFA
- Leakage (see Sect. 2.3.7.1):
    - Hyperfluorescence caused by leakage of fluorescein molecules from the inner (retinal vascular endothelium) and outer blood retinal barriers (RPE)
    - Fluorescence increases in intensity as FFA increases but its original borders become increasingly blurred as the FFA progresses
- Pooling (see Sect. 2.3.7.2):
    - Hyperfluorescence caused by fluorescein accumulating and filling a distinct anatomic space (e.g subretinal space or sub-RPE space)
    - Fluorescence increases in intensity as FFA progresses with distinct borders in the late phase of FFA
- Staining (see Fig. 2.47):
    - Hyperfluorescence caused by the diffusion of fluorescein into a tissue or material (e.g. drusen or scar tissue)
    - Fluorescence increases in intensity as FFA progresses and persists in late phases, but its borders remain the same throughout the FFA

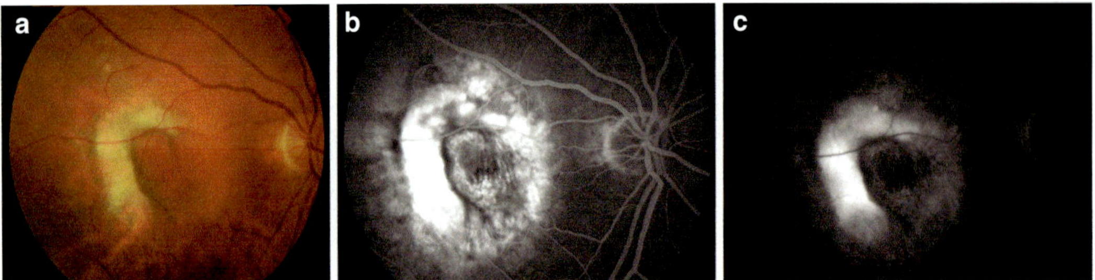

Fig. 2.47 (**a**) Colour fundus image showing a disciform scar associated with a temporal macular RPE tear depicted by the pigmented edge adjacent to the pale crescent temporal to the fovea. (**b**) Venous phase of a fluorescein angiogram showing hyperfluorescence from staining and a hypofluorescent margin corresponding to the folded margin of the RPE tear. (**c**) Re-circulation phase of a fluorescein angiogram showing that the borders of the hyperfluorescence from staining of the disciform scar and temporal 'bare sclera' shown in image (**a**) remained the same throughout the angiogram

2.3.7 Fluorescein Angioscopic Appearance of Common Macular Disorders

2.3.7.1 Choroidal Neovascular Membrane (CNV) Membrane

Classic CNV Membrane

- Consists of a discrete, well demarcated focal area of hyperfluorescence that can be seen in the early phases of the angiogram (see Fig. 2.48)
- Hyperfluorescence increases in intensity and extends beyond the boundaries of the hyperfluorescent area identified in earlier frames of the angiogram through the mid- and late-phase frames

Occult CNV Membrane

- Refers to 2 hyperfluorescent patterns on FFA:
  - Fibrovascular PED: appears as an irregular elevation of the RPE with stippled hyperfluorescent dots (see Fig. 2.49)
  - Late leakage of an undetermined source: no clearly identifiable classic CNV or fibrovascular PED in the early- or mid-phases of the angiogram to account for an area of leakage in the late phase

2.3.7.2 CSR

'Ink Blot' Leakage Pattern

- Leakage starts as a hyperfluorescent pin point in the early phase and concentrically diffuses out in the late phase and appears like an 'ink blot' (see Fig. 2.50).

Smoke Stack Leakage Pattern

- Leakage starts as a hyperfluorescent pinpoint in the early phase, but it gradually tracks upward and then expands to form a mushroom cloud or umbrella-like appearance.

2.3.7.3 Cystoid Macular Oedema (CMO)

- Cystoid oedema in the macular takes on a stellate form (see Fig. 2.51) due to the oblique nature of the outer plexiform layer

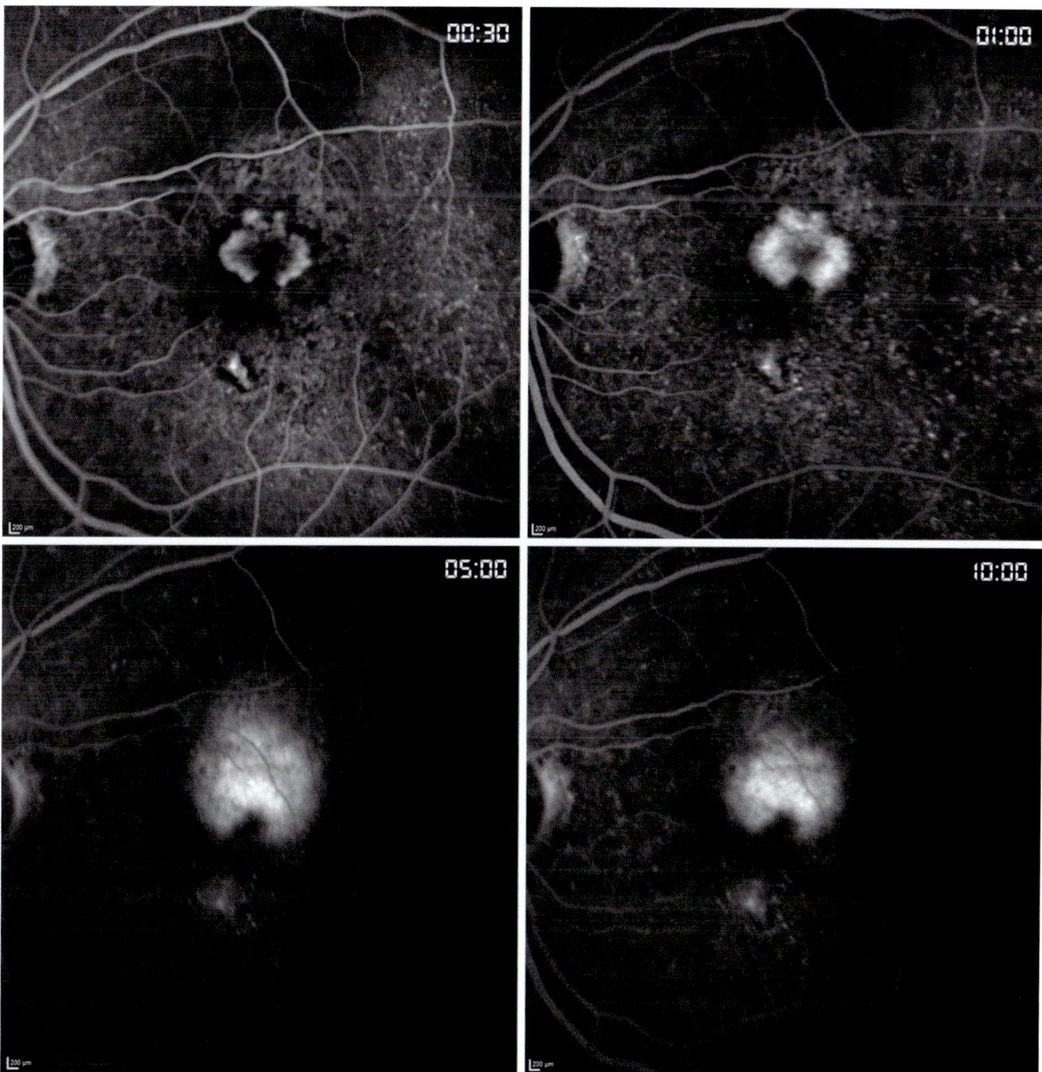

Fig. 2.48 Fluorescein angiogram showing a classic CNV membrane: initial irregular, lacy pattern of leakage which subsequently obliterated by dye leakage

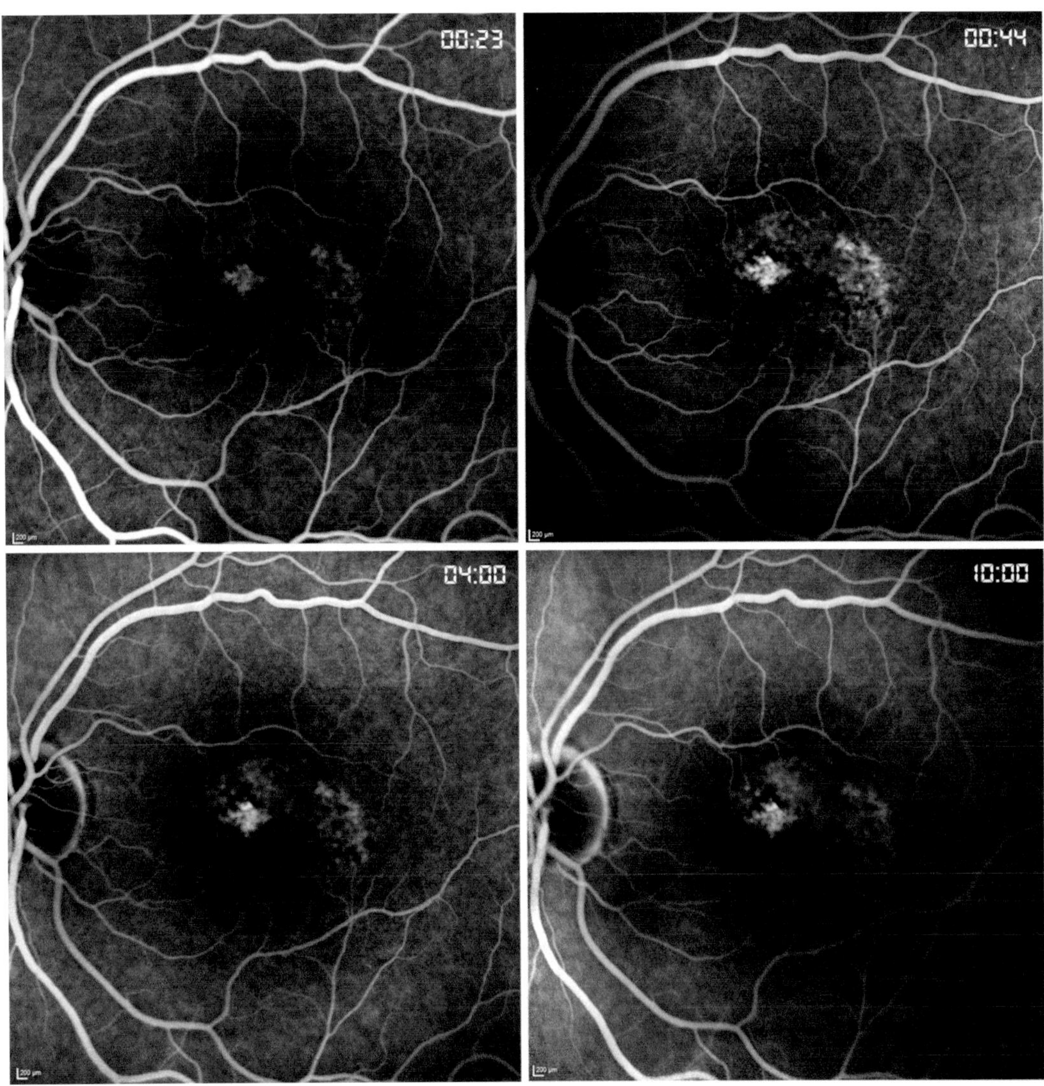

Fig. 2.49 Fluorescein angiogram showing an occult CNV membrane

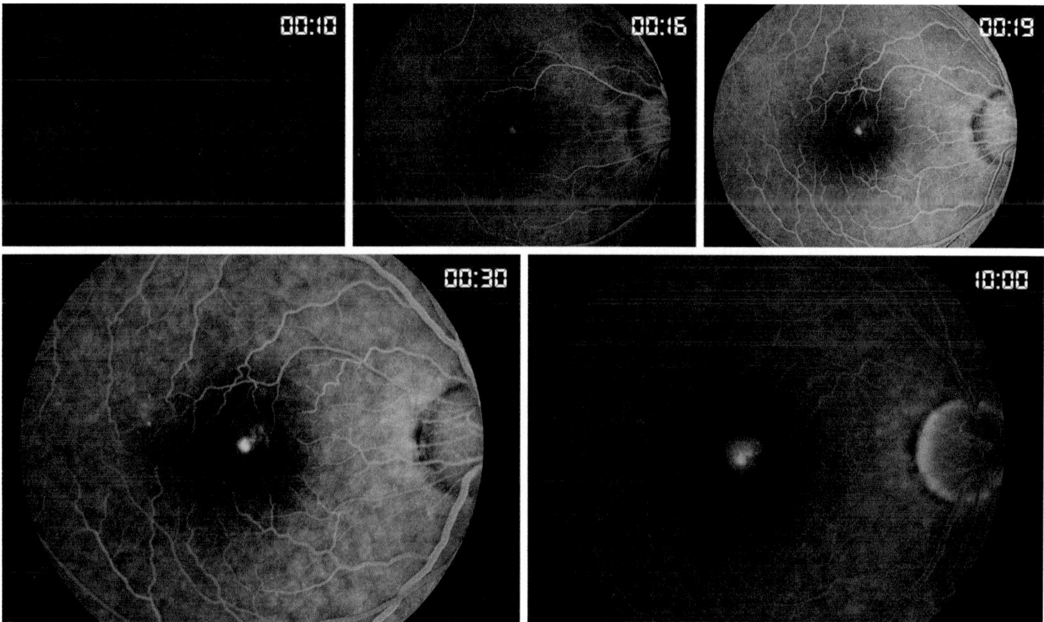

Fig. 2.50 Fluorescein angiogram showing leakage with an inkblot appearance

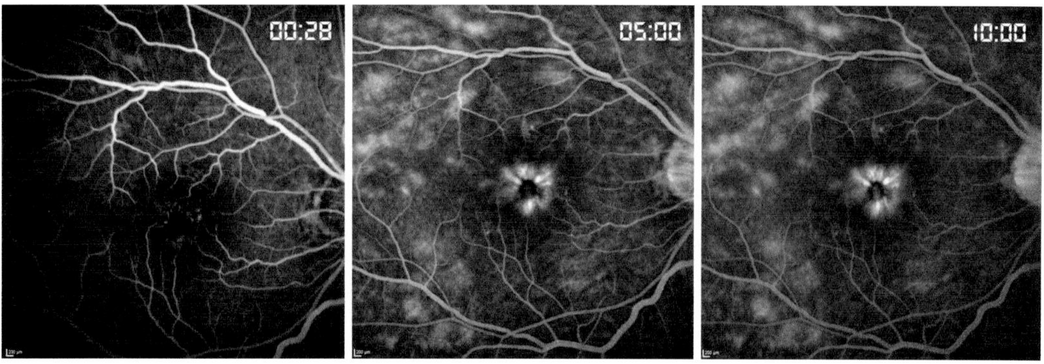

Fig. 2.51 Fluorescein angiogram showing CMO with a petaloid leakage pattern of hyperfluorescence surrounding the fovea. There are scattered hyper-fluorescent (leaking) areas, probably subretinal, in the macula

2.4 Hess Chart

2.4.1 Principles

- Foveal projection in the presence of normal retinal correspondence
- Sherrington's and Hering's law of innervation
- Dissociation of the eyes by means of complementary colour (Hess chart) or a mirror (Lees screen)

2.4.2 Indications

- Help diagnosis for incomitant cases of strabismus
- Monitoring (for improvement or progression)
- Surgical planning and post-operative effects of surgery

2.4.3 Interpretation

- Size:
  - Smallest field denotes the affected eye
  - Underactions are depicted by noting the inward displacement of the dot. Maximum displacement occurs in the direction of the main action of the affected muscle
  - Overactions are noted by the outward displacement of the dots. Maximum displacement occurs in the direction of the main action of the overacting contralateral synergist
  - Other displacements may also be noted, indicating the development of muscle sequelae
- Position:
  - The position of the field reflects the position of the eye e.g. the higher the field the higher the eye
  - The position of the central dot indicates the deviation in primary position, fixing with the opposite eye
  - Each small square represents 5°; therefore an approximate measurement may be made
  - Torsion cannot be assessed unless an adaptation is used (T-bar)
- Shape:
  - Mechanical restrictions will have a much flatter displacement, usually showing reversal of deviation
  - Sloping fields denote the presence of alphabet patterns such as A or V patterns. They do not indicate the presence of torsion
  - Longstanding deviations show the development of muscle sequelae i.e. concomitant fields

2.4.4 Distinguishing Neurogenic Palsies and Mechanical Disorders of Ocular Motility on a Hess Chart

- Neurogenic palsies (see Fig. 2.52, 2.53, 2.54, 2.55, 2.56, 2.57, 2.58, 2.59, 2.60, 2.61 and 2.62):
  - Field of affected eye will be smaller
  - Proportional spacing between the outer and inner fields, with both fields displaced according to the deviation
  - Muscle sequelae: overaction of contralateral synergist (yoke muscle) in the unaffected eye, overaction of ipsilateral antagonist in the affected eye, secondary inhibition of contralateral antagonist in the unaffected eye
- Mechanical disorders (see Figs. 2.63 and 2.64):
  - Outer field of chart will be very close to the inner field in the direction of maximum limitation of movement
  - Field of the affected eye will be very narrow either horizontally or vertically
  - Muscle sequelae: limited, often confined to overaction of the contralateral synergist in the unaffected eye

2.4.5 Hess Charts of Common Ocular Motility Disorders

2.4.5.1 Cranial Nerve III Palsy

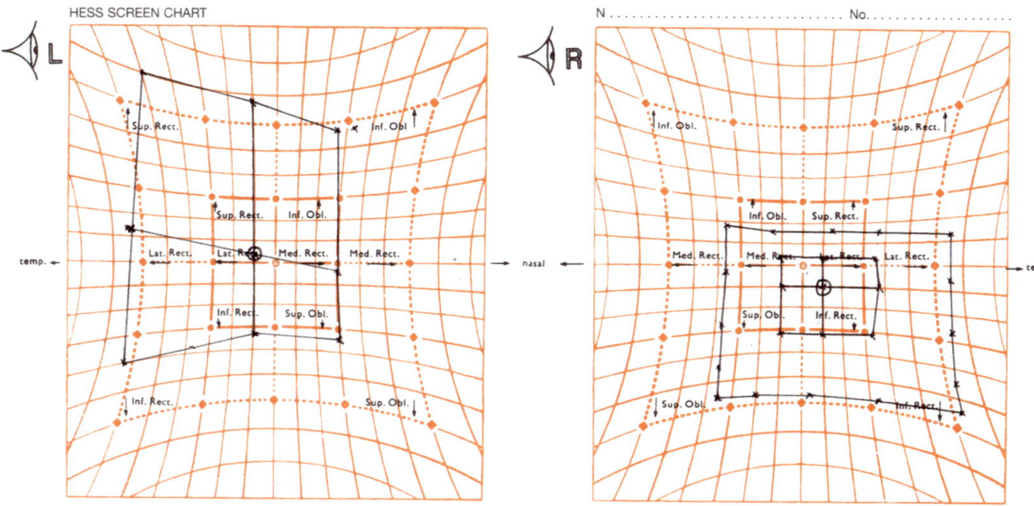

Fig. 2.52 Hess chart of a patient with a right CN III palsy

2.4.5.2 Cranial Nerve IV Palsy

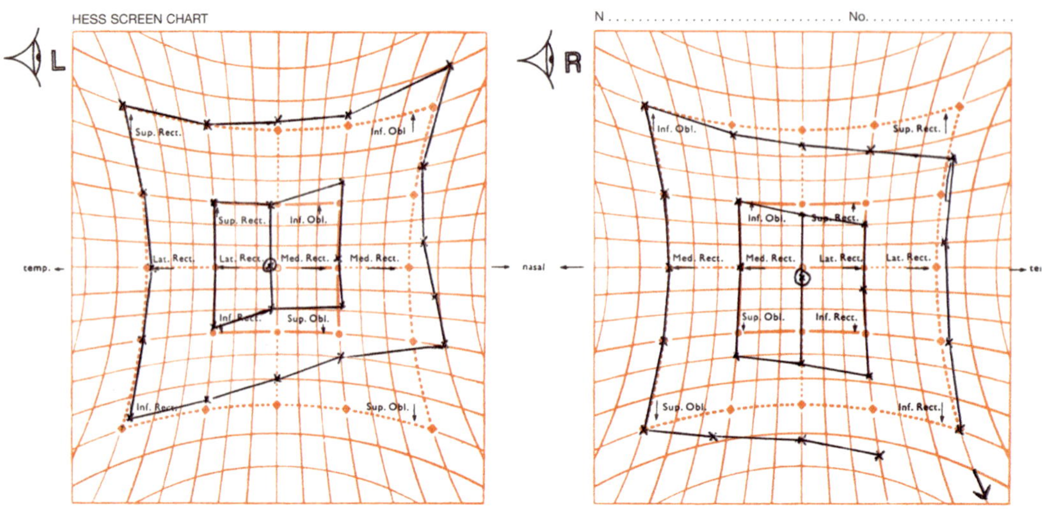

Fig. 2.53 Hess chart of a patient with a left CN IV palsy with muscle sequelae (left IO overaction, right IR overaction, right SR underaction)

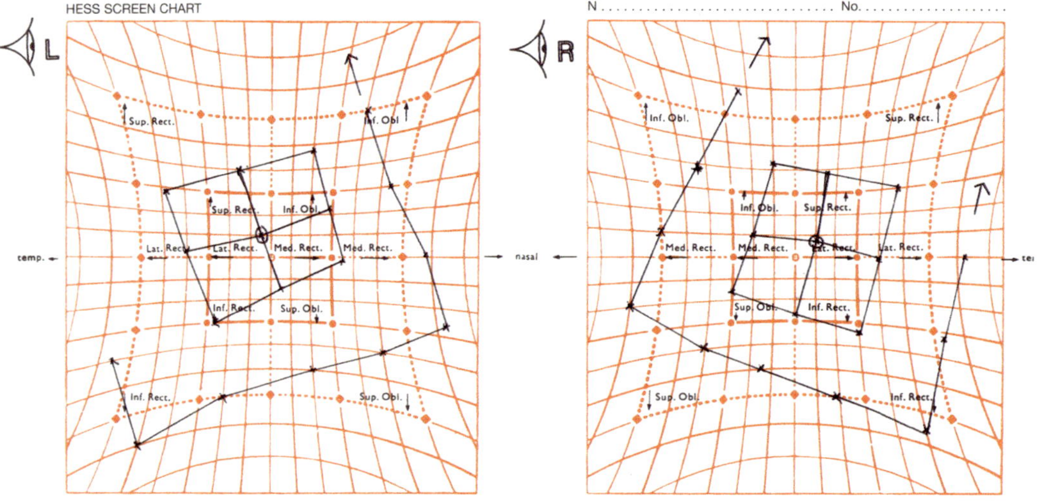

Fig. 2.54 Hess chart of a patient with a bilateral CN IV palsy with a V-pattern

2.4.5.3 Cranial Nerve VI Palsy

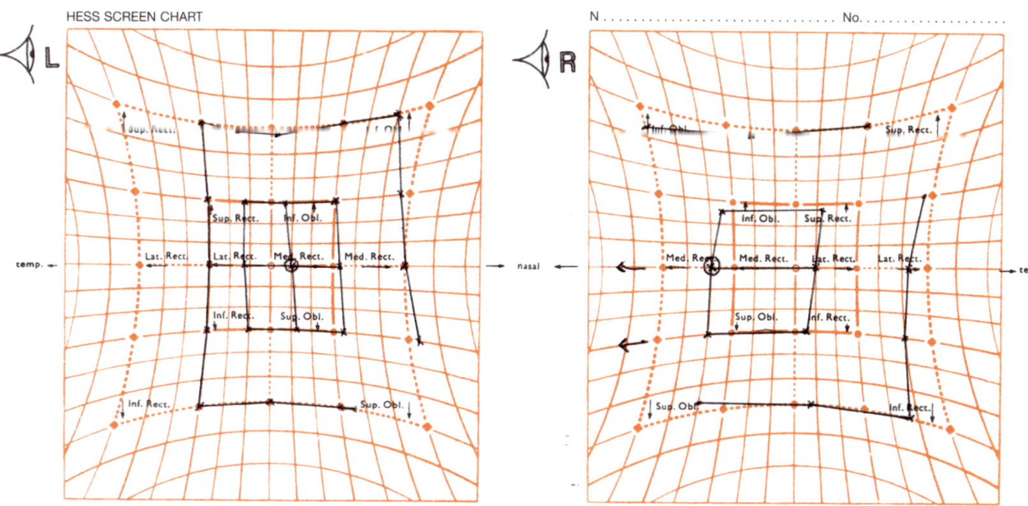

Fig. 2.55 Hess chart of a patient with a left CN VI palsy

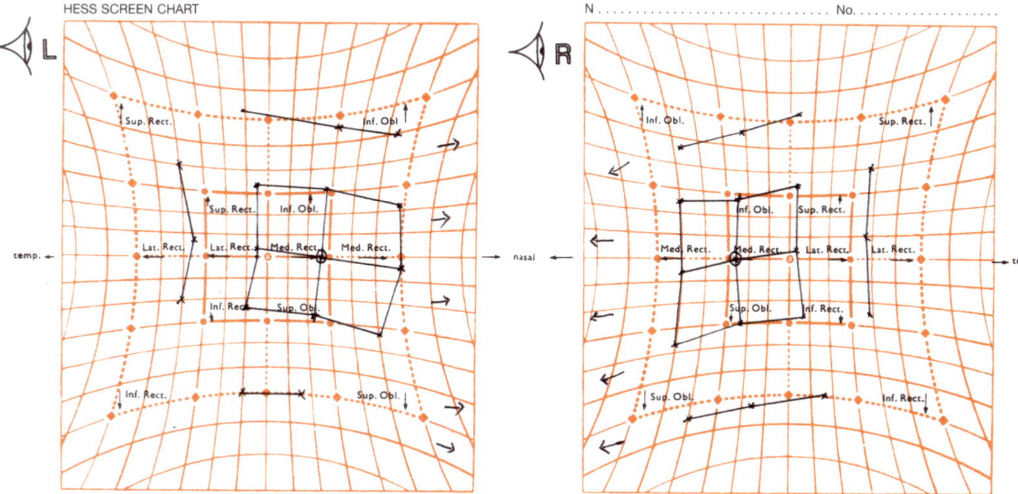

Fig. 2.56 Hess chart of a patient with a bilateral CN VI palsy

2.4.5.4 Brown Syndrome

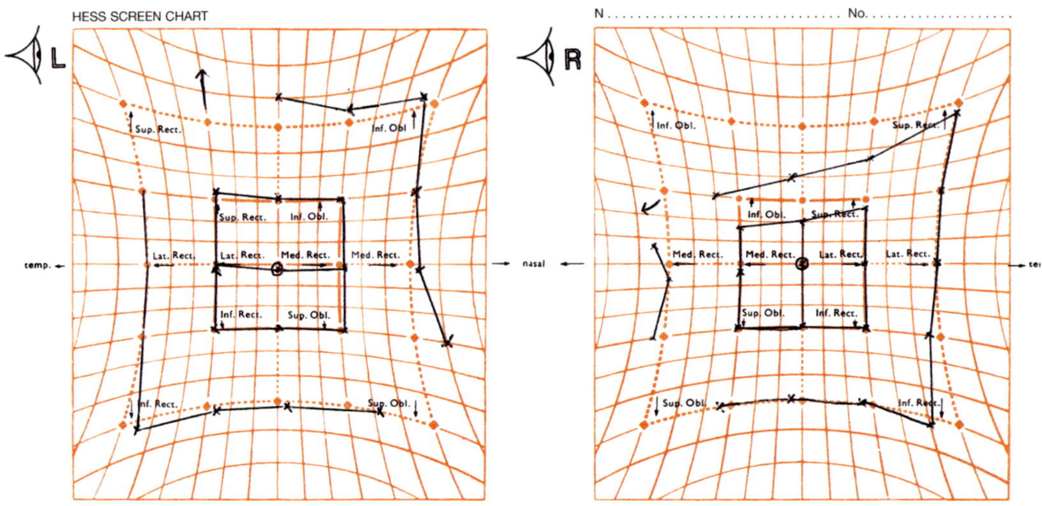

Fig. 2.57 Hess chart of a patient with a right Brown syndrome with limited muscle sequelae of overaction of the right SR muscle

2.4.5.5 Duane's Syndrome

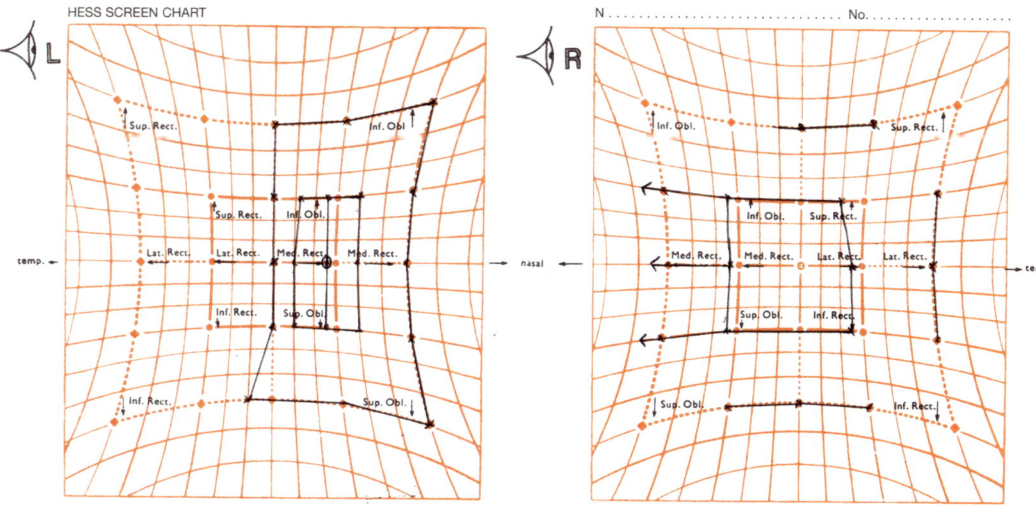

Fig. 2.58 Hess chart of a patient with type I Duane's syndrome

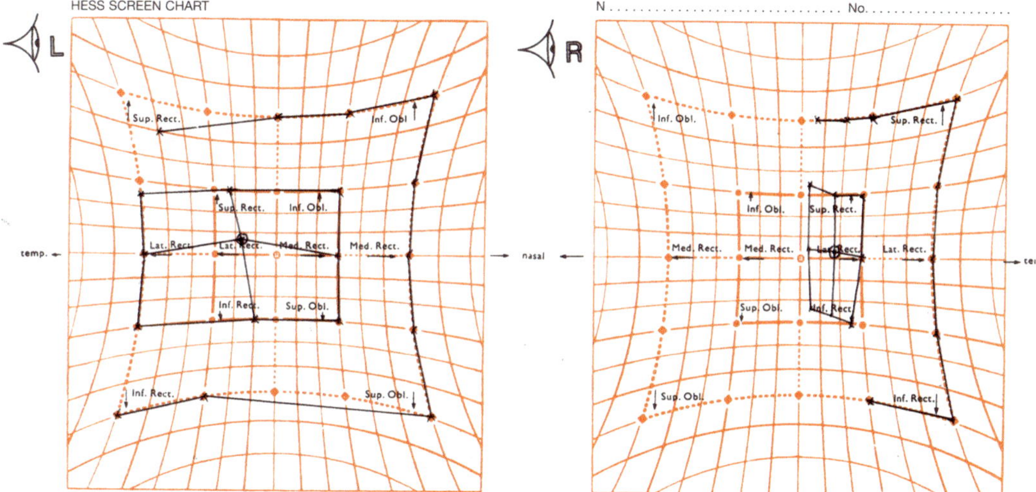

Fig. 2.59 Hess chart of a patient with type II Duane's syndrome

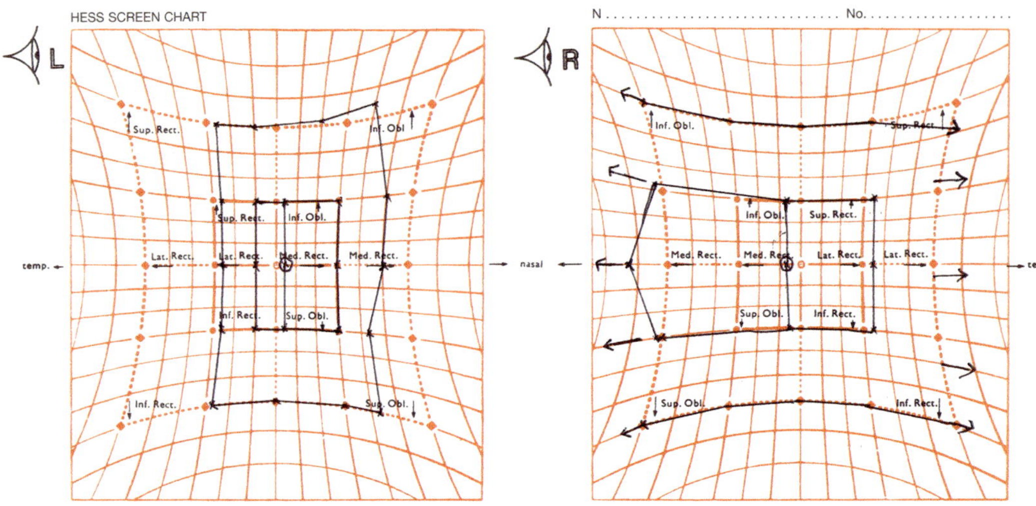

Fig. 2.60 Hess chart of a patient with type III Duane's syndrome

2.4.5.6 Internuclear Ophthalmoplegia (INO)

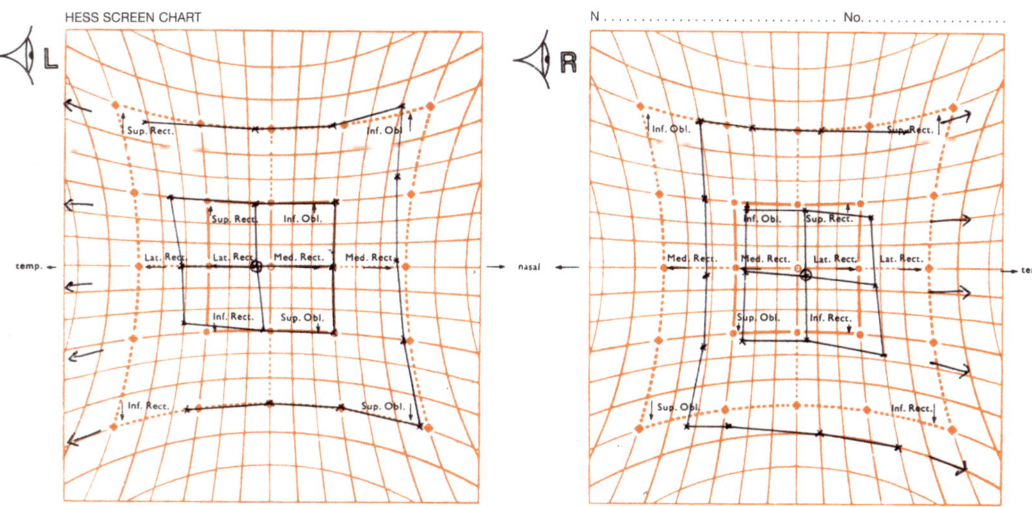

Fig. 2.61 Hess chart of a patient with a right INO

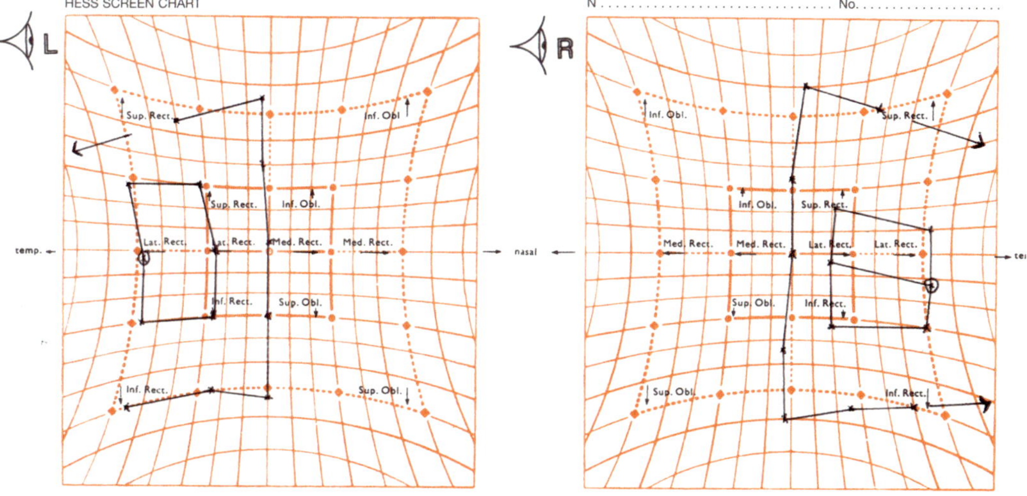

Fig. 2.62 Hess chart of a patient with a walled eye bilateral INO (WEBINO)

2.4.5.7 Thyroid Eye Disease (TED)

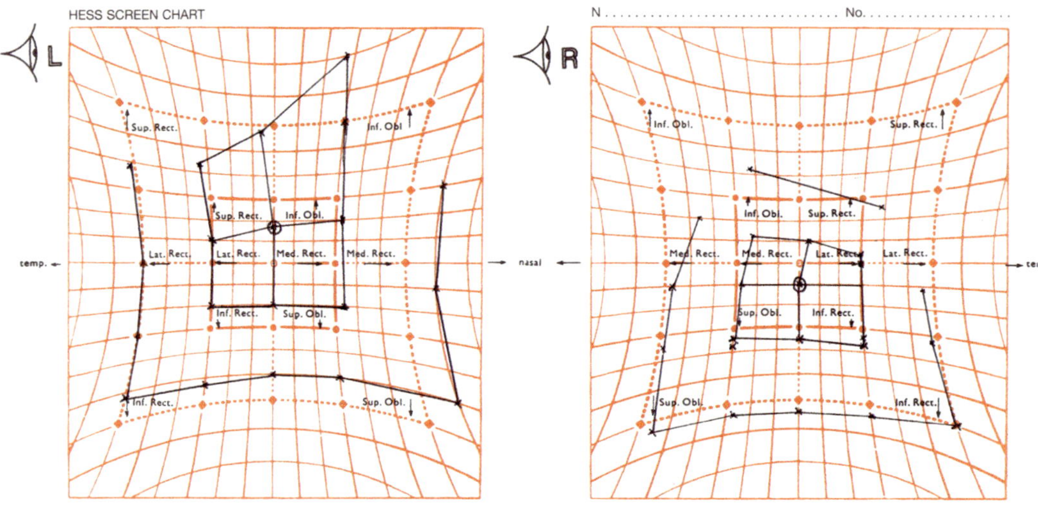

Fig. 2.63 Hess chart of a patient with TED with restriction of elevation of the right eye

2.4.5.8 Orbital Floor Fracture

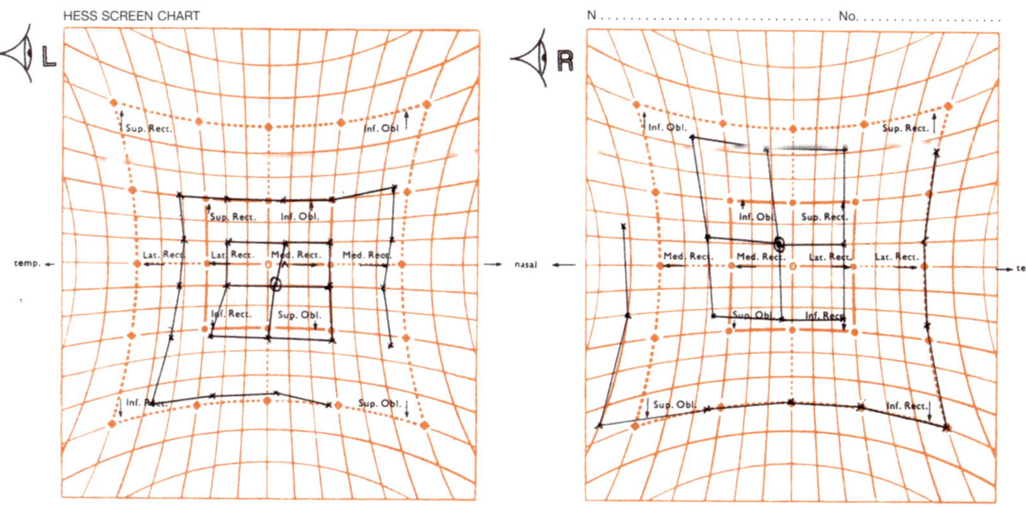

Fig. 2.64 Hess chart of a patient with a left orbital floor fracture

2.5 Computerised Tomography (CT)

2.5.1 Principles

- CT scanner is shaped like a large ring. Thin beams of X-rays are scanned through the patient (located in the centre of the ring) from many different points around the ring, and picked up by detectors on the opposite side (of the ring). As X-rays pass through the patient in a CT scanner, it is partially absorbed by the tissues it encounters. The amount absorbed depends on the density of the tissues traversed. CT scans measure radiographic density of the tissues being studied.
- CT was developed directly from conventional X-ray technology with only 2 differences from conventional X-rays:
  - Rather than taking one view (as in conventional X-ray), the X-ray beam is rotated around the patient to take multiple different views of multiple slices of the patient
  - The X-ray data acquired in this way are reconstructed by a computer to obtain a detailed image of all the structures in the slices (including bone, air, soft tissues)

2.5.2 Indications

- Orbital trauma: fractures, foreign bodies
- Orbital infection

2.5.3 Contraindications

- Pregnancy

2.5.4 Advantages

- Excellent for bony detail
- Quick and readily available
- Minimal patient cooperation required

2.5.5 Disadvantages

- Uses ionising radiation

2.5.6 Interpretation

1. Define image plane: axial, coronal, sagittal
2. Terminology: isodense (structures of intermediate density similar to that of brain tissue and appears grey), hyperdense (structures appear as brighter areas than that of brain tissue), hypodense (structures appear darker than that of brain tissue)
3. Define mass:
   - Tissue of origin: is mass from a normal orbital structure such as the lacrimal gland, optic nerve, or extraocular muscle(s)
   - Position of the mass: intraconal space, extraconal space, subperiosteal space, extraocular muscles, tenon's space, extra-orbital space
   - Imaging clues to the biologic behaviour of a mass: "pusher" (benign well circumscribed lesions)—push adjacent structures aside, "eater" (malignant)—infiltrative lesions
   - Relationship to adjacent bone: slow growing benign masses "push" the bone or cause fossa formation. Aggressive malignant tumours "eat" the bone or cause bone erosion.
   - Shape of the mass: cavernous haemangiomas are usually "round", benign mixed tumours of the lacrimal gland are said to be "oval", "kink" of an enlarged optic nerve (a sharp change in the direction of the nerve) strongly suggests a glioma
   - Size of the mass
   - Internal characteristics of the mass: homogenous (majority of tumours), heterogenous (combination of solid and cystic components in a child's tumour—lymphangioma, layering of fat and keratin debris in a cystic mass—dermoid cyst (see Fig. 2.72), small areas of calcification in a

soft tissue orbital mass—malignancy, "tram tracking" of an optic nerve tumour—optic nerve meningioma, hyperostosis of the sphenoid wing—sphenoid wing meningioma)

– Contrast enhancement of the mass: meningioma, rhabdomyosarcoma, inflammatory lesions such as sarcoidosis

2.5.7 CT Scan Images of Common Orbital Disorders Occurring in Adults

2.5.7.1 TED (Fig. 2.65)

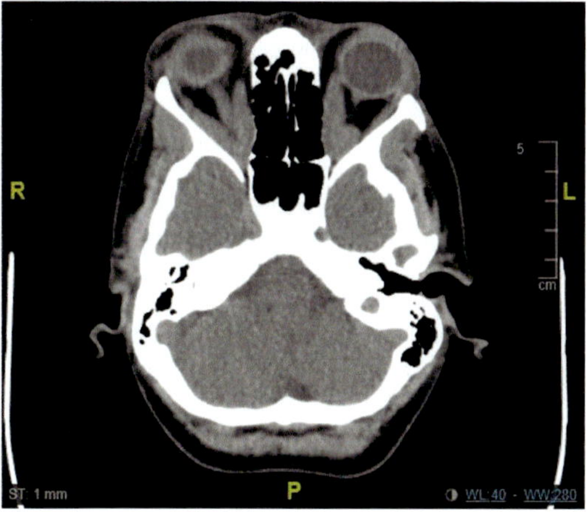

Fig. 2.65 Axial CT scan image of a patient with TED showing multiple enlarged extraocular muscles

2.5.7.2 Orbital Pseudotumour (Idiopathic Orbital Inflammatory Disease) (Fig. 2.66)

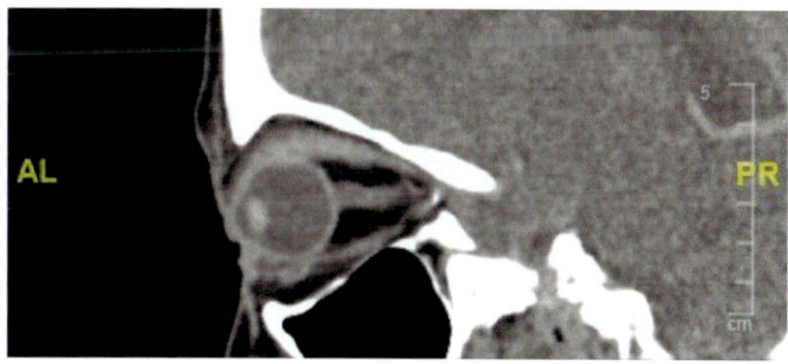

Fig. 2.66 Sagittal CT scan image of a patient with orbital inflammatory disease with an enlarged SR muscle

2.5.7.3 Cavernous Haemangioma (Fig. 2.67)

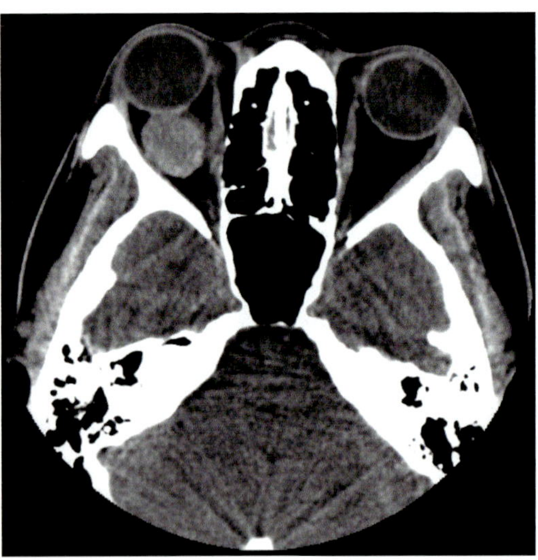

Fig. 2.67 Axial CT scan image of a patient with a right intraconal cavernous haemangioma

2.5.7.4 Lymphoid Lesions of the Orbit (Fig. 2.68 and Tables 2.1, 2.2)

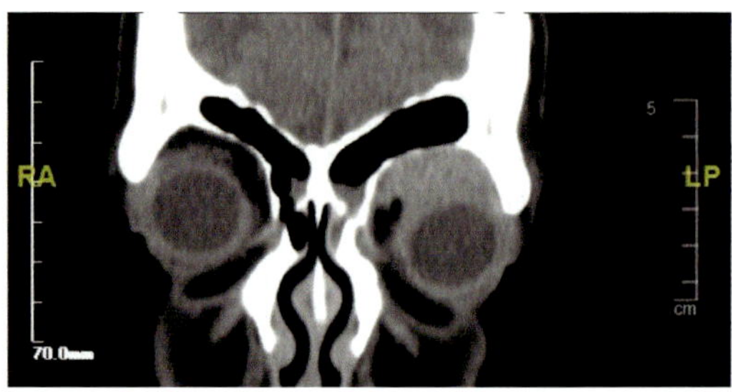

Fig. 2.68 Coronal CT scan image of a patient with a left orbital lymphoma

Table 2.1 Useful information about orbital lymphoid lesions

Lymphoid lesions occur most commonly in elderly patients, but may occur in middle age
In some patients, the disease may present bilaterally (an exception to the rule that orbital tumours are usually unilateral)
A large no. of all orbital lymphoid lesions will eventually be associated with systemic disease
Almost all periocular lymphomas are non-Hodgkin type, almost all of B-cell origin
Most common periocular lymphoma is the MALT type (others include diffuse lymphoplasmacytic, follicle center, diffuse large cell)

Table 2.2 Approach to a patient with an orbital lymphoid lesion

History:

Any pain and rate of progression: gradual onset with slow progression of a painless orbital mass, often anterior and superior

Any previous diagnosis of lymphoma

Examination:

Look for proptosis: axial or non-axial (depending on the position of the mass) – usually non-axial, extraconal and anterior

Look for characteristic salmon patch on the conjunctiva (suggestive of lymphoma)

Palpate for any orbital masses (normally felt anteriorly – smooth, usually mobile, and firm to touch – no tenderness associated with palpation): most commonly, you will see lymphoid tumours arising in the superior orbital quadrants (the extraconal space, especially with involvement of the lacrimal gland, is a common site. Although the inferior orbit is not the most common site, lymphoid lesions are the most common condition presenting there)

Investigations:

FBC with a differential count

CT scan (see Fig. 2.68): smooth mass (lobular or irregular in shape rather than round) that is a typical "pusher", not "eater" of orbital tissues (no infiltration of orbital tissues – lesion is said to mold to the orbital tissues, bone erosion is rare)

Incisional biopsy is required to make the final diagnosis (fresh tissue for immunopathologic staining, and formalin fixed tissue for haematoxylin and eosin staining) – required for all lymphoid lesions as they all look the same on a CT scan

Referral to oncologists/haematologists for evaluation to rule out systemic involvement – chest and abdominal CT scan to identify abnormal nodes, bone marrow aspiration to rule out marrow involvement

Management:

Radiotherapy in the absence of systemic disease

Chemotherapy for poorly differentiated types of lymphoma – follicular, large cell

Monoclonal antibody (Rituximab) +/- chemotherapy protocols (CHOP)

Differential Diagnosis:

Benign – benign reactive lymphoid hyperplasia

Malignant – lymphoma

Indeterminate – atypical lymphoid hyperplasia

2.5.7.5 Metastatic Tumours to the Orbit (Fig. 2.69 and Tables 2.3, 2.4)

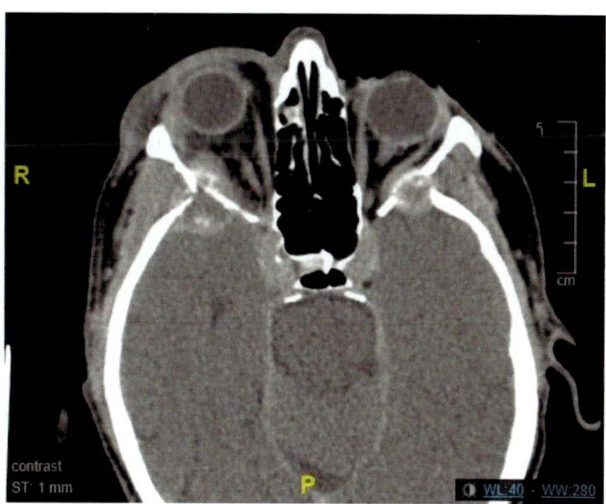

Fig. 2.69 Axial CT scan image of a patient with a metastatic neuroendocrine tumour showing bone erosion

Table 2.3 Useful information about metastatic orbital tumours

Lung cancer is the most common metastatic orbital tumour in men
Breast cancer is the most common metastatic orbital tumour in women

Table 2.4 Approach to a patient with a metastatic orbital tumour

History:
Any pain and rate of progression: onset of proptosis occurring over a few days to a few weeks, sometimes with mild pain or inflammatory signs
Ask about history of any known malignancy: up to 25% of metastatic orbital tumours will not have a known primary tumour
Examinations:
Look for proptosis: often non-axial – areas infiltrated by tumour are often outside the muscle cone, sometimes eroding the bones
Look for enophthalmos – metastatic scirrhous breast cancer resulting from fibrosis of the involved orbital tissues
Look for eyelid swelling and chemosis – often seen with many metastatic tumours
Investigations:
CT scan (see Fig. 2.69): infiltrative mass (tumours are "eaters"—often the tumours extend into more than one of the orbital spaces and infiltrates several orbital structures), bone erosion is commonly seen with any adenocarcinoma, diagnosis of metastatic prostate carcinoma can be made on a CT-scan alone based on the characteristic combination of both osteoclastic (destroyed bone) and osteoblastic (new bone) changes
Incisional biopsy: make definitive diagnosis of a metastatic orbital tumour
Referral to oncologist for systemic work up
Management:
Radiation therapy: if the orbit is the only site of metastasis
Chemotherapy: if other areas of metastatic involvement are found

2.5.7.6 Sphenoid Wing Meningioma (Fig. 2.70 and Table 2.5, 2.6)

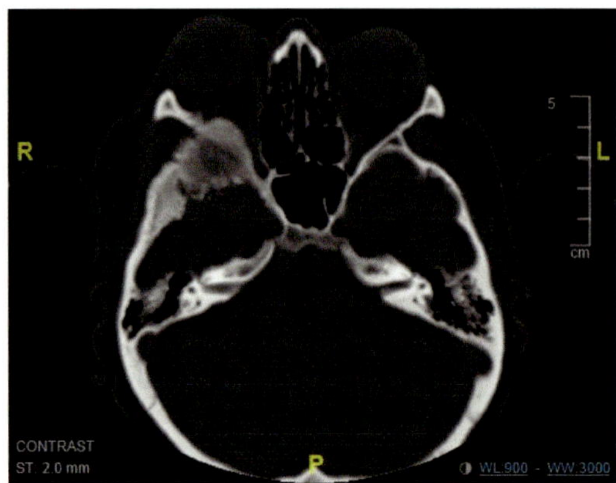

Fig. 2.70 Axial CT scan image of a patient with a right sphenoid wing meningioma

Table 2.5 Useful information about sphenoid wing meningioma

Meningioma arising from the intracranial side of the sphenoid bone and extending into the orbit secondarily

Table 2.6 Approach to a patient with a sphenoid wing meningioma

History:
Ask about any vision loss: suggests optic nerve compression
Examination:
Look for any proptosis: any proptosis and downward displacement of the eye precede vision loss, often by years
Look for any fullness of the temple: hyperostotic bone pushes into the orbit and temporalis fossa
Look for any corneal exposure: advanced meningioma causes disfiguring proptosis and corneal exposure
Check optic nerve function: VA, RAPD, colour vision, VF
Look for optic disc swelling
Investigations:
CT with contrast enhancement (see Fig. 2.70): soft tissue involvement surrounding the hyperostotic sphenoid wing
MRI: usually performed to view the details of the soft tissues in the orbital apex and around the chiasm
Treatment:
Excision: meningioma can be debulked to relieve compression, but complete removal is not possible
Radiation therapy: used as adjunctive therapy although tumour not very radiosensitive

2.5.7.7 Lacrimal Gland Tumours (Fig. 2.71 and Table 2.7)

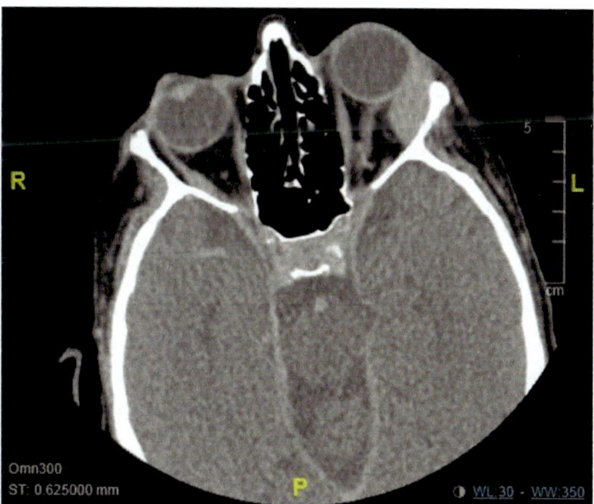

Fig. 2.71 Axial CT scan image of a patient with an enlarged left lacrimal gland

Table 2.7 Approach to a patient with an enlarged lacrimal gland

Differential diagnosis:
Infiltration of abnormal cells into the gland (most common cause of lacrimal gland enlargement): lymphoid tumours, benign reactive lymphoid hyperplasia (benign), lymphoma (malignant), atypical lymphoid hyperplasia (indeterminate)
Sarcoidosis
Idiopathic orbital inflammatory disease
Tumours arising from lacrimal tissue: benign mixed tumour (benign), adenoid cystic carcinoma (malignant), adenocarcinoma (malignant)
History:
Age: elderly (lymphoid lesions), middle age (benign mixed tumour)
Pain: orbital inflammatory disease (acute pain with associated inflammatory signs)
Onset and progression of symptoms: differentiating adenoid cystic carcinoma (rapid progression over a few months, no pain present, symptoms or signs never present for more than 1 year) from benign mixed tumours (slowly progressive over a period of months to years, no pain, no periocular signs, no pulsations), lymphoid lesions/tumours (painless, slowly progressive – weeks to months), sarcoidosis (slowly progressive, painless)
History of sarcoidosis
Examination:
Look for proptosis: non-axial – inferonasal/inferior displacement of the eye (proptosis occurs relatively late with lacrimal gland masses as the lacrimal gland is anterior to the equator of the eye), globe ptosis prominent with benign mixed tumour, globe ptosis less likely with lymphoid lesions
Look for fullness or a palpable mass in the superotemporal quadrant (if you lift the upper eyelid, you may be able to see an enlarged palpebral lobe of the lacrimal gland) – soft anterior mass (lymphoid lesion), firm larger smooth convex mass (benign mixed tumour), firm non smooth mass (adenoid cystic carcinoma)
Look for numbness or paraesthesias in the temporal region as a result of typical neurotrophic spread of adenoid cystic carcinoma
Look for salmon patch: lymphoid lesion
Look for associated inflammatory signs: lid swelling, chemosis (orbital inflammatory disease)
Look for intraocular inflammation/iris nodules (Busacca, Berlin, Koeppe): sarcoidosis
Investigations:
FBC with a differential count: lymphoid lesions/tumours
ACE, Calcium, CXR, CT Chest: sarcoidosis
CT scan (see Fig. 2.71): round or oval well circumscribed mass in the superotemporal quadrant with globe indentation and bony moulding with adjacent fossa formation in the bone as a result of the long standing pressure changes (benign mixed tumour), erosive bone changes (malignancy – adenoid cystic carcinoma), infiltrative superotemporal mass extending across the orbital space (adenoid cystic carcinoma), well circumscribed enlargement of the lacrimal gland with the typical moulding of the mass to the surrounding tissues – a "pusher" – with no bony changes (lymphoid lesions/tumours)
MRI scan: if you suspect intracranial extension based on the clinical examination or CT scan
Incisional biopsy: don't perform if benign mixed tumour (need to keep pseudocapsule intact otherwise increases risk of recurrence – as benign mixed tumour grows within the lacrimal gland, it compresses adjacent glandular and orbital tissue to form a pseudocapsule – no epithelial lining – separating the tumour from the surrounding tissue), non-caseating granulomas in lacrimal tissue (sarcoidosis)
Management:
Complete excision: benign mixed tumour
Exenteration, including bone removal and craniotomy, when necessary, followed by radiation therapy: adenoid cystic carcinoma

2.5.8 CT Scan Images of Common Orbital Disorders Occurring in Childhood

2.5.8.1 Dermoid Cyst (Fig. 2.72)

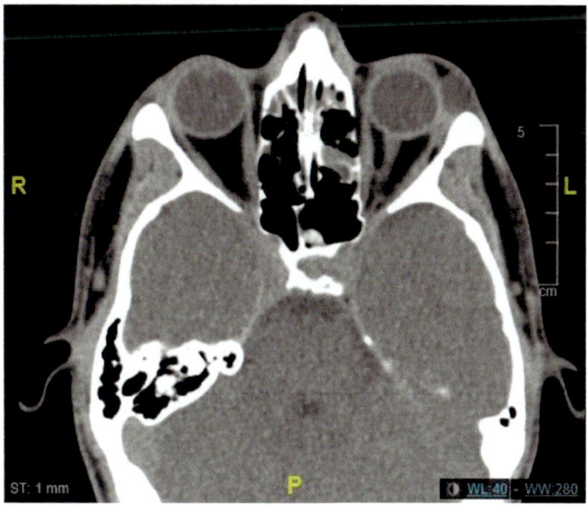

Fig. 2.72 Axial CT scan of a patient showing a left extraconal round mass with a lucent central area. This is consistent with a left orbital dermoid cyst

2.5.8.2 Optic Nerve Glioma (Fig. 2.73)

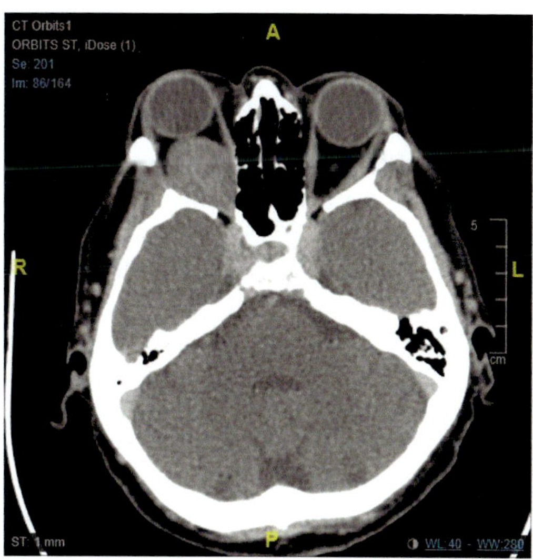

Fig. 2.73 Axial CT scan of a patient with a fusiform enlargement of the right optic nerve. This is consistent with an optic nerve glioma

2.6 Magnetic Resonance Imaging (MRI)

2.6.1 Principles

- An external powerful magnetic field is applied by the MRI scanner to a patient that causes protons in the patient to align their intrinsic spins in parallel with the magnetic field.
- A radio-frequency pulse is generated from an emission-reception coil that excites these protons, causing them to flip their spins away from the direction of the magnetic field. When the pulse stops, the protons spins relax back in parallel with the magnetic field and give off energy in the form of electromagnetic waves that are detected by the same emission-reception coil to generate images.

2.6.2 Indications

- Orbital tumours
- Optic nerve tumours

2.6.3 Contraindications

- Metallic foreign bodies
- Pacemakers
- Claustrophobia
- Cochlear implants
- Aneurysmal clips
- Pregnancy

2.6.4 Advantages

- Excellent soft tissue contrast
- Lack of exposure to radiation

2.6.5 Disadvantages

- Greater patient cooperation required
- Longer examination time
- Less readily available
- More expensive for the trust

2.6.6 Interpretation

- Type of imaging sequence:
  - T1-weighted images: vitreous and CSF appears hypointense (dark) while fatty tissue appears bright. Grey matter of the brain will be hypointense as compared to white matter (grey is grey and white is white)
  - T2-weighted images: vitreous and CSF appears bright while fatty tissue appears dark. White matter is hypointense (dark) compared to grey matter (grey is white and white is grey)
  - FLAIR (T2-weighted image with CSF suppression): vitreous and CSF appears dark. Grey and white matter appearances are similar to T2-weighted images
- Terminology: hyperintense (structures appear as brighter areas than that of brain tissue), hypointense (structures appear darker than that of brain tissue
- Define mass:
  - Tissue of origin: is mass from a normal orbital structure such as the lacrimal gland, optic nerve, or extraocular muscle(s)
  - Position of the mass: intraconal space, extraconal space, subperiosteal space, extraocular muscles, tenon's space, extra-orbital space
  - Imaging clues to the biologic behaviour of a mass: "pusher" (benign well circumscribed lesions)—push adjacent structures aside, "eater" (malignant)—infiltrative lesions
  - Shape of the mass: cavernous haemangiomas are usually "round", benign mixed tumours of the lacrimal gland are said to be "oval", "kink" of an enlarged optic nerve (a sharp change in the direction of the nerve) strongly suggests a glioma
  - Size of the mass
  - Internal characteristics of the mass: homogenous (majority of tumours), heterogenous (combination of solid and cystic components in a child's tumour—lymphangioma, layering of fat and keratin debris in a cystic mass—dermoid cyst, small areas of calcification in a soft tissue orbital mass—malig-

nancy, "tram tracking" of an optic nerve tumour—optic nerve meningioma (see Fig. 2.74)

- Contrast enhancement of the mass: meningioma, rhabdomyosarcoma, inflammatory lesions such as sarcoidosis

2.6.7 MRI Images on Orbital Disorders Occurring in Adulthood

2.6.7.1 Optic Nerve Sheath Meningioma (Fig. 2.74)

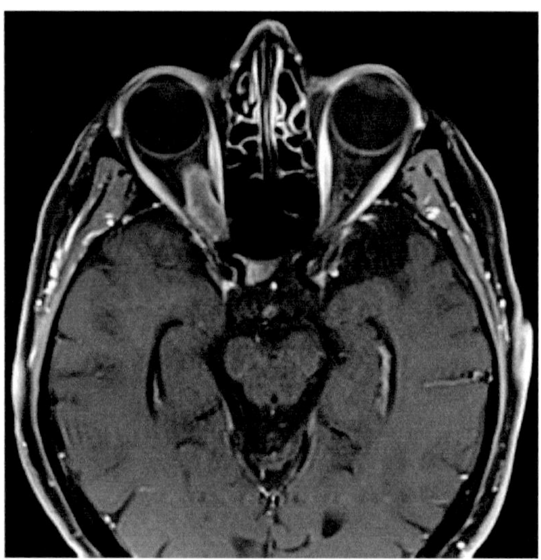

Fig. 2.74 Axial T1-weighted MRI scan image of a patient with a right optic nerve sheath meningioma with the typical 'tram track' sign (tubular thickening and enhancement of the optic nerve sheath)

2.6.8 MRI Images of Orbital Disorders Occurring in Childhood

2.6.8.1 Optic Nerve Glioma (Fig. 2.75)

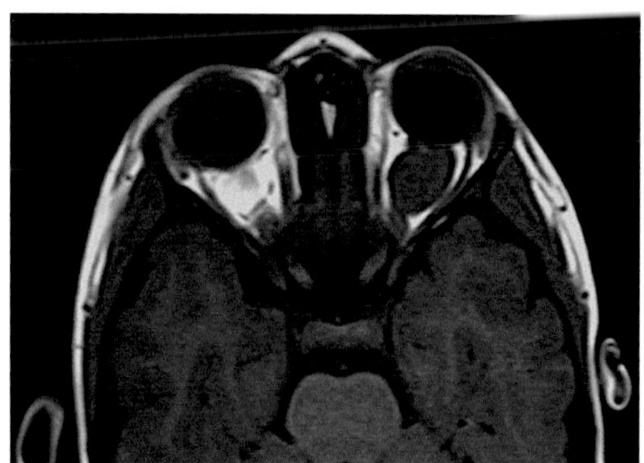

Fig. 2.75 Axial T1-weighted MRI scan image of a patient with a left optic nerve glioma

2.7 Humphrey Visual Field (HVF)

2.7.1 Principles

- HVF is a type of static perimetry that involves the presentation of stationary test objects
- Entire goal of perimetry is to determine a patient's "threshold" sensitivity to a light stimulus at specific locations within the patient's visual field. Threshold refers to the intensity or brightness of the light stimulus that can be detected 50% of the time at that location.

2.7.2 Indications

- Screening, monitoring, and diagnosis of glaucomatous and neuro-ophthalmic conditions

2.7.3 Interpretation

1. **Field parameter**
   - 10-2 HVF (test points 10° around the fovea)
   - 24-2 HVF (test points 24° around the fovea – see Fig. 2.76)
   - 30-2 HVF (test points 30° around the fovea)
2. **Fixation losses—reliability indices**:
   - Fixation plotted, if patient moves and the machine retests and patient see spots, then a fixation loss is recorded
3. **False positives—reliability indices**:
   - Patient presses the button when no actual light stimulus is present
4. **False negatives—reliability indices**:
   - Patient failing to see a bright stimulus in the same spot where they previously detected a dim stimulus
5. **Numerical display**
   - Gives the threshold for all points tested (in dB)
6. **Grey scale**
   - Graphical representation of the data shown in the numerical display
   - Decreasing sensitivity is represented by the darker tones. Grey tone scales correspond to 5 dB change in threshold
7. **Total deviation**
   - Calculated by comparing the patient's measurements with age-matched controls
8. **Pattern deviation**
   - Values adjusted for any generalised depression in the overall field.
   - This highlight focal depressions in the field, which might be masked by generalised depressions in sensitivity (e.g. cataract and corneal opacities)
9. **Glaucoma hemifield test (GHT)**
   - Compares 5 points on the upper field to corresponding 5 points on the lower field.
   - Differences between corresponding superior and inferior fields are compared with differences present in the population of normal controls
   - Outside normal limits: difference in the upper and lower set of points would not be found in 99% of patients without glaucoma
   - Borderline: difference detected would not be found in 97% of patients without glaucoma
10. **Visual field index (VFI)**
    - This index expresses the visual field status as a percent of a normal age-adjusted visual field. Greater weight is given to points closer to fixation to adjust for ganglion cell density and visual function. VFI assigns a number from 0% to 100% (100% being a perfect age-adjusted visual field and 0% representing a perimetrically blind field) and is calculated from pattern deviation plots in eyes with a MD of better than −20 dB and from total deviation plots in eyes with a MD of worse than −20 dB
11. **Mean defect (MD)—global indices**
    - A measure of the overall field loss.
    - An average of deviations across all test locations
12. **Pattern standard deviation (PSD)—global indices**
    - Measure of focal loss or variability within the field, taking into account any generalised depression
13. **Corrected pattern standard deviation (CPSD)—global indices**
    - A measure of variability within the field after correction for SF

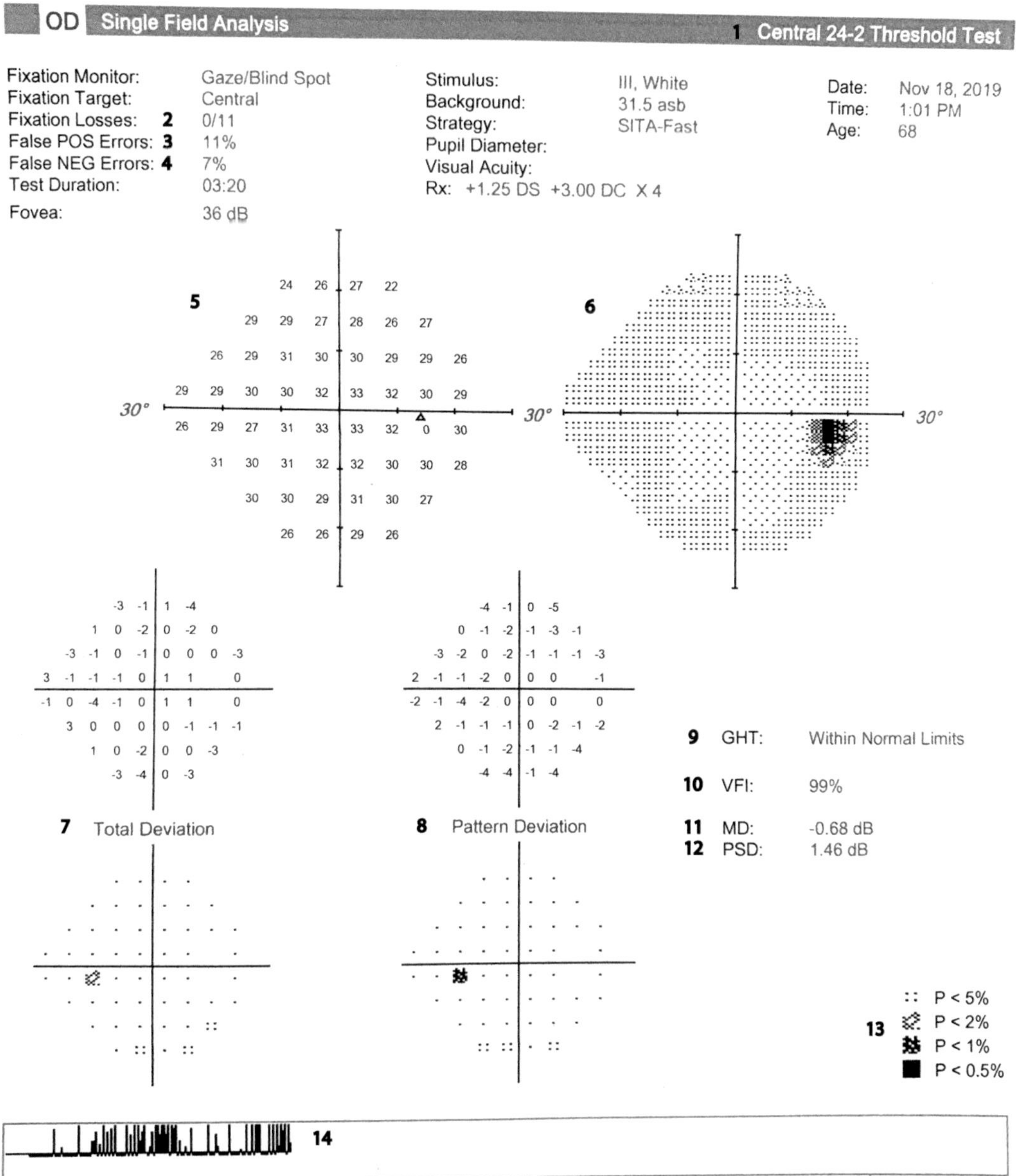

Fig. 2.76 A printout of a normal 24-2 HVF with key features indicated. 1: Field parameter. 2: Fixation losses. 3: False positive errors. 4: False negative errors. 5: Numerical display. 6: Grey scale. 7: Total Deviation. 8: Pattern Deviation. 9: Glaucoma Hemifield Test (GHT). 10: Visual Field Index (VFI). 11: Mean Defect (MD). 12: Pattern Standard Deviation (PSD). 13: Probability display. 14: Gaze tracker.

14. **Short-term fluctuations (SF)—global indices**
    - An indication of the consistency of responses. It is assessed by measuring threshold twice at 10 pre-selected points and calculated on the difference between the first and 2nd measurements (>5 dB difference is abnormal)

15. **Probability display**
    - P < 0.5%: less than 0.5% of the population would attain the result
    - P < 1%: less than 1% of the population would attain the result
    - P < 2%: less than 2% of the population would attain the result
    - P < 5%: less than 5% of the population would attain the result

16. **Gaze tracker**
    - Printed at the bottom of the print out
    - Measures how often and how far from fixation the patient looked away during the test
    - Higher spikes indicate larger eye movements

2.7.4 Detecting Glaucoma Progression

- Trend-based analysis (e.g. PROGRESSOR software and PeriData):
  - Defines progression by monitoring the change over time using regression analysis to provide a rate of progression and corresponding significance level (evaluates slope of measured parameter over time)
- Event-based analysis (e.g. Glaucoma Progression Analyser for the Humphrey Field Analyser):
  - Defines progressive change when a follow up measurement exceeds a pre-established threshold for change from baseline (e.g. loss of three or more test points in the same location on 3 consecutive field tests—EMGT)
  - Glaucoma progression analysis (GPA):
    - Individual test locations in the visual field are flagged as possibly, likely, or probably progressed from baseline if the retinal sensitivity at that location has changed by an amount expected in fewer that 5% of stable glaucoma on 1, 2, or 3 consecutive visual fields, respectively
- Heidelberg Retinal Tomograph (HRT)—Scanning Laser Tomography:
  - A scanning laser ophthalmoscopy (SLO) that allows for 3-D reconstruction of the optic nerve
  - SLO devices employ a confocal (pinhole) aperture, generating a single point of laser light at a specific wavelength that is scanned across the optic nerve in a raster pattern (i.e. series of horizontal parallel lines)
  - Measures:
    - Cup: CDR
    - Rim: rim area, rim volume, Moorfields regression analysis—comparison to normative database and risk of glaucoma assessed
    - RNFL: mean RNFL thickness, height variation contour
- Optic nerve head and peripapillary RNFL OCT:
  - Bruch's membrane opening-minimum rim width (BMO-MRW: measures neuroretinal rim by OCT)—minimum distance between Bruch's membrane opening (BMO—anatomic end of Bruch's membrane) and the inner limiting membrane—uses stable borders and offers a more accurate geometric assessment of neuroretinal rim tissue and may be a better way of detecting glaucomatous damage than circumpapillary RNFL thickness.

2.8 Field of Binocular Single Vision (BSV)

2.8.1 Principles

- The field of binocular single vision is plotted on a perimeter to depict the areas of the binocular field in which binocular single vision is maintained and those in which there is diplopia

2.8.2 Indications

- Monitoring change and progression in a patient's binocular diplopia
- Surgical planning for the management of a patient's binocular diplopia

2.8.3 Interpretation

- Position
- Size:

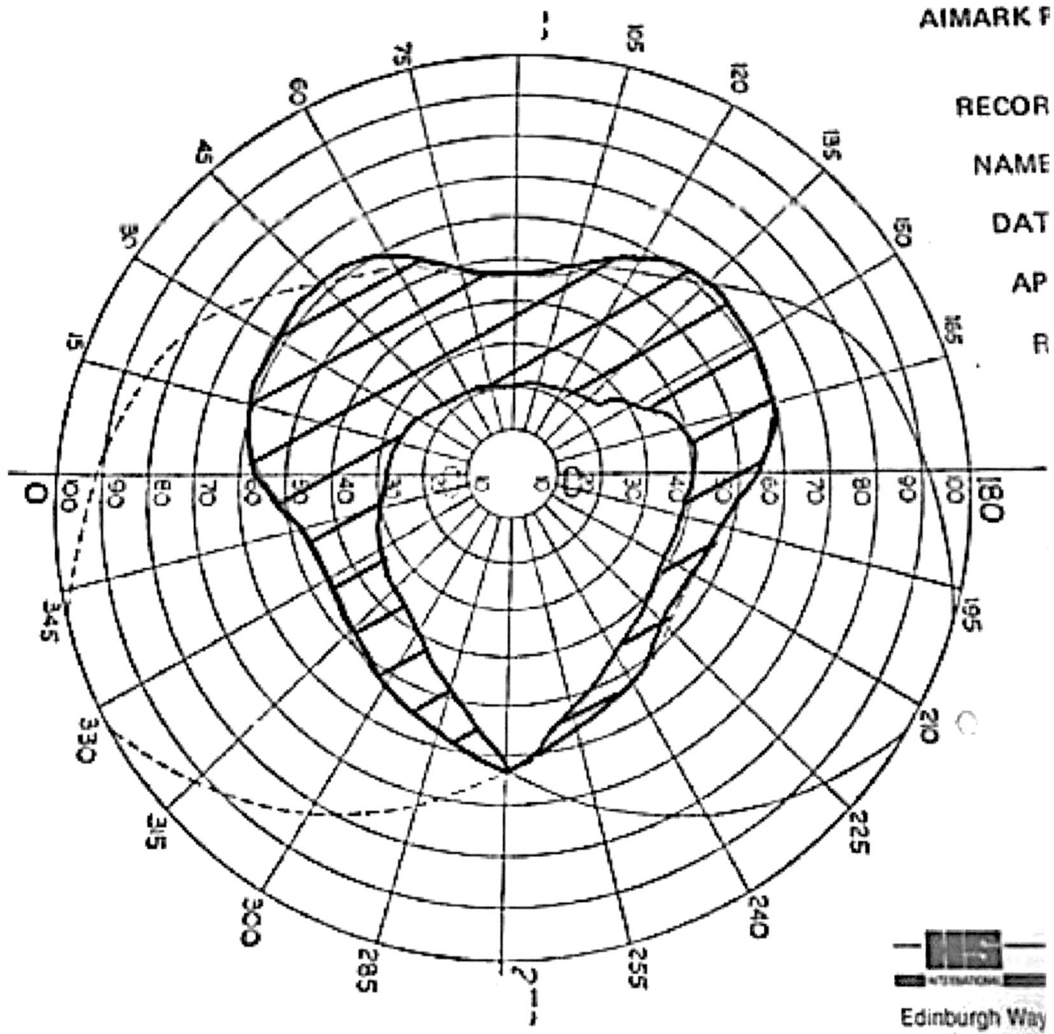

Fig. 2.77 Field of BSV of a patient with TED

- The field of BSV can be measured in degrees from the perimeter chart and these measurements can be compared with those of the normal field
- Influenced by a patient's fusion amplitude; if this is good the field of BSV will be enlarged in patients with TED involving the vertically acting muscles and in congenital vertical muscle palsies
- The greater the limitation of ocular movement, the smaller the field of BSV
- A narrow field of BSV, often relatively centrally placed, is characteristic of mechanically caused limitation of movement in opposing directions (see Fig. 2.77)

• Shape:
  - The field is displaced away from the direction of maximum limitation of movement e.g. the field of BSV will be situated on dextro-elevation in a right CN IV palsy, with diplopia on laevodepression (see Fig. 2.78)

• Crossed out areas represents the patient's areas of diplopia

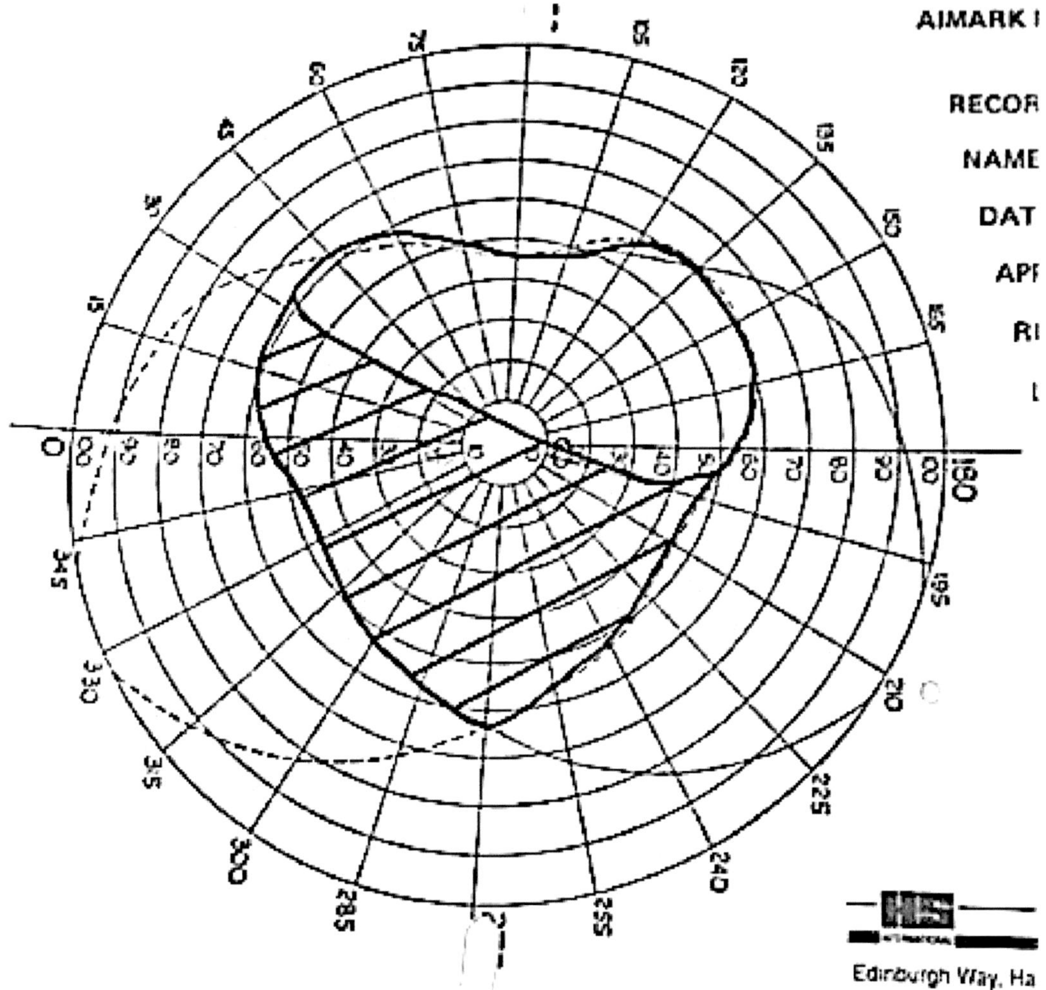

Fig. 2.78 Field of BSV of a patient with a right CN IV palsy

2.9 Corneal Topography

2.9.1 Principles

- Placido disc-based systems:
  - Consists of circular target of alternating concentric light and dark rings and a central aperture for observing the corneal reflections of these light and dark bands over the cornea
  - Examination of the reflected rings gives information about the shape of the cornea
  - The closer the mires the steeper the cornea. The wider the mires the flatter the cornea
  - Advantage: quickly captures data of the anterior corneal surface
  - Disadvantage: misses data on the central cornea as it is only able to acquire limited data points, difficult to focus and align, only captures data about the anterior corneal surface and its premise is based upon the assumption that the cornea is prolate (irregular corneal surfaces are often misdiagnosed), requires an intact epithelial surface and tear film for the instrument to obtain a clear image
- Scanning slit systems (e.g. Orbscan):
  - The scanning slit system is a reflection-based system that measures the triangulation

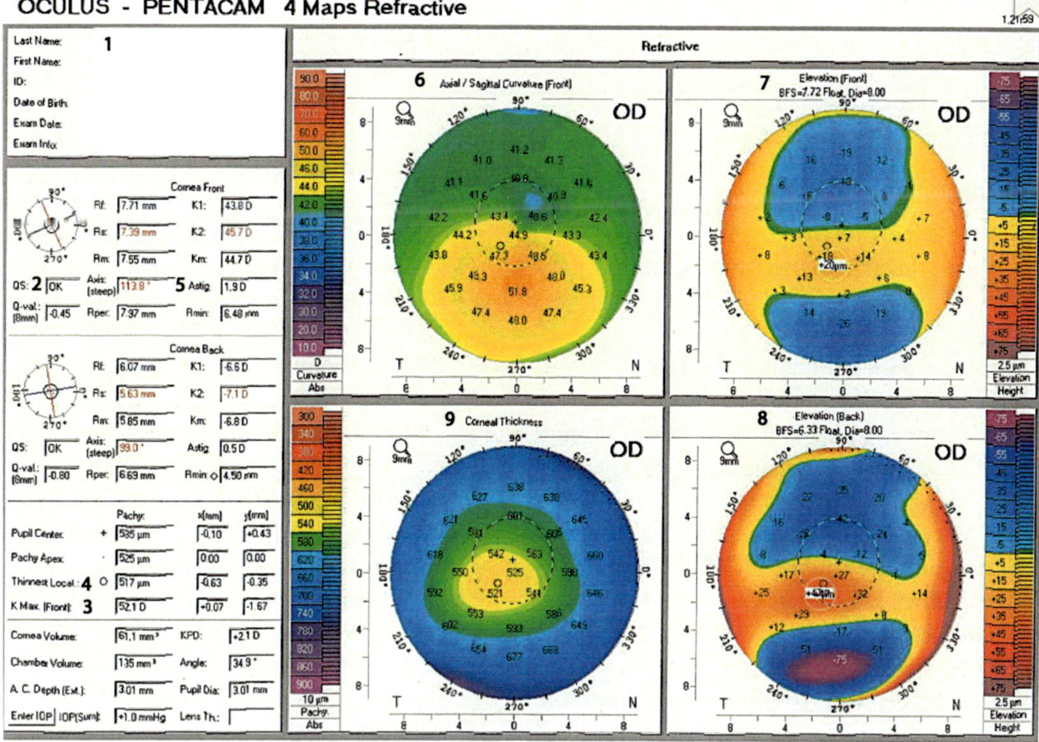

Fig. 2.79 A printout of a Pentacam printout with key features indicated. 1: Patient details. 2: Quality Specification (QS). 3: K Max (Front). 4: Thinnest location. 5: Astigmatism. 6: Axial/Sagittal Curvature [Front] map. 7: Elevation [Front] map. 8: Elevation [Back] map. 9: Corneal Thickness map

between the reference slit beam surface and the reflected beam captured by a camera

- Combines a 3D scanning slit beam system with an added Placido attachment
- Forty slits (20 nasal, 20 temporal) are projected sequentially on the cornea during image acquisition to create an overlapping pattern of scanning slits.
- The light reflected from the multiple slits of light projected through the cornea is interpreted by a camera using triangulation, and the final image is represented as a 3D topographic map including curvature, elevation and pachymetric maps of the entire corneal surface
- Advantages: More user friendly, quicker analysis, captures data about the anterior and posterior corneal surfaces
- Disadvantages: poor/unreliable capture of the corneal data from the periphery caused by the non-planar shape of the cornea, not useful in scarred non-reflective corneas

- Scheimpflug imaging systems (e.g. Pentacam—see Fig. 2.79):
  - Projection based system that is based on the Scheimpflug principle whereby a rotating camera enables the intersection of the object plane, lens plane, and image plane when they are not parallel to each other
  - Advantages: captures data about the anterior and posterior corneal surfaces, can measure scarred and non-reflective corneal surfaces, higher resolution and uniform accuracy across the whole cornea
  - Disadvantages: longer time required for image capture

2.9.2 Indications

- Screening, monitoring and planning treatment for corneal ectasias
- Refractive surgery screening and treatment

- Pre-operative IOL selection
- Post-keratoplasty astigmatism evaluation and management
- Ocular surface disorder evaluation
- CL fitting

2.9.3 General Approach to Interpreting Pentacam Printouts

1. **Ensure patient details are correct**
2. **Quality Specification (QS):**
   - If box is white with "OK" printed inside then all the data collected by the computer was correct. If box is yellow then some data is missing and a repeat scan is needed
3. **Maximum K reading (K Max [Front]):**
   - Normal is ≤47.2D
4. **Thinnest location:**
   - Normal ≥470 μm
5. **Compare topographic vs manifest astigmatism:**
   - Normal ≤1.0D astigmatism and ≤ 15-degree axis
6. **Axial/Sagittal Curvature (Front) Map:**
   - Areas of hot colours indicate areas with steep K readings
   - Cold colours indicate areas with flat K readings
   - Study shapes:
     - Symmetric or central shapes: round, oval, symmetric bowtie (SB)—these shapes are normal if K Max ≤47.2D
     - Asymmetric shapes: superior steep (SS), inferior steep (IS), asymmetric bowtie superior steep (AB/SS), asymmetric bowtie inferior steep (AB/IS)
     - Skew shapes: symmetric bowtie with skewed radial axis (SB/SRAX), asymmetric bowtie with skewed radial axis (AB/SRAX), SRAX reflects the angle between the axis of the inferior segment and the axis of the superior segment and is normal when ≤21°)
     - Special shapes: butterfly, crab claw (suggestive of PMD), vertical D, irregular (suggestive of scar, pterygium or previous refractive surgery)
   - Study values:
     - Compare the value 2 points above and the value 2 points below the center on the vertical meridian (I-S for 9 mm map): the difference between these 2 opposing points should be <2.5D (for SS or AB/SS shapes) and < 1.5D (for IS or AB/IS shapes)
7. **Elevation (Front) Map:**
   - Study shapes using best fit sphere (BFS):
     - Symmetric shapes: central island when no or insignificant astigmatism, hourglass shape when significant astigmatism
     - Asymmetric shapes (skewed hour glass, tongue-like extensions, irregular)
   - Study the values:
     - If using the BFS float mode:
       - Go to the thinnest location symbol displayed on map and click on mouse at that point and see the value: normal for myopes ≤8 and normal for hyperopes ≤7
     - If using the best-fit toric ellipsoid (BFTE) float mode:
       - Look at the highest plus numbers within the central 5 mm zone (black circle): normal if numbers are ≤12
   - If asymmetric shapes are present on Elevation (Front) map, one needs to exclude misalignment (poor fixation of patient during image capture), large angle kappa, exclude dry eye or excess tears, exclude corneal opacity, scar, cataract or other pathologies, exclude previous corneal surgeries
8. **Elevation (Back) Map:**
   - Study the shapes using best fit sphere (BFS):
     - Symmetric shapes: central island when no or insignificant astigmatism, hourglass shape when significant astigmatism
     - Asymmetric shapes: skewed hour glass, tongue-like extensions, irregular
   - Study the values:
     - If using the BFS float mode:
       - Go to the thinnest location symbol displayed on map and click on mouse at that point and see the value: normal for myopes ≤18 and normal for hyperopes ≤28

– If using the BFTE float mode:
  - Look at the highest plus numbers within the central 5 mm zone (black circle): normal if numbers are ≤15
- If asymmetric shapes are present on Elevation (Back) maps, one needs to exclude misalignment (poor fixation of patient during image capture), large angle kappa (look at X-coordinate of pupil center—if ≤0.20 then angle kappa is normal), exclude dry eye or excess tears, exclude corneal opacity, scar, cataract or other pathologies, exclude previous corneal surgeries

9. **Corneal Thickness Map:**
   - Study shapes:
     – Symmetric shapes
     – Asymmetric shapes: horizontal displacement of thinnest location, vertical displacement of thinnest location (dome shape, bell shape with inferior thinning for PMD, globus shape with generalised thinning to limbus)
   - Check values:
     – Compare the value 2 points above the center with the value 2 points below the center and the I-S difference should be ≤30 μm
   - If asymmetrical shapes on thickness map, need to exclude misalignment (poor fixation of patient during image capture), large angle kappa (look at X-coordinate of pupil center—if ≤0.20 then angle kappa is normal), exclude dry eye or excess tears, exclude corneal opacity, scar, cataract or other pathologies, exclude previous corneal surgeries
10. **Thickness profile diagram** (see Fig. 2.80):
   - Describes the change of corneal thickness in relation to location

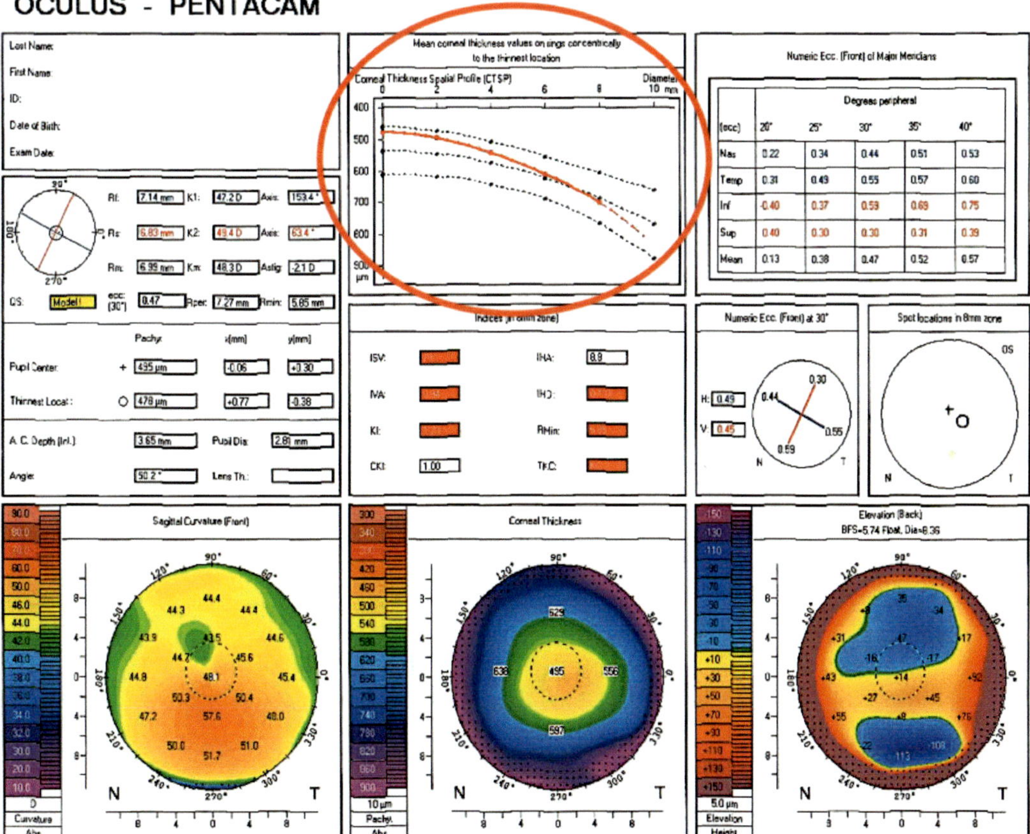

Fig. 2.80 Corneal topography with the thickness profile diagram shown in the red circle. Deviation of the red curve before the 6 mm point is an indicator of a relatively thin corneal center, commonly seen in ectatic corneal disorders

- Study shapes:
  – Normal shape: red line takes normal slope passage and does not leave it before 6 mm zone and average of progression is <1.2
  – Abnormal shapes:
    - Quick slope: red lines leave normal slope passage before 6 mm zone with high average
    - S-shape: red line leaves normal slope and then returns to slope again
    - Flat shape: red line is horizontal and implies cornea is oedematous like in FED or PBK
    - Inverted or upwards shape: red line slopes upwards and implies PMD

2.9.4 Corneal Topography of Ectatic Disorders (Table 2.8)

Table 2.8 Features on corneal topography suggestive of an ectatic pathology

A cornea can be considered highly suspect for ectatic pathology if the following parameters are present:
The highest curvature point (on Sagittal Curvature [Front] map) and thinnest point (on Corneal Thickness map) coincide: highly suspect cornea
The highest curvature point (on Sagittal Curvature [Front] map) coincides with the highest anterior (front) and posterior (back) points on the elevation maps: highly suspect cornea
The highest curvature point (on Sagittal Curvature [Front] map), the thinnest point (on Corneal Thickness map), and the highest anterior and posterior points of the corneal surface on the elevation maps all coincide: diagnosis of ectasia can be made

2.9.4.1 Keratoconus (KC) (Fig. 2.81)

Corneal Topography Findings to Look for Specifically in KC

- Rabinowitz-McDonnell indices [12]:
  – Central corneal power ≥47.2D:
    - <47.2D: normal cornea
    - 47.2–48.7D: forme fruste KC
    - >48.7D: KC
  – Inferior-superior dioptric asymmetry (I-S value) >1.2
  – Sim-K astigmatism >1.5D
  – Skewed radial axes (SRAX) >21°
- The Rabinowitz-McDonnell indices identifies 98% of patients with KC [12]
- Form fruste KC (FFKC) differs from KC in that the latter can be diagnosed clinically with use of the slit-lamp examination and characteristic pattern on corneal topography. FFKC has no identifiable slit-lamp signs, but corneal topography does.

2.9.4.2 Pellucid Marginal Degeneration (PMD)

Corneal Topography Findings to Look for Specifically in PMD

- Sagittal curvature [Front] map (see Fig. 2.82): low corneal power along central vertical axis, increased power as the inferior cornea is approached, and high corneal power along the inferior oblique meridians (crab-claw appearance)
- Elevations maps: location of the cone and the "kissing birds" sign (this sign is absent

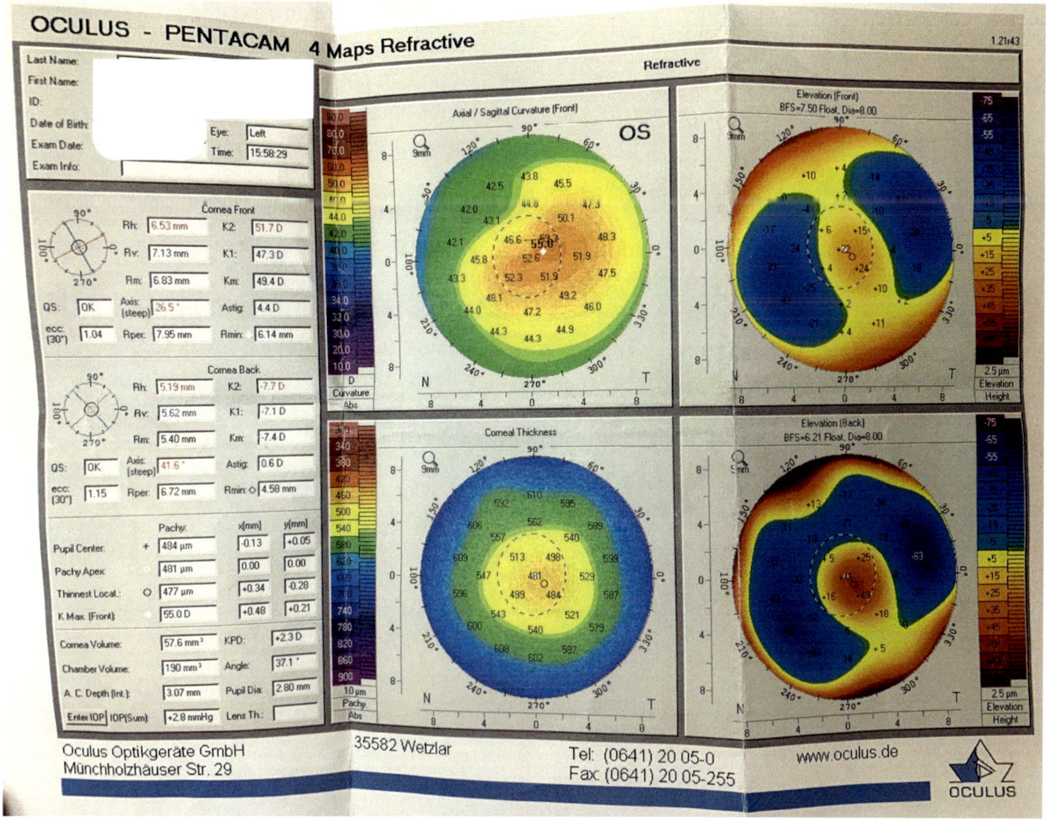

OCULUS - PENTACAM 4 Maps Refractive

Last Name:			
First Name:			
ID:			
Date of Birth:		Eye:	Left
Exam Date:		Time:	15:58:29
Exam Info:			

Cornea Front

Rh:	6.53 mm	K2:	51.7 D
Rv:	7.13 mm	K1:	47.3 D
Rm:	6.83 mm	Km:	49.4 D
QS: OK	Axis (steep): 26.5°	Astig:	4.4 D
ecc (30°): 1.04	Rper: 7.95 mm	Rmin:	6.14 mm

Cornea Back

Rh:	5.19 mm	K2:	-7.7 D
Rv:	5.62 mm	K1:	-7.1 D
Rm:	5.40 mm	Km:	-7.4 D
QS: OK	Axis (steep): 41.6°	Astig:	0.6 D
ecc (30°): 1.15	Rper: 6.72 mm	Rmin:	4.58 mm

	Pachy:	x[mm]	y[mm]
Pupil Center: +	484 µm	-0.13	+0.05
Pachy Apex:	481 µm	0.00	0.00
Thinnest Locat.: ○	477 µm	+0.34	-0.28
K Max. (Front):	55.0 D	+0.48	+0.21

Cornea Volume:	57.6 mm³	KPD:	+2.3 D
Chamber Volume:	190 mm³	Angle:	37.1°
A. C. Depth (Int.):	3.07 mm	Pupil Dia:	2.80 mm
Enter IOP IOP(Sum):	+2.8 mmHg	Lens Th.:	

Refractive

Axial / Sagittal Curvature (Front) OS

Elevation (Front) BFS=7.50 Float, Dia=8.00

Corneal Thickness

Elevation (Back) BFS=6.21 Float, Dia=8.00

Oculus Optikgeräte GmbH Münchholzhäuser Str. 29 35582 Wetzlar Tel: (0641) 20 05-0 Fax (0641) 20 05-255 www.oculus.de OCULUS

Fig. 2.81 Corneal topography of a patient with keratoconus. Note how the highest curvature point, the thinnest point, and the highest anterior and posterior points of the corneal surface on the elevation maps all coincide with each other

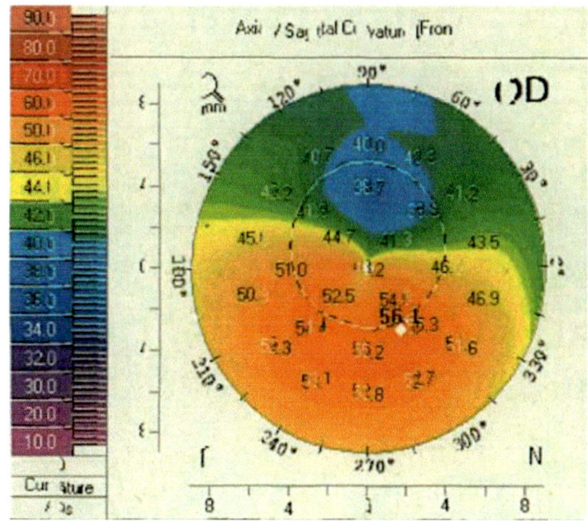

Fig. 2.82 Sagittal curvature map of a patient with PMD showing a crab-claw appearance

when the cone is central or paracentral and is present when the cone is peripheral, sign only appears when the BFS float mode is used)

- Corneal thickness map: cornea thickens from the center to the periphery. If any part of the peripheral cornea is thinner than the center, this is a cause for concern. In PMD, the corneal thickness may reveal a thinning of the inferior cornea. This thinning is characterised with a special sign called the "bell" shape, which is a hallmark of PMD
- Thickness profile: in advance cases of PMD, the curve usually takes an inverted passage

2.10 Biometry

2.10.1 Optical Biometry

2.10.1.1 Principles

- Non-contact method of biometry using the IOL Master
- Axial length measured from cornea to RPE
- Utilises 2 coaxial partially coherent laser beams (partial coherence interferometry) from the infrared spectrum (780 nm wavelength)
- Device can measure axial length, keratometry, AC depth, corneal white to white distance
- Unable to carry out adequate measurements in dense cataracts, especially with posterior subcapsular cataracts

2.10.1.2 Indications

- IOL power calculations for cataract surgery

2.10.1.3 Interpretation (Fig. 2.83)

1. Ensure **patient details** are correct
2. Check correct **formula** has been used:

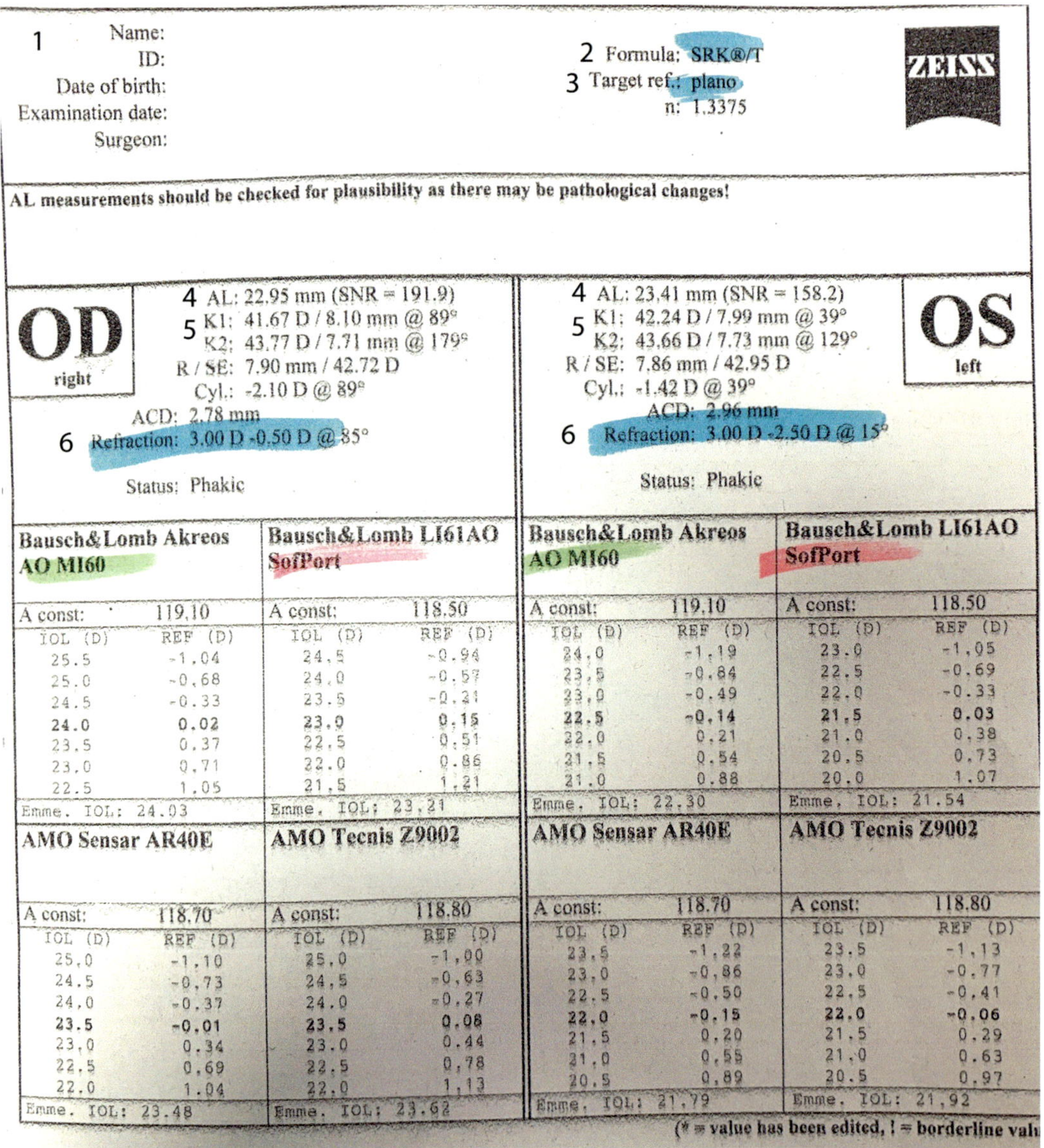

1 Name:
ID:
Date of birth:
Examination date:
Surgeon:

2 Formula: SRK®/T
3 Target ref.: plano
n: 1.3375

ZEISS

AL measurements should be checked for plausibility as there may be pathological changes!

OD right

4 AL: 22.95 mm (SNR = 191.9)
5 K1: 41.67 D / 8.10 mm @ 89°
K2: 43.77 D / 7.71 mm @ 179°
R / SE: 7.90 mm / 42.72 D
Cyl.: -2.10 D @ 89°
ACD: 2.78 mm
6 Refraction: 3.00 D -0.50 D @ 85°

Status: Phakic

Bausch&Lomb Akreos AO MI60		Bausch&Lomb LI61AO SofPort	
A const:	119.10	A const:	118.50
IOL (D)	REF (D)	IOL (D)	REF (D)
25.5	-1.04	24.5	-0.94
25.0	-0.68	24.0	-0.57
24.5	-0.33	23.5	-0.21
24.0	**0.02**	**23.0**	**0.15**
23.5	0.37	22.5	0.51
23.0	0.71	22.0	0.86
22.5	1.05	21.5	1.21
Emme. IOL: 24.03		Emme. IOL: 23.21	

AMO Sensar AR40E		AMO Tecnis Z9002	
A const:	118.70	A const:	118.80
IOL (D)	REF (D)	IOL (D)	REF (D)
25.0	-1.10	25.0	-1.00
24.5	-0.73	24.5	-0.63
24.0	-0.37	24.0	-0.27
23.5	**-0.01**	**23.5**	**0.08**
23.0	0.34	23.0	0.44
22.5	0.69	22.5	0.78
22.0	1.04	22.0	1.13
Emme. IOL: 23.48		Emme. IOL: 23.62	

OS left

4 AL: 23.41 mm (SNR = 158.2)
5 K1: 42.24 D / 7.99 mm @ 39°
K2: 43.66 D / 7.73 mm @ 129°
R / SE: 7.86 mm / 42.95 D
Cyl.: -1.42 D @ 39°
ACD: 2.96 mm
6 Refraction: 3.00 D -2.50 D @ 15°

Status: Phakic

Bausch&Lomb Akreos AO MI60		Bausch&Lomb LI61AO SofPort	
A const:	119.10	A const:	118.50
IOL (D)	REF (D)	IOL (D)	REF (D)
24.0	-1.19	23.0	-1.05
23.5	-0.84	22.5	-0.69
23.0	-0.49	22.0	-0.33
22.5	**-0.14**	**21.5**	**0.03**
22.0	0.21	21.0	0.38
21.5	0.54	20.5	0.73
21.0	0.88	20.0	1.07
Emme. IOL: 22.30		Emme. IOL: 21.54	

AMO Sensar AR40E		AMO Tecnis Z9002	
A const:	118.70	A const:	118.80
IOL (D)	REF (D)	IOL (D)	REF (D)
23.5	-1.22	23.5	-1.13
23.0	-0.86	23.0	-0.77
22.5	-0.50	22.5	-0.41
22.0	**-0.15**	**22.0**	**-0.06**
21.5	0.20	21.5	0.29
21.0	0.55	21.0	0.63
20.5	0.89	20.5	0.97
Emme. IOL: 21.79		Emme. IOL: 21.92	

(* = value has been edited, ! = borderline val

Fig. 2.83 IOL master biometry printout 1 with key features indicated. 1: Patient details. 2: Formula. 3: Target refraction. 4: Axial length values. 5: Keratometry values. 6: Refraction

NICE guideline [NG77] [11]:
- Hoffer Q: AL <22 mm
- SRK-T or Barrett Universal II: AL 22-26 mm
- SRK-T or Haigis: AL >26 mm
- Special formulas for eyes that have had previous laser refractive surgery e.g. Haigis-L

3. Check **target refraction:**
   - Consider using 50% of first-eye refractive outcome prediction error to guide second-eye power calculation (The Royal College of Ophthalmologists [14] Correct IOL implantation in cataract surgery guideline)
4. Check **axial length (AL)** and **signal-to-noise ratio (SNR)** measurements
   - When checking the quality of AL values, look for a sharp centralised peak and an even baseline on the axial length measurement signal (see Fig. 2.84)
   - The SNR is a measure of scan quality and indicates the height of the highest peak above the baseline. A good quality scan will have an SNR >2.0
5. Check **keratometry (K)** readings
6. Check **refraction** of eyes

2.10.1.4 Indications for Repeating Biometry Measurements

The Royal College of Ophthalmologists [13] Cataract Surgery Guideline suggest repeating biometry when:

- AL <21.20 mm or >26.60 mm
- Difference in axial length between fellow eyes of >0.7 mm
- Mean corneal power <41D or >47D
- Difference in mean corneal power of >0.9D
- Delta K is >2.5D

The Royal College of Ophthalmologists [14] Correct IOL implantation in cataract surgery guideline suggest repeating biometry when:

- Previous biometry measurements are more than 4 years old
- IOL exchange is required
- Patient has had previous corneal surgery or a progressive corneal disease
- Major eye operation since last biometry
- AL may have changed due to eye disease

2.10.1.5 Contact Lens Wear andBiometryMeasurements (The Royal College of Ophthalmologists[14] Correct IOL Implantation in Cataract Surgery Guideline)

- The following types of contact lenses should be left out before biometry for the following time periods:
  - Rigid gas permeable lenses: 2–4 weeks
  - Soft lenses: 1 week

2.10.2 Ultrasound (A-Scan) Biometry

2.10.2.1 Principles

- 10 mHz probe
- Estimation of axial length (measured from cornea to ILM) assumes that the speed of US has a constant value of 1540 m/s in the anterior chamber, 1641 m/sec in the lens and 1540 m/sec in the posterior chamber
- Immersion technique: saline filled scleral shell, avoiding corneal indentation
- Contact applanation technique: indentation of the cornea with possible shallowing of the AC and subsequent overestimation of the IOL power (myopic shift)

2.10.2.2 Indications

- IOL power calculations for cataract surgery if biometry results are unobtainable with optical biometry

2.10.2.3 Interpretation (Fig. 2.85)

1. Ensure **patient details** are correct
2. Check correct **formula** is used:

   NICE Guidance [NG77] [11]:
   - Hoffer Q: AL <22 mm
   - SRK-T or Barrett Universal II: AL 22-26 mm
   - SRK-T or Haigis: AL >26 mm
   - Special formulas for eyes that have had previous laser refractive surgery e.g. Haigis-L

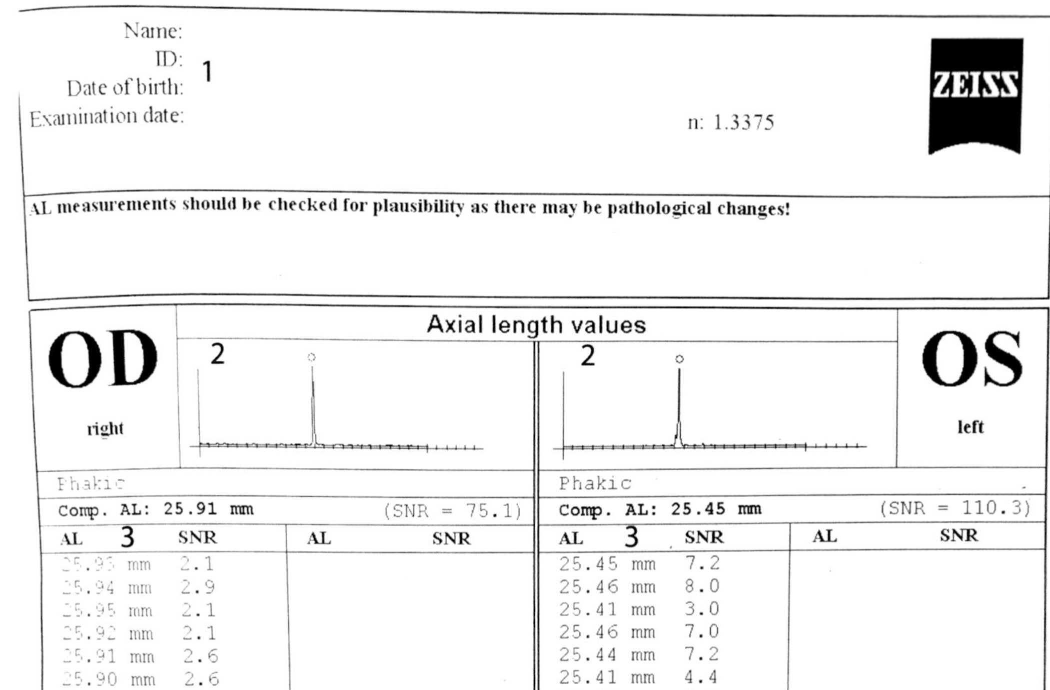

Name:
ID: 1
Date of birth:
Examination date:

n: 1.3375

ZEISS

AL measurements should be checked for plausibility as there may be pathological changes!

Axial length values

OD right	2	2	OS left

Phakic				Phakic			
Comp. AL: 25.91 mm			(SNR = 75.1)	Comp. AL: 25.45 mm			(SNR = 110.3)
AL 3	SNR	AL	SNR	AL 3	SNR	AL	SNR
25.93 mm	2.1			25.45 mm	7.2		
25.94 mm	2.9			25.46 mm	8.0		
25.95 mm	2.1			25.41 mm	3.0		
25.92 mm	2.1			25.46 mm	7.0		
25.91 mm	2.6			25.44 mm	7.2		
25.90 mm	2.6			25.41 mm	4.4		
25.89 mm	2.2			25.46 mm	3.5		
25.90 mm	2.6			25.46 mm	16.6		
				25.44 mm	4.6		
				25.45 mm	7.2		

4 Keratometer values

MV: 44.82/45.98 D	SD: 0.00 mm	MV: 44.58/45.98 D	SD: 0.00 mm
K1: 44.82 D x 178°	7.53 mm	K1: 44.58 D x 21°	7.57 mm
K2: 45.98 D x 88°	7.34 mm	K2: 45.92 D x 111°	7.35 mm
ΔK: -1.16 D x 178°		ΔK: -1.34 D x 21°	
K1: 44.82 D x 0°	7.53 mm	K1: 44.58 D x 22°	7.57 mm
K2: 45.98 D x 90°	7.34 mm	K2: 45.98 D x 112°	7.34 mm
ΔK: -1.16 D x 0°		ΔK: -1.40 D x 22°	
K1: 44.82 D x 179°	7.53 mm	K1: 44.53 D x 22°	7.58 mm
K2: 45.92 D x 89°	7.35 mm	K2: 45.98 D x 112°	7.34 mm
ΔK: -1.10 D x 179°		ΔK: -1.45 D x 22°	

Anterior chamber depth values

ACD: 3.32 mm					ACD: 3.53 mm				
3.33 mm	3.31 mm	3.33 mm	3.31 mm	3.31 mm	3.55 mm	3.53 mm	3.53 mm	3.53 mm	3.53 mm

White-to-white values

WTW : 12.2 mm	Pup: 6.4 mm	WTW : 12.0 mm	Pup: 6.9 mm
Ix:+0.0mm Iy:+0.2mm	Px:-0.2mm Py:+0.2mm	Ix:-0.8mm Iy:+0.1mm	Px:-0.5mm Py:+0.1mm
WTW : 12.3 mm	Pup: 6.4 mm	WTW : 12.0 mm	Pup: 6.9 mm
Ix:+0.0mm Iy:+0.3mm	Px:-0.1mm Py:+0.3mm	Ix:-0.8mm Iy:+0.1mm	Px:-0.5mm Py:+0.1mm
WTW : 12.2 mm	Pup: 6.4 mm	WTW : 12.0 mm	Pup: 6.9 mm
Ix:-0.0mm Iy:+0.3mm	Px:-0.2mm Py:+0.3mm	Ix:-0.8mm Iy:+0.1mm	Px:-0.5mm Py:+0.1mm

Reference image capture

No image	No image

(* = value has been edited, ! = borderline value)

Fig. 2.84 IOL master biometry printout 2 with key features indicated. 1: Patient details. 2: Axial length measurement signal. 3: Axial length (AL) and signal-to-noise ratio (SNR) values. 4: Keratometer (K) values

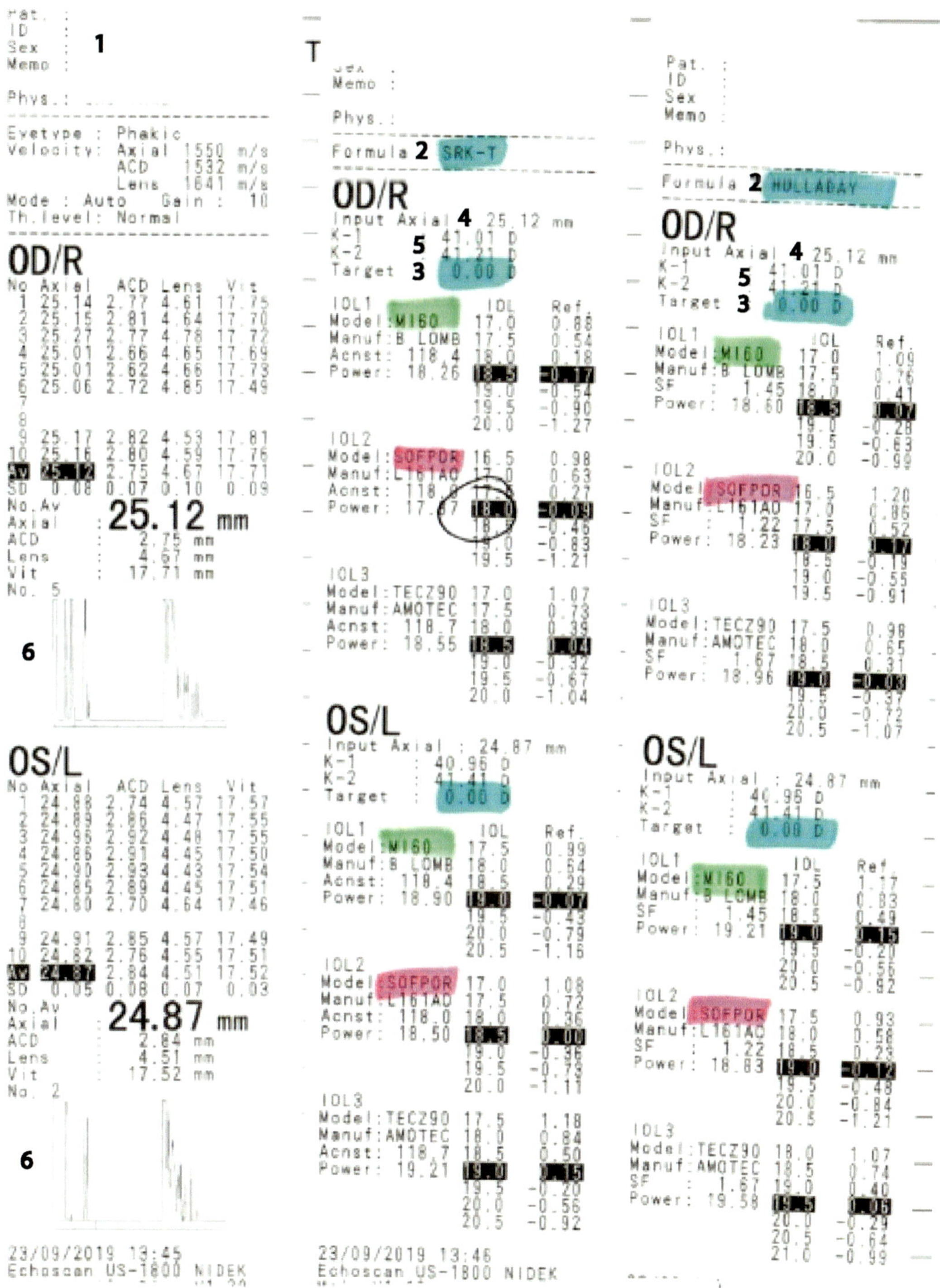

Pat. :
ID :
Sex : **1**
Memo :

Phys. :

Eyetype : Phakic
Velocity: Axial 1550 m/s
ACD 1532 m/s
Lens 1641 m/s
Mode : Auto Gain : 10
Th.level: Normal

OD/R

No	Axial	ACD	Lens	Vit
1	25.14	2.77	4.61	17.75
2	25.15	2.81	4.64	17.70
3	25.27	2.77	4.78	17.72
4	25.01	2.66	4.65	17.69
5	25.01	2.62	4.66	17.73
6	25.06	2.72	4.85	17.49
7				
8				
9	25.17	2.82	4.53	17.81
10	25.16	2.80	4.59	17.76
Av	25.12	2.75	4.67	17.71
SD	0.08	0.07	0.10	0.09

No.Av
Axial : 25.12 mm
ACD : 2.75 mm
Lens : 4.67 mm
Vit : 17.71 mm
No. 5

6

OS/L

No	Axial	ACD	Lens	Vit
1	24.88	2.74	4.57	17.57
2	24.89	2.86	4.47	17.55
3	24.95	2.92	4.48	17.55
4	24.86	2.91	4.45	17.50
5	24.90	2.93	4.43	17.54
6	24.85	2.89	4.45	17.51
7	24.80	2.70	4.64	17.46
8				
9	24.91	2.85	4.57	17.49
10	24.82	2.76	4.55	17.51
Av	24.87	2.84	4.51	17.52
SD	0.05	0.08	0.07	0.03

No.Av
Axial : 24.87 mm
ACD : 2.84 mm
Lens : 4.51 mm
Vit : 17.52 mm
No. 2

6

23/09/2019 13:45
Echoscan US-1800 NIDEK

T

Memo :

Phys. :

Formula **2** SRK-T

OD/R
Input Axial **4** 25.12 mm
K-1 **5** 41.01 D
K-2 41.21 D
Target **3** 0.00 D

IOL1
Model: MI60
Manuf: B LOMB
Acnst: 118.4
Power: 18.26

IOL	Ref.
17.0	0.88
17.5	0.54
18.0	0.18
18.5	-0.17
19.0	-0.54
19.5	-0.90
20.0	-1.27

IOL2
Model: SOFPOR
Manuf: L161AO
Acnst: 118.[illegible]
Power: 17.87

IOL	Ref.
16.5	0.98
17.0	0.63
[illegible]	0.27
18.0	-0.09
18.5	-0.46
19.0	-0.83
19.5	-1.21

IOL3
Model: TECZ90
Manuf: AMOTEC
Acnst: 118.7
Power: 18.55

IOL	Ref.
17.0	1.07
17.5	0.73
18.0	0.39
18.5	0.04
19.0	-0.32
19.5	-0.67
20.0	-1.04

OS/L
Input Axial : 24.87 mm
K-1 : 40.96 D
K-2 : 41.41 D
Target : 0.00 D

IOL1
Model: MI60
Manuf: B LOMB
Acnst: 118.4
Power: 18.90

IOL	Ref.
17.5	0.99
18.0	0.64
18.5	0.29
19.0	-0.07
19.5	-0.43
20.0	-0.79
20.5	-1.16

IOL2
Model: SOFPOR
Manuf: L161AO
Acnst: 118.0
Power: 18.50

IOL	Ref.
17.0	1.08
17.5	0.72
18.0	0.36
18.5	0.00
19.0	-0.36
19.5	-0.73
20.0	-1.11

IOL3
Model: TECZ90
Manuf: AMOTEC
Acnst: 118.7
Power: 19.21

IOL	Ref.
17.5	1.18
18.0	0.84
18.5	0.50
19.0	0.15
19.5	-0.20
20.0	-0.56
20.5	-0.92

23/09/2019 13:46
Echoscan US-1800 NIDEK

Pat. :
ID :
Sex :
Memo :

Phys. :

Formula **2** HOLLADAY

OD/R
Input Axial **4** 25.12 mm
K-1 **5** 41.01 D
K-2 41.21 D
Target **3** 0.00 D

IOL1
Model: MI60
Manuf: B LOMB
SF : 1.45
Power: 18.60

IOL	Ref.
17.0	1.09
17.5	0.76
18.0	0.41
18.5	0.07
19.0	-0.28
19.5	-0.63
20.0	-0.99

IOL2
Model: SOFPOR
Manuf: L161AO
SF : 1.22
Power: 18.23

IOL	Ref.
16.5	1.20
17.0	0.86
17.5	0.52
18.0	0.17
18.5	-0.19
19.0	-0.55
19.5	-0.91

IOL3
Model: TECZ90
Manuf: AMOTEC
SF : 1.67
Power: 18.96

IOL	Ref.
17.5	0.98
18.0	0.65
18.5	0.31
19.0	-0.03
19.5	-0.37
20.0	-0.72
20.5	-1.07

OS/L
Input Axial : 24.87 mm
K-1 : 40.96 D
K-2 : 41.41 D
Target : 0.00 D

IOL1
Model: MI60
Manuf: B LOMB
SF : 1.45
Power: 19.21

IOL	Ref.
17.5	1.17
18.0	0.83
18.5	0.49
19.0	0.15
19.5	-0.20
20.0	-0.56
20.5	-0.92

IOL2
Model: SOFPOR
Manuf: L161AO
SF : 1.22
Power: 18.83

IOL	Ref.
17.5	0.93
18.0	0.58
18.5	0.23
19.0	-0.12
19.5	-0.48
20.0	-0.84
20.5	-1.21

IOL3
Model: TECZ90
Manuf: AMOTEC
SF : 1.67
Power: 19.58

IOL	Ref.
18.0	1.07
18.5	0.74
19.0	0.40
19.5	0.06
20.0	-0.29
20.5	-0.64
21.0	-0.99

Fig. 2.85 A-scan biometry printout using the contact applanation method with key features identified. 1: Patient details. 2: Formula. 3: Target refraction. 4: Axial length. 5: Keratometry readings. 6: Identifiable peaks

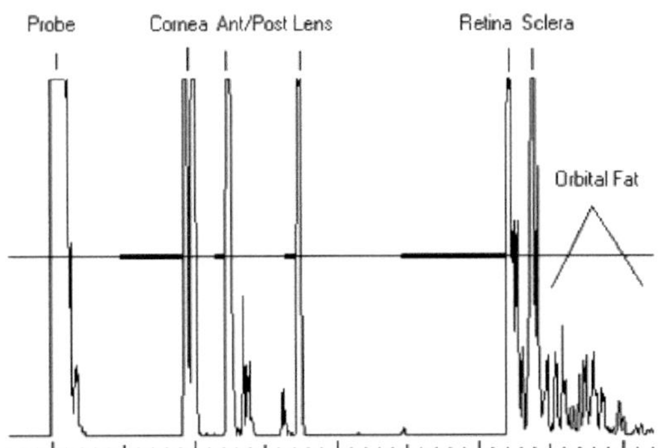

Fig. 2.86 Series of peaks that should be seen in a phakic eye on an A-scan printout

3. Check **target refraction:**
   - Consider using 50% of first-eye refractive outcome prediction error to guide second-eye power calculation (The Royal College of Ophthalmologists [14] Correct IOL implantation in cataract surgery guideline)
4. Check **axial length (AL)** measurements
5. Check **keratometry (K)** readings
6. Check **identifiable peaks** (see Fig. 2.86)
7. Check **refraction** of eyes

2.10.2.4 Improving the Accuracy of the A-Scan

- Immersion method rather than contact applanation technique
- Adjust velocity settings for silicone oil filled eyes
- Ensure perpendicular positioning of probe on eye with following characteristics present:
  - Equal height double corneal peaks
  - 5 high, sharply rising echoes
  - Descending orbital fat behind the scleral echo
  - Reproducibility
- Optimising the IOL constants for each IOL model for the method of axial length measurements (optical or acoustic) has a much greater impact on the predictability of the refractive outcome than choosing between modern IOL formulae.
- Optimising A constants for each IOL model according to the method of axial length measurement is much more important than optimising A constants for each surgeon when using the same method of axial length measurement

2.11 Dacryocystography (DCG) (Fig. 2.87)

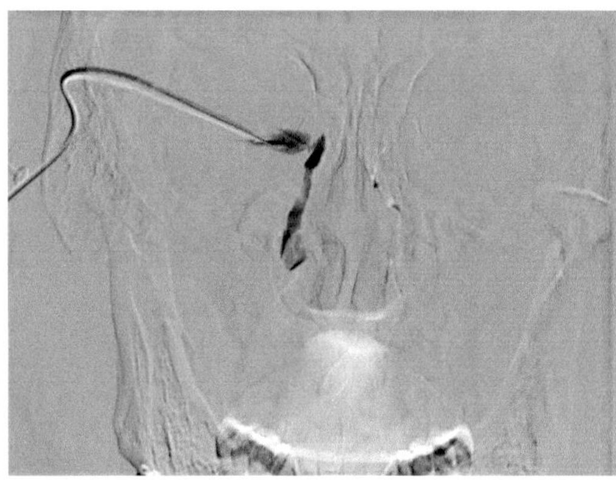

Fig. 2.87 DCG image showing a patent lacrimal drainage system on the right side

2.11.1 Principles

- A fluoroscopic contrast examination of the nasolacrimal apparatus.
- With the patient supine, a drop of topical anaesthesia is placed into the palpebral aperture in both eyes.
- A control film is taken after intubation of both lower puncta with Portex intravenous cannulae that were fixed 5 mm into the lower canalicular systems by taping.
- A volume of 1–2 ml of an iodised oil-based contrast medium is injected simultaneously into both lacrimal systems and a series of macroradiographs are taken.
- The patient is then sat upright for 5 m before a final delayed erect oblique radiograph is taken.
- Functional NLDO is diagnosed if there was poor emptying, such that residual contrast was present in the lacrimal sac or NLD of the delayed radiograph.

2.11.2 Indications

- Functional obstruction of the lacrimal drainage system: incomplete obstructions and intermittent tearing with no anatomic pathology—location of stenosis, diverticuli, stones
- Failed lacrimal surgery—size of the sac
- Suspicion of sac tumours

2.11.3 Interpretation

- Look for any filling defects in the lacrimal drainage system

2.11.4 DCG Images of Common Pathologies of the Lacrimal Drainage System (Figs. 2.88, 2.89, 2.90, 2.91 and 2.92)

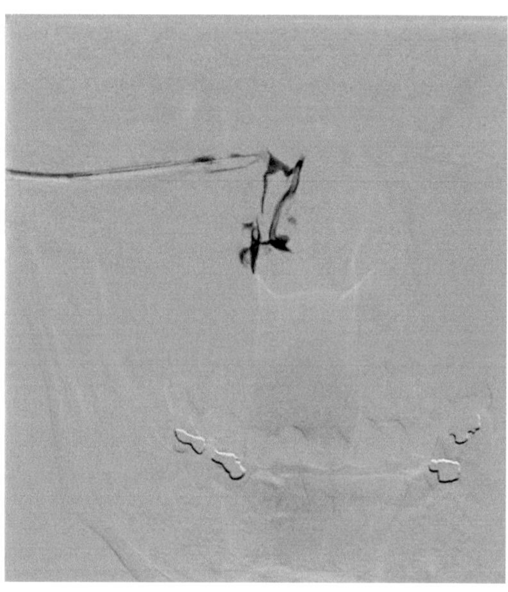

Fig. 2.88 DCG image of a patient with a patent right DCR showing a Y-shaped configuration (result of dye entering directly from the lacrimal sac into the nasal cavity)

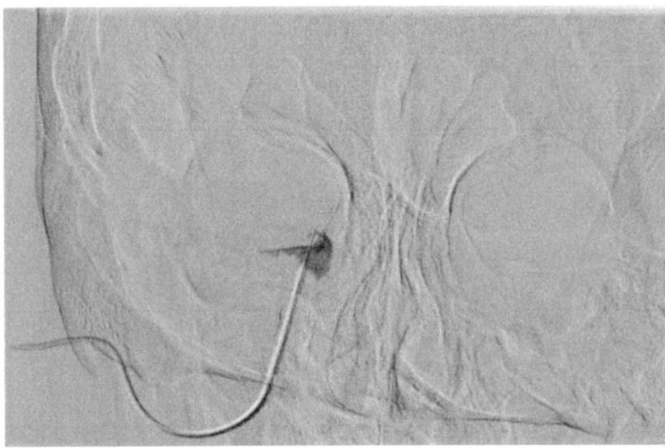

Fig. 2.89 DCG image of a patient with a complete obstruction of the right superior and inferior canaliculus with no flow of dye into the lacrimal drainage system and overflow of dye into the tear lake

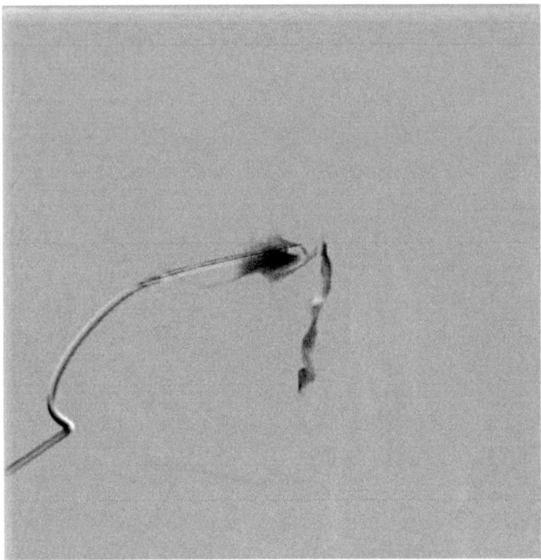

Fig. 2.90 DCG image of a patient with a right common canaliculus stenosis

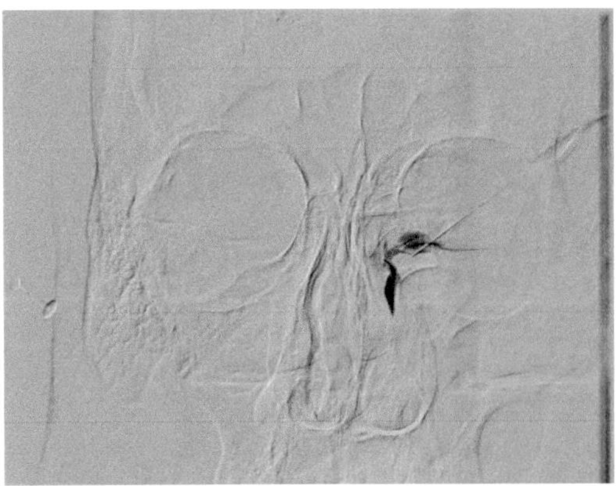

Fig. 2.91 DCG image of a patient with a left distal nasolacrimal duct obstruction

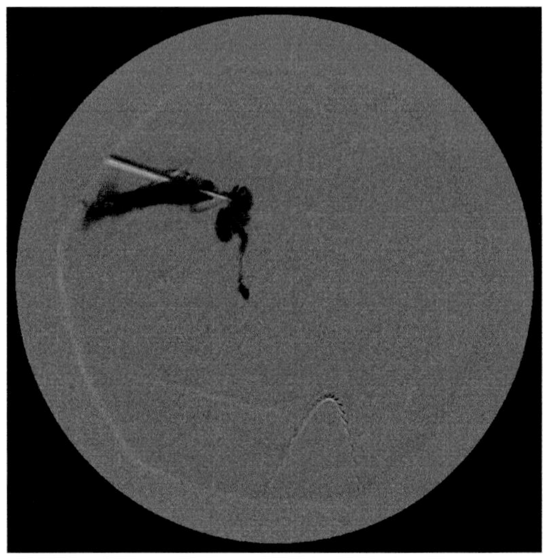

Fig. 2.92 DCG image of a patient with a complete obstruction at the level of the right nasolacrimal duct inferiorly with gross dilation of the right lacrimal sac

2.12 Dacryoscintigraphy (DSG)

2.12.1 Principles

- Nuclear medicine procedure used as a diagnostic tool for "functional" NLDO (patients who complain of epiphora without tear overproduction, whom an increased tear line is associated with patent lacrimal systems but show easy passage on syringing)
- Useful as a physiological test of tear flow through the lacrimal system
- Patient is seated upright in front of the pinhole collimator of the gamma camera, and a drop of Technetium-99 m pertechnetate (radioactive tracer isotope) is placed into the inferior fornix of both eyes and the patient is requested to blink normally.
- A dynamic study is performed initially with the tracer distribution imaged every 10 s for the first 160 s. Static views were then taken routinely at 5, 10, 15, and 20 m.
- When radiotracer flows from the conjunctival sac to the nose, drainage is considered to be normal, and when it fails to reach the nose, the drainage is abnormal.

2.12.2 Indications

- Functional obstruction of the lacrimal drainage system
- Surgical planning (patient selection)

2.12.3 Interpretation

- Look for delays in the flow of the radioactive tracer isotope in the lacrimal drainage system [16]:
  - Presac delay (canalicular problem)—hold up at the inner canthus or failure of the tracer to reach the lacrimal sac by the end of the dynamic study
  - Preductal delay (NLD problem)—early filling of lacrimal sac, but no sign of sac emptying on the first static image at 5 m
  - Intraduct delay (NLD problem)—nuclide in the upper part of the NLD at 5 m, but no further drainage over the next 15 m.
- Better prognosis for DCR with preductal and intraductal delay.

2.13 Electrodiagnostic Tests

2.13.1 Full Field Electroretinogram (ERG) (Fig. 2.93)

2.13.1.1 Principles

- Records the mass electrical activity from the retina when stimulated by a light stimulus. The light stimuli may be either a flash stimulus or a pattern stimulus
- The rod and cone responses may be functionally dissected with ERG in the light of International Society for Clinical of Vision (ISCEV) recommendations [9]

2.13.1.2 Indications

- To confirm or exclude a specific diagnosis e.g. hereditary retinal or macular disorders
- Monitor the progress and treatment of a known condition e.g. Birdshot chorioretinopathy
- To provide an indication of visual potential in a diseased or injured eye

2.13.1.3 Interpretation

- ERG waveforms:
  - Negative A wave: response of photoreceptors
  - Positive B wave: response of bipolar and muller cells
  - Oscillatory potentials: response of amacrine cells
- Scotopic (dark-adapted) ERG:
  - Dim white flash: rod response only—B wave
  - Bright white flash (maximal ERG): mixed rod and cone response—A & B wave
- Photopic (light-adapted) ERG:
  - 30 Hz white light flicker stimulus: cone response
  - Photopic single flash: cone response
- Negative ERG (reduced scotopic B wave and normal A wave):
  - CRAO
  - X-linked retinoschisis
  - Congenital stationary night blindness (CSNB)
  - Myotonic dystrophy
  - Melanoma associated retinopathy (MAR)
  - Quinine toxicity
  - Birdshot chorioretinopathy
- Reduced A- and B-waves:
  - Rod-cone dystrophies (e.g. RP)
  - Drug toxicity e.g. phenothiazines
  - Total RD
  - Cancer associated retinopathy (CAR)
- Abnormal photopic and normal scotopic ERG:
  - Achromatopsia
  - Cone dystrophy
- Reduced oscillatory potentials:
  - Drug toxicity e.g. vigabatrin

2.13.2 Pattern ERG (PERG)

2.13.2.1 Principles

- Objective assessment of macular function
- A reversing checkerboard evokes small potentials that arise from the inner retina

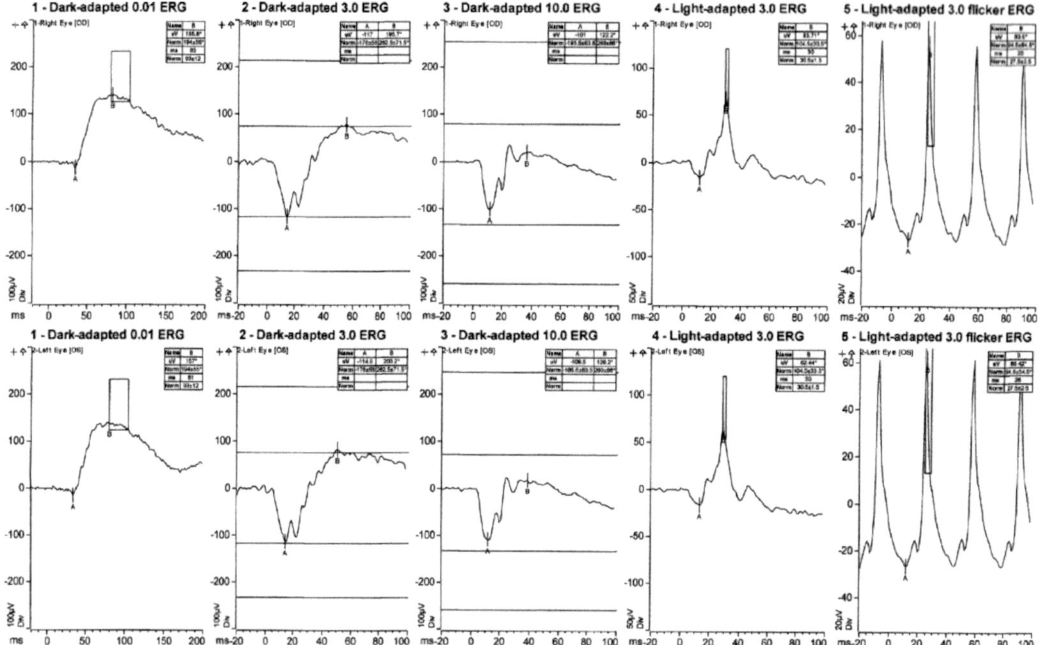

Fig. 2.93 A normal full-field ERG display. 1: Dark-adapted 0.01 ERG (rod response). 2: Dark-adapted 3.0 ERG (mixed rod and cone response—maximal ERG). 3: Dark-adapted 10.0 ERG (mixed rod and cone response with enhanced a-waves reflecting photoreceptor function). 4: Light adapted 3.0 ERG (single flash cone response). 5: Light adapted 30 Hz flicker ERG (cone response)

2.13.2.2 Indications

- Macular dystrophies e.g. Stargardt's disease
- PERG can help facilitate the electrophysiological differentiation between macular and optic nerve dysfunction
- PERG serves to determine which diagnostic path to follow in patients who present with unexplained visual acuity reduction. A normal PERG is followed by VEP. If VEP is completely normal then visual loss is likely to be non-organic. If the VEP is abnormal, there is optic nerve/ganglion cell dysfunction

2.13.2.3 Interpretation

- PERG waveforms (see Fig. 2.94):
  - Small negative component at 35 ms (N35)
  - Prominent positive component at 50 ms (P50): originates from photoreceptors
  - Larger negative component at 95 ms (N95): originates from ganglion cells
- A marked reduction in the PERG P50 component amplitude, or less commonly an increase in the PERG P50 component latency, suggests dysfunction of the macular anterior to the ganglion cells. A full field ERG will then determine whether there is generalised retinal dysfunction or whether the pathology is confined to the macula:
  - Abnormal PERG P50, normal ERG: indicates disease is confined to the macular (e.g macular dystrophies or localised maculopathy) and excludes generalised retinal dysfunction
  - Abnormal PERG P50, Full-field ERG A-wave abnormality: may be suggestive of a rod-cone or a cone-rod dystrophy
  - Abnormal PERG P50, Full-field ERG B-wave abnormality (negative ERG): abnormalities of the PERG (reflect abnormal function within the central retina) can occur with causes of a negative full-field ERG. See Sect. 2.13.1.3 for possible causes of a negative ERG
- A selective reduction in the PERG N95 (with a normal PERG P50) abnormality suggests optic nerve/ganglion cell dysfunction from

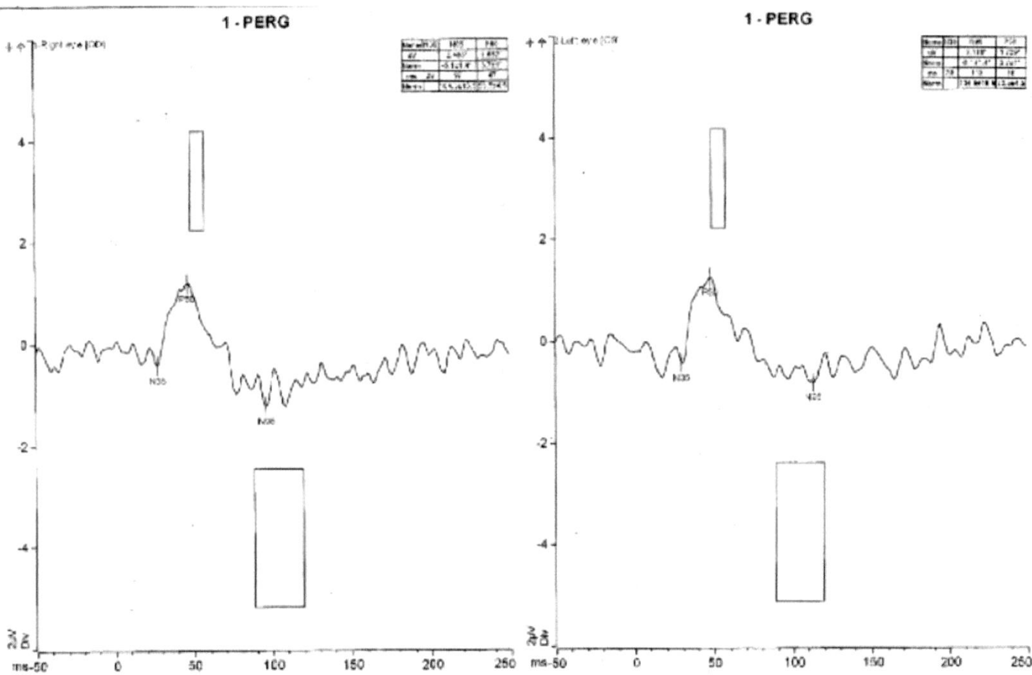

Fig. 2.94 PERG showing reduced responses affecting the N95 component (ganglion cell) more than the P50 component (retinal) in both eyes. The P50 component is of short latency in both eyes

numerous causes including optic nerve demyelination, ischaemic optic neuropathy, tobacco-alcohol amblyopia, optic nerve and chiasmal compression from pituitary tumours or craniopharyngiomas, Leber Hereditary Optic Neuropathy (LHON) and Kjer-type dominant optic atrophy (DOA). A VEP may assist in the discrimination between different types of optic nerve or chiasmal dysfunction

2.13.3 Multifocal ERG (mfERG)

2.13.3.1 Principles

- A map demonstrating the topographical variation in ERG responses across the retina (multiple small areas of the retina are stimulated)

2.13.3.2 Indications

- Detecting early outer retinal disease (pathology before the ganglion cells) that are not sufficiently extensive to significantly reduce the full-field ERG
- Decide whether a visual field defect is due to damage to the outer retina (before the ganglion cells) or damage to the optic nerve/ganglion cells:
  - An abnormal mfERG provides strong evidence for an outer retinal lesion (since damage to the ganglion cells or optic nerve does not decrease the amplitude of the mfERG)
  - Seeing abnormal mfERG's in the same regions of the visual field that are abnormal of perimetry provides reassurance of the retinal origin of the defect
- Following disease progression:
  - mfERG shows good repeat reliability and hence can be used to follow the progression of a disease. This is particularly helpful in patients who are poor visual field takers
- Differentiating organic from non-organic disorders:
  - The advantage of the mfERG over the conventional full-field ERG is that is provides a topographical representation that can be compared with the patient's visual field

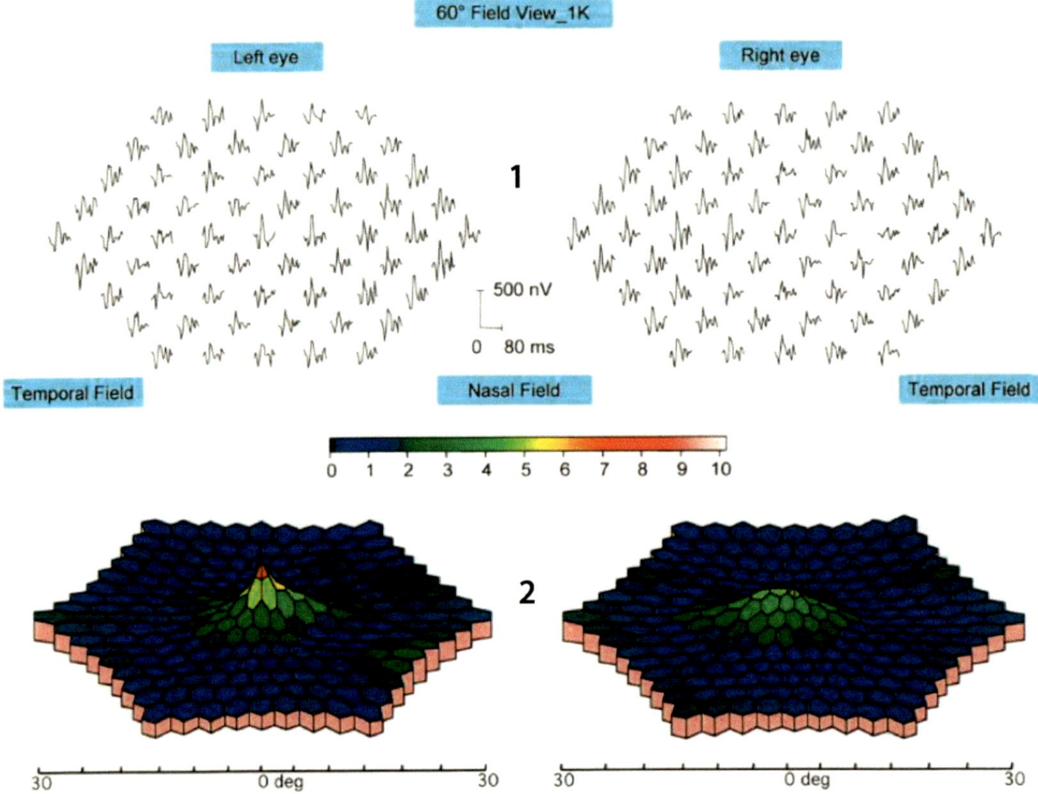

Fig. 2.95 A multifocal ERG printout display with key features identified. 1: Trace arrays. 2: Topographic response density plots

  - A normal mfERG does not, by itself, establish a visual deficit as non-organic. If the mfERG is normal, then a multifocal VEP should be performed to rule out damage to the optic nerve/ganglion cells

2.13.3.3 Interpretation

- mfERG waveforms:
  - Initial negative deflection (N1) followed by a positive peak (P1). There may be a second negative deflection (N2) after the positive peak
- To optimise the value of the mfERG, it is important to compare the results of the mfERG to automated visual fields obtained concurrently:
  - Reduced mfERG amplitudes that correspond to areas of visual field defects suggest an outer retinal pathology as the cause of the VF defect
- Look at the printout display options (see Fig. 2.95):
  - Trace arrays:
    - An array of mfERG traces from different regions of the retina
    - Useful for observing areas of variation and abnormality
  - Topographic (3-D) response density plots:
    - Plots show the overall signal strength per unit area of retina (combining N and P components) in a 3-D figure
    - Sometimes useful as an overview or demonstration of certain types of pathology

2.13.4 Electrooculogram (EOG)

2.13.4.1 Principles

- Measures the standing potential at the RPE-photoreceptor interface: gives information regarding RPE function

2.13.4.2 Indications

- Early detection and diagnosis of Best's disease

2.13.4.3 Interpretation

- Results are expressed based on the Arden ratio (light peak/dark trough × 100): result is abnormal if Arden ratio is less than 1.4

2.13.5 Visual Evoked Potential (VEP)

2.13.5.1 Principles

- Gross electrical response recorded from the visual cortex in response to a changing visual stimulus such as multiple flash or reversing checkerboard pattern stimulus

2.13.5.2 Indications

- Rule out non-organic visual loss: a normal VEP can be useful to prove good vision in a patient suspected of non-organic visual loss
- Diagnosing and following demyelinating optic neuritis
- To provide an approximate objective measurement of visual acuity (using the reversing checkerboard pattern stimulus)
- To provide an indication of the maturity of the visual system in infants
- Detection of misrouting of optic nerve fibers in ocular albinism (using the reversing checkerboard pattern stimulus): fibers from the temporal retina which would normally project to the ipsilateral hemisphere instead decussate in the chiasm and project to the contralateral hemisphere

2.13.5.3 Interpretation

- VEP waves:
  - Negative deflection occurs at 75 ms (N75)
  - Positive deflection occurs at about 100 ms (P100): macular dominated response
  - Negative deflection occurs at 135 ms (N135)
- In acute demyelination, the VEP is usually undetectable (Fig. 2.96 and Fig. 2.97). When VA has returned to normal, the VEP tends to show almost normal amplitudes but permanently delayed peak time
- In the detection of misrouting of optic nerve fibers in ocular albinism, stimulation of the left eye will result in a response predominantly over the right occipital lobe and vice versa.

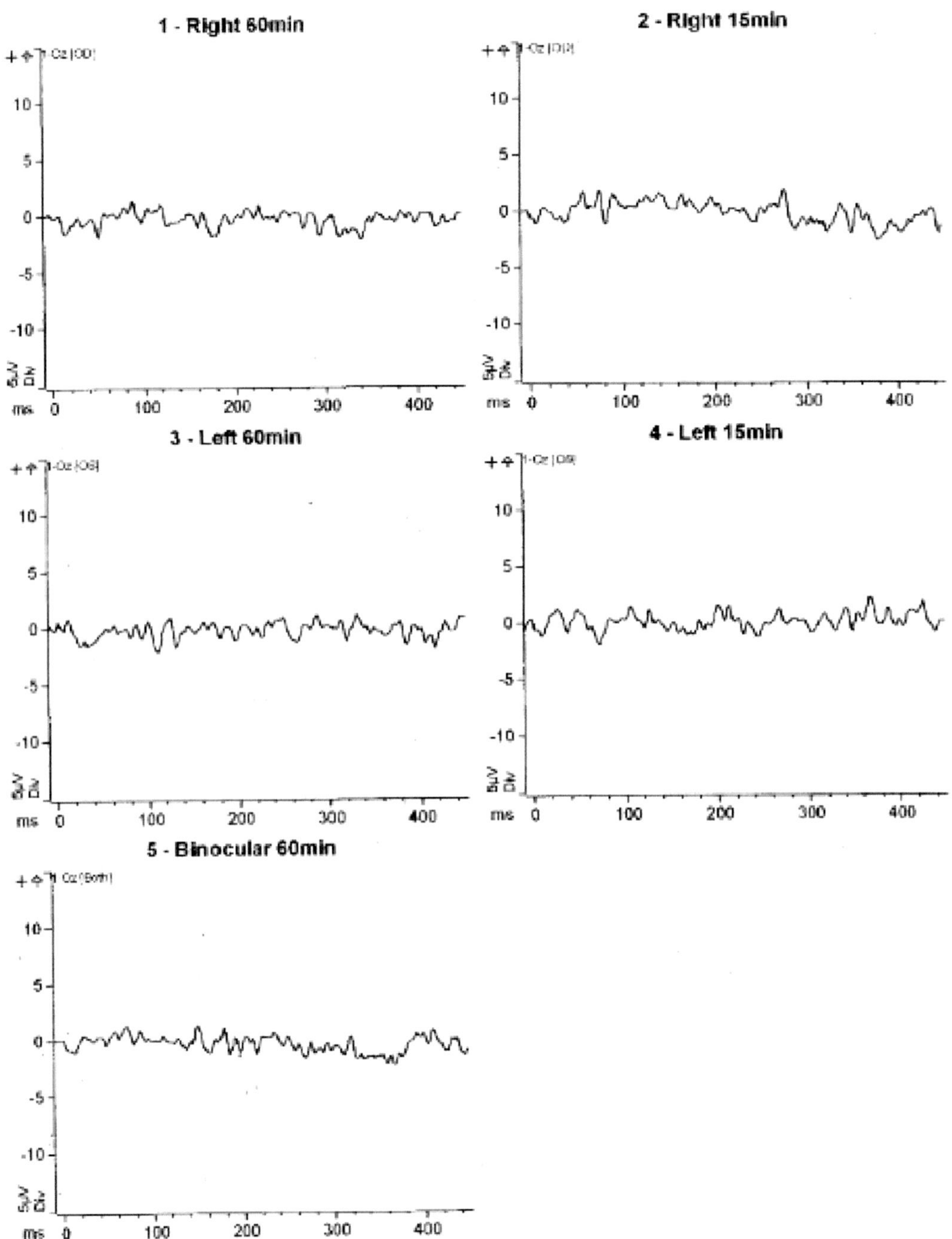

Fig. 2.96 Pattern reversal VEP of a patient with a bilateral atypical optic neuritis showing markedly reduced responses that were not measurable bilaterally

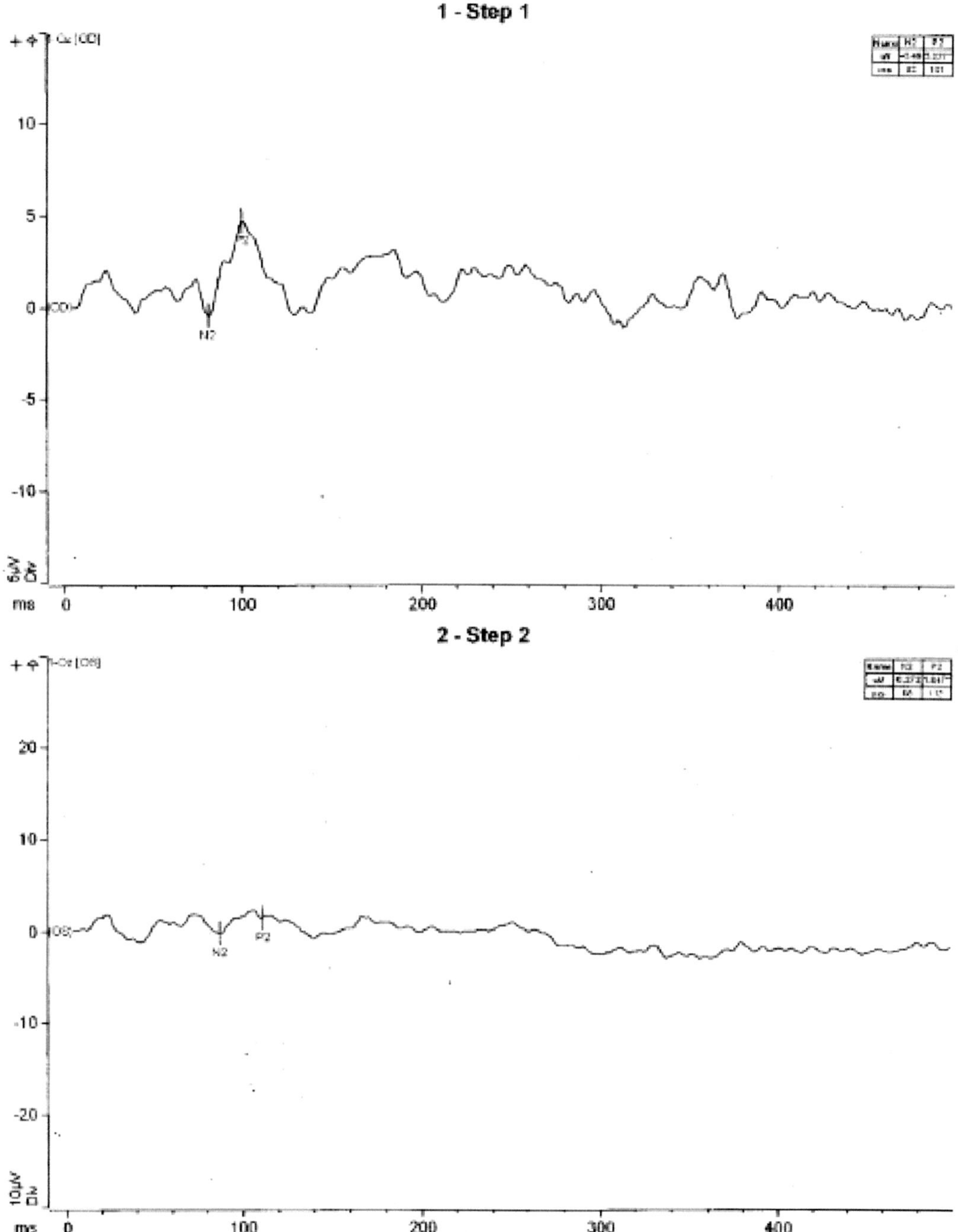

Fig. 2.97 Flash VEP of a patient with bilateral atypical optic neuritis showing low amplitude with normal latency in the right eye and markedly reduced and difficult to measure responses in the left eye

References

1. Casswell AG, Kohen D, Bird AC. Retinal pigment epithelial detachments in the elderly: classification and outcome. Br J Ophthalmol. 1985;69:397–403.
2. Chen JJ, Kardon RH. Avoiding clinical misinterpretation and artifacts of optical coherence tomography analysis of the optic nerve, retinal nerve fiber later, and ganglion cell layer. J Neuroophthalmol. 2016;36:417–38.
3. Cherfan GM, Michels RG, de Bustros S, Enger C, Glaser BM. Nuclear sclerotic cataract after vitrectomy for idiopathic epiretinal membranes causing macular pucker. Am J Ophthalmol. 1991;111:434–8.
4. Cukras C, Agron E, Klein ML, Ferris FL 3rd, Chew EY, Gensler G, Wong WT. Natural history of drusenoid pigment epithelial detachment in age-related macular degeneration: Age-Related Eye Disease Study Report No.28. Ophthalmology. 2010;117:489–99.
5. de Bustros S, Thompson JT, Michels RG, Rice TA, Glaser BM. Vitrectomy for idiopathic epiretinal membranes causing macular pucker. Br J Ophthalmol. 1988;72:692–5.
6. Haritoglou C, Gandorfer A, Gass CA, Schaumberger M, Ulbig MW, Kampik A. The effect of indocyanine-green on functional outcome of macular pucker surgery. Am J Ophthalmol. 2003;135:328–37.
7. Hood DC, Raza AS, Moraes CGV, Liebmann JM, Ritch R. Glaucomatous damage of the macula. Prog Retin Eye Res. 2012;17:1–21.
8. Malmqvist L, Bursztyn L, Costello F, Digre K, Fraser A, Fraser C, Katz B, Lawlor M, Petzold A, Sibony P, Warner J, Wegener M, Wong S, Hamann S. The optic disc drusen studies consortium recommendations for diagnosis of optic disc drusen using optical coherence tomography. J Neuroophthalmol. 2018;38:299–307.
9. Marmor MF, Fulton AB, Holder GE, Miyake Y, Brigell M, Bach M. ISCEV standard for full-field clinical electroretinography (2008 update). Doc Ophthalmol. 2009;118:69–77.
10. Michels RG, Gilbert HD. Surgical management of macular pucker after retinal reattachment surgery. Am J Ophthalmol 1979; 88: 925–9.
11. National Institute for Health and Care Excellence. Cataracts in adults: management [NG77]. London: NICE; 2017. Available at https://www.nice.org.uk/guidance/ng77. Accessed 30 Nov 2019.
12. Rabinowitz YS. Videokeratographic indices to aid in screening for keratoconus. J Refract Surg. 1995;11:371–9.
13. The Royal College of Ophthalmologists. Cataract surgery guidelines. London: The Royal College of Ophthalmologists; 2010. Available at https://www.rcophth.ac.uk/wp-content/uploads/2014/12/2010-SCI-069-Cataract-Surgery-Guidelines-2010-SEPTEMBER-2010-1.pdf. Accessed 30 Nov 2019
14. The Royal College of Ophthalmologists. Ophthalmic Service Guidance for Correct IOL implantation in cataract surgery. London: The Royal College of Ophthalmologists; 2018. Available at https://www.rcophth.ac.uk/wp-content/uploads/2018/03/Correct-IOL-implantation-in-cataract-surgery-quality-standard.pdf. Accessed 30 Nov 2019.
15. The Royal College of Ophthalmologists. Retinal Vein Occlusion (RVO) Guidelines. London: The Royal College of Ophthalmologists; 2022. Available at https://www.rcophth.ac.uk/wp-content/uploads/2015/07/Retinal-Vein-Occlusion-Guidelines-2022.pdf. Accessed 6 Nov 2024.
16. Wearne MJ, Pitts J, Frank J, Rose GE. Comparison of Dacryocystography and lacrimal scintigraphy in the diagnosis of functional nasolacrimal duct obstruction. Br J Ophthalmol. 1990;83:1032–5.

Patient Management in Clinical Practice

3

Timothy H. M. Fung and Winfried M. K. Amoaku

Abstract

Examination candidates must possess the knowledge to effectively manage various ophthalmic pathologies encountered in clinical practice. This chapter provides essential information on the management of these conditions.

3.1 Non-Proliferative Diabetic Retinopathy (NPDR)

3.1.1 Other Diagnoses to Consider

- Retinal vein occlusion
- Hypertensive retinopathy
- Ocular ischaemic syndrome
- Radiation retinopathy

3.1.2 Risk Factors for Diabetic Retinopathy (DR)

The Royal College of Ophthalmologists (RCOphth) Diabetic Retinopathy Guidelines 2012 [119]:

- Non-modifiable:
  - Genetic factors
  - Gender
  - Duration of diabetes
- Modifiable:
  - Glycaemia (HbA1C)
  - BP
  - Lipid levels
- Other:
  - Carotid arterial disease
  - Pregnancy
  - Renal impairment
  - Smoking

3.1.3 Classification

- Proposed International Clinical Diabetic Retinopathy Severity Scale 2003 [128]:
  - Mild NPDR (see Fig. 3.1):
    Microaneurysms (Mas) only
  - Moderate NPDR:
    More than just Ma but less than severe NPDR
  - Severe NPDR (4-2-1 rule)—one or more of the following features are present:
    More than 20 intraretinal haemorrhages in each of 4 quadrants
    Definite venous beading in in 2 or more quadrants
    Prominent intraretinal microvascular abnormalities (IRMA) in 1 or more quadrants

T. H. M. Fung (✉)
University Hospitals of Derby & Burton NHS Foundation Trust, Royal Derby Hospital, Derby, UK
e-mail: timothy.fung@nhs.net

W. M. K. Amoaku
Eye, Ear, Nose and Throat Centre, Queens Medical Centre, Nottingham University Hospitals NHS Trust, Nottingham, UK

T. H. M. Fung, W. M. K. Amoaku (eds.), *Viva and OSCE Exams in Ophthalmology*,
https://doi.org/10.1007/978-3-031-97401-4_3

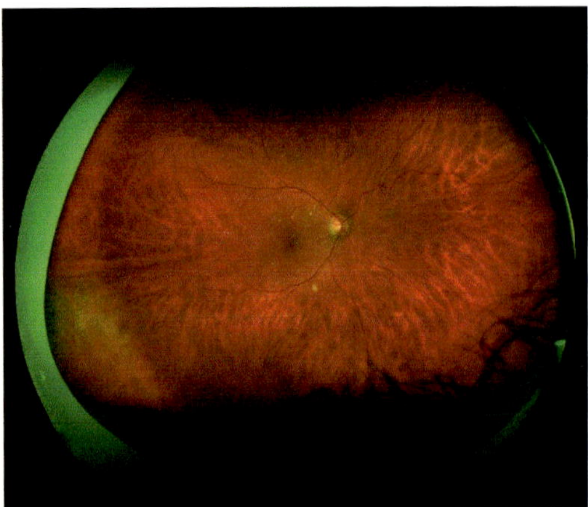

Fig. 3.1 Optos pseudocolour fundus image of a patient with mild NPDR

- Very severe NPDR:
  2 or more features of severe NPDR are present
- Public Health England NHS Diabetic Eye Screening Programme Grading Definitions 2017 [89]:
  - R0: No retinopathy
  - R1 (Background DR / mild NPDR):
    Venous loop
    Microaneurysms
    Retinal haemorrhage
    Any exudate or cotton wool spot in presence of other non-referable DR features
  - R2 (pre-proliferative DR/moderate NPDR):
    Venous beading
    Venous reduplication
    Multiple blot haemorrhages (if uncertain, refer only in the presence of IRMA that are definitely seen)
    - Blot haemorrhages (located in OPL and INL) are larger than the width of the smallest of the 4 branches of the central retinal vein as it crosses the edge of the disc

    IRMA (check that they can still be seen on the colour image as well as the red-free image that has not been enlarged)
  - R3 (proliferative DR):
    R3A (active proliferative retinopathy): newly presenting proliferative retinopathy; previous treatment that has not been deemed stable by the treating ophthalmologist; new features indicating reactivation of proliferative or potentially sight-threatening change from fibrous proliferation can be seen with respect to a previously obtained reference image set
    R3S (stable treated proliferative retinopathy): evidence of peripheral retinal laser treatment; a stable retina with respect to reference images taken at or shortly after discharge from HES

3.1.4 Examination

- Microaneurysms (Mas): small red dots
- Intraretinal haemorrhages: dot and blot haemorrhages, flame haemorrhages
- Exudates: sharply demarcated yellow-white deposits within the retina
- Cotton wool spots (CWS—patches of relative ischaemia affecting the NFL of the retina): small white patches with wispy borders situated in the inner retina
- Venous beading: localised areas of change in vessel calibre with alternating regions of relative dilation and constriction
- Venous loops
- Intraretinal microvascular abnormalities (IRMA): segments of dilated and tortuous retinal vasculature without crossing both arterioles or veins in the underlying retina
- Subretinal fibrosis

3.1.5 Investigations

- Blood test for diagnosis of diabetes mellitus:
  - Venous fasting glucose ≥7.0 mmol/L &/or
  - Oral glucose tolerance test (75 g anhydrous glucose) with a 2-hour value ≥11.1 mmol/L &/or
  - Random venous glucose ≥11.1 mmol/L
- FFA:
  - Mas appear as hyperfluorescent dots visible during the arteriovenous transit phase

- Intraretinal haemorrhages appear hypofluorescent blocking normal fluorescence from the underlying choroid
- Exudates appear hypofluorescent
- CWS appear hypofluorescent
- IRMA appear hyperfluorescent during the arteriovenous transit phase and are often situated at the borders of areas of capillary non-perfusion

3.1.6 Treatment

- When making decisions about ophthalmic interventions, the persons stage of DR, HbA1C level, renal function **and** BP should be taken into account (NICE Guidance NG242 [79])
- Modification of life-style:
  - Smoking cessation
  - Weight loss
  - Exercise
- Modification of systemic risk factors:
  - Hyperglycaemia control
    - (a) **DCCT** [24]: Type 1 DM—tight control of HbA1C at mean of 7.2% was associated with 76% reduction in onset of retinopathy and slowed progression of DR by 54%, 60% reduction in onset of neuropathy, and 54% reduction in onset of nephropathy at 6.5 years
    - (b) **UKPDS** [126]: Type 2 DM—tight control of HbA1C at mean of 7% was associated with a 25% reduction in the onset of microvascular disease
    - (c) **ACCORD** [104]: Type 2 DM—intensive control of HbA1C reduced progression of DR by 42% and reduced development of PDR from 10.2% to 6.5%: avoid Pioglitazone in the presence of macular oedema, personalized HbA1c target should be set, usually between 48–58 mmol/mol (6.5–7.5%)
    - (d) **NICE Guidance [NG242]** [79]: if a diabetic treatment is likely to result in a rapid, substantial drop in a person's HbA1C, an ophthalmologist should assess a person's eyes before treatment begins and check for changes afterwards
    - (e) **NICE Guidance [NG28]** [83]: for adults whose type 2 DM is managed either with lifestyle and diet, or lifestyle and diet combined with a single drug not associated with hypoglycaemia, aim for a HbA1C level of 48 mmol/mol (6.5%). For adults on a drug associated with hypoglycaemia, aim for a HbA1C level of 53 mmol// mol (7.0%)
  - BP control:
    - (a) **UKPDS** [126]: Type 2 DM—tight control of BP at mean of 144/82 was associated with a 37% reduction in the onset of microvascular disease and 32% reduction in diabetes related deaths
    - (b) **NICE Guidance [NG136]** [80]: For adults with hypertension aged under 80 with type 1 or type 2 DM, reduce clinic BP to below 140/90 mmHg and ensure it is maintained below that level. For adults with hypertension aged 80 and over with type 1 or type 2 DM, reduce clinic BP to below 150/90 mmHg and ensure it is maintained below that level
  - Lipid control:
    - (a) **ACCORD** [104]: Type 2 DM—40% reduction in the odds of having progression of DR over 4 years in patients allocated to fenofibrate in combination with a statin, compared to simvastatin alone): consider adding fenofibrate to a statin for NPDR in type 2 DM, avoid statins in pregnancy
    - (b) **NICE Guidance [NG242]** [79]: Ophthalmologists should consider fenofibrate for people with NPDR and type 2 DM to reduce the progression of DR

3.1.7 Follow-Up

- Mild NPDR: discharge to community for DRSS screening or 12 months follow up if seen in hospital eye service (HES)
- Moderate NPDR: every 6 to 12 months (NICE Guidance [NG242]) [79]

- Severe or very severe NPDR: every 3 to 6 months (NICE Guidance [NG242]) [79]

3.1.8 Prognosis

- In the Diabetic Retinopathy Study (DRS) [112], 50% of untreated severe DR will develop proliferative diabetic retinopathy (PDR) within 15 months
- In the Early Treatment Diabetic Retinopathy Study (ETDRS) [27]:
  - 6.2% risk of progression to PDR at 1 year for mild NPDR
  - 11.3% risk of progression to PDR at 1 year for moderate NPDR
  - 20.7% risk of progression to PDR at 1 year for severe NPDR

3.2 Diabetic Macular Oedema (DMO)

3.2.1 Other Causes of Macular Oedema to Consider

- Inflammatory disorders: post-operative (cataract, VR, corneal), post-laser (PI, PRP), post-cryotherapy, uveitis
- Retinal vascular diseases: DR, RVO, OIS, hypertensive retinopathy, radiation retinopathy, MacTel
- Choroidal vascular disease: CNV
- Drugs: latanoprost, topical adrenaline, glitazones, niacin, chemotherapy agents (e.g paclitaxel)
- Inherited retinal dystrophies: RP, autosomal dominantly inherited CMO
- Disorders of vitreoretinal interface: VMT, ERM
- Optic nerve head abnormalities: optic disc pit, optic disc coloboma
- Tumours of the choroid/retina

3.2.2 Classification

- Proposed International Clinical Diabetic Macular Edema Severity Scale, 2003 [128]:
  - Mild DME:
    Some retinal thickening or exudates in the posterior pole, distant from the center of the macula
  - Moderate DME:
    Retinal thickening or exudates near the center of the macula but not involving the center
  - Severe DME:
    Retinal thickening or exudates involving the center of the macula
- Public Health England NHS Diabetic Eye Screening Programme (DESP) Grading Definitions 2017 [89]:
  - M0: No maculopathy
  - M1:
    Exudate within 1-disc diameter of the centre of the fovea (see Fig. 3.2)
    Circinate or group of exudates within the macula:
    - A group of exudates is an area of exudates that is greater than or equal to half the disc area and this area is all within the macular area

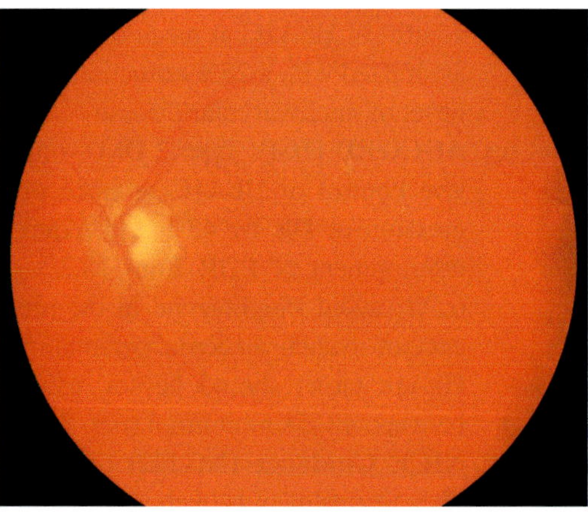

Fig. 3.2 Colour fundus image of a patient with DMO

- To work out the area, the outer points of the exudates are joined and compared to half the area of the optic disc
- Any Ma or haemorrhage within 1-disc diameter of the centre of the fovea only if associated with a best VA of 6/12 or worse

- NICE Guidance (NG242) [79]:
  - Centre-involving diabetic macular oedema (based on OCT):
    Clinically significant macular oedema (CSMO) that involves the central subfield of the ETDRS grid, which has a diameter of 1 mm
  - Non-centre involving diabetic macular oedema (based on OCT):
    CSMO that does not involve the central subfield of the ETDRS grid, which has a diameter of 1 mm

3.2.3 Examination

- Exudates within the macular
- Mas or retinal haemorrhages within the macular
- CSMO [26] is present when any of the following signs are present, based on slit-lamp biomicroscopy and stereopsis:
  - Retinal thickening at or within 500 μm of the centre of the macula &/or
  - Exudates at or within 500 μm of the centre of the macula, if associated with thickening of the adjacent retina &/or
  - Zone or zones of retinal thickening 1-disc area or larger, any part of which is within 1-disc diameter of the center of the macula

3.2.4 Investigations

- OCT:
  - Exudates appear as hyperreflective foci within the retina
  - Macular oedema
  - Traction from ERM or VMT causing underlying macular oedema in the absence of retinal vascular leakage demonstrable by FFA
- OCT-A:
  - Quantify foveal avascular zone and non-perfused areas
- FFA:
  - Petaloid pattern of leakage from macular oedema
  - Enlarged foveal avascular zone from ischaemic diabetic maculopathy

3.2.5 Treatment

- Offer treatment to people with CSMO (centre-involving and non-centre involving) and discuss the benefits and potential side-effects of macular laser treatment, intravitreal anti-VEGF treatment, intravitreal steroid treatment, vitrectomy and observation (NICE Guidance [NG242]) [79]
- Focal/grid laser:
  - Indications: offer macular laser treatment to people with non-centre involving CSMO (NICE Guidance [NG242]) [79]. Consider macular laser treatment for people with centre-involving CSMO and good vision (79 ETDRS letters or better) (NICE Guidance [NG242]) [79]. For people with centre-involving CSMO, visual impairment (78 ETDRS letters or worse / snellen acuity of 6/9 or worse) and CMT < 400 μm, consider macular laser treatment (NICE Guidance [NG242]) [79]
  - Clinical trial:
    ETDRS [26]: focal/grid laser reduced the risk of moderate vision loss (loss of ≥15 letters from baseline) by 50% at 3 years in eyes with mild or moderate NPDR with CSMO
- Anti-VEGF therapy:
  - Indications (NICE Guidance [NG242]) [79]: offer anti-VEGF treatment for people with centre-involving CSMO, visual impairment (78 ETDRS letters or worse / snellen acuity of 6/9 or worse) and CMT ≥ 400 μm. Consider anti-VEGF treatment for people with centre-involving CSMO, visual impairment and CMT < 400 μm

- Anti-VEGF treatment options (see also Table 3.1):
  1. Faricimab (Vabysmo)
  - NICE Guidance [TA799] [81]: option for treatment of DMO if CMT ≥ 400 μm at the start of treatment
  - Regimen: a single injection every 4 weeks for 4 months, followed by 1 injection every 4–16 weeks
  - Clinical trials:
    - **YOSEMITE** study [130]
    - **RHINE** study [130]
  2. Brolucizumab (Beovu)
  - NICE Guidance [TA820] [82]: option for treatment of DMO if CMT ≥ 400 μm at the start of treatment
  - Regimen: a single injection every 6 weeks for the first 5 doses, followed by 1 injection every 8–12 weeks
  - Clinical trials:
    - **KITE** study [12]
    - **KESTREL** study [12]
  3. Aflibercept (eylea, aflibercept biosimilars)
  - NICE Guidance [TA346] [71]: option for treatment of DMO if CMT ≥ 400 μm at the start of treatment
  - Regimen: a single injection every month for 5 consecutive months, followed by 1 injection every 2 months with no requirement for monitoring between visits for the first 12 months
  - Clinical trials:
    - **VIVID** study [11]
    - **VISTA** study [11]
  4. Ranibizumab (lucentis, ranibizumab biosimilars)
  - NICE Guidance [TA274] [67]: option for treatment of DMO if CMT ≥ 400 μm at the start of treatment
  - Regimen: given monthly and continued until maximum VA is reached—VA stable for 3 consecutive months:
  - Clinical trials:
    - **RISE** study [10, 86]
    - **RIDE** study [10, 86]
    - **RESTORE** study [63]
- Assessing response (NICE Guidance [NG242]) [79]: after the loading phase of anti-VEGF treatment, assess response and consider using macular laser as adjuvant treatment if the response is suboptimal. Treatment response is suboptimal if there is reduced vision or increased macular oedema or no change or increase in retinal thickness. Twelve months after starting anti-VEGF treatment, assess response to treatment and consider switching to an intravitreal steroid implant if the response is suboptimal. At any time after the start of treatment, if a person does not want to continue with regular anti-VEGF treatment, consider switching treatment to an intravitreal steroid implant

• Steroid therapy:
  - Indications (NICE Guidance [NG242]) [79]: consider an intravitreal steroid implant when people with centre-involving CSMO have visual impairment and cannot have non-corticosteroid therapy
  - Intravitreal steroid implants:

Table 3.1 Biosimilars in Ophthalmology

As the patent for original biologics used to treat conditions such as DMO, neovascular AMD, retinal vein occlusions and uveitis approach expiration, numerous companies strive to replicate these biologics with biosimilars
A biosimilar medicine is a biological medicine which has been shown not to have any clinically meaningful differences from the originator medicine in terms of quality, safety and efficacy, although they do not have the same identical active ingredients
Where NICE has already recommended the originator biological medicine, the same guidance will normally apply to a biosimilar of that originator or innovator molecule
Commonly used biosimilar medicines in ophthalmology include:
Ongavia, Ximluci, Byooviz: biosimilar versions of ranibizumab
Yesafili, Opuviz: biosimilar versions of aflibercept
Benepali: biosimilar version of etanercept
Yuflyma, Amgevita, Hyrimoz, Idacio, Imraldi: biosimilar versions of adalimumab
Inflectra, Remsima: biosimilar versions of infliximab

1. Dexamethasone intravitreal steroid implant (Ozurdex)
   - NICE Guidance [TA349] [73]: option for treatment of DMO if eye is pseudophakic and CSMO does not respond to non-corticosteroid treatment or such treatment is unsuitable
   - Regimen: A single implant is injected into the vitreous and remains in the vitreous for up to 270 days before fully dissolving
   - Clinical trials:
     - **PLACID** study [13]
     - **BEVORDEX** study [38]
     - **MEAD** study [7]
2. Fluocinolone intravitreal steroid implant (Iluvien)
   - NICE Guidance [TA301] [69]: option for the treatment of chronic CSMO that is insufficiently responsive to available therapies if an eye is pseudophakic
   - Regimen: A single 190 μm of Fluocinolone Acetonide implant is injected with daily release of 0.2 μg/day for 36 months
   - Clinical trials:
     - **FAME** study [21]

- Vitrectomy:
  - Indications (NICE Guidance [NG242]) [79]: for people with CSMO that do not respond to anti-VEGF treatment and also have either VMT or ERM. Check for warning signs of permanent damage (photoreceptor cell loss, macular atrophy or lamellar macular holes) and consider vitrectomy before any permanent damage occurs
- Observation:
  - Consider observation for people with good vision (79 ETDRS letters or better) and centre-involving macular oedema (NICE Guidance [NG242]) [79]

3.2.6 Follow-Up

- Center involved DMO: 1–3 months
- Non-center involved DMO: 3–6 months
- Stable treated DMO: 3–6 months
- For people whose macular oedema has resolved (presence of isolated or sparse, small, intraretinal cysts with no other features as seen from OCT scans) after treatment, monitor under the care of the HES for the first 12 months after the end of treatment (NICE Guidance [NG242]) [79]
- For people whose macular oedema has resolved after treatment, after the first 12 months following the end of treatment, discharge the person to the DESP if they are eligible for it. If the persons retina has features that makes it ineligible for the screening programme, monitor them under the care of HES, and consider seeing the person every 12 months (NICE guidance [NG242]) [79]

3.2.7 Focal & Grid Laser Techniques

Diabetic Retinopathy Clinical Research Network (DRCR.net) laser techniques [129]:

- Focal treatment:
  - Topical anaesthetic
  - Spot size: 50 μm
  - Burn duration: 0.05 to 0.1 second
  - Burn intensity: mild grey-white burn evident beneath all Mas
  - Directly treat all leaking Mas in areas of retinal thickening between 500 and 3000 μm from the center of the macula
  - Follow up: 3–4 months
- Grid treatment:
  - Topical anaesthetic
  - Spot size: 50 μm
  - Burn duration: 0.05 to 0.1 second
  - Burn intensity: light grey burn
  - Burn separation: 2 visible burn widths apart
  - Apply to all areas with oedema not associated with Mas: 500–3000 μm superiorly, nasally and inferiorly from center of macula; 500–3500 μm temporally from macular center; no burns placed within 500 μm of optic disc
  - Follow up: 3–4 months
  - Complications: pain, worsened VA, choroidal detachment or RD, CNV membrane, vitreous haemorrhage

3.3 Proliferative Diabetic Retinopathy (PDR)

3.3.1 Other Causes of Neovascularisation to Consider

- Retinal vein occlusion
- Ocular ischaemic syndrome
- Radiation retinopathy
- Occlusive retinal vasculitis—MS, sarcoid, Behcet's disease

3.3.2 High-Risk PDR

- Defined by the Diabetic Retinopathy Study [112] with patients at higher risk of visual loss and requires prompt PRP treatment:
  - Neovascularisation of the disc (NVD—new vessels on or within 1-disc diameter of the optic disc): NVD ≥ one quarter to one third the disc area in size or any size NVD with a vitreous &/or preretinal haemorrhage
  - Neovascularisation elsewhere in the retina (NVE): NVE ≥ one half the disc area in size with a vitreous &/or preretinal haemorrhage (see Fig. 3.3)

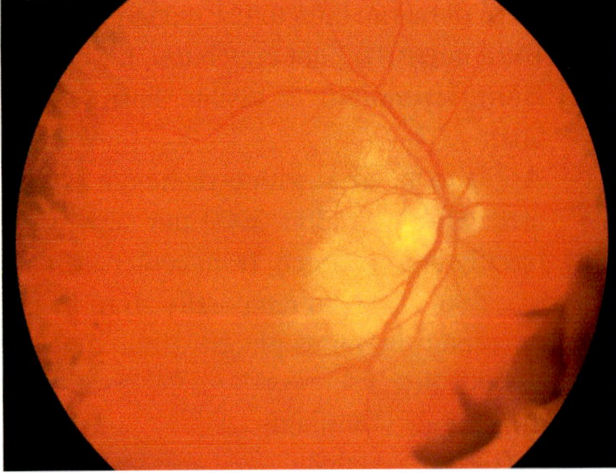

Fig. 3.3 Colour fundus image of a patient with PDR with an active NVE and a vitreous haemorrhage

3.3.3 PDR in Pregnancy

NICE Guidance [NG3] [72]

- Diabetic patients planning pregnancy should be informed on the need for assessment of DR before and during pregnancy
- Statins and drugs blocking the renin-angiotensin system should be discontinued before conception and always at first antenatal booking if still being taken
- Ideally, all patients with PDR should be identified and treated prior to conception
- Rapid optimisation of poor glycaemic control should be deferred at least until after retinal assessment
- Retinal assessment during and after pregnancy:
  - Newly pregnant women with pre-existing DM should be offered retinal assessment by digital imaging following their first antenatal clinic (i.e. first trimester, typically 8–12 weeks) appointment (unless they have had a retinal assessment in the last 3 months) and again at 28 weeks (third trimester) if the first assessment is normal. If any DR is present, an additional retinal assessment should be performed at 16–20 weeks (second trimester)
  - At term, DR should not be considered a contraindication to vaginal birth
  - Women who have NPDR diagnosed during pregnancy should have ophthalmological follow up for at least 6 months following the birth of the baby
  - Tropicamide alone should be used if mydriasis is required during pregnancy
- Women with gestational DM are not at increased risk for the development of DR and do not need such monitoring.

3.3.4 Treatment

- Modification of life-style (see Sect. 3.1.6)
- Modification of systemic risk factors (see Sect. 3.1.6)
- NICE Guidance [NG242] [79]: discuss with the person with PDR the benefits and potential

side effects of each of the following options: PRP, anti-VEGFs, vitrectomy and no treatment (observation)

- Pan-retinal photocoagulation (PRP)
  - Indications (The Royal College of Ophthalmologists Diabetic Retinopathy Guideline 2012) [119]: presence of NVD/NVE/NVI/NVA—PRP performed on same day or within 2 weeks of diagnosis, consider PRP for severe/very severe NPDR in older patients with type 2 DM, where retinal view is difficult, prior to cataract surgery, in only eye where first eye lost to PDR, where regular clinic attendance is likely to be poor, difficult to examine patient for other reasons
  - NICE Guidance [NG242] [79]: Offer PRP to people when they are first diagnosed with PDR. If possible, start treatment within 4 weeks of offering. If it cannot be started within 4 weeks, start it within 6 weeks of offering. Complete PRP within 4 weeks of starting treatment. For people with high-risk characteristics or who have difficulty attending appointments, offer to start PRP on the same day.
  - Prognosis [112]: PRP reduces severe vision loss (<5/200 at 2 consecutive visits) from high-risk PDR by 50% at 2 years
- Anti-VEGF therapy
  - In August 2024, the only anti-VEGF treatment licensed for PDR was ranibizumab and use of any other anti-VEGF treatment would be off-label (NICE Guidance [NG242]) [79]
  - Indications (NICE Guidance [NG242]) [79]: offer anti-VEGF treatment for people whose PDR remains active after complete PRP. Consider anti-VEGF treatment as a temporary treatment for people with PDR who have vitreous haemorrhage that is preventing PRP and/or need cataract surgery and the severity of the cataract is preventing PRP.
- Vitrectomy
  - Indications [119]: non-clearing (within 3 months for type 2 diabetic and 1 month for a type 1 diabetic) severe vitreous haemorrhage (confirmation of attached retina not possible with ophthalmoscopic examination), significant recurrent vitreous haemorrhage despite maximal PRP, tractional RD involving or threatening the fovea, combined tractional rhegmatogenous RD which involves or threatens to involve the fovea, diffuse CSMO associated with posterior hyaloidal traction
  - NICE Guidance [NG242] [79]: consider vitrectomy for people with PDR and vitreous haemorrhage that has not cleared within 3 months. Perform vitrectomy within 3 months of offering it. Offer vitrectomy to people with PDR and macula involving or macula-threatening RD. Consider vitrectomy for people with non-macula-involving or non-macula-threatening RD who, despite complete PRP, have PDR that is active or recurring vitreous haemorrhages related to active PDR or VMT
  - Prognosis [111]: early vitrectomy (for those with severe vitreous haemorrhage with VA 5/200 or worse) increased chance of 20/40 vision from 12% to 36% in type 1 diabetics

3.3.5 Follow-Up

- NICE Guidance [NG242] [79]:
  - Consider using ultrawide-field fundus imaging alongside clinical examination when assessing eyes for the presence of PDR
  - Assess disease regression in people who have received treatment of PDR. Conduct this assessment 2 to 3 months after the end of treatment. Disease regression is defined by (1) regressing or disappearance of new vessels as seen on fundus examination or fundus imaging or FFA, (2) fibrosis developing in areas of new vessels, and (3) absence of new vitreous or preretinal haemorrhages
  - For people whose disease has regressed after treatment for PDR, monitor under the

care of HES for 12 months after the end of treatment
  – For people whose disease has regressed after treatment for PDR, after the first 12 months following the end of treatment, discharge the person to the DESP if they are eligible for it. If the person is ineligible for the DESP, monitor the persons eyes under the care of HES, and consider seeing them every 12 months

3.3.6 Prognosis

- 25% with type 1 DM and 16% with type 2 DM will develop PDR after 15 years of DM [55]

3.3.7 PRP Laser Technique

RCOphth Diabetic Retinopathy Guideline 2012 [119]

- Topical anaesthetic
- Spot size: 400 μm spot size (if 200 μm is preselected on laser interface, a mainster 165 PRP lens with a spot magnification factor of 1.96 will produce a theoretical retinal spot size of 392 μm)
- Burn duration: 20 ms
- Burn intensity: barely visible grey-white burn (titrate power down by up to 50 mW in the periphery)
- Burn separation: 1 visible burn width apart for early or moderate PDR, 0.5 burn width apart for severe PDR
- Retinal surface coverage: burns applied as far peripheral as possible up to the ora serrata, no closer than 3000 μm temporal to fovea, no closer than 500 μm nasal to the optic disc, no further posterior than 1 burn within the temporal arcades
- No. of sessions to complete full primary PRP: 1–2 sessions within 2 weeks for mild (NVD or NVE <1/3 disc area and flat) and moderate (NVD or NVE >1/3 disc area) PDR, 2–3 sessions in 3–4 weeks for severe (NVD or NVE with tractional RD) PDR, 3–4 sessions within 4 weeks for young patients with type 1 diabetes with PDR (increased risk of developing macular oedema post PRP)
- Follow up: 4 months for early PDR, 3 months for moderate PDR, 2 weeks for PDR in pregnancy. Regression of new vessels is characterised by blunting of the NV growing tips or replacement with fibrosis
- Complications:
  (a) Related to damage to posterior ocular structures:
    – Retinal tear
    – Choroidal haemorrhage
    – Choroidal neovascularisation
    – Vitreous, preretinal or subhyaloid haemorrhage
    – Inadvertent optic disc or foveal damage
  (b) Related to loss of visual function:
    – Diminished or loss of peripheral visual field—implications for driving
    – Diminished colour vision and contrast sensitivity
    – Reduced or loss of dark adaptation—effect on night vision
  (c) Related to the destructive nature of the procedure:
    – Pain during and shortly after treatment
    – Corneal epithelial defects and recurrent erosions
    – Mydriasis
    – Iris burns and damage/Lenticular burns or opacification
  (d) Related to contraction of fibrovascular tissue:
    – Progressive traction RD
  (e) Related to break down of blood-retinal barrier breakdown:
    – Exudative RD/choroidal detachment / choroidal effusion
    – Macular oedema

NICE Guidance (NG242) [79]

- PRP is complete when all of the midperipheral retina and peripheral retina (from 2-disc diameters away from the fovea to the equator) has been treated with PRP, leaving one-size burn space in between burns **and** for people whose PDR had remained active after this original treatment, additional fill-in laser has been applied, if appropriate, adding burns in the spaces left by the original treatment.

3.4 Branch Retinal Vein Occlusion (BRVO)

3.4.1 Other Diagnoses to Consider

- Macular telangiectasia
- Diabetic retinopathy
- Radiation retinopathy
- Susac syndrome: small BRAO (may be multiple) and capillary occlusions, sensorineural hearing loss, subacute encephalopathy, hyperintense lesions in the corpus callosum on T2 MRI
- Behcet's disease
- Sarcoidosis

3.4.2 Risk Factors

- Arteriosclerosis: HTN, DM, smoking, hyperlipidaemia (including secondary to hypothyroidism)
- Glaucoma
- Ocular inflammatory disease: Behcet's disease, PAN, sarcoidosis, SLE
- Haematological: Protein C, protein S or antithrombin deficiency, activated protein C resistance, factor V Leiden, myeloma, Waldenstrom's macroglobulinaemia, antiphospholipid syndrome

3.4.3 Examination

- Acute BRVO: wedge shaped segmental distribution of intraretinal haemorrhage in a quadrant of the fundus, narrowed branch retinal vein passing under a retinal artery, dilated and tortuous retinal vein, cotton wool spots
- Chronic BRVO (see Fig. 3.4): telangiectatic vessels (dilation of capillaries) forming collaterals that cross the horizontal raphe, microaneurysms, exudates, sclerosed retinal vein +/− NVE gt; NVD gt; NVI

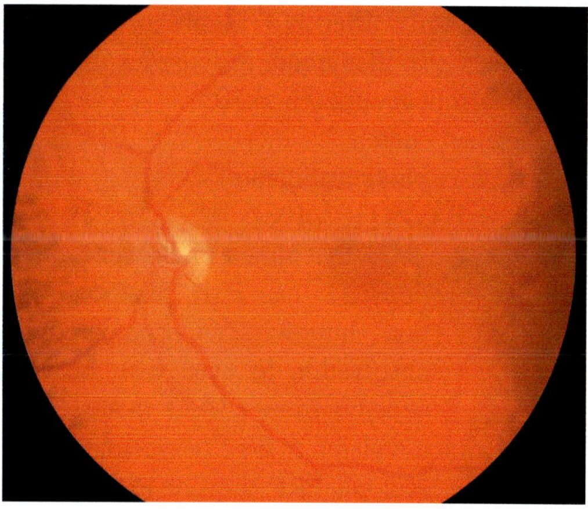

Fig. 3.4 Colour fundus image of a patient with a chronic non-ischaemic BRVO

- Check for RAPD
- Check the IOP
- Look for NVI on anterior segment examination
- Perform gonioscopy for NVA

3.4.4 Investigations

RCOphth Retinal Vein Occlusion (RVO) Guidelines 2022 [120]:

- BP
- Bloods: FBC (leukaemia/lymphoproliferative disorders), ESR (paraprotein), glucose
- OCT: CMO
- FFA (if uncertain diagnosis): delayed filling of the occluded retinal vein, capillary non-perfusion—>5 DD is defined as an ischaemic BRVO [107, 108], macular ischaemia, telangiectatic vessels forming collaterals that cross the horizontal raphe
- OCTA is recommended to assess retinal non-perfusion

3.4.5 Treatment

- Control of cardiovascular risk factors: HTN, hyperlipidaemia, smoking, DM
- Neovascularisation: sectoral PRP—branch vein occlusion study—BVOS [107, 108] recommended that laser photocoagulation be

applied only after NV is observed, which reduces the likelihood of vitreous haemorrhage from about 60% to 30%

- Macular oedema:
  (a) Laser photocoagulation
    - **BVOS** [107, 108]:
      An RCT that aimed to answer 3 questions: (1) can laser photocoagulation improve VA compared to observation in eyes with macular oedema from BRVO that reduces the vision to 6/12 or worse; (2) Can sectoral PRP prevent the development of NV; (3) Can sectoral PRP prevent vitreous haemorrhage
      Wait for at least 3/12 if VA 6/12 or worse before considering laser therapy to allow clearing of intraretinal haemorrhages to permit FFA and evaluation of macular oedema and macular ischaemia
      If perfused macular oedema accounts for the visual loss, and vision continues to be 6/12 or worse without spontaneous improvement, consider grid macular photocoagulation (0.1 s duration, 100 μm spot size, power titrated to produce a "medium" white burn) to the leaking area demonstrated by FFA
      After 3 years of follow-up, 65% of treated eyes gained 2 or more lines of vision compared to 37% of untreated eyes
    - RCOphth RVO Guidelines 2022 [120]:
      If laser photocoagulation is contemplated, it should be performed in those eyes with macular oedema secondary to BRVO of at least 3 months duration with VA of 6/12 or worse and without significant macular haemorrhage and with a FFA showing capillary perfusion in the absence of blood involving the fovea.
      Those with severe visual loss (less than 6/60 vision) and those in whom symptoms have been present for more than 1 year are unlikely to benefit from the treatment
  (b) Dexamethasone intravitreal steroid implant (Ozurdex)
    - NICE Guidance [TA 229] [66]: recommend as an option for treatment of macular oedema due to a BRVO when treatment with laser photocoagulation has not been beneficial or treatment with laser photocoagulation is not considered suitable because of the extent of retinal haemorrhages
    - **GENEVA** study [42]: A RCT that evaluated the effects of a single dexamethasone implant compared to sham injection for the treatment of macular oedema secondary to BRVO and CRVO. Increase in BCVA of ≥15 ETDRS letters was achieved in 30% of the Ozurdex 0.7 mg group, 26% of the Ozurdex 0.35 mg group, and 13% of the sham group 60 days after injection (peak response) and was maintained through day 90 in BRVO patients. There was no difference between either Ozurdex groups and the sham group at day 180.
  (c) Faricimab
    - NICE Guidance [TA1004] [84]: recommended as an option for treatment of visual impairment caused by macular oedema following BRVO
    - **BALATON** study [102]: A RCT to evaluate the 24-week efficacy and safety of faricimab versus aflibercept in patients with treatment-naïve foveal center-involved macular oedema resulting from BRVO. Patients were randomised 1:1 to faricimab 6.0 mg or aflibercept 2.0 mg every 4 weeks for 24 weeks. The best-corrected visual acuity gains (BCVA) from the baseline to week 24 with faricimab were noninferior versus aflibercept. The adjusted mean BCVA change from baseline at week 24 was +16.9 ETDRS letters in the faricimab arm versus +17.5 ETDRS letters in the aflibercept arm.

(d) Ranibizumab (lucentis, ranibizumab biosimilars)
   - NICE Guidance [TA283] [68]: recommend as an option for treatment of macular oedema due to a BRVO when treatment with laser photocoagulation has not been beneficial or treatment with laser photocoagulation is not considered suitable because of the extent of retinal haemorrhages
   - **BRAVO** study [14]: A RCT to evaluate the efficacy and safety of Lucentis in the treatment of macular oedema from BRVO. Patients were randomised into 3 groups: (1) sham injection; (2) 0.3 mg Lucentis; and (3) 0.5 mg Lucentis. In the first 6/12, injections were given monthly. At 6/12, both Lucentis groups gained +16.6 and + 18.3 ETDRS letters (0.3 mg and 0.5 mg groups, respectively) compared with a gain of +7.3 letters in the control group. At 6/12, 55.2% and 61.1% of patients receiving Lucentis 0.3 mg and 0.5 mg gained ≥3 ETDRS lines compared to 28.8% in the sham injection group

(e) Aflibercept (eylea, aflibercept biosimilars)
   - NICE Guidance [TA409] [74]: recommend as an option for treatment of visual impairment caused by macular oedema following BRVO
   - **VIBRANT** study [15]: A RCT that evaluated the efficacy and safety of Eylea compared to macular grid laser in the treatment of macular oedema from BRVO or HRVO. After 6/12 of treatment, 26.7% of the laser group gained ≥3 ETDRS lines compared to 52.7% in the Eylea group. Mean change in letters from baseline was +6.9 letters in the laser group compared to +17.0 letters in the Eylea group.

3.4.6 RCOphth RVO Guidelines 2022 Treatment Algorithm [120]

3.4.6.1 Non-ischaemic BRVO

- Treatment of risk factors by patient's physician
- Baseline assessment:
  - Measure VA, OCT, colour fundus photography
  - FFA+/− OCTA can be helpful for assessing the presence and degree of ischaemia, reasons for poor vision after initial anti-VEGF treatment, to distinguish new vessels from collaterals or if laser is planned for new vessels
- For a centre involving macular oedema start intravitreal therapy (anti-VEGF injections or dexamethasone implant)
- For a macular BRVO with no oedema follow up with repeat OCT can be performed
- For a non-macular involving BRVO follow up may or may not be required depending on the degree of ischaemia. Grid laser is an option

3.4.6.2 Ischaemic BRVO

- Watch carefully for NV
- If NVE: consider sector laser PRP applied to all ischaemic quadrants +/− off license avastin
- Follow up at 3 monthly intervals for up to 24 months

3.4.7 Prognosis

- BVOS [107, 108]:
  - Only eyes with ischaemic BRVO (> 5 DD of retinal capillary non-perfusion) are at risk of developing NV—40% of these eyes develop NV, and of these 40%, 60% will experience periodic vitreous haemorrhage
  - Retinal or disc NV, or both, may develop at any time within the first 3 years after an occlusion but are most likely to appear

within the first 6–12 months after the occlusion
- Up to 10% of patients with BRVO in one eye will develop any type of RVO in the fellow eye

3.5 Central Retinal Vein Occlusion (CRVO)

3.5.1 Other Diagnoses to Consider

- Diabetic retinopathy
- Ocular ischaemic syndrome
- Radiation retinopathy
- Hypertensive retinopathy

3.5.2 Risk Factors

- Arteriosclerosis: HTN, DM, smoking, hyperlipidaemia (including secondary to hypothyroidism)
- Glaucoma
- Ocular inflammatory disease: Behcet's disease, PAN, sarcoidosis, SLE
- Haematological: Protein C, protein S or antithrombin deficiency, activated protein C resistance, factor V Leiden, multiple myeloma, Waldenstrom's macroglobulinaemia, antiphospholipid syndrome
- Pharmacological: oral contraceptive pill
- Eye disease case-control study group [90]: HTN, DM (ischaemic CRVO), glaucoma, cardiovascular disease (ischaemic CRVO)

3.5.3 Examination

- Acute CRVO (see Fig. 3.5): retinal haemorrhages (flame shaped and deep blot type) in all 4 quadrants of the fundus with a dilated tortuous retinal venous system, cotton wool spots, optic disc swelling, CMO
- Chronic CRVO: optociliary shunt vessels (collateral vessels connecting the choroidal and the retinal vasculature—do not leak on FFA), telangiectatic capillary bed, persistent dilatation and tortuosity, perivenous sheathing, NVI > NVD > NVE, CMO, glaucomatous optic neuropathy
- Check for a RAPD
- Check the IOP
- Look for NVI on anterior segment examination
- Perform gonioscopy for NVA

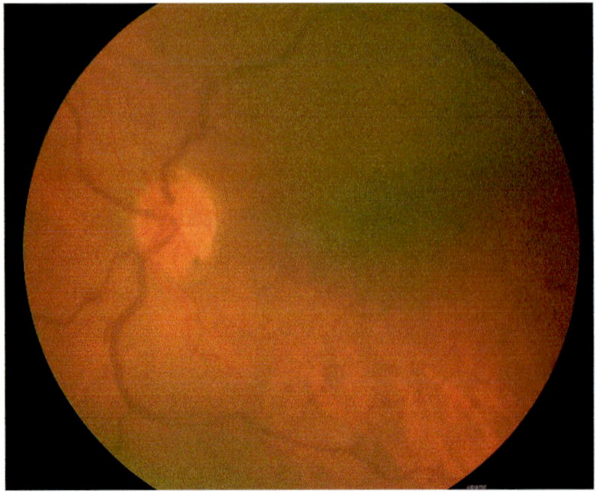

Fig. 3.5 Colour fundus image of a patient with an acute CRVO

3.5.4 Investigations

RCOphth RVO Guidelines 2022 [120]

- BP
- Bloods: FBC (leukaemia / lymphoproliferative disorder), ESR (paraprotein), glucose
- OCT: CMO
- FFA (if uncertain diagnosis): delayed filling of the occluded retinal vein, capillary non-perfusion, macular ischaemia, telangiectatic vessels forming collaterals that cross the horizontal raphe
- Widefield OCTA where available is recommended to assess macular ischaemia or posterior pole non-perfusion to aid the identification of eyes with ischaemic CRVO

3.5.5 Treatment

- Control of cardiovascular risk factors: HTN, hyperlipidaemia, smoking cessation, DM

- Neovascularisation:
  (a) Full scatter PRP: central vein occlusion study—**CVOS** [110] recommended that laser photocoagulation be applied only after NV is observed, with greater resolution of NVI/NVA by 1 month after PRP in 56% of no early treatment eyes (no NVI or NVA present) compared with 22% of early treatment eyes (NVI or NVA present)
- Macular oedema:
  - Delay in initiating treatment up to 6 months results in fewer visual gains compared to immediate initiation of treatment. Therefore, treatment should be initiated as soon as the diagnosis is established (RCOphth RVO Guidelines 2022) [120]
  - Anecdotal clinical experience indicates that eyes with Snellen VA less than 6/96 can do well with treatment providing there is no gross afferent pupillary defect. Careful consideration should be given to further therapy in such eyes that do not improve in terms of Snellen VA or OCT central subfield thickness after 3 loading injections at monthly intervals and treatment is not recommended if no response occurs after 6 injections (RCOphth RVO Guidelines 2022) [120]
  - No robust data on outcomes of switching steroid to an anti-VEGF agent or switching between anti-VEGF agents or combining steroids with anti-VEGF agents for macular oedema due to CRVO
  - Intravitreal therapies:
    (a) Ozurdex
      - NICE Guidance [TA229] [66]: recommend as an option for the treatment of macular oedema following CRVO
      - **GENEVA** study [42]: A RCT that evaluated the effects of a single dexamethasone implant compared to sham injection for the treatment of macular oedema secondary to BRVO and CRVO. Increase in BCVA of ≥15 ETDRS letters was achieved in 29% of the Ozurdex 0.7 mg group and 9% of the sham group 60 days after injection but not at 90 or 180 days.

    (b) Faricimab (Vabysmo)
      - NICE Guidance [TA1004] [84]: recommended as an option for treatment of visual impairment caused by macular oedema following CRVO
      - **COMINO** study [102]: A RCT to evaluate the 24-week efficacy and safety of faricimab versus aflibercept in patients with treatment-naïve foveal center-involved macular oedema resulting from CRVO or HRVO. Patients were randomised 1:1 to faricimab 6.0 mg or aflibercept 2.0 mg every 4 weeks for 24 weeks. The best-corrected visual acuity gains (BCVA) from the baseline to week 24 with faricimab were noninferior versus aflibercept. The adjusted mean BCVA change from baseline at week 24 was +16.9 ETDRS letters in the faricimab arm versus +17.3 ETDRS letters in the aflibercept arm.

    (c) Ranibizumab (lucentis, ranibizumab biosimilars)
      - NICE Guidance [TA283] [68]: recommend as an option for treatment of visual impairment caused by macular oedema following CRVO
      - **CRUISE** study [9]: A RCT to evaluate the efficacy and safety of Lucentis in the treatment of macular oedema from CRVO. Patients were randomised into 3 groups: (1) sham injection; (2) 0.3 mg Lucentis; and (3) 0.5 mg Lucentis. In the first 6/12, injections were given monthly. At 6/12, both Lucentis groups gained +12.7 and +14.9 ETDRS letters (0.3 mg and 0.5 mg groups, respectively) compared with a gain of +0.8 letters in the control group. At 6/12, 46.2% and 47.7% of patients receiving

Lucentis 0.3 mg and 0.5 mg gained ≥3 ETDRS lines compared to 16.9% in the sham injection group

(d) Aflibercept (eylea, aflibercept biosimilars)
- NICE Guidance [TA305] [70]: recommend as an option for treatment of visual impairment caused by macular oedema following CRVO
- **CORPERNICUS** study [6]: comparison of Eylea and sham injection—the proportion of patients who gained ≥15 letters from baseline in the Eylea and sham groups was 56.1% and 12.3% at week 24, respectively
- **GALILEO** study [48]: comparison of Eylea and sham injection—the proportion of patients who gained ≥15 letters from baseline in the Eylea and sham groups was 60.2% and 22.1% at week 24, respectively

3.5.6 Follow Up

- Non-ischaemic CRVO (may resolve completely without any complications): follow up every 3 months is recommended in the first 6 months in eyes not requiring treatment. Discharge from HES can be considered after a minimum of 18 months if no intervention is required or 18 months from the last intravitreal injection (RCOphth RVO Guidelines 2022) [120].
- Ischaemic CRVO: monthly monitoring recommended for 6 months and subsequently every 3 months for a year if anti-VEGF therapy is not commenced. Follow-up can be extended in the second and third year. In eyes that received anti-VEGF therapy, 1–2 monthly reviews are recommended in the first year. Follow up is recommended for 3 years from the last intervention, if any (RCOphth RVO Guidelines 2022) [120]
- RCOphth RVO guidelines 2022 [120] recommends that oestrogen containing HRT and OCP should not be commenced in women with history of RVO. However, the continued use in a patient who develops RVO does not appear to be associated with a higher rate of recurrence.

3.5.7 RCOphth RVO Guidelines 2022 Treatment Algorithm [120]

3.5.7.1 Non-ischaemic CRVO

- Treatment of risk factors by patient's physician
- Baseline assessment:
  - Measurements: VA, RAPD, OCT, IOP
  - Colour fundus photography and FFA should be performed when the diagnosis is uncertain
  - If VA is 6/96 or better—commence on intravitreal anti-VEGF therapy
  - If VA less than 6/96—offer treatment, high risk of NV
  - If VA better than 6/12—reasonable to observe for spontaneous resolution
- Choice of agent: anti-VEGF preferred in eyes with previous hx of glaucoma and younger pt's who are phakic, Ozurdex may be better choice in pt's with recent cardiovascular events and in those who do not favour monthly injections
- Re-treatment: monthly intravitreal anti-VEGF injections are continued until maximum VA is achieved (defined as stable VA for 3 consecutive monthly assessments), once maximum VA is achieved monitor and resume treatment if VA loss occurs due to macular oedema (or treat and extend)
- Stopping treatment: consider stopping anti-VEGF therapy if after 3 consecutive monthly treatments, VA has not improved by at least 5 letters and CMT has not reduced from baseline / recommend stopping anti-VEGF therapy is recommended after 6 consecutive monthly treatments, VA has not improved by at least 5 letters and CMT has not reduced from baseline
- Switching agents: no RCT that provides evidence that switching to another anti-VEGF agent or intravitreal steroids may be effective.

Consider switching from anti-VEGF to steroids or vice versa if response is poor or suboptimal.

3.5.7.2 Ischaemic CRVO

- Features suggestive of an ischaemic CRVO (RCOphth RVO Guidelines 2022) [120]:
  - Poor VA
  - RAPD
  - Presence of multiple dark deep intraretinal haemorrhages
  - Presence of multiple cotton wool spots
  - Degree of venous dilation and tortuosity
  - FFA showing greater than 10-disc areas of capillary non-perfusion on 7 field FFA
  - ERG: reduced b wave amplitude, reduced b:a ratio (negative ERG) and prolonged b-wave implicit time
- Treatment of risk factors by patient's physician
- Baseline (RCOphth RVO Guidelines 2022) [120]:
- Measurements: VA, RAPD, OCT, IOP, gonioscopy
  - Colour fundus photography and FFA should be performed when the diagnosis is uncertain.
  - Angiography (FFA or widefield OCTA) performed at baseline or at a later stage (if anti-VEGF therapy is commended) is recommended to assess the extent of retinal non-perfusion in suspected ischaemic CRVO cases
  - If no NVI or NVA and CMO present on OCT:

    If VA is 6/96 or better—commence on intravitreal anti-VEGF therapy

    If VA less than 6/96—offer treatment with a guarded significant visual acuity improvement, high risk of NV (monitor for NVI/NVA)

    If VA better than 6/12—reasonable to observe for spontaneous resolution
- If NV occurs and AC angle is open:
  - Urgent intravitreal anti-VEGF with PRP within the same day (prior to anti-VEGF treatment) or within 2 weeks initially (RCOphth RVO Guidelines 2022) [120].
  - PRP + intravitreal bevacizumab (off-license) can be repeated if NVI/NVA persist (RCOphth RVO Guidelines 2022) [120]
- If NV occurs and AC angle is closed + raised IOP:
  - Seek early specialist glaucoma opinion
  - Topical and medical management of IOP in addition to urgent PRP with cyclodiode/GDI (RCOphth RVO Guidelines 2022) [120]. GDI is preferable if the angle closure is established.
  - If IOP is normal or normalises with treatment, intravitreal bevacizumab can be considered (RCOphth RVO Guidelines 2022) [120]
  - If vitreous haemorrhage precludes a view of the fundus, cyclodiode therapy and retinal cryotherapy can be used (RCOphth RVO Guidelines 2022) [120]
- Consider prophylactic PRP in ischaemic CRVO without NV if angiography shows >10-disc areas of posterior pole non-perfusion (RCOphth RVO Guidelines 2022) [120].

3.5.8 Prognosis

- At 3 years, there was a 45% chance of developing neovascular glaucoma after onset of ischaemic CRVO—highest risk if VA <6/60 or >10 DD of non-perfusion on FFA [110]
- Overall, 34% of initially perfused eyes converted to non-perfused status after 3 years [110]
- Risk of CRVO in contralateral eye is 5% by 1y (RCOphth RVO Guidelines 2022) [120].

3.6 Cilioretinal Artery Occlusion (CLRAO) in a Young Patient

3.6.1 Causes

- Embolic: cardiac valvular disease, arrhythmias, cardiac septal defects, cardiac myxoma, intravenous drug use (talc)

- Coagulopathies: antiphospholipid syndrome, protein C & S deficiency, lupus anticoagulant, anti-thrombin III deficiency, activated protein C resistance, factor V Leiden, leukaemia, lymphoma
- Collagen vascular diseases: SLE, PAN, Wegener's granulomatosis
- Pharmacological: cocaine, OCP
- Infective: syphilis, toxoplasmosis, mucormycosis, lyme disease
- Retinal migraines (vasospasm): ≥2 attacks of a fully reversible monocular positive &/or negative visual phenomena with migraine without aura begins during the visual symptoms or follows them within 60 minutes

3.6.2 Examination

- Retinal whitening secondary to inner retinal oedema extending from the temporal disc into the macula in the distribution of cilioretinal artery perfusion (see Fig. 3.6)

3.6.3 Investigations

- Hypercoagulability evaluation for young patients with a suggestive history (e.g. FHx, prior Hx, miscarriage): factor V Leiden mutation, protein C/S and anti-thrombin deficiencies, homocysteine levels, antiphospholipid antibodies
- Syphilis serology: VDRL
- Vasculitis screen: ANA, ANCA
- Transthoracic/trans-oesophageal echocardiography
- ECG
- Carotid doppler US
- OCT: inner retinal oedema (acute) and inner retinal atrophy (chronic)
- FFA: look for filling of the cilioretinal artery during the choroidal phase

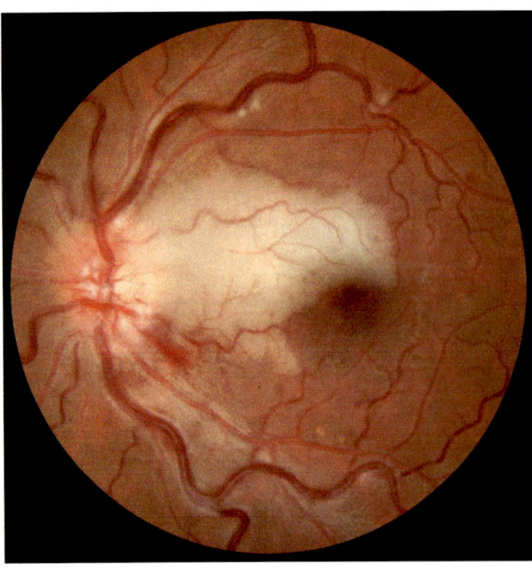

Fig. 3.6 Colour fundus image of a patient with a cilioretinal artery occlusion

3.6.4 Treatment

- No proven treatments for CLRAO exist
- Refer to stroke (TIA) clinic for carotid doppler +/− echocardiography if embolus identified
- Treat neovascularisation with PRP

3.6.5 Prognosis

- Isolated CLRAO: 90% of eyes achieve 6/12 or better vision
- CLRAO associated with CRVO: 70% of eyes achieve 6/12 or better vision
- CLRAO in conjunction with AION: 0% of eyes achieve 6/12 or better vision

3.7 Usher Syndrome (Table 3.2)

3.7.1 Other Diagnoses to Consider

- RP
- CSNB
- Vitamin A deficiency
- Choroideraemia
- Gyrate atrophy
- MAR
- CAR

Table 3.2 Useful facts about Ushers syndrome

AR condition that results in RP with associated congenital hearing loss
Occurs in 1 of every 10 deaf children (5% of all cases of congenital deafness)
Subdivided into 3 groups:
Type 1: most severe form, associated with delayed sitting and walking due to abnormal vestibular function
Type 2: normal vestibular function
Type 3: sensorineural hearing loss is postlingual (as opposed to the prelingual loss in USH1 and USH2) with patients acquiring normal speech

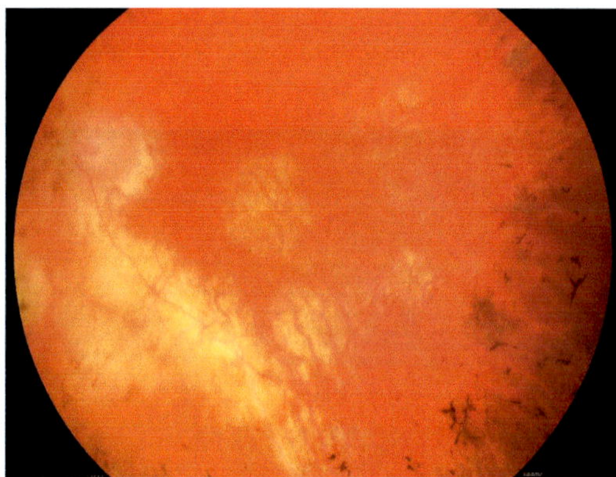

Fig. 3.7 Colour fundus image of a patient with Ushers syndrome showing RP changes

3.7.2 History

- Night blindness
- Positive FHx

3.7.3 Examination

- Peripheral retinal atrophy with bone spicule like pigmentation (see Fig. 3.7)
- Retinal arteriolar attenuation
- Waxy pallor of the optic disc

3.7.4 Investigations

- VF: constricted (ring scotoma)
- EDTs: abnormal ERG
- Audiogram: sensorineural hearing loss

3.7.5 Treatment

- Cochlear implantation for sensorineural deafness
- Visual impairment registration and referral to low vision aids service
- Sensory visual impairment service (specialist schools)
- Sense Usher service
- Royal National Institute of Blind people (RNIB) website/telephone helpline

3.8 Rhegmatogenous Retinal Detachment (RD) (Table 3.3)

3.8.1 Risk Factors

- Hereditary/congenital/developmental/degenerative
  - Myopia
  - Retinal breaks (see Fig. 3.8)
  - Male gender
  - Hereditary vitreoretinopathies e.g. Sticklers syndrome

Table 3.3 Useful facts about rhegmatogenous RD

Incidence of RD is approximately 10 in 100,000 [93]
Approximately 90% of patients with acute symptoms of PVD have a retinal tear at the time of initial examination. Approximately 10% of retinal tears are not seen at initial presentation or develop later [95]

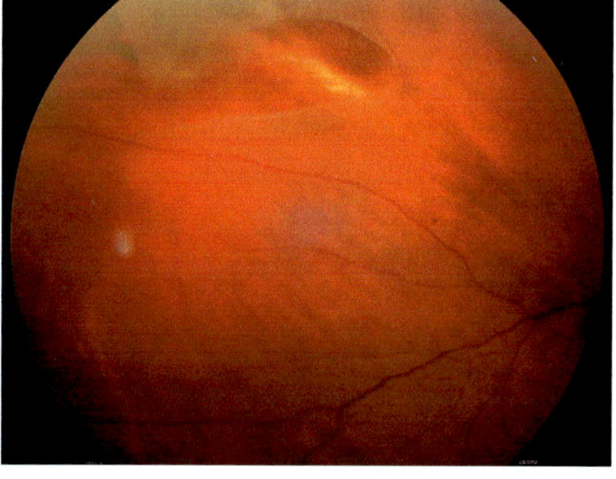

Fig. 3.8 Colour fundus image of a patient with an acute rhegmatogenous retinal detachment secondary to a large horse-shoe retinal tear

  - Lattice degeneration
  - Cystic retinal tuft
  - Degenerative retinoschisis
- Prior ocular surgery
  - Aphakia/pseudophakia
  - Nd:YAG posterior capsulotomy
  - Other surgery involving vitreous gel
- Prior ocular trauma
- Inflammatory
  - CMV retinitis
  - ARN
- Other
  - Fellow eye non-traumatic RD e.g. giant retinal tear (GRT)
  - Treatment: observation if signs of chronicity (e.g. tidemarks and retinal cysts) present, laser demarcation if limited RD, segmental scleral buckles if extensive RD
- Giant retinal tear (GRT)
  - A retinal tear of more than 3 clock hours of circumferential extent (see Fig. 3.10)
  - Posterior vitreous is detached (hence posterior flap has a tendency to fold over) and the vitreous gel is adherent to the anterior flap
  - Associated with high myopia, Marfan syndrome, Stickler syndrome, trauma

3.8.2 Retinal Tears

- 15% of eyes with a symptomatic PVD develop retinal tears (full thickness defects in the retina) of various types
- 60% of retinal tears occur in the superotemporal quadrant
- Tears with persistent vitreoretinal traction
  - Symptomatic horseshoe-shaped retinal tears: treatment required
  - Symptomatic operculated retinal tear with vitreoretinal traction on a nearby retinal vessel: treatment required
- Tears without persistent vitreoretinal traction
  - Symptomatic operculated retinal tears without vitreoretinal traction on a nearby retinal vessel: no treatment required unless the possibility of vitreoretinal traction cannot be excluded
- Retinal holes
  - Asymptomatic atrophic retinal holes within areas of lattice degeneration or in the outer layers of degenerative retinoschisis: no treatment required
- Retinal dialysis
  - Tear of the retina from its insertion at the ora serrata (see Fig. 3.9)
  - Vitreous adherent to the posterior retina (no tendency for posterior flap to fold over)
  - Most secondary to trauma and are most commonly found in the inferotemporal quadrant

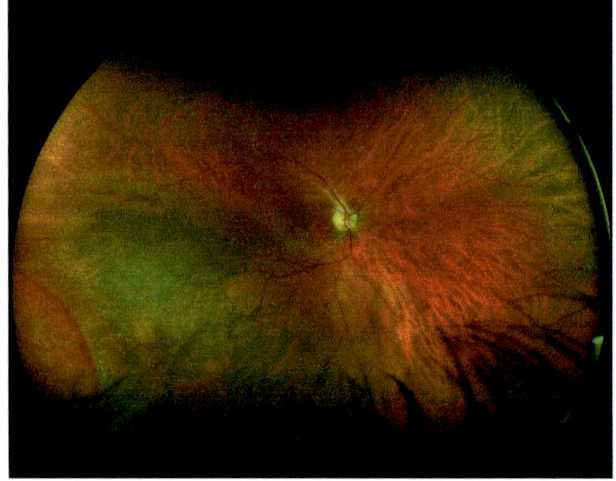

Fig. 3.9 Ultra-widefield pseudocolour fundus image of a patient with a RD secondary to an inferotemporal retinal dialysis

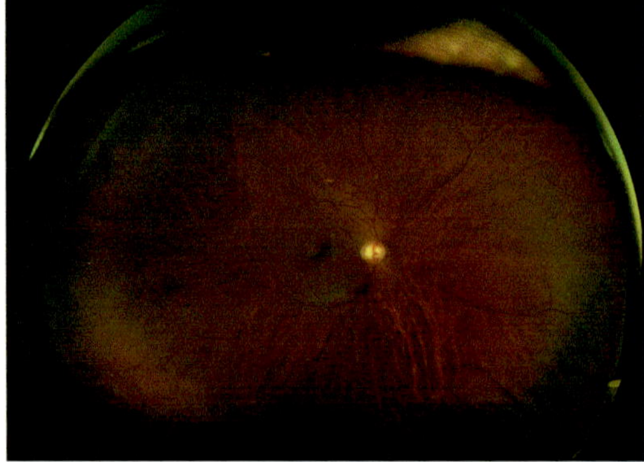

Fig. 3.10 Ultra-widefield pseudocolour fundus image of a patient with a GRT extending from superotemporally to inferotemporally

- Treatment: vitrectomy of affected eye +/– prophylactic 360-degree laser to fellow eye.

3.8.3 Lincoff Rules

- Describes how the location of a retinal break determines the distribution of subretinal fluid [58]
  (1) For superotemporal or superonasal RDs, the primary break lies within 1.5 clock hours of the highest border of the RD
  (2) For total or superior RDs that cross the 12 o'clock position, the primary break is at 12 o'clock or in a triangle with the apex at the ora serrata at 12 o'clock and sides extend 1.5 clock hours to either side
  (3) For inferior RDs, the higher side of the RD indicates on which side of the optic disc the primary break is located
  (4) For inferior bullous RDs, the primary break is located superiorly.

3.8.4 History

- Symptoms (flashes/floaters) and signs (Weiss ring: detachment at optic disc) of PVD
- Visual field defect for RD that has progressed sufficiently posteriorly.

3.8.5 Examination

- Pigmented cells ("tobacco dust") in the vitreous—sign associated with a high chance of associated retinal tear
- Dilated fundus exam with 360-degree indentation with indirect ophthalmoscopy (for patients who present acutely with flashes and floaters) to exclude the presence of tractional retinal tears (RCOphth Guidelines) [121]
- Subclinical RD: SRF extending more than 1-disc diameter from the break but not posterior to the equator
- Signs of chronicity: tidemarks (present from 3 months: imply stability of the extent of the detachment) (see Fig. 3.11), intraretinal cysts (present from 1 year), PVR (see Figs. 3.12 and 3.13).

3.8.6 Investigations

- B-scan (see Fig. 3.14): if poor fundal view present

3.8.7 Treatment

- Round hole RD
  - Laser demarcation:
    For asymptomatic RD's or those with minimal symptoms
  - Segmental scleral buckling
- Detachment due to retinal dialysis
  - Laser demarcation
  - Segmental scleral buckling (see Fig. 3.15)
- Detachment secondary to U (horseshoe) tears
  - Laser demarcation:
    Small asymptomatic peripheral detachment
    Although laser photocoagulation creates an instant adhesion this is not up to full strength for up to 14 days—rapidly progressing fluid may extend through the area of demarcation before a strong enough adhesion develops

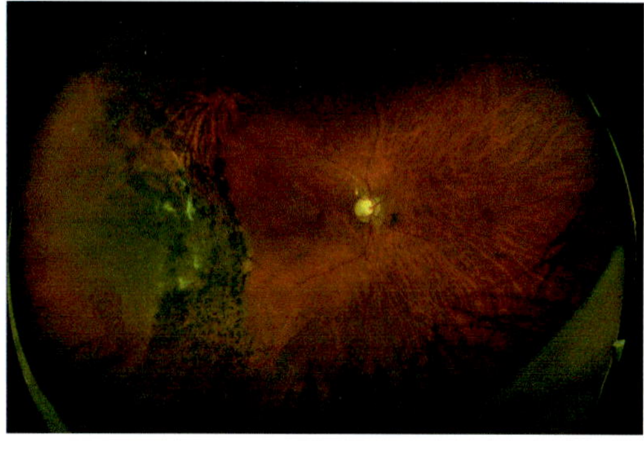

Fig. 3.11 Ultra-widefield pseudocolour fundus image of a patient with a temporal chronic RD with a tidemark demarcating the extent of the RD

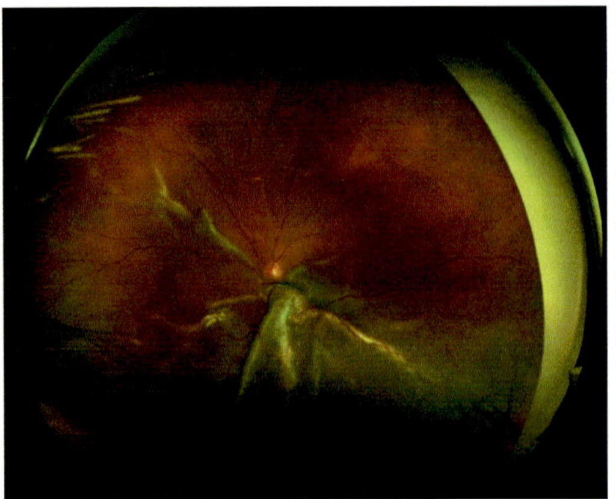

Fig. 3.12 Ultra-widefield pseudocolour fundus image of a patient with a rhegmatogenous RD with the presence of PVR

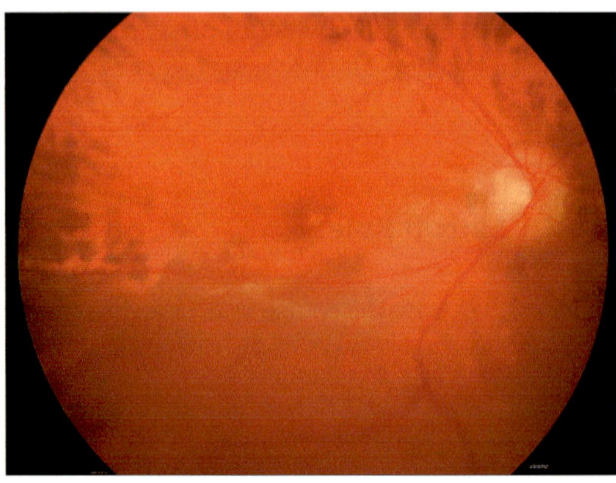

Fig. 3.13 Colour fundus image of a patient with a chronic rhegmatogenous RD with the presence of a subretinal band

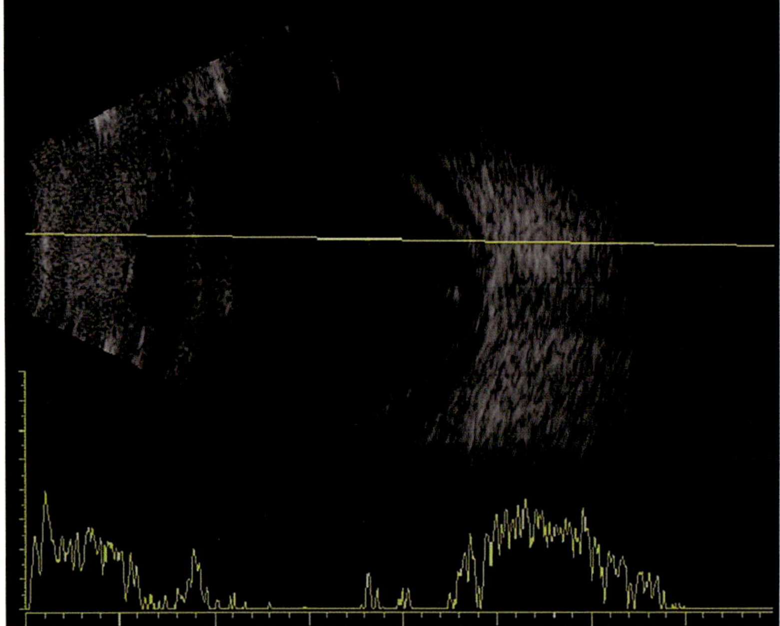

Fig. 3.14 B-scan of a patient with a total rhegmatogenous RD

- Pneumatic retinopexy

  Suitable for detachments with a single or group of breaks no larger than one clock hour in detached retina and all breaks in detached retina lie above the 8 and 4 o'clock meridian [47]
- Scleral buckling

  Young patients

  Anteriorly located small holes with localised RD in phakic patients
- Vitrectomy

  Older patients with a liquefied vitreous

  Wide and bullous RD

  Presence of breaks in multiple quadrants

  Presence of RD with marked traction with different anterior posterior depth of breaks

  Absence of an apparent retinal break in a pseudophakic patient

  GRT RD

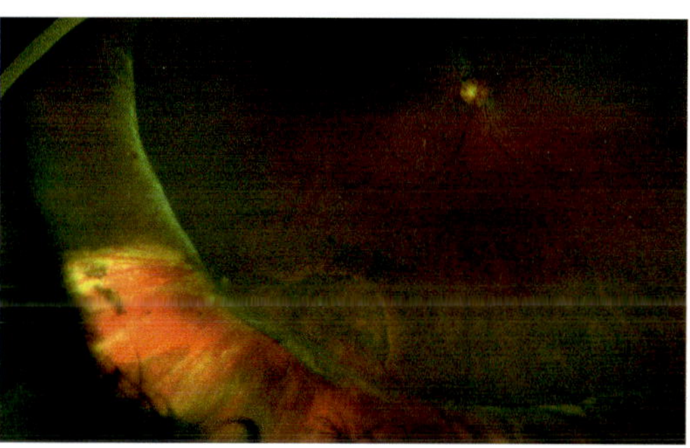

Fig. 3.15 Ultra-widefield pseudocolour fundus image showing the presence of a scleral buckle indent in a patient who previously had an inferotemporal retinal dialysis

Macular hole RD

- Prophylactic therapy for asymptomatic retinal tears in phakic non-fellow eyes is usually not recommended except for an inferior retinal dialysis and for a non-traumatic GRT that occurred in the first eye
- Maximum strength of chorioretinal adhesion following laser photocoagulation is achieved between 3 and 14 days later (stronger adhesion than normal appears within 24 hours of the application of treatment).

3.8.8 The RCOphth Ophthalmic Services Guidance for the Management of Acute Retinal Detachment 2010 [121]

- Retinal tears
  - Tractional (horseshoe) retinal tears should be treated urgently with laser photocoagulation or cryotherapy
  - Asymptomatic retinal breaks and atrophic round holes do not require any treatment
  - Asymptomatic retinal breaks and atrophic round holes with localised subretinal fluid may require treatment (localised RD is often asymptomatic, progresses very gradually if at all) but does not need to be treated as an emergency—non urgent referral is recommended to a local retinal specialist or department to determine what management is best tailored to the patient needs
- Reduce progression of RD
  - Bed rest
  - Dependent posturing: posture with tear at the lowest location
- RD surgery
  - Urgent surgery required if RD is reaching within 1-disc diameter of the fovea, particularly with a superior bullous detachment
  - Where there is imminent danger of foveal detachment and expertise and facilities to operate urgently are unavailable locally, a transfer should be agreed to a suitably equipped and staffed unit with an available VR surgeon.

3.9 Macular Hole (MH) (Table 3.4)

3.9.1 Differential Diagnosis

- Lamellar macular hole (LMH)
  - The mandatory criteria [49] for the diagnosis of LMH (see Fig. 3.17) are the presence of:
    (1) Irregular foveal contour (i.e. abnormal, non-linear shape of the foveal pit contour)
    (2) Foveal cavity with undermined edges (the angle formed between the retinal surface and the edges of the hole should be less than 90°)
    (3) Presence of at least one other sign evoking a loss of foveal tissue, that is, pseudo-operculum, thinning of the foveal at its centre, or around.

Table 3.4 Key facts about macular holes

Round opening in the foveal center (see Fig. 3.16)
Occurs in middle-aged or elderly patients. Incidence of idiopathic full-thickness MHs peaks between age 60 to 70 on average [125]
More common in females
Incidence of idiopathic full thickness MHs is approximately 7.8 per 100,000 of the general population per year [61]
Prevalence of idiopathic MHs is up to 1 in 200 in the over 60-year-old age group [100]
Bilateral idiopathic MHs can occur in up to 10% of patients [100]

  - Associated pathological changes can include: (1) epiretinal proliferation (the OCT appearance of thick, homogenous and isoreflective epiretinal material over the ILM); (2) foveal bump; and (3) ellipsoid line disruption

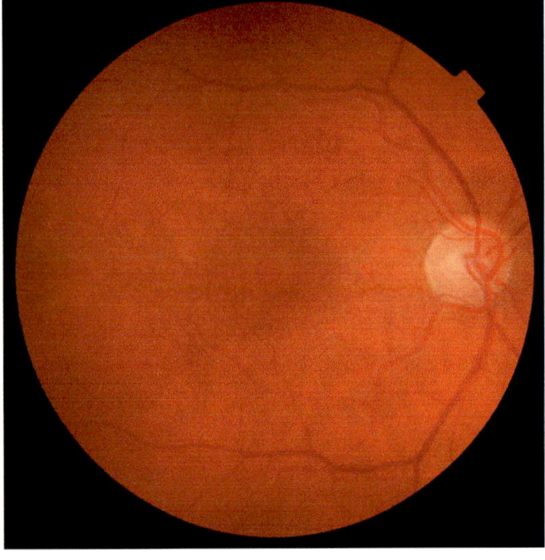

Fig. 3.16 Colour fundus image of a patient with a full thickness macular hole

3.9.2 Risk Factors

- Age ≥ 65 years old
- Female sex
- Asian Americans have an increased risk of idiopathic full thickness MHs compared to white individuals [125].
- Increased axial length

3.9.3 Causes

- Idiopathic: due to abnormal vitreofoveal traction
- Secondary
  - Trauma: sudden axial compression of the eye resulting in equatorial expansion and retinal rupture of the fovea
  - Pathological myopia
  - VMT
  - Chronic CMO

3.9.4 Classification

- Biomicroscopy (Gass Classification)
  - Stage 1a (impending MH): focal central yellow spot, loss of foveal depression
  - Stage 1b (occult MH): yellow foveolar ring

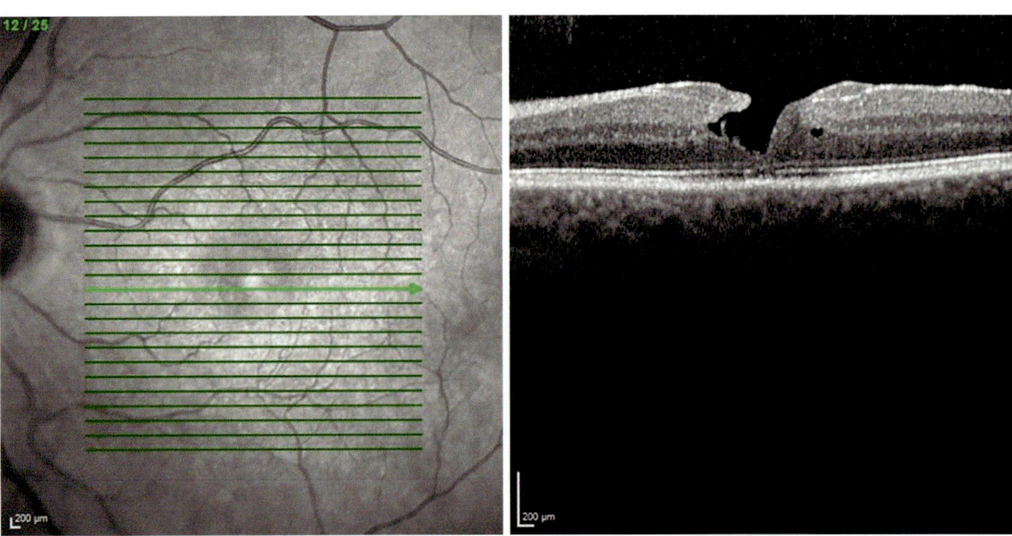

Fig. 3.17 OCT image showing a lamellar macular hole with associated epiretinal proliferation

  - Stage 2 (full thickness MH): central round <400 μm diameter retinal defect
  - Stage 3 (full thickness MH): central round ≥400 μm diameter retinal defect, no Weiss ring
  - Stage 4 (full thickness MH): stage 3 with Weiss ring (PVD)
- OCT (see Fig. 3.18)
  - Stage 1a: inner foveal cyst
  - Stage 1b: inner foveal cyst completed by disruption of the outer retina up to the RPE, posterior hyaloid still attached to the intact roof of the cyst
  - Stage 2: disruption in roof of the cyst with a partially detached operculum from hole edge

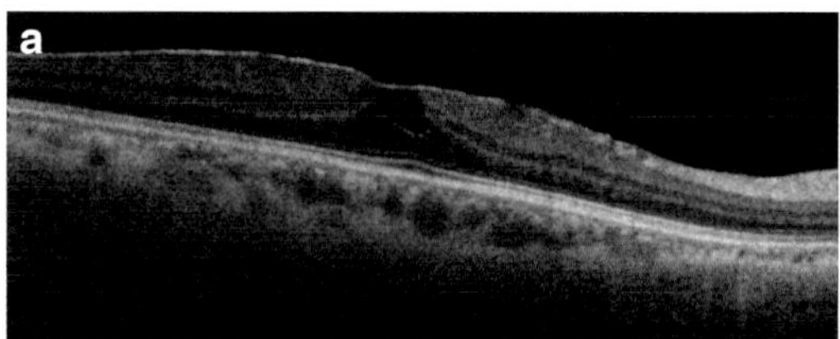

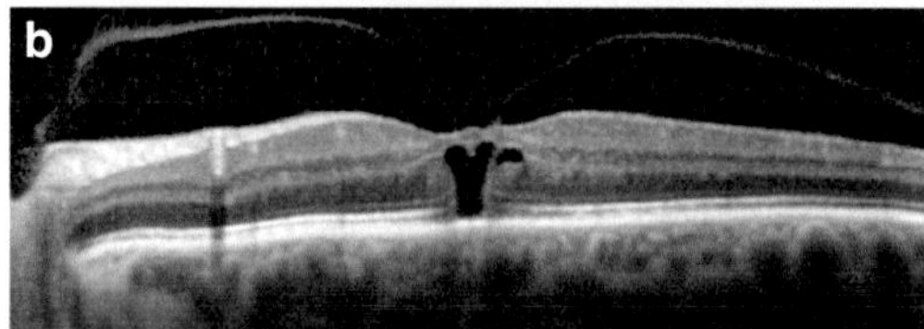

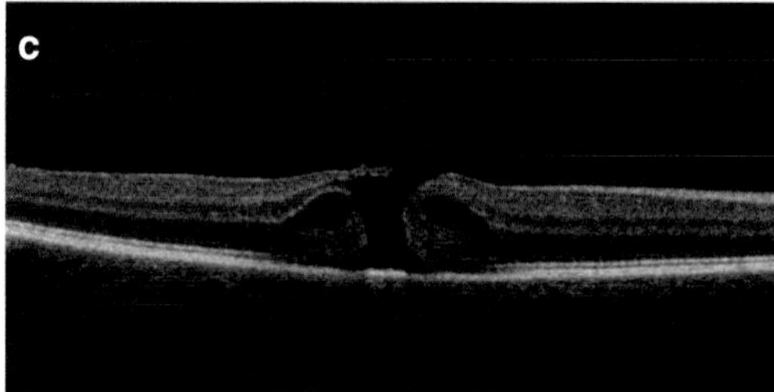

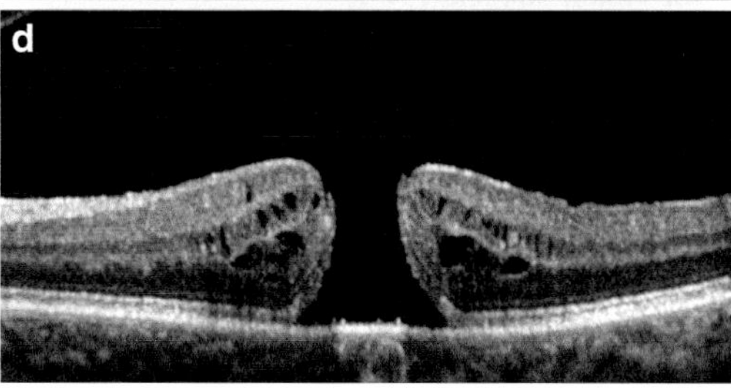

Fig. 3.18 OCT staging of macular holes (**a**) Stage 1a (**b**) Stage 1b (**c**) Stage II (**d**) Stage III

  - Stage 3: complete absence of the roof with vitreous completely detached form the retinal surface over the posterior pole and is not connected to the hole edge
  - Stage 4: OCT unable to diagnose stage 4 MH, stage 4 MH remains a diagnosis from biomicroscopy with the presence of a Weiss ring.
- The International Vitreomacular Traction Study (IVTS) classification system [25]
  - Vitreomacular adhesion (VMA): vitreous adhesion to central macula with no demonstrable retinal morphologic changes
  - Vitreomacular traction (VMT): vitreous adhesion to central macula with demonstrable changes by OCT but no full thickness tissue dehiscence; may include the following: cystoid changes in macula, elevation of the fovea above RPE, tissue cavitation, loss of foveal contour
  - Full thickness MH: full thickness foveal lesion that interrupts all macular layers from the ILM to RPE
  - Small full thickness MH: minimum linear diameter (MLD) of hole ≤250 μm, may be round or have a flap adherent to vitreous; operculum may or may not be present
  - Medium full thickness MH: MLD of hole >250 μm but ≤400 μm; may be round or have a flap adherent to vitreous; operculum may or may not be present
  - Large full thickness MH: MLD of hole >400 μm; vitreous more likely to be fully separated from macula
  - Impending MH: term used when a full thickness MH is observed in one eye and VMA or VMT is observed on OCT in the fellow eye
  - Lamellar MH: partial thickness foveal defect that typically appears on biomicroscopy as a round or oval, well-circumscribed, reddish lesion. Anatomic OCT-based features of lamellar MH include the following: (1) a defect in the inner fovea (may or may not have actual loss of tissue); (2) maintenance of an intact photoreceptor layer (lamellar MH can be distinguished from full thickness MH on OCT by the presence

of intact photoreceptors at the base); (3) an irregular foveal contour; (4) intraretinal splitting (schisis), typically between the outer plexiform and outer nuclear layers
 - Macular pseudohole: anatomic OCT-based features of macular pseudohole include the following: (1) invaginated or heaped foveal edges; (2) steep macular contour to the central fovea with near-normal central foveal thickness; (3) concomitant ERM with central opening; (4) no loss of retinal tissue

3.9.5 Examination

- Yellow spot (stage 1a)
- Yellow foveal ring (stage 1b)
- Central red round area at the fovea (stage 2–4)
- Positive Watzke-Allen test: shine a vertical thin beam of light using the slitlamp over the macular hole—narrowing or gap in the beam of light is seen in macular holes [103].

3.9.6 Investigations

- OCT: measurements in MH include base diameter (BD—widest linear dimension of MH at the level of the RPE layer) and minimum linear diameter (MLD—minimum horizontal diameter at approximately the mid area of the hole in an area excluding the operculum). MLD should be used to measure hole sizes due to its practicality and strong association to surgical outcomes [125]

3.9.7 Treatment

- Idiopathic MH
  (a) Observation:
    - For stage 1 MH: high rate of spontaneous resolution. Surgery has shown no benefit [23, 96]
  (b) Surgical
    - Initial surgery: vitrectomy + ILM peeling + gas tamponade +/− lens extraction
    - For holes that don't close with initial surgery, assuming an ILM peel has been performed, simple procedures with either insertion of gas or enlarging the ILM peel result in closure in 50–90% of persistent holes [125]. Positive prognostic indicators for success with these relatively simple procedures include holes that reduce in size after initial surgery, an increasing Macular Hole Index (MHI: height of hole divided by base diameter), the presence of an elevated fluid cuff around the hole and repeat surgery within 3 months of primary surgery
- Traumatic MH
  - High spontaneous closure rate (50%). Recommended to wait 4 months from the trauma before surgical intervention [131].

3.9.8 Prognostic Factors for Treatment of Idiopathic MH

- Preoperative VA: eyes with better preoperative VA achieve higher rates of visual success (logMAR ≤0.30 or Snellen 6/12) [100]
- Preoperative hole size: smaller holes are associated with better visual outcomes and closure rates [100].
- Duration of symptoms: the chance of visual success is halved in those with durations longer than 4 months [100]
- Presence of AMD: eyes with a MH and without the presence of AMD achieve higher rates of visual success [100]

3.9.9 Face Down Posturing for Idiopathic MH

- A cochrane review [20] of eight RCT's showed low certainty evidence that face-down posturing may have little or no effect on macular hole closure after surgery. However, the studies were not directly comparable due to differences in the surgical techniques used and the durations of post-operative posturing advised

3.9.10 Development of Idiopathic MH in Fellow Eyes

- A fellow eye with PVD has a <1% risk of progressing to a MH [32]
- A fellow eye without a PVD has a 15.6% risk of progressing to a MH over 5 years [31]
- A fellow eye with the presence of VMT has a 20–35.5% risk of progressing to a MH (The RCOphth Idiopathic Full Thickness Macular Holes Clinical Guideline 2025) [125]
- A fellow eye with the presence of an outer foveal defect has a 27.8–100% risk of progressing to a MH (The RCOphth Idiopathic Full Thickness Macular Holes Clinical Guideline 2025) [125]
- A fellow eye with the presence of an inner foveal cyst has a 16.7–57% risk of progressing to a MH [125]

3.9.11 Success Rates for Idiopathic MH Closure

- 88% anatomical hole closure for stage 2 macular holes [92]
- 69% anatomical hole closure for stage 3 and 4 macular holes [34]
- Holes <400 μm have a 94% chance of closure compared with 56% for those 400 μm or more [52].
- The strongest predictor of hole closure was hole size. Hole closure remains fairly constant at approximately 97–98% until a size of around 500 μm in MLD, and then reduces to around 90% for holes between 500 μm and 599 μm and 87% for holes greater than 600 μm [100]

3.9.12 Post-Operative Complications of Surgery

- Intraoperative:
  - Retinal tears during surgery: 12.7% with PVD induction and 3.1% without PVD induction [18]
  - Retinal/RPE/choroidal damage secondary to instrument trauma during ILM peeling
  - Suprachoroidal haemorrhage
  - Lens damage due to inadvertent touch of the lens capsule
- Early post-operative:
  - Raised IOP
  - Transient posterior, star-shaped, feathery cataract—usually clears within 2–3 weeks
  - Retinal detachment: 6.6–14% [39]
  - Visual field defects
  - Cystoid macular oedema
  - Endophthalmitis
- Late post-operative:
  - Cataract
  - Re-opening of the hole: 11% [5] especially in those who have postoperative cataract extraction
  - Sympathetic ophthalmia

3.10 Toxoplasmosis

3.10.1 Other Diagnoses to Consider

- Infectious: TB, syphilis, rubella, CMV retinitis, herpes simplex, toxocariasis
- Non-infectious: sarcoidosis

3.10.2 History

- Symptoms: asymptomatic, floaters, reduced vision
- Immunocompromised: post organ transplantation, HIV positive, therapeutic immunosuppression for systemic disease (e.g. SLE, RA, GPA).

3.10.3 Examination

- Acute lesions: intensely white focal lesions with overlying vitreous inflammatory haze adjacent ("headlight in the fog") to old hyperpigmented scars (satellite lesions), periphlebitis
- Chronic lesions: hyperpigmented scars with an atrophic center devoid of all retinal and choroidal elements (see Fig. 3.19)—the

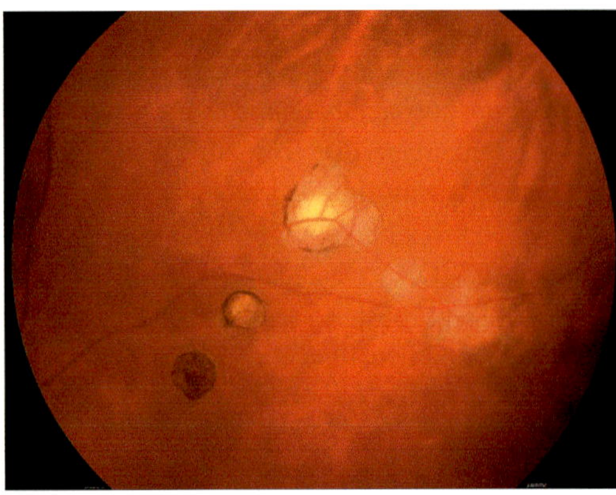

Fig. 3.19 Colour fundus image of a patient with a chronic toxoplasmosis scar

underlying sclera gives the lesion its white center
- Check the IOP
- Perform an anterior segment examination to look for any visually significant cataract.

3.10.4 Investigations

- VDRL: rule out syphilis
- ACE, CXR: rule out sarcoidosis
- HIV serology: rule out HIV
- Pregnancy test
- Anti-toxoplasma IgM & IgG antibodies:
  - Negative IgG and negative IgM antibodies implies infection has not occurred
  - Positive IgG and negative IgM antibodies implies an infection that was in the distant past
  - Positive IgM antibodies may suggest a recently acquired infection.
- PCR: detection of T gondii DNA by PCR in both aqueous humour and vitreous humour fluid is both sensitive and specific

3.10.5 Treatment

- Inflammation
  (a) In immunocompetent patients, the disease is self-limiting and does not require treatment unless sight threatening
  (b) Indications for treatment:
    - Lesions involving the disc, macula, or papillomacular bundle
    - Lesions threatening a major vessel
    - Marked vitritis
    - Any lesion in an immunocompromised patient
  (c) No corticosteroids if patient is immunocompromised
  (d) Triple therapy: pyrimethamine, sulfadiazine, folinic acid, corticosteroids
  (e) Co-trimoxazole (trimethoprim + sulfamethoxazole) + corticosteroids
  (f) Intravitreal dexamethasone + clindamycin
  (g) Oral clindamycin
  (h) Spiramycin or atovaquone if maternal infection acquired during pregnancy (15% in the first trimester and 60% in the third trimester risk of fetal transmission if acquired during pregnancy)
- Cataract extraction once uveitis is inactive for ≥3 months.

3.11 Vogt-Koyanagi-Harada (VKH) Syndrome (Table 3.5)

3.11.1 Other Diagnoses to Consider

- Sympathetic ophthalmia: history of penetrating eye injury
- Sarcoidosis
- Posterior scleritis: T-sign on B-scan
- Uveal effusion syndrome: lacks intraocular inflammation
- Acute posterior multifocal placoid pigment epitheliopathy (APMPPE)

Table 3.5 Key facts about VKH syndrome

VKH syndrome is a bilateral granulomatous inflammatory panuveitis often associated with exudative RD and with extraocular manifestations
No history of penetrating ocular trauma or surgery preceding initial onset of uveitis

3.11.2 Examination

- Systemic features
  - Cutaneous not preceding ocular/CNS disease:
    Vitiligo
    Poliosis
    Alopecia
  - Neurological
    Sterile meningism: headaches, neck stiffness, photophobia
    Encephalitis
    CN palsies
  - Auditory
    Tinnitus
    Deafness
    Vertigo
- Ocular features
  - Prodromal stage:
    Non-specific viral like illness
    Meningism
  - Acute uveitic stage:
    Bilateral panuveitis: anterior uveitis, multifocal choroiditis
    Multiple serous RDs (see Fig. 3.20)
    Optic disc swelling
  - Chronic uveitic stage (convalescent phase):
    Vitiligo
    Perilimbal vitiligo—Sugiura sign
    Poliosis
    Choroidal depigmentation: pale optic disc with bright red-orange choroid (sunset glow fundus)
    Small yellow well circumscribed areas of chorioretinal atrophy
  - Chronic recurrent stage:
    Acute episodic exacerbations of granulomatous anterior uveitis
    Subretinal choroidal neovascular membrane
    Cataracts (posterior subcapsular) / glaucoma

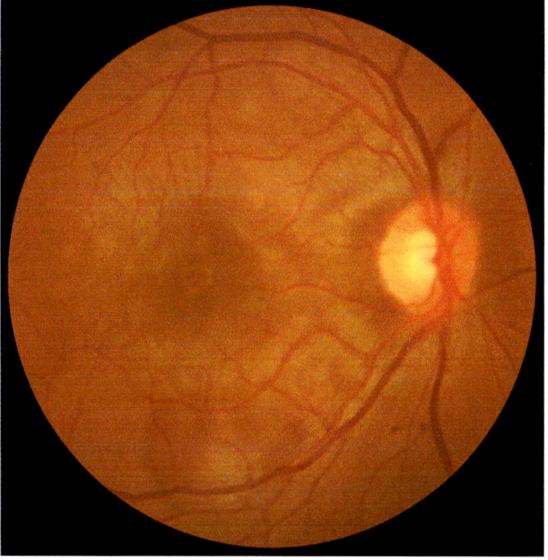

Fig. 3.20 Colour fundus image of a patient with VKH syndrome showing multiple serous RDs

3.11.3 Investigations

- B-scan: choroidal thickening
- OCT: serous RD
- OCT-A: detect CNV membrane
- FFA: multifocal areas of pinpoint leakage, focal areas of delay in choroidal perfusion, large placoid areas of hyperfluorescence
- LP: CSF pleocytosis

3.11.4 Treatment

- Inflammation: high dose systemic corticosteroids +/− immunosuppresants
- CNV membrane: anti-VEGF agents (bevacizumab or ranibizumab)
- Cataracts: cataract extraction if VA reduced and uveitis absent for a minimum of 3 months
- Glaucoma: drops, surgery

3.12 Malattia Leventinese / Doyne Honeycomb Retinal Dystrophy

3.12.1 Other Diagnoses to Consider

- AMD
- Fundus flavimaculatus: flecks do not hyperfluoresce on FFA, subnormal EOG, ERG & dark adaptation normal
- Sorsby macular dystrophy

- Pattern dystrophies
- Best disease (in its later stages)

3.12.2 Examination

- Presence of multiple elongated yellow-white deposits between the RPE and inner collagenous zone of Bruch's membrane in a radiating pattern throughout the macula that is present early in life (often by the second decade) (see Fig. 3.21)
- These elongated drusen may also be found outside the arcades, especially nasal to the disc, which is unusual in other types of macular degeneration
- These drusen may also be found in some patients in a peripapillary pattern or on the margin of the disc itself
- Coalescence of drusen may simulate a vitelliform lesion
- RPE atrophic changes +/− chorioretinal atrophy

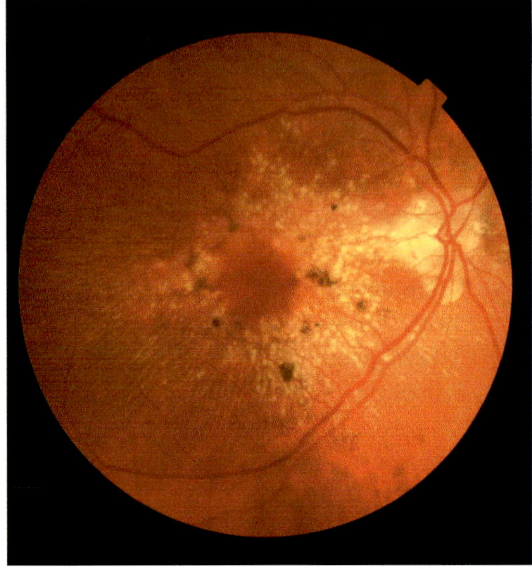

Fig. 3.21 Colour fundus photo of the right eye of a patient with malattia leventinese

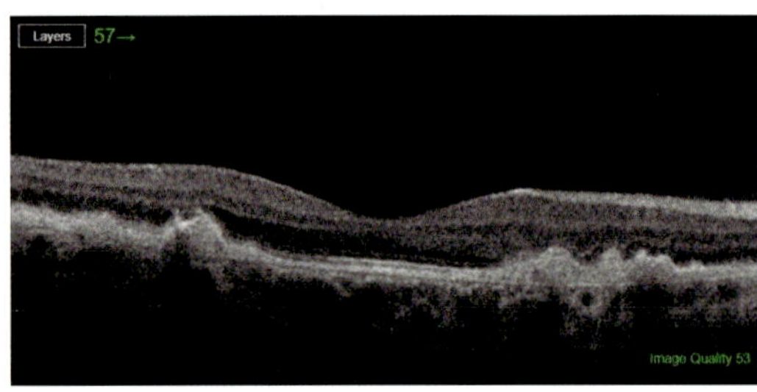

Fig. 3.22 OCT image of the same eye of the same patient as shown in Fig 3.21 showing areas of hyperreflective thickening of the RPE-Bruch membrane complex, associated with localised dome-shaped elevations

3.12.3 Investigations

- OCT: hyperreflective thickening of the RPE-Bruch membrane complex, associated with localised dome-shaped elevations (see Fig. 3.22)
- OCT-A: detect CNV membranes
- FFA: during the arterial phase, multiple, round, sharply defined fluorescent spots corresponding to the lesions observed at ophthalmoscopy, no leakage of fluorescein is seen
- EDTs: ERG, EOG, dark adaptation normal in the initial stages
- Genetic testing: single mutation in the fibulin-3 gene

3.12.4 Treatment

- Genetic counselling and discussion with patient
- CNV: anti-VEGF agents

3.13 Approach to the Adult Watering Eye

3.13.1 History

- "Do the tears flow down your cheek or do they stay in your eye?": watery eye (no spilling of tears onto the cheek) vs tearing eye (tears overflow onto the cheek)
- "Do the tears flow down your cheek inside when you are resting or mainly when you are outside in cold or wind?": partial obstruction (if tearing only present in the wind and cold) vs complete obstruction

- "Is the problem unilateral or bilateral?": tearing eye (i.e. obstruction in lacrimal drainage system) usually unilateral, watery eye usually bilateral
- Ask about findings suggestive of obstruction of the lacrimal system: unilateral symptoms, epiphora, history of dacryocystitis, onset after conjunctivitis (obstruction of puncta or canaliculi), facial fracture (damage to NLD), or nasal surgery (Hx of nasal surgery—damage to NLD)
- Ask about any pro-secretory drugs e.g. oral pilocarpine for Sjogren Syndrome

3.13.2 Differential Diagnosis of a Watery Eye in an Adult

- Poor tear film: blepharitis/MGD
- Reflex tearing: entropion, trichiasis, reduced or incomplete blinking from parkinsonism, incomplete eyelid closure from CN VII palsy
- Inadequate lacrimal pump: ectropion, CN VII palsy (reduced strength of eyelid closure), lid laxity

3.13.3 Differential Diagnosis of a Tearing Eye in an Adult

- Result of canalicular or NLD obstruction
  - Children: congenital NLDO
  - Young adults: trauma (canalicular laceration or facial trauma), canalicular obstruction (post viral conjunctivitis with scarring of each canaliculus)
  - Middle-aged adult: dacryolith (episodes of recurrent epiphora which resolves spontaneously +/− signs of acute dacryoadenitis)
  - Older adults: primary NLDO (PANDO): scarring in distal portion of NLD, symptoms include: epiphora, chronic mucopurulent discharge (chronic dacryocystitis) and acute cellulitis of the lacrimal sac (acute dacryocystitis)

3.13.4 Examination

- Examine for possible causes of a watery eye
  - Eyelid problems:
    (a) Ectropion and entropion
    (b) Lacrimal pump problems—CN VII palsy, lid laxity—lid distraction test (manually pulling lower eyelid away from eyeball: more than 6 mm off eyeball implies lid laxity) & snap test (measure horizontal lid laxity by pulling the lower eyelid inferiorly toward the inferior orbital rim. Eyelid with no laxity will spring back into position without a blink. Can be quantified by counting no. of blinks before eyelid returns to normal position)
    (c) Punctal problems—eversion of punctum, canaliculitis (swelling and erythema of the canalicular portion of the eyelid, pouting punctum with dilated punctum, pressure on canaliculus expresses pus), congenital punctal atresia (1 or more punta are absent), stenosis of punctum (antiglaucoma drops, phospholine iodide, following eyelid eversion such as with an ectropion—stenosis resolves once lid position restored)
  - Eyelash problems—trichiasis secondary to marginal entropion, blepharitis/MGD (keratin plugging, posterior lid telangiectasia, hyperaemia of eyelid margin)
  - Tear film abnormalities—meniscus high/low, faster TBUT (<10 s), Schirmer's test
- Examine for possible causes of a tearing eye
  - Lacrimal examination:
    (a) Rule out dacryocystitis first: diagnosis of NLDO is made if signs of acute dacryocystitis (erythema, swelling, and tenderness in the medial canthus) are present, you can express pus/mucoid from lacrimal sac, or a mucocele is present (palpable cystic mass present in medial canthus caused by obstruction at both the NLD below and common internal punctum above causing lacrimal sac to fill with mucus)

(b) Evaluate tear lake with slit lamp: enlarged if obstruction present—mucoid/pus in tear lake if NLD obstructed, no debris in tear lake if punctum or canaliculi obstructed
(c) Evaluate cornea—rule out any pathologic changes, watch patient blink spontaneously to see how much cornea is covered with a blink
(d) Evaluate lid margins for signs of blepharitis or marginal entropion
(e) Evaluate position of punctum—normal punctum not easily visible without slight manual eversion of the eyelid
(f) Check lacrimal system vital signs:
Dye disappearance test: 2% fluorescein into each fornix. After 5 minutes, check to see how much dye is retained in eye. Normal result documented as spontaneous symmetric dye disappearance. An abnormal result is recorded as dye retained in right or left eye,
Lacrimal probing to demonstrate patency of upper and lower canaliculi using a lacrimal probe: probe should be placed vertically in the punctum for 1–2 mm. Lid pulled temporally and probe directed towards the canthal angle. Probe should pass easily to lacrimal sac where a hard stop (lacrimal bone) is felt. A soft stop indicates canalicular obstruction.
Lacrimal irrigation: using a lacrimal irrigation cannula in the lower canaliculus, not the sac, you should be able to irrigate saline easily into the nose without any reflux around the cannula or out the upper canaliculus (normal NLD). If you can't irrigate with pressure on syringe then the duct is closed (anatomic obstruction—regurgitation through same canaliculus irrigated through if obstruction in upper or lower canaliculus, regurgitation through opposite canaliculus than the one irrigating through if common canaliculus obstruction). If you can irrigate with pressure on syringe then duct is partially obstructed (functional obstruction)
(g) Perform a nasal examination—nasal endoscopy if possible, to rule out intranasal tumours or mucosal abnormalities

3.13.5 Investigations

- Dacryoscintigraphy (DSG): indicated for functional NLDO (patient gives hx typical of PANDO but you cannot demonstrate an obstruction) and gives an estimate of the physiologic drainage of tears. If any delay is noted (delayed filling of NLD), a DCR is recommended (DCR not recommended if no filling of NLD seen)
- Dacryocystogram (DCG): useful if previous trauma, destructive disease (inflammatory) or suspected tumour
- Jones testing—considered in cases of partial obstruction to determine level of block:
  (a) Jones I—physiological without syringing—2% fluorescein into lower fornix, after 5 minutes, assess dye recovery with a cotton bud placed at NLD opening at inferior meatus, positive if dye recovered and implies normal patency, negative if no dye recovered and implies partial obstruction or lacrimal pump failure
  (b) Jones II—non-physiological after syringing—wash out fluorescein from fornix, insert lacrimal cannula into the lower canaliculus and irrigate, assess dye recovery from nose as before, positive if dye recovered and implies partial obstruction of NLD, negative if no dye recovered and implies partial obstruction above the lacrimal sac (punctal or canalicular obstruction)

3.13.6 Treatment

- In all cases, eyelid and eyelash problems should be treated before lacrimal surgery
- Poor tear film: lid hygiene, lubricants, punctal plugs, punctal cautery
- Reflex tearing: treat entropion, lubricants
- Lacrimal pump problems: ectropion / laxity of lower eyelid—LTS, CN VII palsy—lubricants, LTS, gold weight placement in upper eyelid
- Punctal stenosis: discontinue treatment with any known offending eye drop, two- (vertical cut of punctum and horizontal cut of canaliculus) or three-snip (excision of a small triangle of the posterior wall of the vertical and horizontal portion of the canaliculus) punctoplasty
- Punctal eversion: if no lid laxity present—medial spindle procedure (combination of a posterior lamella shortening procedure and a mechanical inversion of the lid margin) only, if lid laxity present—LTS +/− medial spindle procedure (LTS alone may return punctum to normal position—check at slit-lamp to assess for this)
- Canaliculitis: curette the canaliculus through a dilated punctum +/− punctoplasty (keep curetting until you do not retrieve any more sulfur granules or "stones")—topical antibiotic drops post-operatively
- Canalicular obstruction: canalicular reconstruction over stents (lacerations or localised obstructions following trauma), DCR with Lester-Jones tube placement (Pyrex tube that carries the tears from the conjunctival cul-de-sac through a DCR ostium into the nose, bypassing the obstructed canaliculi—see Table 3.6)
- Acute dacryocystitis: do not probe or irrigate, oral or IV antibiotics, if lacrimal sac abscess (see Fig. 3.23) is present—incision and drainage of the lacrimal sac through an external incision will speed recovery but risks formation of a fistula, DCR (external/endonasal) delayed until inflammation has settled

Table 3.6 Key facts about a Lester-Jones tube

Anatomy:
The proximal end of the tube lies at the medial commissure and the distal end lies within the middle meatus of the nose
Indications:
Symptomatic epiphora secondary to extensive scarring of both upper and lower canaliculi
Congenital atresia or complete absence of the canaliculi with epiphora
Symptomatic epiphora secondary to lacrimal pump failure e.g. chronic facial palsy
Failed re-do DCR
Chronic epiphora due to eyelid malpositions which eyelid surgery has failed to or is unable to control, e.g. ichthyosis, severe chronic eczema
Complications:
Tube displacement—scleritis from local scleral indentation and irritation
Tube obstruction
Lacrimal sac infection

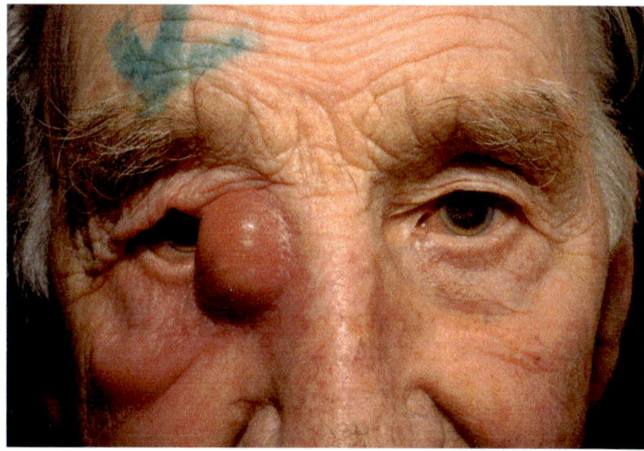

Fig. 3.23 Facial photo of a patient with a lacrimal sac abscess

- Chronic dacryocystitis (mucopurulent discharge but with no signs of cellulitis): topical antibiotics and DCR (external/endonasal), do not probe or irrigate
- Suspected dacryolith: if more than 2 episodes occur within a year, a DCR (external/endonasal) is a reasonable therapeutic option.
- Functional NLDO (anatomically the NLD is open on irrigation but the tears do not seem to pass into the nose spontaneously under normal conditions): DCR or silicone stent intubation of the NLD (remove stents at 6/12 post op—success about 75%)

3.13.7 Dacryocystorhinostomy (DCR)

- Treatment for congenital (when blockage sufficient to prevent passage of a probe) and acquired NLD obstruction
- External DCR (gold standard): the obstructed NLD is by-passed by forming an anastomosis of the lacrimal sac and nasal mucosa through a nasal ostium created by an external skin incision.
- Endonasal DCR: the ostium and anastomosis are made from the inside of the nose, using an endoscope

3.14 Approach to the Paediatric Watering Eye

3.14.1 History

- Onset: soon after birth or if it is more recent
- Photophobia: suggests congenital glaucoma, uveitis, corneal disease (e.g. cystinosis), FB in conjunctival sac
- Eye rubbing or poking: suggests a retinal dystrophy such as LCA
- Watery nose on same side as the watery eye: suggests excessive lacrimation rather than blocked tear drainage

3.14.2 Examination

- External examination
  - Tearing, red macerated skin, stickiness may be seen
  - In NLDO, tear lake is thickened, brimming the lower lid margin—measures 2 mm or more with fluorescein staining of the tear film (normally <1 mm)
  - Secondary bacterial conjunctivitis with generalised conjunctival redness
  - Perilimbal conjunctival injection more specific for keratitis or uveitis
  - Generalised corneal haze with secondary corneal epithelial oedema may be a sign of glaucoma—estimate horizontal corneal diameter using a ruler held close to the lid
  - Congenital swelling over the nasolacrimal sac is probably a dacryocystocele
- Slit lamp examination
  - Puncti: presence or absence, ectropion
  - Lid: epiblepharon with inturned eyelashes, blepharitis
  - Conjunctiva: inspect inferior conjunctival fornix looking for diffuse redness and swelling of the conjunctiva—suggesting chlamydia conjunctivitis
  - Cornea: crystals, abrasions, FB, ulcers, KP's, Haab striae and corneal oedema
  - AC: hypopyon,
  - Iris: posterior synechiae
  - Lens: cataract
- Fluorescein testing
  - Staining with abrasions or epithelial oedema
  - Dye disappearance test
- IOP
- Fundus examination
  - Disc cupping in glaucoma
  - Posterior segment pathology e.g. retinoblastoma (can present as a red watery eye with a pseudo-hypopyon)
- Cycloplegic refraction, fundus examination
  - Unilateral myopia in a child with unilateral glaucoma

3.14.3 Differential Diagnosis

- Reflex tearing (lacrimation)
  (a) Lids:
    - Blepharitis
    - Epiblepharon (see Fig. 3.24): irritation from inturned eyelashes
  (b) Conjunctiva:
    - Conjunctivitis: infective (viral, bacterial), allergic, chemical
    - Conjunctival sac or subtarsal FB
  (c) Cornea:
    - Corneal FB
    - Corneal abrasion
    - Keratitis
    - Cystinosis

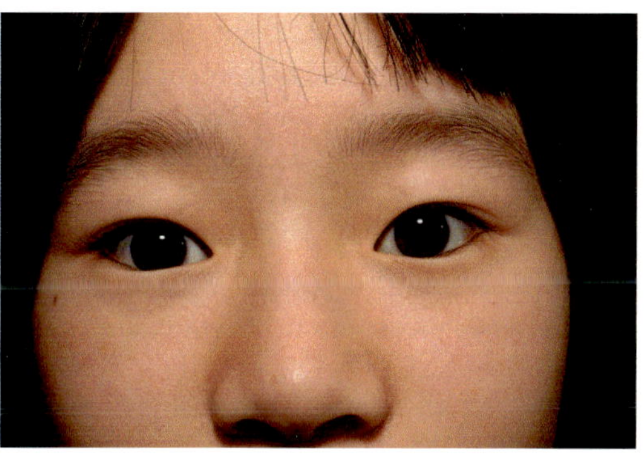

Fig. 3.24 Facial photo of a patient with an epiblepharon

(d) Congenital glaucoma (see Sect. 9.4): horizontal corneal enlargement, Haab striae, buphthalmos, increased CDR, raised IOP
(e) Anterior uveitis

- Decreased lacrimal drainage
  (a) NLDO
  (b) Lid malposition
  (c) Punctal malposition
  (d) Punctal occlusion (punctal atresia)
  (e) Anomalous drainage system (blocked or absent) with craniofacial abnormalities

3.14.4 Congenital Nasolacrimal Duct Obstruction (CNLDO) (Table 3.7)

Table 3.7 Key facts about CNLDO

Caused by a persistent membranous obstruction at the valve of Hasner—in more than 90% of patients, this membrane will spontaneously rupture within the first year of life
Diagnosis is made on a history of a watery eye that has been present from the first few weeks of birth—usually unilateral but may be asymmetrically bilateral

Examination

- Child is well with no evidence of irritation or photophobia
- Periocular skin may become red and excoriated
- Stickiness or crusting of the lashes
- Eye remains white without evidence of active infection, although conjunctivitis may complicate the condition
- Increased tear meniscus
- Mucocele may develop—contents can be expressed into the conjunctival sac

Investigations

- Dye disappearance test (see Fig. 3.25):
  - Fluorescein 1% is instilled into each lower conjunctival fornix and cobalt blue light from the slitlamp illuminates the eyes

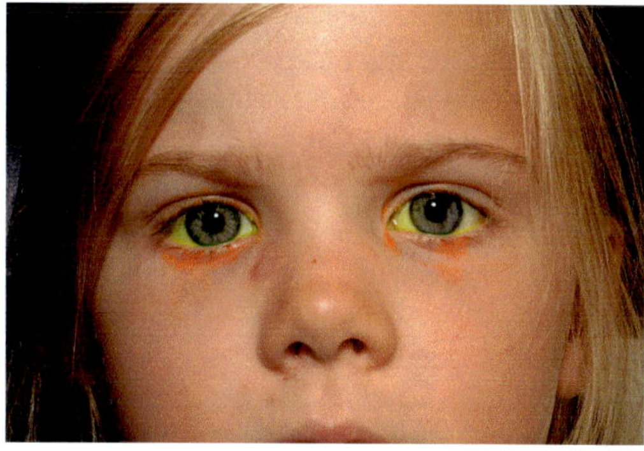

Fig. 3.25 Facial photo of a patient with a congenital NLDO showing a positive 'fluorescein dye disappearance test'

  - Tear meniscus evaluated at 5 minutes
  - Normally fluorescein disappears from tear meniscus by 5 minutes but remains present in children with obstruction
  - Grading [59]:
    0 = no fluorescein
    1 = thin fluorescing marginal tear strip
    2 = more fluorescein persists, higher tear film
    3 = wide, brightly fluorescing tear strip, spillage

Treatment

- Conservative (for the first year of life as high rate of spontaneous resolution):
  - Crigler massage: must push index finger posterior to the anterior lacrimal crest to empty the sac, idea is to massage as often as necessary to empty the sac—massage may build up enough pressure in the sac so that the membrane is broken
  - Antibiotics if conjunctivitis present (avoid antibiotics in watery white eyes)
- Syringing and probing (performed when spontaneous resolution of the tearing and mat-

tering does not occur by 1year of age)—90% success rate:
  - Procedure performed under GA in an outpatient setting
  - Patient preparation—spray a vasoconstricting agent in the nose
  - Dilation of the punctum using a Nettleship dilator
  - Passage of probe into the sac until a "hard" stop is felt
  - Rotation of the probe 90° and passage of the probe into the NLD about 15 mm aiming slightly posteriorly and laterally
  - Fluorescein-stained saline irrigation using a disposable cannula
  - Confirmation that probe is in the nose (suction fluorescein-tinged saline irrigation fluid—suction is in nose whilst canaliculus is irrigated with fluorescein-stained saline)
  - Apply topical antibiotic ointment
- NLD intubation with silicone stents (performed when probing fails):
  - The upper and lower canalicular stents are tied so that the knot lies underneath the inferior turbinate
  - Leave stents in place for 6/12
  - A small amount of tearing will often remain with the stents in place, especially when child has a cold (no discharge should be seen however)
  - Remind parents that tears do not flow through the stents and that any residual tearing usually resolves when the stents are removed
  - If prolapse of stents occur—stents cannot be repositioned because the knot is up in the duct so just tape the loop to the cheek
- DCR (indicated with persistent epiphora despite probing and intubation)

3.15 Approach to the Patient with Proptosis

3.15.1 History

- Pain: caused by inflammation, infection, acute pressure changes (haemorrhage), and a highly malignant tumour growing into bone or nerves (neoplasms in general do not cause pain until a complication related to the neoplasm arises)
- Progression: rapid (hours to days—suggest inflammation or infection), intermediate (weeks to months—suggests more chronic types of inflammatory processes such as thyroid disease), slow (months to years—suggests a benign neoplasm or lymphoma)
- Past medical history: any previous neoplasm elsewhere such as lymphoma or breast carcinoma, any past trauma of the face (caused facial asymmetry that may accentuate or diminish the appearance of a proptotic eye), any history of thyroid disease

3.15.2 Examination

- Orbital examination: start by evaluating the change in the position of the eye in terms of axial and non-axial displacement, next palpate the orbital rims and soft tissues to see if any abnormality is present, then you will check briefly for any pulsations, last you will search for other clues in the periocular area that may give you information to develop a differential diagnosis
- Proptosis: axial displacement in anterior direction (thyroid orbitopathy with enlargement of the EOM, optic nerve tumours or a benign cavernous haemangioma). Measure axial displacement with Hertel exophthalmometer.
  1. Inferior displacement (problems arising in the area of the lacrimal gland, defects in the orbital roof due to trauma, encephalocele, or frontal sinus mucocele formation)
  2. Lateral displacement (problem in the ethmoid sinus—subperiosteal abscess—an acute process—arising in the ethmoid sinus and extending into the subperiosteal space, sinus carcinomas—slowly progressive process, mucocele—very slowly progressive process)
  3. Upward displacement (lymphoid lesion, maxillary sinus tumours)
  4. Medial displacement (enlarged lacrimal gland).

- Measure non-axial displacement with a Ruler or McCoy Tri-Square
- Palpation: start with palpation of the orbital rims and then move toward the eye, palpating the superior and inferior fornix for any anterior masses—if present determine size, shape and position, determine if there is any tenderness in the area of the lesion (infectious or inflammatory disorders will often cause the skin to be erythematous and warm to touch)
- Pulsation: pulsations of the eye suggests either an arterial vascular malformation in the orbit (if high flow you may be able to hear a bruit or feel a thrill) or the absence of orbital bone that allows the normal pulsations of the brain to push on the eye (e.g. absence of sphenoid wing in NF-1), venous lesions do not pulsate but they will usually show enlargement with the Valsalva manoeuvre (orbital or conjunctival varix) or with the head in a dependent position
- Periocular changes: temporal flare of the lateral position of the upper lid and lid lag seen on downgaze (thyroid orbitopathy), conjunctival salmon patch (orbital lymphoma), fullness of the temple (sphenoid wing meningioma), periocular skin malignancy (intraorbital spread of cutaneous carcinoma)

3.15.3 Investigations

- Orbital imaging serves two purposes—providing diagnostic information (what the mass is) and providing information used to plan orbitotomy (want to know the best surgical approach to biopsy the mass)
- CT for bony orbital trauma
- MRI for imaging of the orbital apex, chiasm, optic nerve tumours, FLAIR sequence for optic neuritis due to demyelinating disease, STIR sequence for thyroid orbitopathy

3.15.4 Orbital Disease Occurring in Adults

3.15.4.1 Differential Diagnosis

- Axial displacement:
  - Enlarged EOMs—thyroid orbitopathy, orbital pseudotumour
  - Intraconal mass—cavernous haemangioma
  - Optic nerve tumour—optic nerve meningioma
- Nonaxial displacement:
  - Inferior displacement—lacrimal gland (benign mixed or lymphoid tumour), frontal sinus (mucocele), orbital roof (sphenoid wing meningioma)
  - Lateral displacement—ethmoid sinus (abscess or mucocele)
  - Superior displacement—maxillary sinus (carcinoma), orbital fat (lymphoid tumour)
  - Medial displacement (rare)—benign mixed tumour of lacrimal gland
- Enophthalmos:
  - Scirrhous carcinoma of the breast—infiltrative sclerosing tumour

3.15.4.2 Thyroid Eye Disease (Table 3.8)

Other diagnoses to consider

- Allergic conjunctivitis—acute in onset from a new exposure, causes itching, papillary conjunctival reaction, not associated with eyelid retraction or proptosis
- Myasthenia gravis—diplopia worsens throughout the day and improves after rest

Table 3.8 Key facts about TED

Most common cause of unilateral or bilateral proptosis
Affects women 5 to 6 times more often than men
Onset most common in the early 40s and mid-60s
TED is most commonly associated with Graves disease (90%) but may occur in 3% of Hashimoto's thyroiditis, 6% euthyroid, and 1% primary hypothyroidism

(not variable in TED), may present with ptosis (not associated with TED)

- Orbital myositis—causes enlargement and inflammation of the muscle body and tendon insertion (muscle body only in TED), not associated with eyelid retraction, usually unilateral (bilateral presentation unlikely for orbital myositis, TED can present unilaterally or bilaterally)
- Orbital tumours—typically unilateral in presentation causing proptosis and ocular motility disturbances, unlikely to cause eyelid retraction or lid lag
- Carotid-cavernous fistula—patient may hear pulse-synchronous tinnitus, presentation may include pulsatile proptosis, dilated conjunctival and episcleral vessels, elevated IOP, enlarged EOM, would not cause eyelid retraction or temporal flare
- CPEO—slowly progresses over 5–15 years with most patients presenting with ptosis, all cardinal directions of gaze are affected, with downgaze most likely spared (TED conversely typically affects downgaze and nasal gaze)
- Inflammatory orbitopathy (e.g. GPA)—GPA typically presents with a mix of upper and lower respiratory tract and renal pathologies. Patients may have conjunctivitis, episcleritis, scleritis, and/or uveitis (other than conjunctivitis, these findings are uncommon in TED patients)
- IgG4-related orbitopathy—painless swelling of the EOM's, lacrimal glands, and infraorbital nerves in combination with paranasal sinus disease, multi-organ fibrosis and sclerosis (pancreas, liver, salivary glands, retroperitoneum) may co-exist

History

- Any pain and rate of progression: gradual onset, slow progression without pain. No pain is associated, but discomfort, more like pressure or orbital fullness, is often present
- Any diplopia (restrictive strabismus) or blurred vision (optic nerve compromise)
- Ask about symptoms of hyper- or hypo-thyroidism
- Past medical history often reveals systemic thyroid disease
- A family history is common
- Ask about risk factors for TED: smoking, history of thyroid disease (hyper- or hypothyroidism), poor control of thyroid function is a risk factor for reactivating TED

Examination

- Check lids (see Fig. 3.26):
  - Measure the eyelid position and function (PA, MRD1, LF)
  - Look for lid swelling and erythema
  - Look for upper and lower lid retraction
  - Look for temporal flare of the upper eyelid—lid just keeps getting higher toward the lateral canthus (peak of normal eyelid is just nasal to the pupil)
  - Look for lid lag in downgaze.
  - Look for lagophthalmos
- Check proptosis:
  - Measure the degree of proptosis using an exophthalmometer
  - Axial, usually bilateral, but can be quite asymmetric
- Check optic nerve function for compressive optic neuropathy:
  - VA
  - RAPD
  - Colour vision: first sign of early optic nerve compression is reduced colour vision
  - 24-2 HVF

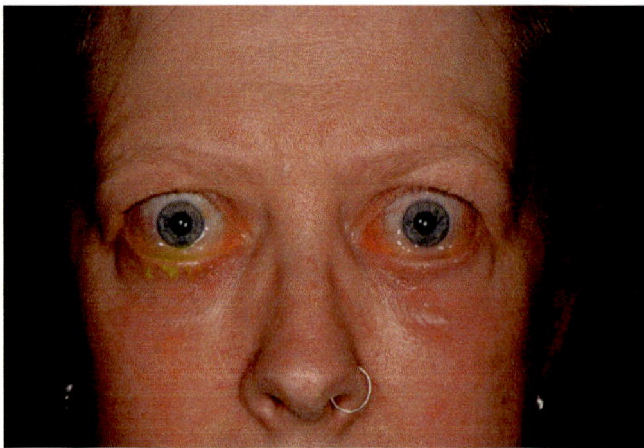

Fig. 3.26 Facial photo of a patient with TED showing superior and inferior lid retraction, proptosis, chemosis, caruncular oedema and upper lid oedema

- Serial visual evoked potentials (VEP—provides objective assessment of optic nerve function—important to know that patient is euthyroid before evaluating the result, as hypothyroid patients without optic nerve compression can show a delay in the P100 component of the VEP)
- Slit lamp examination:
  - Check corneal sensation
  - Look for conjunctival and caruncular injection and/or chemosis
  - Look for signs of corneal exposure, superior limbic keratoconjunctivitis
  - Check IOP in primary position and upgaze (more than 5 mmHg difference)
  - Perform a dilated fundus exam to look for optic disc swelling or pallor and choroidal folds
- Check extraocular muscle involvement:
  - Mechanical restriction of ocular movement +/− pain on looking in the direction of limited movement
  - Retraction of the globe occurs when movement away from the site of the restriction is attempted (commonly seen on upgaze)
  - In order of decreasing frequency, the muscles involved are: IR muscle (restricted up gaze), MR muscle (restricted abduction), SR muscle (restricted downgaze), LR muscle (restricted adduction although LR is usually spared even when enlargement is evident on CT scan)
  - Common ocular posture is hypotropia of the more affected eye, sometimes with associated ET
  - An abnormal head posture, commonly chin elevation, is often adopted, +/− face turn: purpose is to avoid an uncomfortable position of gaze, to centralise a field of binocular single vision
  - Enlarged vertical fusion amplitude
- Systemic examination:
  - Examine for goitre, palmar erythema, atrial fibrillation, and pretibial myxedema
  - Look for signs of hyperthyroidism (warm peripheries, tachycardia, atrial fibrillation, hair loss) or hypothyroidism (bradycardia, dry thin hair, dry coarse skin)

Investigations

- Thyroid functions tests (TSH, T4—most patients will have a high T4 and a low TSH level, although in 5–10% of patients, thyroid orbitopathy will be associated with a euthyroid condition) and thyroid autoantibodies (anti-TSH receptor, anti-thyroid peroxidase, anti-thyroglobulin antibodies)
- In some patients, the diagnosis is so obvious that no imaging is necessary
- CT scan with axial and coronal cuts (see Fig. 2.65): enlarged extraocular muscles, proptosis (>1/3 of eye in front of imaginary line from medial to lateral canthus), CT is preferred imaging modality for planning orbital decompression
- MRI (T2 STIR): better soft tissue resolution and used for grading disease activity, enlarged muscle bellies with sparing of the tendons
- Orthoptic review: Hess/Lees chart, field of binocular single vision, field of uniocular fixation
- Serial visual evoked potentials (VEP—provides objective assessment of optic nerve function—important to know that patient is euthyroid before evaluating the result, as hypothyroid patients without optic nerve compression can show a delay in the P100 component of the VEP)
- Forced duction test: confirm presence and extent of mechanical restrictions

Disease Stratification

- If TED is suspected, determine disease activity and disease severity in order to assess the urgency of treatment
- Disease activity—grade disease activity using the Clinical Activity Score—CAS [65]—at initial visit, patients are given a CAS score of 1–7, 1 point for each sign or symptom (ocular pain at rest in the last 4 weeks, ocular pain on eye movement in the last 4 weeks, eyelid swelling that is considered to be due to active TED, eyelid erythema, conjunctival injection considered to be due to active TED, chemosis, inflammation of caruncle or plica semilunaris); At follow-up visits, add the 3 following criteria (increase of at least 2 mm proptosis

during a period of 1–3/12, decrease in uniocular motility in any one direction of at least 5° during a period of 1–3/12, decrease in VA equivalent to 1 Snellen line during a period of 1–3/12) for a potential CAS score of 10 (1 point for each sign or symptom)

- TED is considered "active" if the CAS is 3 or more at the initial visit or 4 or more at the follow up visits
- Disease severity:
  - EUGOGO classification scheme [3]:
    Mild TED: lid retraction less than 2 mm, exophthalmos less than 3 mm above normal, mild soft tissue involvement, transient or no diplopia, corneal exposure responsive to lubricants—insufficient to justify immunosuppressive/surgical treatment
    Moderate-severe TED: lid retraction at least 2 mm, exophthalmos at least 3 mm above normal, moderate to severe soft tissue involvement, constant diplopia—sufficient impact on QOL to justify immunosuppression if active or surgical intervention if inactive
    Sight threatening TED: optic nerve neuropathy &/or corneal breakdown—warrant immediate intervention
  - NOSPECS:
    No signs or symptoms
    Only signs no symptoms
    Soft tissue involvement
    Proptosis
    EOM involvement
    Cornea involvement
    Sight loss

Rundle's curve

- Depicts schematically the typical course of disease severity with time
- Characterised by an active phase of increasing severity, a regression phase of decreasing severity, and an inactive plateau phase

Treatment

- Achieve a euthyroid state without post-treatment hypothyroidism—seek consultation with an endocrinologist if the patient is not seeing one. Treatment of hyperthyroidism—carbimazole or propylthiouracil, radioactive iodine—short course of prophylactic oral steroid to prevent new onset or progression of TED, thyroidectomy. Treatment of hypothyroidism—levothyroxine
- Promotion of smoking cessation
- Before initiating treatment, determine where the patient's condition falls in the natural history of the disease. Try to determine whether patient is in the "active" stage (swelling or redness of the orbital, lid, and conjunctival tissues—eyelids look "wet" as though you could squeeze oedema fluid out, eyelid swelling and any diplopia are much worse in the mornings) or "chronic" stage (morning eyelid swelling and diplopia are gone, signs of acute inflammation are no longer present, any remaining proptosis and lid retraction probably will not change) of the disease
- Mild TED / CAS < 3—most patients will require only medical management during the active stage—monitor patients for corneal exposure and treat irritation with lubricating drops and ointment, elevate head of the bed to reduce morning swelling or diplopia, sunglasses to decrease photophobia and feelings of dryness, prisms for diplopia
- Moderate-severe TED / CAS ≥ 3—consider immunosuppression (systemic corticosteroids—IV methylprednisolone or oral prednisolone, rituximab, etanercept, AZT) or orbital radiotherapy (2000 cGy—for patients with restrictive myopathy but not for acute optic nerve compression—contraindications include hx of skin cancer, age less than 35 years old)
- Sight threatening TED—admit patient, IV methylprednisolone 1 g every day for 3/7 (maximum total dose of 8 g—if dose exceeds measure LFT's as small risk of acute liver damage). Surgical decompression (fat &/or bony decompression) if the steroid therapy fails and if systemic steroid therapy is contraindicated or has intolerable side effects.
- Surgical (decompression then strabismus surgery then lid surgery)—when you have confirmed that there has been no change over

3–6 months, the patient may want to consider procedures to improve the remaining proptosis, lid retraction, and strabismus (to correct diplopia: conservative—prisms, botulinum injection, and Bangerter foils, surgical—indicated when there is diplopia in primary gaze and downgaze and stable inactive TED with stable myopathy for at least 6/12)

Prognosis

- Poor prognostic factors: smoker, male, older age at onset, diabetes, reduced vision, rapid progression at onset, longer duration of active disease

3.15.4.3 Orbital Pseudotumour (Table 3.9)

Other Diagnoses to Consider

- Bacterial orbital cellulitis—patient usually sick (febrile, weak, etc.), onset usually takes place over a few days, pain usually less than with orbital pseudotumour
- Orbital haemorrhage—onset usually more sudden, with progression occurring over a few minutes, rather than hours

History

- Any pain and rate of progression—acute/abrupt onset of pain with rapid progression occurring over hours to a day or at most two
- Past medical history is only helpful for children in whom a viral syndrome may precede the onset

Examination

- Look for proptosis
- Look for periocular signs of acute inflammation predominate—lid swelling, chemosis
- Look for limited motility
- With palpation, the tissues are tense and warm, but no distinct mass will be present. The inflamed areas are tender to touch. There are no pulsations.

Investigations

- FBC, CRP: normal
- CT scan (see Fig. 2.66): poorly circumscribed (poorly defined margins) mass may be present in any orbital space, dacryoadenitis, myositis (diagnosis can usually be made clinically if the onset and pain are typical)

Management

- Rapid response to oral prednisolone (80 mg/day) is characteristic. Treatment should be continued for 6–8/52 with a tapering schedule.

Table 3.9 Key facts about orbital pseudotumour

Key facts
Any of the orbital tissues may become infiltrated with inflammatory cells (dacryoadenitis or myositis)
Both young and old people are affected

3.15.4.4 Cavernous Haemangioma (Table 3.10)

History

- Any pain and rate of progression—painless and slow progression

Examination

- Vision: not affected unless the mass pushes directly on the eye causing a hyperopic shift
- Look for proptosis: unilateral, axial
- The typical cavernous hamangioma is too far posterior to be palpable
- There are no associated periocular signs
- Although lesion is vascular, there is low flow so no pulsations are seen

Investigations

- CT scan (see Fig. 2.67): well circumscribed oval or round mass, usually in the muscle cone (intraconal)

Management

- Observation: repeat CT scan at 3–4/12 or sooner if any visual loss, pain or change in proptosis occurs

Table 3.10 Key facts about cavernous haemangioma

Key facts
Most common benign orbital tumour in adults
Most common around age 40

- Removal via orbitotomy: if diagnosis is uncertain, vision loss is present, or the patient does not want observation, excisional biopsy (removal) is recommended.

3.15.4.5 Optic Nerve Meningioma (Table 3.11)

History

- Any pain and rate of progression—no pain, rate of progression is very slow over months to years
- Any vision loss—patient's usually note vision loss from compression of the nerve before tumour is large enough to cause proptosis

Examination

- Look for proptosis—usually minimal at the time of presentation—if present, the proptosis is axial
- No external signs of disease are present
- Palpation of the orbit is normal
- No abnormal pulsations of the eye are seen
- Look for optic disc swelling—may be present
- Look for optociliary shunt vessels—compression of the CRA can occur so that blood flow is shunted to the retina via the ciliary vessels

Investigations

- CT scan: enlargement of the optic nerve, calcification of the arachnoid (parallel radiodense lines on the sides of the nerve—tram tracking)
- MRI scan (see Fig. 2.74): to determine extent of the tumour into the orbital apex and chiasm—will be able to see posterior extent of the tumour without the artefact of the bones in the apex obscuring the soft tissue detail as on a CT scan
- Incisional biopsy: if diagnosis cannot be made clinically

Table 3.11 Key facts about optic nerve meningioma

Most often seen in middle-aged adults
Benign tumour originates in the arachnoid villi of the meningeal sheath of the optic nerve

Treatment

- Observation: recommended if VA is good
- Excision: debulking of an optic nerve meningioma cannot be done without damage to the vision, so no attempt to excise is usually done until useful vision is lost (blind eye) or the tumour is extending toward the optic canal as seen on serial MRI examination
- Meningiomas in patients younger than 35 behave more aggressively, suggesting that earlier excision should be considered

3.15.5 Orbital Diseases Occurring in Childhood

- Malignancy is a less common cause of proptosis
- Congenital abnormalities are more common causes—choristoma (normal tissue in an abnormal anatomic location e.g. dermoid cyst), and hamartoma (normal tissue in abnormal quantity e.g. haemangioma or glioma)
- Thyroid orbitopathy is a rare cause of proptosis in children
- Infection is a common cause of proptosis in children
- Rhabdomyosarcoma must be considered in any child with rapidly progressive proptosis

3.15.5.1 Differential Diagnosis

- Dermoid cyst
- Capillary haemangioma
- Orbital cellulitis
- Lymphangioma
- Rhabdomyosarcoma
- Optic nerve glioma

3.15.5.2 Dermoid Cyst (Table 3.12)

Other diagnoses to consider

- Lateral anterior dermoid: lacrimal gland mass, lipodermoid, teratoma, plexiform neurofibroma
- Medial anterior dermoid: mucocele, haemangioma, encephalocele
- Cyst with spontaneous rupture: orbital cellulitis, orbital pseudotumour

Table 3.12 Key facts about dermoid cysts

A choristoma containing skin and skin appendages such as hair and oil glands
In utero, a bit of skin is "pinched" in a suture line where the tissue gradually forms a cyst. The lining of the cyst is normal skin. The contents of the cyst include keratin, oil and hair
If the cyst wall does not contain skin appendages, it is called an epidermal cyst

- Deep dermoid with mass effect: primary cranial nerve palsy

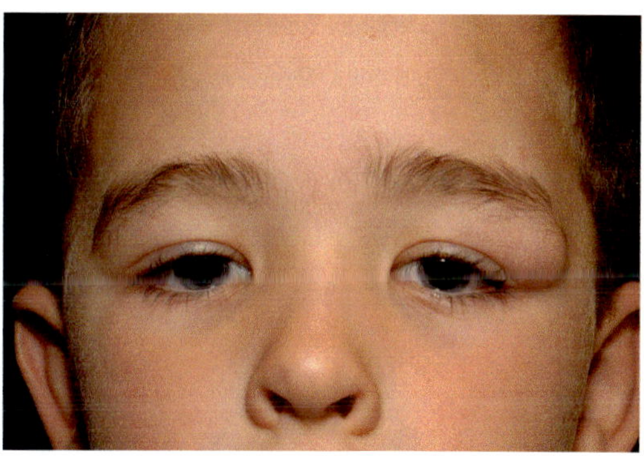

Fig. 3.27 Facial photo of a patient with a left dermoid cyst

History

- Onset—first few months of life, deep orbital dermoid cysts, such as those originating from the sphenozygomatic suture, present later, usually in young adults
- Pain—painless
- Progression—mass increases in size very slowly
- Diplopia—mass effect of a deep dermoid cyst

Examination

- Location of cyst (forms differentials): cyst can occur at any suture line, but it is most commonly seen at the frontozygomatic suture line (frontonasal suture next most common) (see Fig. 3.27)
- Palpate cyst: smooth to palpation, can be either freely moveable or attached firmly to the bone. No mass palpable for a deep orbital dermoid cyst
- Displacement of globe/proptosis: mass effect of a deep orbital dermoid cyst
- Ocular motility: deficits caused by a deep orbital dermoid cyst

Investigations

- Imaging of the typical frontozygomatic dermoid cyst in an infant is *not* required if you can feel around the equator of the mass, suggesting that the entire mass is outside of the orbital cavity
- If the mass is firmly fixed to the bone or you cannot feel around the mass, there may be a component of the cyst extending into the bone or in the orbit itself. Imaging is not absolutely necessary, but it may help you to plan your operation because some bone removal may be required in rare patients.
- If mass is nasal (differentials—haemangioma, encephalocele), order a scan if you are not absolutely sure that the mass is a dermoid cyst
- CT scan (see Fig. 2.72): well circumscribed round mass adjacent to the bone, contents of the cyst may give the density of water or oil, occasionally one can see an interface between the oil and water layers (dermoid cyst), deep orbital dermoid cyst usually diagnosed on CT (as large well circumscribed mass within an area of bone moulding to accommodate the slow growth of the cyst) as there are no characteristics in the history or examination to make a definitive diagnosis.

Treatment

- Excision of cyst: rupture during removal may lead to recurrence

3.15.5.3 Capillary Haemangioma (Table 3.13)

History

- Onset and pain—not present at birth but appears in the first few months of life, painless

Examination

- Look for a blush of red or blue to skin with little elevation (cutaneous haemangioma) &/ or bluish elevation with no surface vasculari-

Table 3.13 Key facts about capillary haemangiomas

The most common orbital hamartoma.
Haemangiomas, if untreated, have 3 phases: initial growth phase (ends before 6/12 of age), stable phase, spontaneous involution phase (begins at 1 year of age up until age 8)

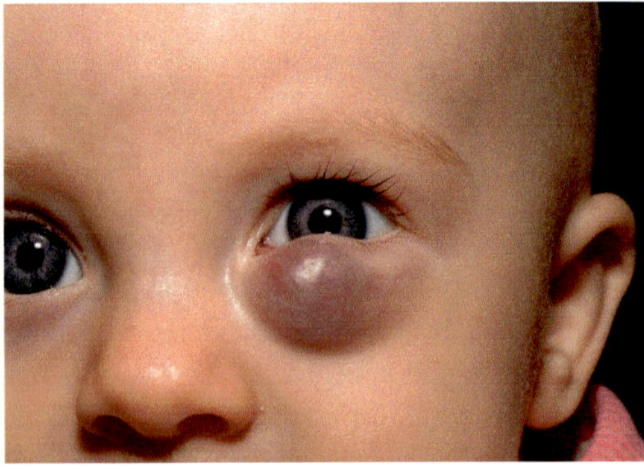

Fig. 3.28 Facial photo of a patient with a lower eyelid capillary haemangioma

sation (subcutaneous haemangioma) on the lid / forehead (see Fig. 3.28)

- Look for proptosis: subcutaneous portion of haemangioma may extend into the orbit causing displacement of the eye inferiorly or proptosis
- Look for ptosis: any large eyelid lesion can cause ptosis
- Cycloplegic refraction: during the growth phase look for astigmatism and amblyopia
- Slight changes in size occur with crying, probably as a result of vascular engorgement (low flow lesion so no pulsations are present)

Treatment

- Indications—amblyopia, astigmatism, or bony orbital asymmetry develops
- Intralesional steroid injection (kenalog 40 mg/ml + betamethasone 6 mg/ml)—helpful if an upper eyelid mass causes amblyopia—follow up 6/52 post injection
- Oral prednisolone—1-2 mg/kg/day—if a mass is in the orbit causing proptosis or if the haemangioma is very large—include paediatrician in this treatment
- Systemic propranolol [56]—3 mg/kg/day for 6 months
- Surgical excision with subsequent reconstruction of the resultant skin defect

3.15.5.4 Orbital Cellulitis (Table 3.14)

Differential Diagnosis of Inflammatory Proptosis

- Inflammation:
  - Orbital inflammatory disease: onset over days or weeks, afebrile, children are more likely to have anterior/posterior uveitis, normal FBC
  - Sarcoidosis: anterior/posterior uveitis, arthropathy, skin rash
  - Wegener's granulomatosis: bilateral, globe displacement with orbital mass, nasal blockage/discharge/bleeds, hearing loss, pain over paranasal sinuses
  - Ruptured dermoid cyst: globe displacement
- Penetrating orbital trauma
- Neoplasia:
  - Benign orbital tumours—lymphangioma, haemangioma
  - Malignant orbital tumours—rhabdomyosarcoma, leukaemia, metastatic disease
- Endocrine:
  - TED: lid retraction

Table 3.14 Key facts about orbital cellulitis

Infection of the ethmoid sinus (sinusitis) spilling into the orbit is the usual cause
Other causes: dacryocystitis, dental abscess, penetrating orbital trauma (septal perforation), surgical (strabismus and retinal surgery)
Preseptal cellulitis—in younger children, in whom the orbital septum is not fully developed there is a high risk of progression and so should be treated similarly to orbital cellulitis. Unless there is an obvious cause for the preseptal cellulitis, such as an insect bite, you should consider the possibility of an ethmoid infection causing the eyelid swelling. Preseptal inflammation without evidence of a skin wound should be considered sinus in origin until proven otherwise. Order a CT scan to find out

Classification

Chandler classification of orbital complications of sinusitis [16]:

- Class I: Inflammatory oedema (preseptal cellulitis)
- Class II: Orbital cellulitis
- Class III: Subperiosteal abscess (SPA)
- Class IV: Orbital cellulitis
- Class V: Cavernous sinus thrombosis

History

- Any pain and rate of progression—proptosis develops over a few days with associated pain
- Recent history of URTI
- History of sinus disease
- History of any dental abscess
- History of dacryocysitis
- History of trauma—septal perforation
- History of surgery—lacrimal procedure, orbitotomy, lid operation, strabismus operation
- History of diabetes or immunocompromised (more for adults)—fungal orbital cellulitis

Examination

- Child looks sick (unlike with orbital pseudotumour)—weak, tired, and febrile—check temperature
- Mild to advanced signs of orbital inflammation (similar to orbital pseudotumour)—proptosis, swollen, red, tender and warm lids, chemosis, limited extraocular movements (mechanical limitation)
- Look for optic nerve compromise—VA, RAPD, Colour vision
- Look for dacryocystitis
- Look for an insect bite/FB from trauma

Investigations

- FBC (raised WCC), CRP, Blood cultures
- CT orbits and sinus (see Fig. 3.29) —sinus disease, abscess formation in the orbit (subperiosteal/intraorbital abscess) +/− intracranial, cavernous sinus thrombosis

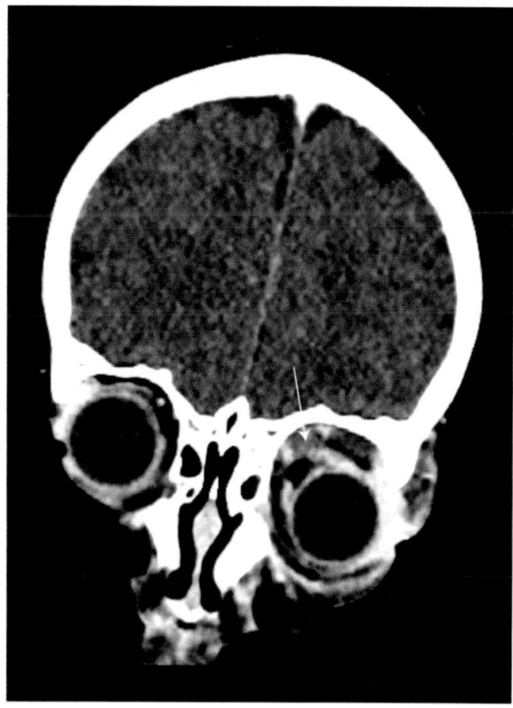

Fig. 3.29 Coronal CT scan image of a patient with an orbital cellulitis showing a superior subperiosteal abscess (white arrow)

Treatment

- Consult with ENT (sinus drainage) and paediatricians
- Broad-spectrum IV antibiotics and nasal decongestants (ephedrine) +/− IV fluid: improvement should occur within 24–48 hours. Daily review.
- Any Intraconal/orbital abscess should be drained
- Indications for early drainage of a SPA [37]: age more than 9, presence of frontal sinusitis, non-medial location of SPA, large SPA, suspicious of anaerobic infection (e.g. presence of gas in abscess on CT), recurrence of SPA after prior drainage, evidence of chronic sinusitis (e.g. nasal polyps), acute optic nerve compromise, infection of dental origin

Complications

- Subperiosteal and orbital abscess
- Cavernous sinus thrombosis: CN III, IV, V_1, VI CN palsies, retinal venous dilatation + optic disc swelling
- Meningitis
- Septicemia
- Brain abscess
- Optic neuropathy
- CRAO

3.15.5.5 Optic Nerve Glioma (Table 3.15)

History

- Pain and rate of progression: slowly progressive, no pain
- History of NF-1/Family history of NF-1 (first degree relative)

Examination

- Look for axial proptosis: suggests an Intraconal mass
- Check optic nerve function: VA, RAPD, Colour vision—optic nerve compromise
- Look for signs of NF-1: café-au-lait spots, plexiform neurofibroma, lisch iris nodules (see Fig. 3.30), axillary/inguinal freckling
- Look for optic disc swelling

Investigation

- CT scan (see Fig. 2.73): enlarged nerve, often fusiform in shape, mass causes eccentric enlargement of the nerve, no calcification
- MRI scan (see Fig. 2.75): to delineate posterior extent of tumour—optic nerve tumour is characteristically bright on a T2-weighted scan—chiasm can be involved in up to 50% of cases of optic nerve glioma
- Incisional biopsy: only if diagnosis is in question

Table 3.15 Key facts about optic nerve glioma

Occurs primarily in children in the first decade of life. Most tumours are unilateral
Gliomas originate within the optic nerve tissue itself

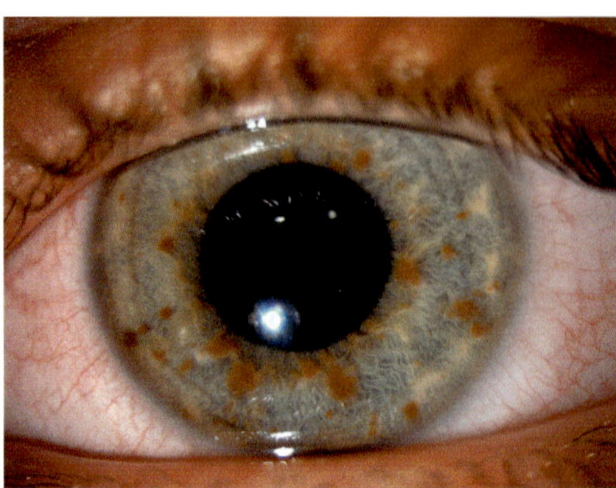

Fig. 3.30 Anterior segment image of a patient with NF-1 showing lisch iris nodules

Treatment

- Observation with serial MRI scans performed every 6 months or so—majority of optic nerve gliomas are benign (hamartomas) and little or no growth posteriorly along the nerve will be seen over time
- Excision: only recommended for blind eyes with disfiguring proptosis or posterior spread threatening the chiasm, usually performed through a transcranial orbitotomy, removing the entire nerve
- Chemotherapy/radiotherapy: for chiasmal or midbrain involvement

3.15.5.6 Rhabdomyosarcoma

History

- Pain and rate of progression: rapidly progressive painless proptosis over a period of several days to a few weeks. 70% occur in the first decade of life

Examination

- Look for proptosis: typically non-axial with the superonasal quadrant being involved most commonly, typically proptosis is relatively advanced somewhat out of scale to the short duration of symptoms
- Look for periocular ecchymosis (differential: neuroblastoma metastatic to orbit—bilateral periocular ecchymoses are typical)

- Look for enlarged preauricular or cervical lymph nodes
- Palpate for smooth mass in the anterior orbit, sometimes fixed to bone. No abnormal pulsations.
- Tumour may involve facial structures outside the orbit so look for masses elsewhere, including in the nose

Investigations

- CT scan: well circumscribed orbital mass with associated bone destruction, if mass extends outside orbit—you will see extensive soft tissue involvement and bone destruction
- MRI scan: if any of the cranial bones are involved, an MRI scan will be necessary to determine the extent of intracranial involvement
- Incisional biopsy

Treatment

- Early oncology consultation for systemic work up
- Combination of chemotherapy and radiotherapy

3.16 Approach to the Patient with Ptosis

3.16.1 Classification of Ptosis

- Simple congenital ptosis (see Fig. 3.31)
  - Eyelid is ptotic because of a dystrophy of the levator muscle itself (muscle is fibrotic and infiltrated with fat)—"simple" implies that the only problem causing the ptosis is the dystrophic levator muscle
  - Almost always bilateral, often asymmetric
  - Ranges from mild to severe
  - Reduced levator function
  - Weak or absent skin crease
  - Lid hang up on downgaze
- Involutional ptosis (aponeurotic ptosis)
  - Ptosis is caused by the aponeurosis separating from the tarsal plate
  - The term "disinsertion" is used, implying a slippage of aponeurosis off the tarsal plate or thinning of the aponeurosis ("dehiscence") itself

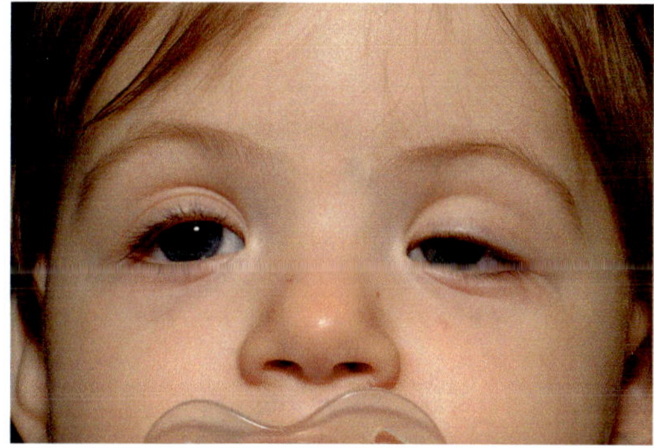

Fig. 3.31 Facial photo of a patient with a simple congenital ptosis

  - Associated with normal, or near normal, levator function (muscle is normal)
  - A high skin crease is the result of the levator fibers to the skin being dragged upward with the disinserted aponeurosis
  - Lid margin remains low throughout downgaze: lid drop on downgaze
  - Ranges from mild to severe
  - May be bilateral or unilateral
- "Unusual" types of ptosis
  - "Unusual" types of ptosis are usually associated with reduced levator function, but levator function also can be normal
  - Congenital causes:
    1. Superior rectus weakness:
       - Congenital ptosis associated with SR weakness in 5% of cases but has little clinical implication
    2. Marcus Gunn jaw winking (see Fig. 9.36):
       - Miswiring of CN V (pterygoid muscles) to CN III causing the drooping upper eyelid to elevate with movements of the mouth
    3. Blepharophimosis syndrome (see Fig. 3.32):
       - Ptosis (bilateral, symmetric, poor levator function),
       - Epicanthus inversus (medial canthal fold of skin extending from lower eyelid to upper eyelid)
       - Telecanthus

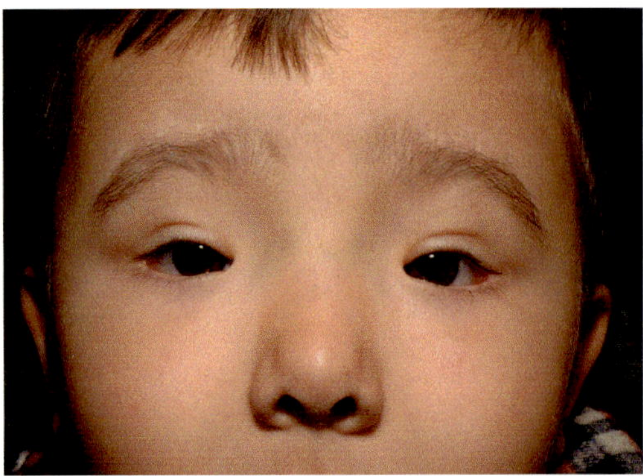

Fig. 3.32 Facial photo of a patient with BPES

- Blepharophimosis of the eyelids (horizontal aperture of eyelid narrowed laterally and medially)
- Acquired causes:
  A. Neurogenic (abnormal innervation & normal muscle):
  1. Myasthenia Gravis (see Figs. 9.37 and 9.38):
     - Reduced Ach receptors at neuromuscular junction
     - Diplopia
     - Variable ptosis: change in lid position from minute to minute or changes occurring throughout the day
     - Test fatigability: ask patient to look up for 30–60 seconds and eyelid will fatigue and slowly drop
     - Investigate with edrophonium testing: IV injection of Tensilon results in temporary elevation of the ptotic eyelid
     - Investigate with ice pack test: cooling of eyelid allows eyelid to elevate temporarily
     - Treatment with systemic oral pyridostigmine, thymectomy, immunosuppression, surgical ptosis correction if medical treatment unsuccessful although variability remains (presence of diplopia precludes possibility of successful eyelid elevation)
  2. CN III palsy:
     - Ptosis with normal or reduced levator function
     - Non-comitant strabismus
     - Mydriasis
     - Aberrant regeneration with the ptotic eyelid elevating with contraction of the MR or IR muscle, pupil constriction with eye movements
  3. Horner's syndrome:
     - Mild ptosis with normal levator function, miosis, lower lid elevation

  B. Myogenic (normal innervation & abnormal muscle—reduced levator function is typical, facial muscle activity and ocular motility are also reduced):
  1. Oculopharyngeal dystrophy (see Fig. 3.33):
  - Autosomal dominant inheritance
     - Progressive bilateral ptosis (good levator function initially) with facial weakness and difficulty swallowing (ask patient to drink glass of water rapidly)
  2. Myotonic dystrophy:
     - Autosomal dominant inheritance
     - Slowly progressive bilateral mild or moderate ptosis
     - Failure of muscles to relax after a sustained contraction

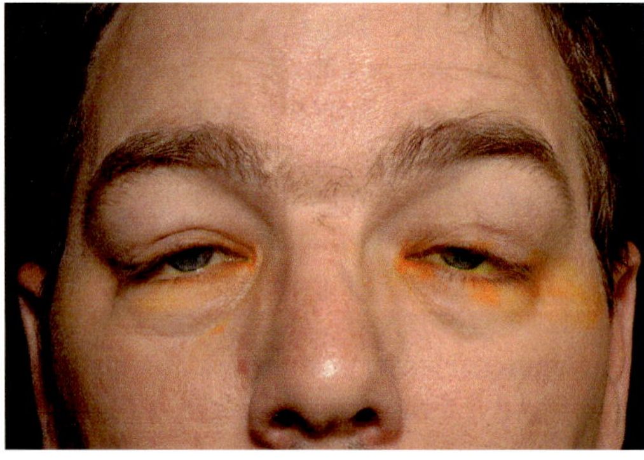

Fig. 3.33 Facial photo of a patient with oculopharyngeal dystrophy

- Facial and peripheral skeletal muscle weakness
- Associated abnormalities in other organ systems (frontal balding, christmas tree cataract, testicular atrophy, weak cognitive function)

3. Chronic Progressive External Ophthalmoplegia (CPEO):
   - Mitochondrial inheritance
   - Bilateral symmetrical ptosis with poor levator function
   - Facial weakness
   - An extreme loss of ocular motility (often to the point of no movement—frozen globe) with no diplopia
   - Pupils are spared
   - Kearns-Sayre syndrome: CPEO, heart block, pigmentary retinopathy
4. Post-traumatic (damage to levator muscle)

C. Post traumatic (damage to levator aponeurosis):
1. Lid swelling
2. Blepharochalasis:
   - Recurrent bouts of idiopathic lid swelling with secondary dermatochalasis

D. Pseudoptosis (MRD1 and levator function are normal):
1. Hemifacial spasm
2. CN VII palsy with aberrant regeneration
3. Contralateral lid retraction

3.16.2 History

- Adult patients
  - Questions to identify type of ptosis:
    Is the diagnosis involutional ptosis?
    - Indefinite onset
    - Gradual progression
    - No other associated eye or systemic problems
    - Ptosis usually about the same severity throughout the day

    Is the ptosis acquired or has it been present since birth? When was the onset? What is the rate of progression?
    - Most adults will have an acquired form of ptosis, usually the common involutional type. The onset is difficult to identify, as the progression is usually so gradual over several years that no particular time can be identified as the exact onset. An acute onset suggests a diagnosis other than involutional ptosis—an exception to this is the onset of involutional ptosis after cataract surgery
    - Occasionally an adult will have preexisting congenital ptosis that has slowly gotten worse over time or may have asymmetric congenital ptosis that can no longer be ignored because the "normal" side has progressively drooped more—physical exam will confirm the reduced levator function of congenital ptosis
  - Questions to identify factors that may modify the treatment plan:
    Is there a history of previous ptosis operations?
    - History of previous lid operations may be a warning sign that the levator aponeurosis has already been shortened so that further tightening may cause lagophthalmos

    Does the patient have symptoms of "dry" eye?
    Is there a history of facial nerve palsy?
    - A history of CN VII palsy signals the potential for poor blinking and lagophthalmos after surgery
  - Questions to identify an "unusual" type of adult ptosis:
    Positive family history
    Associated diplopia
    Variation in degree of ptosis: minute to minute, with eye movements, better after naps

Associated facial movement problems: history of facial nerve palsy, history of facial spasms

- Paediatric patients
  - Questions to identify type of ptosis:
    Is the diagnosis simple congenital ptosis?
    - Simple congenital ptosis involves only a ptotic upper eyelid in an otherwise healthy child with no abnormal eye finding

    Is the ptosis congenital?
    - When a ptosis is seen in a child, it is almost always congenital. Any onset after birth suggests a different diagnosis

    Is the ptosis unilateral or bilateral?
    - Congenital ptosis is usually bilateral, but often asymmetric

    Does the lid change position? Is the lid ever open all the way?
    - Wide variations in the day are not typical of simple congenital ptosis

    Does the lid position change with chewing or sucking?
    - Variation of lid position from movement to movement suggests a synkinetic form of ptosis.
    - Ptosis associated with abnormal lid movements caused by chewing, sucking, or other changes in jaw position is known as Marcus-Gunn jaw winking
    - Ptosis associated with abnormal lid movements caused by changes in eye position is seen in CN III palsy with aberrant regeneration

    Is there a family history of ptosis?
    - Strict inheritance of simple congenital ptosis is rare
    - A positive family history (autosomal dominant inheritance) may suggest the presence of blepharophimosis syndrome
    - Congenital ptosis is not commonly associated with any ocular or systemic abnormalities. Dystophy of the levator muscle is the only abnormality present
  - Questions to identify factors that may modify the treatment plan:
    Is the eyelid open above the pupil? During which part of the day? (how many times is the eyelid above the pupil?): assess risk of amblyopia

    Surgical repair of a simple congenital ptosis is usually done before the child starts school (age 4). Features in the history suggesting the possibility of amblyopia should alter the timing of treatment

    History of previous ptosis surgery:
    - Previous ptosis repair, especially levator aponeurosis advancement procedures, puts the patient at risk for corneal exposure after more advancement
  - Questions to identify an "unusual" type of congenital ptosis:
    Associated strabismus

    Family history: blepharophimosis syndrome

    Developmental delay: many syndromes associated with ptosis

    Extreme variation of ptosis from minute to minute or throughout the day: lid movement associated with chewing or sucking, lid movement associated with eye movements

3.16.3 Examination

- Adult patients
  - Measure eyelid vital signs:
    Palpebral aperture (PA): measure from upper lid margin to lower lid margin in mm (normal 9-10 mm). For the PA measurement to be meaningful in describing the upper lid position, the lower lid must be in the normal position

    Marginal reflex distance 1 (MRD1): distance of upper lid margin from the corneal light reflex (normal 4-5 mm), measures degree of ptosis, with patient at your eye level, ask him/her to look straight ahead at a distance target, shine the penlight at the patient's eye

Marginal reflex distance 2 (MRD2): distance of lower lid margin from the corneal light reflex

Levator function (LF): block action of the brow with your thumb and don't allow the head to tip up with eye elevation

Skin crease height: distance from upper lid margin to the skin crease (normal 8-10 mm in women and 6-8 mm in men)

– Does the patient have normal facial expression?

Weakness of the facial muscles is associated with the myogenic types of unusual ptosis

Is there hyperkinetic movement of the face suggesting hemifacial spasm or aberrant regeneration of the facial nerve?

– Measure the motility:

Eye movements should be normal for the patients age in involutional ptosis

Any reduction in motility or symptoms of diplopia suggest a diagnosis of other than involutional ptosis (MG, CN III palsy, CPEO)

Any bizarre association of the upper eyelid position (ptosis or lid retraction) with eye movements should suggest aberrant regeneration of the third nerve

– Is the pupil normal? Are there signs of Horner's syndrome? Do you see any miosis or lower eyelid elevation to suggest that a loss of sympathetic tone is responsible for the patient's mild ptosis (Horner's syndrome—upper lid ptosis, lower lid elevation, miosis, and anhidrosis of the ipsilateral side of the face)

– Look for risk factors that increase the chance of post-operative corneal exposure:

Bell's phenomenon—a poor Bell's phenomenon is only a relative contraindication for ptosis repair

Look for lagophthalmos—possibly from previous ptosis surgery, look for lower eyelid retraction from any cause,

Slit lamp examination to evaluate the tear film and if minimal do a Schirmer's test—if corneal exposure is present preoperatively it will be worse after elevating the lid, use the maximal treatment of any corneal exposure before proceeding with ptosis repair—consider the use of punctal plugs

- Paediatric patients
  – Measure eyelid vital signs:

  Palpebral aperture (PA): measure from upper lid margin to lower lid margin in mm (normal 9-10 mm). For the PA measurement to be meaningful in describing the upper lid position, the lower lid must be in the normal position

  Marginal reflex distance 1 (MRD1): distance of upper lid margin from the corneal light reflex (normal 4-5 mm), measures degree of ptosis, with patient at your eye level, ask him/her to look straight ahead at a distance target, shine the penlight at the patient's eye

  Marginal reflex distance 2 (MRD2): distance of lower lid margin from the corneal light reflex

  Levator function (LF): block action of the brow with your thumb and don't allow the head to tip up with eye elevation

  Skin crease height: distance from upper lid margin to the skin crease (normal 8-10 mm in women and 6-8 mm in men)

  – Measure VA:

  Fixation should be steady and maintained

  Check for amblyopia: if amblyopia, due to deprivation or astigmatism, is present, consider earlier surgery to correct ptosis

  – External appearance of child:

  Appearance should be normal for simple congenital ptosis

  Most common abnormal facies are seen in blepharophimosis syndrome

  Many other syndromes can have ptosis as one of the associated findings

  – Measure the motility:

  Normal motility is associated with simple congenital ptosis

  Most common motility disturbance seen in children with ptosis is a localised weakness of the superior rectus muscle (occurs in 5% of patients born with ptosis)

Any bizarre movement of the upper lid associated with eye movement should suggest aberrant regeneration of CN III

- Ask the child to open and close the mouth and move the jaw around:
  No movement of the eyelid should occur with simple congenital ptosis
  Any lid movement will diagnose a Marcus Gunn jaw winking ptosis
- Look for risk factors that increase the chance of corneal exposure (rare in children): facial nerve palsy, poor Bell's phenomenon, lagophthalmos (previous ptosis surgery), poor tear film, corneal exposure

3.16.4 Investigations

- Bloods: anti-Ach receptor/muscle-specific receptor tyrosine kinase (MuSK) antibodies if myasthenia gravis suspected
- Genetic testing: oculopharyngeal dystrophy, myotonic dystrophy
- CT angiography: indicated if partial CN III palsy (rule out a posterior communicating artery aneurysm) or a painful Horner's syndrome (rule out ICA dissection) is identified
- Skeletal muscle biopsy: look for red ragged fibers in CPEO

3.16.5 Treatment

- Adult patients
  - Indications for surgical correction of eyelid ptosis:
    Symptoms: decreased central or peripheral vision, heaviness of the lids, brow ache or headache, difficulty reading, and neck ache (from chronic lifting of the chin)
    Examination findings: elevated or arched eyebrows, prominent forehead furrows, and a chin up position
  - Preoperative considerations:
    Stop aspirin or clopidogrel (7–10 days before operation), NSAIDS (24–72 hours before operation), warfarin (5 days before operation), rivaroxaban (at least 24 hours before operation), apixaban (at least 48 hours before operation)
  - Choice of surgical procedure:
    For simple congenital ptosis with levator function greater than 4 mm, a levator aponeurosis advancement (see Table 3.16) is the correct treatment
    For simple congenital ptosis with levator function less than 3 mm, a frontalis sling (see Table 3.17) is appropriate
    For simple ptosis with levator function between 3 and 4 mm, a generous advancement is usual, with the resection extending high above Whitnall's ligament into the muscle itself
    For involutional ptosis with a normal levator function, a levator aponeurosis advancement is the procedure of choice
    Decide if additional procedures such as a blepharoplasty or browplasty are neces-

Table 3.16 Levator advancement procedure

Procedure of choice for adults with involutional ptosis
Tightening the levator muscle doesn't improve the levator function or movement of the eyelid; it essentially only resets the lid height
Operation most easily done using a local anaesthetic under the skin (allows operation on aponeurosis but does not paralyse the deeper levator muscle—makes intraoperative adjustment of lid height and contour possible)
Operation includes:
(a) Patient preparation: mark upper lid skin crease, inject local anaesthetic with epinephrine
(b) Skin incision: open orbicularis muscle
(c) Identification of the levator aponeurosis: dissect orbicularis off orbital septum, open septum, dissect septum off preaponeurotic fat, dissect preaponeurotic fat off aponeurosis
(d) Dissection of the levator aponeurosis off Muller's muscle: disinsert levator aponeurosis from anterior surface of tarsus, dissect aponeurosis free from Muller's muscle
(e) Levator aponeurosis advancement
(f) Intraoperative adjustment to height and contour: aim for 1 mm overcorrection
(g) Closure: reform skin crease, running suture to close skin)

Table 3.17 Frontalis sling procedure

Procedure of choice for any type of ptosis with poor levator function
Eyelid is surgically "connected" to the brow with the action of the frontalis muscle lifting the upper eyelid
Operation includes:
(a) Patient preparation
(b) Skin incisions
(c) Suturing of the fascia to tarsus
(d) Passing the fascia to the brow
(e) Skin crease closure
(f) Adjustment of height and contour
(g) Closure of forehead incisions

sary. Older patients often have dermatochalasis and brow ptosis accompanying involutional ptosis

- Paediatric patients
  - Indications for surgical correction of eyelid ptosis:
  - Choice of surgical procedure:
    Ptosis with poor levator function (1-3 mm) requires a frontalis sling operation
    Ptosis with medium to good levator function (>4 mm: lowest amount of levator function that will allow eyelid to lift without creating corneal exposure) can be corrected with a levator aponeurosis advancement operation

3.17 Approach to the Patient with Vertical Diplopia

3.17.1 Diagnoses to Consider for Monocular Vertical Diplopia

- Tear film abnormalities
- Uncorrected refractive error
- Corneal irregularity (e.g. keratoconus, refraction surgery) or scar
- Cataract
- Polycoria
- Dislocated lens
- Macular distortion (e.g. ERM)
- Non-organic

3.17.2 Diagnoses to Consider for Binocular Vertical Diplopia

- Neurogenic:
  - CN III palsy
  - CN IV palsy
- Mechanical:
  - TED
  - Myasthenia gravis
  - Orbital floor fracture
  - Congenital and acquired Brown's syndrome
  - Orbital inflammatory disease (myositis)
- Other:
  - Skew deviation
  - Ocular surgery e.g. scleral buckling surgery
  - Decompensated hyperphoria
  - Superior oblique myokymia

3.17.3 History

- "Does the double vision resolve when either eye is covered?": In binocular diplopia, one of the images disappear when one eye is covered. In contrast, monocular diplopia ceases when covering the affected eye but persists when occluding the unaffected eye
- Patients with binocular diplopia should be asked the following questions:
  - "Is the double vision intermittent, constant, or variable?"
    Double vision that is worse in the mornings may suggest TED
    Double vision that is worse in the evenings or with fatigue could indicate myasthenia gravis or a decompensated phoria
  - "Does the double vision depend upon direction of gaze (left, down, distance, near)?"
  - Ask for old photographs to look for an anomalous head posture: suggests a chronic ocular misalignment
  - If patient 50 years or older, ask about headaches, jaw claudication, scalp tenderness and weight loss to rule out giant cell arteritis (GCA)

- Ask about dysphagia, dyspnea, dysarthria, or proximal muscle weakness: suggests myasthenia gravis
- Ask about oscillopsia: suggests a nystagmus or superior oblique myokymia
- Ask about eyelid malpositions (retraction or ptosis): suggests myasthenia gravis, CN III palsy, or TED
- Past medical and ocular history should include the following questions:
  Head or ocular trauma
  Thyroid disease
  Vasculopathic risk factors (including smoking history)
  Childhood strabismus or amblyopia
  Previous eye muscle surgery

3.17.4 Examination

- Monocular vertical diplopia:
  - Examine anterior segment for any tear film abnormalities (early tear-film break up time, abnormal Schirmer test), areas of corneal thinning or cataract
  - Examine posterior segment for macular pathologies such as an ERM
  - Full ocular motility
- Binocular vertical diplopia:
  - Examine for an abnormal head posture: head tilt (e.g. CN IV palsy), chin-up position (e.g. TED)
  - Examine eyelid position
  - Perform exophthalmometry
  - Examine pupils
  - Examine ocular motility:
    Examine pursuits and saccades of the eyes individually (ductions) and together (versions):
    - Ophthalmoplegia secondary to a myopathy, neuropathy, or neuromuscular junction disorder reveals slowed saccades +/− abnormal pursuits (
    - Restrictive ophthalmoplegia demonstrates normal saccadic velocity

    Ocular alignment should be evaluated in primary position, upgaze, downgaze, and horizontal gaze positions, including distance and near:
    - Cover-uncover test: distinguish phorias from tropias
    - Alternate cover test: reveals full deviation of tropia plus latent phoria

3.17.5 Investigations

- Monocular vertical diplopia:
  - Refraction: reveal any unidentified or irregular astigmatism from corneal or lenticular causes
  - Corneal topography: detect an irregular corneal surface or contour
  - OCT: detect macular pathology
- Binocular vertical diplopia:
  - Bloods tests: anti-Ach receptor/ MuSK antibodies (myasthenia gravis), TSH/T3/T4 levels (TED), glucose levels (vasculopathic CN palsies), FBC/CRP/ESR (if patient 50 years or older to rule out GCA)
  - Blood pressure: vasculopathic CN palsies
  - ICE pack test/Tensilon test: myasthenia gravis
  - Repetitive stimulation electromyography (EMG): myasthenia gravis
  - Hess chart: for incomitant strabismus
  - CT scan: if orbital fracture is suspected, sight threatening TED is suspected, partial CN III palsy (rule out a posterior communicating artery aneurysm) is identified or multiple cranial nerves are involved
  - Forced duction testing: verify a restrictive process

3.17.6 Restriction of Extraocular Motility in Orbital Fractures

3.17.6.1 Differential Diagnosis of Enophthalmos

- Bony defects: orbital fractures, congenital orbital wall defects
- Small globe: microphthalmos, nanophthalmos, phthisis bulbi, orbital implant

- Soft tissue atrophy: post-irradiation, scleroderma, cicatrizing tumours

3.17.6.2 Classification of Blow Out Fractures

- Orbital rim remains intact: fracture affects the floor (antral blowout), medial wall (ethmoidal blow out), combined antral and ethmoidal blow out
- Orbital rim fractured in addition to an antral, ethmoidal, or combined blow out

3.17.6.3 Classification of Orbital Floor Blow Out Fractures

- Type I: limited elevation of affected eye from mechanical restriction
- Type II: limited depression of affected eye from IR muscle palsy
- Type III: combined limited elevation and depression from mechanical restriction and IR muscle palsy, respectively

3.17.6.4 Examination

- Orbital floor fracture: vertical diplopia with limitation of both upgaze and downgaze (upgaze is commonly more affected than downgaze resulting in downward displacement of the small field of BSV)
- Type I orbital floor blow out fracture:
  - Limitation of ocular movement on up gaze
  - Positive FDT for mechanical restriction with the greatest limitation in elevation and abduction
  - Field of BSV is reduced in upgaze
- Type II orbital floor blow out fracture:
  - Limitation of ocular movement on down-gaze
  - Negative FDT for mechanical restriction on depression
- Type III orbital floor blow out fracture:
  - Limitation of ocular movement on up-gaze with positive FDT for mechanical restriction, with the greatest restriction in elevation and abduction
  - Limitation of ocular movement on downgaze with negative FDT for mechanical restriction on depression
  - Patient often has small central island of BSV, but is considerably handicapped by diplopia on downgaze
- Medial wall fracture (most often seen in association with a blowout fracture of the orbital floor): horizontal diplopia with restriction of abduction (mechanical restriction) and adduction (either mechanical restriction or to a neurogenic palsy of the MR)
- Backwards (enophthalmos) +/− downward displacement (herniation of fat from the inferior part of the orbit into the antrum) of the globe
- Retraction of the globe (on elevation in a floor blow out fracture and on abduction in medial wall blow out fracture): occurs when the eye moves away from the site of entrapment
- Infraorbital anaesthesia (damage to infraorbital nerve): loss of sensation to ipsilateral cheek and upper teeth
- >5 mm difference in IOP in primary position and in position of gaze in which movement is restricted

3.17.6.5 Investigations

- CT scan: tear drop sign (small clump of soft tissue lying outside the orbit), missing rectus sign (absence of IR above orbital floor), muscle rounding sign (rounding of IR muscle)
- Hess chart: mechanical restriction
- Field of binocular single vision (BSV)
- Force duction testing (FDT)

3.17.6.6 Treatment

- Advise patients to refrain from nose blowing
- Antibiotic prophylaxis
- Type I orbital floor blow out fracture:
  (a) Conservative treatment: prisms, occlusion
  (b) Surgical treatment (avoid if it puts the field of BSV in the primary position and downgaze at risk): recession of contralateral IO muscle +/− contralateral SR muscle
- Type II orbital floor blow out fracture:
  (a) Conservative treatment (continued for at least 9–12 months from the time of injury

to allow spontaneous recovery of IR muscle function): prisms, occlusion
  (b) Surgical treatment: recession of contralateral SR +/− inverse Knapp procedure
- Type III orbital floor blow out fracture:
  (a) Conservative treatment: occlusion
  (b) Surgical treatment: IR and SR recessions of the unaffected eye
- Medial wall blow-out fracture:
  (a) Conservative (continued for at least 9–12 months from the time of injury to allow spontaneous recovery of IR muscle function): prisms, occlusion
  (b) Surgical treatment: limitation of adduction due to MR muscle palsy is corrected by an ipsilateral MR resection/LR recession if palsy is partial and by a transposition of the SR and IR to the MR + LR weakening by Botox if palsy is complete

3.17.6.7 Indications for Surgical Intervention in Orbital Floor Fractures

- Immediate:
  - Persistent oculocardiac reflex
  - Young patient with "white eyed" trapdoor fracture
  - Significant facial asymmetry
- Early (<2 weeks):
  - Persistent symptomatic diplopia (diplopia within 30° of fixation)
  - Significant enophthalmos (>2 mm)
  - Hypoglobus
  - Progressive infraorbital anesthesia
  - Fracture involving >50% of the orbital floor
- Observation:
  - Minimal diplopia (e.g. just in upgaze)
  - Minimal restriction
  - Minimal enophthalmos

3.17.7 Restriction of Extraocular Motility in TED

3.17.7.1 Examination (See Sect. 3.15.4.2)

3.17.7.2 Investigation (See Sect. 3.15.4.2)

3.17.7.3 Treatment

- Conservative:
  (a) Treatment of diplopia: prisms, Botox, occlusion (last resort)
- Surgical:
  (a) Aims of extraocular muscle surgery are to improve the patient's appearance and to establish a field of binocular single vision in the primary position and on down-gaze, extending the area into other fields of gaze if possible
  (b) Patient should be euthyroid and the ocular muscle imbalance should have remained stable for at least 3 months before considering surgery
  (c) Categorise the ocular motility disturbances into recognisable patterns:
    (1) Unilateral or grossly asymmetrical bilateral restriction of elevation
      - Incomitant (increase in vertical deviation on upgaze and a reduction on downgaze, usually with an intact inferior field of BSV): mechanical restriction of ipsilateral IR—treat with ipsilateral IR recession
      - Concomitant (vertical deviation that is the same on upgaze and which decreases minimally or not at all on downgaze, usually with no field of BSV): mechanical restriction of ipsilateral IR + con-

tralateral SR—treat with IR recession +/− SR recession

(2) Unilateral or grossly asymmetric bilateral restriction of abduction
   - Incomitant (ET which increases in the direction of mechanical restriction and reduces in the opposite field of gaze + face turn away from the side with the mechanical restriction + intact field of BSV): mechanical restriction of ipsilateral MR—treat with ipsilateral MR recession
   - Concomitant (ET in all positions of gaze): bilateral mechanical restriction of both MR—treat with unilateral or bilateral MR recession

(3) Unilateral or grossly asymmetric bilateral restriction of both elevation and abduction: management is the same as for pattern (1) and (2)

(4) Bilateral symmetric restriction of elevation
   - Neither eye is able to maintain fixation in primary position
   - Asymmetrical mechanical restriction of elevation, with a −2 to −3 restriction in the more mobile eye
   - A pattern ET is present on upgaze, with a convergence retraction movement as the eyes attempt to move into the field of maximum restriction
   - Contraction of the SR, if present, will restrict movement on down-gaze
   - Treat with bilateral IR recession

(5) Bilateral restriction of both elevation and abduction

(6) Mechanical restriction of the superior rectus muscles resulting in limited down-gaze
   - Limitation of depression that is greatest in abduction
   - Treat with SR recession

3.18 Angle Closure (Table 3.18)

3.18.1 Risk Factors for Angle Closure

- Inuit/South east asians/Chinese
- Hyperopia with short axial length
- Older age: reduced depth and volume of the AC
- A Shallow central and peripheral AC
- Anterior lens vault (see Fig. 3.34): perpendicular distance between the anterior pole of the lens and the horizontal line joining the 2 scleral spurs on horizontal anterior segment OCT—eyes with angle closure have greater lens vault compared with normal eyes
- Retinitis pigmentosa and Best Vitelliform Macular Dystrophy are associated with angle-closure (The RCOphth Management of Angle Closure Glaucoma Guidelines 2021 [123])

3.18.2 Mechanisms of Angle Closure

- Pupil-block (most common mechanism—75% of cases): strong apposition of iris sphincter to anterior lens capsule (mid-dilated pupil), increased fluid pressure in posterior chamber causes a forward shift of the iris, anterior movement of iris results in closure of AC angle
  (a) Acute angle closure +/− glaucoma
  (b) Sub-acute angle closure +/− glaucoma: symptoms intermittent (colour halos

Table 3.18 Angle closure terminology

Angle closure is characterised by apposition of the peripheral iris against the trabecular meshwork, resulting in obstruction of aqueous outflow
Primary angle closure suspect (PACS) / Occludable angle: ≥2 quadrants (180°) of iridotrabecular contact (ITC), normal IOP, no PAS, normal optic nerve (ZAP Trial—see Table 3.22)
Primary angle closure (PAC): ≥2 quadrants (180°) of ITC, raised IOP (>21 mmHg) and/or PAS, normal optic nerve (EAGLE Study—see Table 3.21)—30% in 5 years develop PACG
Primary angle-closure glaucoma (PACG): PAC with disc or reproducible field defects consistent with glaucoma (EAGLE Study—see Table 3.21)

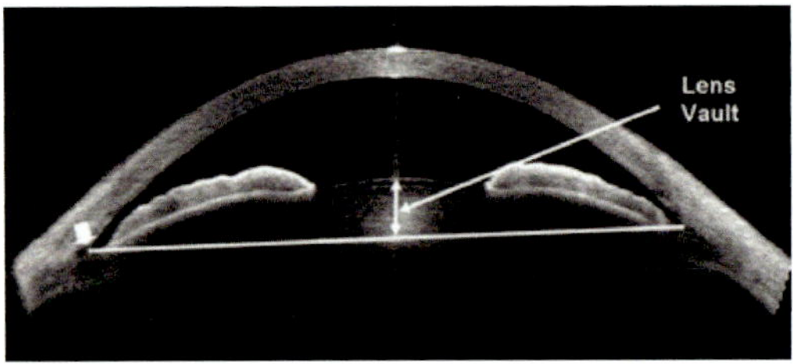

Fig. 3.34 Anterior lens vault

around lights from corneal epithelial oedema—blue-green central halo and yellow-red peripheral halo) or absent

(c) Chronic angle closure +/− glaucoma: IOP chronically elevated with varying degree of PAS (usually broad based and starts in the superior quadrant—narrowest)

(d) Combined mechanisms glaucoma: angle initially closed, PI performed, angle open but IOP remains high

- Plateau iris:
  - Plateau iris configuration (see Fig. 3.35): pre-iridotomy anatomic appearance, anterior position of ciliary body and processes, flat iris plane, closed AC angle, normal central AC depth, gonioscopy (double-hump sign on indentation gonioscopy—central iris moves posteriorly, peripheral hump created from anterior ciliary body pushing iris root forward, central hump created by iris sitting on anterior lens capsule)
  - Plateau iris syndrome: angle closure in eye with plateau iris configuration despite presence of a patent PI
- Secondary angle closure (at the level of the lens or resulting from lens intumescence or behind the lens, within the vitreous, the retina or the choroid)

3.18.3 History

- Ask about risk factors for angle closure (see Sect. 3.18.1)

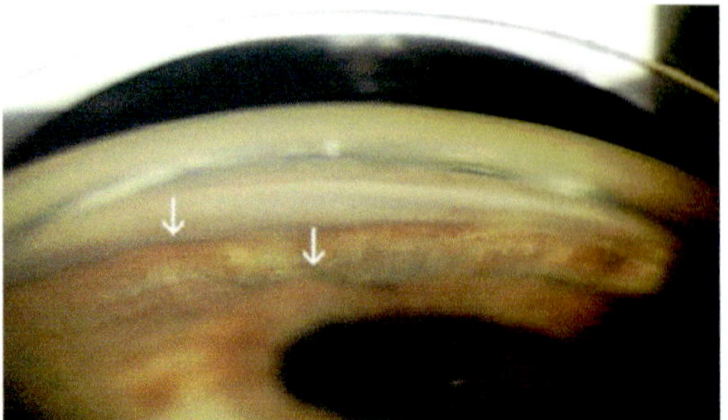

Fig. 3.35 Gonioscopic view of a patient with a plateau iris configuration showing the double hump sign (white arrows) on indentation gonioscopy

3.18.4 Examination

- Bilateral (PAC) or unilateral (secondary angle closure e.g. phacomorphic) shallow peripheral AC: Van Herick's method—direct a narrow-slit beam at 60° onto the cornea just anterior to the limbus, AC considered narrow if distance between the anterior iris and posterior cornea is < ¼ of the corneal thickness
- Normal Central AC depth
- Fixed semi-dilated pupil with diffuse iris atrophy/transillumination defects: suggestive of previous acute angle closure attack
- Glaucomflecken: small anterior subcapsular opacities (lens epithelial necrosis) suggestive of previous acute angle closure attack
- Check IOP
- Perform gonioscopy: open or closed angle, PAS
- Examine the optic disc for signs of glaucoma:
  - Generalised signs: CDR 0.7 or more, asymmetry of CDR of 0.2 or more, progressive enlargement of cup
  - Focal signs: rim thinning/notching (ISNT rule), regional pallor, NFL haemorrhage, NFL loss

3.18.5 Investigations

- HVF: early: paracentral defect, nasal step (IT or ST rim thinning), temporal wedge (nasal disc thinning)/late: arcuate defect, double arcuate defect, central vision only
- AS-OCT can be a useful supplement for showing ITC

3.18.6 Treatment

- If IOP raised: reduce IOP (see also Sect. 3.18.8)
- PACS (See Tables 3.21, 3.22, and 3.23): Yag PI only advisable if patients have additional risk factor(s) (PACS-Plus) (The RCOphth Management of Angle Closure Glaucoma Guidelines 2021 [123]) (see Table 3.19). Risk of an AAC crisis from PACS is around 1/1000 per year
- PAC: Yag PI (see Table 3.20), strong recommendation to perform phacoemulsification/clear lens extraction if IOP ≥30 mmHg (The RCOphth Management of Angle Closure Glaucoma Guidelines 2021) [123], trabeculectomy/GDI
- PACG (see Table 3.21): Yag PI, strong recommendation to perform phacoemulsification/clear lens extraction if IOP ≥30 mmHg (The RCOphth Management of Angle Closure Glaucoma Guidelines 2021) [123], trabeculectomy/GDI
- Plateau iris syndrome: iridoplasty, lens extraction

Table 3.19 YAG PI in PACS

Laser PI is advised for people with PACS who have one or more of the following risk factors (The RCOphth Management of Angle Closure Glaucoma Guidelines 2021):
1. An only eye
2. Vulnerable adults who may not report ocular or vision symptoms
3. A family history of significant angle closure disease
4. High hypermetropia (greater than + 6.00 dioptres)
5. Diabetes or another condition requiring regular pupil dilation
6. Use of antidepressants or medication with an anticholinergic action
7. Living or working in remote locations (such as armed forces stationed overseas, oil rig workers, or foreign aid workers) where accessing emergency ophthalmic care is not possible

Table 3.20 Yag PI procedure

Indications: therapeutic—angle closure with pupil block, prophylactic—PACS-Plus, fellow eye in AACG (approximately 50% to 75% of pts who develop acute angle closure in one eye will have an attack in the fellow, unoperated eye within 5 to 10 years)
Consent: risks—bleeding, inflammation, pressure spike, monocular diplopia, failure/need for retreatment, corneal burns (if shallow AC)
Pre-procedure: instill topical pilocarpine 2% (tightens the iris), topical Iopidine 1% (prevents IOP spike + reduce bleeding), topical anaesthetic, set up laser—2 to 3 pulses of 3-6 mJ, angle the beam (beam should not be perpendicular), position the Abraham CL
During procedure: identify suitable iridotomy site—temporal or superior (hidden by normal lid position) location, peripheral, and ideally in an iris crypt, focus and fire laser—success indicated by a forward gush of pigment loaded aqueous. There is no consistent evidence for PI location influencing dysphotopsia (The RCOphth Management of Angle Closure Glaucoma Guidelines 2021)
Post-procedure: check IOP at 30–60 minutes post PI, topical steroid, follow-up in outpatient's clinic in 2/52

3.18.7 Other Diagnoses to Consider

- Trauma (surgical or non-surgical): sectoral iris atrophy/transillumination defects, mydriasis

3.18.8 Management of Acute Angle Closure (AAC) Attack / Crisis

The RCOphth recommends the following approach when dealing with an AAC attack/crisis with a pupillary block or plateau iris mechanism (The RCOphth Management of Angle Closure Glaucoma Guidelines 2021) [123]:

- Analgesia and anti-emetics if required
- Examination to confirm elevated IOP from angle-closure and to identify/exclude secondary lenticular / retro-lenticular causes
- Identify any prior allergies/contraindictations

3.19 Normal Tension Glaucoma (NTG) (Table 3.24)

3.19.1 History

- History of Raynaud's disease
- History of migraines

3.19.2 Examination

- Check VA, colour vision, RAPD
- Check IOP: <21 mmHg
- Perform gonioscopy: open angle
- Examine the optic nerve for signs of glaucoma:
  - Generalised signs: CDR 0.7 or more, asymmetry of CDR of 0.2 or more, progressive enlargement of cup
  - Focal signs: rim thinning/notching (ISNT rule), regional pallor, NFL haemorrhage, NFL loss

3.19.3 Investigations

- HVF: early: paracentral defect, nasal step (IT or ST rim thinning), temporal wedge (nasal disc thinning) / late: arcuate defect, double arcuate defect, central vision only
- Phasing: look for IOP spikes (diurnal fluctuations in IOP)
- 24-hour BP monitoring: nocturnal hypotension
- Ensure correlation between optic nerve head findings and VF defects (see Figs. 3.36 and 3.37)
- Neuro-imaging (see Table 3.25 for indications)

3.19.4 Treatment

- Reduce IOP by 30% (see Table 3.26): medical tx initially and surgical tx (laser trabeculoplasty, trabeculectomy, GDI) after failure of maximal tolerated medical therapy (MTMT)
- Avoid drug induced nocturnal systemic hypotension: liaise with GP/physicians

Table 3.24 Definition of NTG

Open normal appearing angles who have glaucomatous optic nerve head and VF damage despite pressures that have never been documented above 21 mmHg

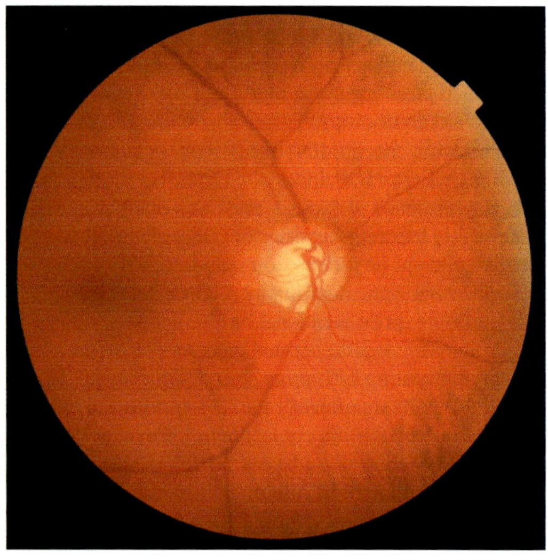

Fig. 3.36 Colour fundus image of a patient with NTG showing increased optic disc cupping and prominent inferior notching with loss of normal sheen of NFL radiating temporally from notch

3.19.5 Risk Factors for Progression of NTG

- Female sex
- Hx of migraines
- Disc haemorrhages at diagnosis

3.19.6 Other Diagnoses to Consider

- POAG
- Secondary open angle glaucomas: steroid induced, PDS, PXF
- PACG
- Ischaemic optic neuropathy
- Compressive lesions of the optic nerve and tract
- Optic neuritis
- Trauma

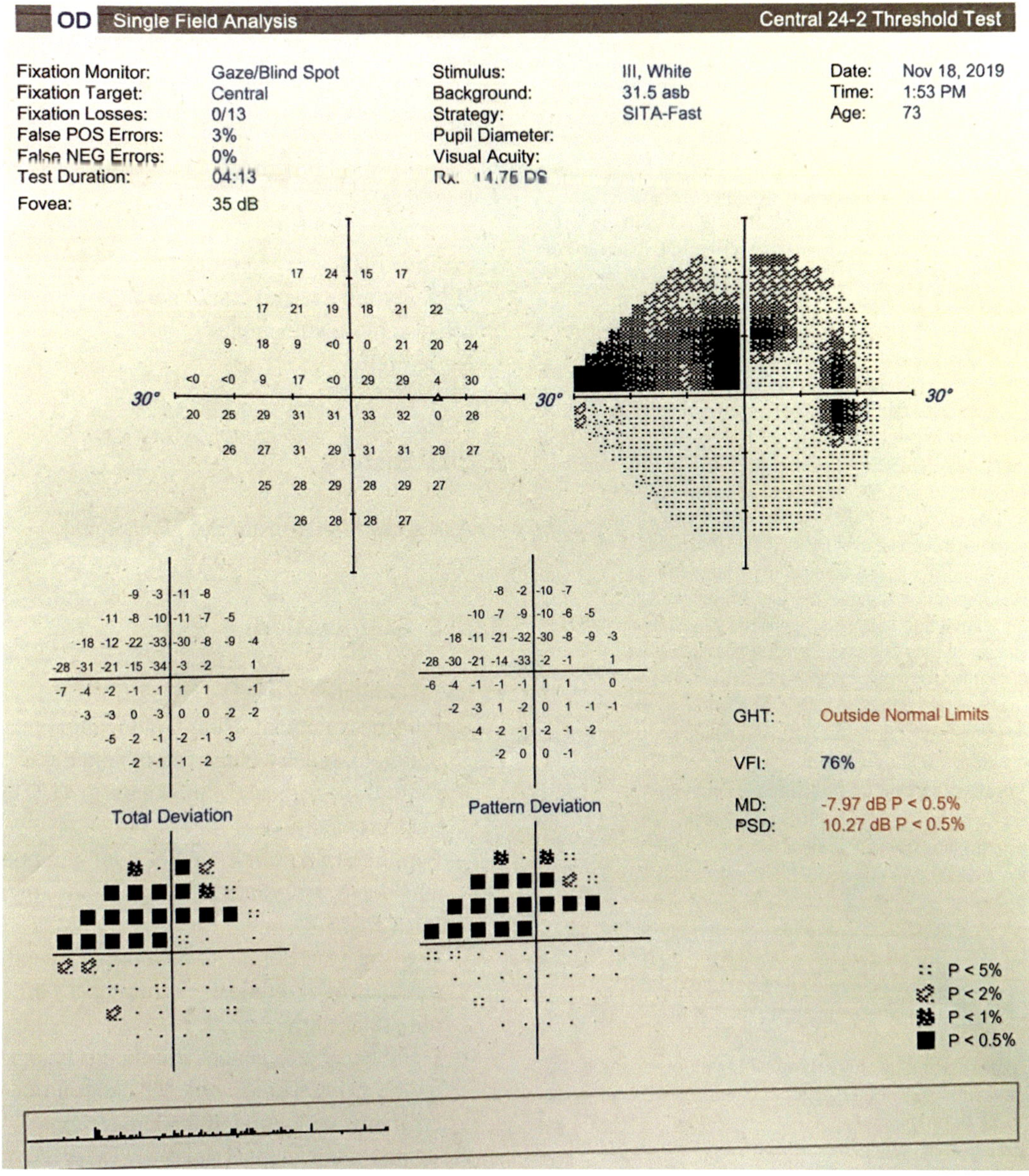

Fig. 3.37 30–2 HVF of the same patient as in Fig. 3.36 showing a superior arcuate scotoma which correlates to the prominent inferior optic disc notching as shown in Fig. 3.36

Table 3.25 Indications for neuro-imaging

General factors: age < 50, new onset or increased severity of headaches, localising neurologic symptoms other than migraines
Ocular factors: positive visual symptoms, colour vision abnormalities, lack of disc and VF correlation, VF defect respecting the vertical midline, optic disc pallor, unexplained VA reduction, RAPD

Table 3.26 Summary of the Collaborative Normal Tension Glaucoma Study [19]

Primary outcome: An RCT conducted to determine whether IOP played a part in the pathogenic process of NTG
Methods:
(a) Inclusion criteria: unilateral or bilateral NTG with optic disc abnormalities and VF defects characteristic of glaucoma, no single IOP reading of >24 mmHg with median IOP reading (from 10 baseline IOP readings) of ≤20 mmHg, age > 20 years and < 90 years, pupil diameter ≥ 2.5 mm
(b) Exclusion criteria: pts taking systemic β-blockers or clonidine, eyes with previous laser tx, previous ocular surgery, or cyclodestructive procedures, non-glaucomatous conditions that might later affect the visual field, narrow angles or advanced field loss, BCVA <20/30
(c) Groups: One eye of each patient was randomised to either the untreated control arm or to the 30% IOP reduction (from the mean of the last 3 pre-randomisation pressure readings) arm by medical (pilocarpine) or surgical (ALT or trabeculectomy) intervention. Randomisation began if eye had VF defect that threatened fixation, VF progression was demonstrated, a change in the optic nerve head appearance was confirmed, or a disc haemorrhage was noted.
(d) Primary end points: VF progression, change in degree of glaucomatous optic disc damage, or both
(e) Follow up: 5 years (initial report)
Results: 145 eyes of 145 patients
(a) Lowering of IOP by 30% reduces the rate of VF progression from 35% to 12%
(b) 12% of eyes showed VF progression despite an IOP reduction of 30%
(c) 65% of pt's showed no progression during follow up of 5 years or more
(d) 30% IOP reduction could be achieved and maintained in 57% of pt's with topical medications, ALT, or both
(e) Females, especially those with a hx of migraine and pt's with disc haemorrhages at diagnosis were all more likely to progress
Conclusions: IOP is part of the pathogenic process of NTG. Therapy that is effective in lowering IOP and free of adverse effects would be expected to be beneficial in patients who are at risk of disease progression

3.20 Chronic Open Angle Glaucoma (COAG) (Table 3.27)

3.20.1 Risk Factors for COAG

- Age
- African-Caribbean: more frequent, younger onset, more severe

Table 3.27 Useful information about COAG

Adult-onset optic neuropathy with glaucomatous optic disc and/or VF changes, open angles, IOP > 21 mmHg and no other underlying disease
Prevalence (proportion of a population with the disease at a given time point) of 1% greater than 40 years old / prevalence of 10% greater than 75 years old + Caucasian

- Positive FHx
- High myopia: scleral canal morphology making disc more vulnerable
- Raised IOP

3.20.2 History

- Ask about family history of glaucoma

3.20.3 Examination

- NICE Guidance [NG81] [75]:
  - IOP measurement using Goldmann applanation tonometry (slit-lamp mounted)
  - Central corneal thickness (CCT) measurement
  - Peripheral anterior chamber configuration and depth assessments using gonioscopy: open angle
  - Use the van Herick peripheral AC depth assessment if clinical circumstances rule out gonioscopy
  - Optic nerve assessment and fundus examination using stereoscopic slit lamp biomicroscopy, with pupil dilatation.
- Optic disc signs in glaucoma:
  - Generalised signs: CDR 0.7 or more, asymmetry of CDR of 0.2 or more, progressive enlargement of cup
  - Focal signs: rim thinning/notching (ISNT rule not obeyed), regional pallor, NFL haemorrhage, NFL loss

3.20.4 Investigations

- NICE Guidance [NG81] [75]:
  - Visual field assessment using standard automated perimetry (central threshold testing)

- Optic nerve head (ONH) image for baseline documentation (for example, OCT or a stereoscopic optic nerve head image)
- HVF signs in glaucoma:
  - Early: paracentral defect, nasal step (IT or ST rim thinning), temporal wedge (nasal disc thinning)
  - Late: arcuate defect, double arcuate defect, central vision only
  - Ensure correlation between optic nerve head findings and VF defects

3.20.5 Diagnosis

- NICE Guidance [NG81] [75]:
  - Ocular hypertension (OHT): baseline IOP 24mmHg or more and a normal optic nerve head and VF
  - Suspected COAG: any IOP, suspicious of possible glaucoma on ONH, normal or uncertain VF
  - COAG: any IOP, ONH damage, normal/uncertain/defects on VF

3.20.6 Treatment (see Tables 3.28, 3.29, 3.30, and 3.31)

NICE Guidance [NG81] [75]:

People with OHT:

- At the time of diagnosis of OHT, assess the risk of future visual impairment taking into account risk factors such as level of IOP, CCT, family history, life expectancy
- Do not offer treatment to people with OHT who are not at risk of visual impairment within their lifetime.
- Offer 360° SLT to people with newly diagnosed OHT with IOP of 24 mmHg or more (excluding cases associated with PDS) if they are at risk of visual impairment within their lifetime
- Consider a second 360° SLT for people with OHT if the effect of an initial successful SLT has subsequently reduced over time
- Offer a generic prostaglandin analogue (PGA) to people with OHT with IOP of 24 mmHg or more if they are at risk of visual impairment within their lifetime and:
  - Patient chooses not to have SLT **or**
  - 360° SLT is not suitable (e.g. they have PDS) **or**
  - They are waiting for an 360° SLT and need an interim treatment **or**

Table 3.28 Summary of the Early Manifest Glaucoma Trial [44]

Primary outcome: Compare the effect of immediate therapy to lower the IOP, vs no treatment or later treatment, on the progression of newly detected open-angle glaucoma (OAG) as measured by increasing VF loss or optic disc changes
Methods:
(a) Inclusion criteria: diagnosis of early manifest open angle glaucoma (POAG, NTG, PXF glaucoma), age between 50 and 80 years, reproducible glaucomatous VF defects in at least one eye
(b) Exclusion criteria: advanced VF loss (MD > -16 dB) or a threat to fixation, VA < 20/40, mean IOP > 30 mmHg or any IOP > 35mmmHg in at least one eye, any condition precluding reliable results of perimetry or optic disc photography, the use of study interventions, or 4 years of follow up, cataractous lens changes exceeding gradings of N1, C2, or P1 according to the lens opacification classification system (LOCS) II
(c) Groups: Treatment group—360-degree ALT + betaxolol 0.5% BD (reduced mean IOP by 25%, a reduction maintained throughout follow up—IOP reduction was larger in eyes with a baseline IOP of ≥21 mmHg [29%] than in eyes with a baseline IOP of less than 21 mmHg [18%])/ non-treatment group
(d) Primary endpoints: Progression of either glaucomatous VF defects or optic disc cupping
(e) Follow up: median 6 years (initial report)
Results: 255 patients
(a) Primary endpoints: After a median of 6 years of follow-up, progression was less frequent in the treatment group (45%) than in controls (62%) and occurred significantly later in treated patients (median time to progression was 18 months longer in the treatment group than the control group). Each 1 mmHg of decreased IOP was related to an approximately 10% lowering of risk.
(b) Safety / complications: Nuclear cataract developed faster in the treated group and 6 had surgery (compared to 2 controls)
(c) Risk factors for progression (in decreasing order of risk): PXF, bilateral glaucoma, higher baseline IOP (≥21 mmHg), worse baseline MD (more than -4 dB), older age, frequent disc haemorrhages post treatment (not associated with IOP or treatment)
Conclusion of study: Clear beneficial effects of lowering IOP on delaying the onset of progression, with lower rates of progression in the treatment group than the control group

Table 3.29 Summary of the Advanced Glaucoma Intervention Study (The AGIS Investigators 1997; [106])

Primary outcome: Assess the effects of two surgical intervention sequences in patients with advanced POAG after the failure of medical therapy.
Methods:
(a) Inclusion criteria: eyes with either advanced (glaucoma not controlled adequately despite MTMT in the presence of glaucomatous VF defect) POAG without previous surgery or advanced POAG in a phakic eye 4 weeks or more after PI, phakic VA better than 20/80 [6/24]), age 35–80 years old, reproducible glaucomatous VF defects in at least one eye, a table of specific combinations of elevated IOP & VF defect was used to define uncontrolled glaucoma & was used to determine if a second or third operation was required
(b) Exclusion criteria: secondary glaucoma or congenital angle anomalies, other active eye diseases that cause field loss or previous surgery
(c) Groups: A-T-T group: ALT followed if necessary by trabeculectomy, followed if necessary by repeat trabeculectomy / T-A-T group: trabeculectomy followed if necessary by ALT, followed if necessary by repeat trabeculectomy
(d) Primary endpoints: VA and/or VF (score 0 normal to-20 blind)
(e) Follow up: 7 years (initial report)
Results: 332 black patients, 249 white patients, 10 patients of other races
(a) Low post intervention IOP is associated with reduced progression of VF defect
Predictive analysis (IOP averaged over the first three 6-month visits: designed to assess whether IOP during early follow up is predictive of subsequent change from baseline in VF defect score): Initial mean IOP < 14 mmHg over the first 18 months after surgery had a mean VF score deterioration of less than 1 point from baseline and those with an initial IOP ≥ 18 mmHg had a mean score deterioration of 3 points over 7 years
Associative analysis (% of visits over the first 6 years of follow up for which an eye presented with IOP < 18 mmHg): IOP < 18 mmHg on 100% of follow up visits over 6 years resulted in a mean score deterioration of close to zero, but those achieving IOP <18 mmHg on <100% of visits had a mean deterioration of 2 to 3 points
(b) After 7 years of follow-up, overall (both races) the mean decrease in IOP from baseline is greater in eyes assigned to T-A-T than in those assigned to A-T-T
(c) In white patient's VF was better preserved by T-A-T only after the first year of follow-up and thereafter favour the A-T-T sequence, and acuity was better preserved by A-T-T throughout follow up.
(d) For black patients, VF and acuity loss were less for eyes in the A-T-T sequence
(e) Complications of trabeculectomy: relative risk of cataract in the 5 years after trabeculectomy was 1.78 compared to those participants who avoided trabeculectomy. Youth and high IOP were key risk factors for failure of either ALT or trabeculectomy. Diabetes mellitus or persistent postop inflammation were also significant risk factors for trabeculectomy failure
Conclusion of study: Low IOP reduces risk of VF progression. Data supports the use of the A-T-T sequence for all black patients. For white patients the data supports the use of the T-A-T sequence

Table 3.30 Summary of the Collaborative Initial Glaucoma Treatment Study [57]

Primary outcome: Determine whether patients with newly diagnosed OAG are best treated by initial treatment with topical medications or by immediate trabeculectomy
Methods:
(a) Inclusion criteria: newly diagnosed OAG (POAG, PXF glaucoma, pigmentary glaucoma); one of three combinations of qualifying IOP (IOP ≥ 20 mmHg), VF changes, and optic disc findings; BCVA of 20/40 or better in both eyes; age 25–75 years; no prior ocular surgery; little (≤14 cumulative days of topical therapy) or no prior treatment of glaucoma
(b) Exclusion criteria: use of glaucoma medication >14 cumulative days; CIGST VF score > 16 in either eye; ocular disease that might affect measurement of IOP, VA, or VF; undergone ophthalmic laser, refractive, conjunctival, or intraocular surgery in either eye; PDR, DMO, or NPDR with >10 MA's by clinical count; current or expected chronic use of corticosteroids; likely require cataract surgery within 1 year of randomisation
(c) Groups: topical medication group—escalating drops, if further treatment was required start with ALT, then trabeculectomy +/− 5-FU drops, then trabeculectomy + anti-fibrotic agent, then medication / trabeculectomy group—trabeculectomy +/− 5-FU, if further treatment was required start with ALT, then escalating drops, then repeat trabeculectomy + anti-fibrotic agent, then medication
(d) Primary endpoint: increasing CIGST VF score reflecting increased VF loss
(e) Secondary endpoints: change in VA, change in IOP, occurrence of cataract extraction, QOL (questionnaire)
(f) Follow up: 5 years (initial report)
Results: 607 patients
(a) Primary endpoint: no significant difference in VF scores at 5 years in both groups

(continued)

Table 3.30 (continued)

(b) Secondary endpoints: initial VA decrease in the trabeculectomy group that was not observed in the topical medication group, resulted in lower mean VA in the trabeculectomy group that persisted through 3.5 years after surgery. After that time, mean VA levels were comparable in the 2 treatment groups up to 5 years of follow up (VA less in trabeculectomy group compared to topical medications group); there were no significant differences in the QOL between the 2 groups; both groups had significantly decreased mean IOP after treatment initiation (3 mmHg better reduction with trabeculectomy) although the amount of decrease was greater in the trabeculectomy group (48% in trabeculectomy group vs 35% in the topical medication group), and the difference was maintained over 5 years of observation; the trabeculectomy group had a higher cataract extraction probability over time; Risk factors for VF progression: older age, non-white race, DM, development of cataract, maximal IOP, IOP fluctuation between visits
Conclusion of study: CIGTS clinical outcomes do not suggest a change in the way ophthalmologists currently manage their patients with newly diagnosed OAG

- They have previously had 360° SLT but need additional treatment to reduce IOP sufficiently to prevent the risk of visual impairment

- Offer another pharmacological treatment to people with an IOP of 24 mmHg or more who cannot tolerate their current treatment. The first choice should be an alternative generic PGA, and if this is not tolerated, offer a beta-blocker. If neither of these options is tolerated, offer a non-generic PGA, carbonic anhydrase inhibitor, sympathomimetic, miotic or a combination of treatments
- Offer a medicine from another therapeutic class (beta-blocker, carbonic anhydrase inhibitor or sympathomimetic) to people with an IOP of 24 mmHg or more whose current treatment is not reducing IOP sufficiently to prevent the risk of progression to sight loss. Topical medicines from different therapeutic classes may be needed at the same time to control IOP
- Offer preservative-free eye drops to people who have an allergy to preservatives or people with clinically significant and symptomatic ocular surface disease, but only if they are at high risk of conversion to POAG

Table 3.31 Summary of the selective laser trabeculoplasty versus eye drops for first-line treatment of ocular hypertension and glaucoma (LiGHT) trial [40]

Primary outcome: To compare eye drops versus selective laser trabeculoplasty (SLT) as first line treatment for OAG or OHT Methods:
(a) Inclusion criteria: newly diagnosed untreated OAG or OHT in 1 or both eyes; qualified for treatment according to NICE guidelines; VF loss with MD not worse than -12 dB in the better eye or -15 dB in the worse eye with corresponding damage to the optic nerve for those with OAG; VA 6/36 or better in eyes to be treated; no previous intraocular surgery except uncomplicated phacoemulsification at least 1 year prior to randomisation
(b) Exclusion criteria: patients with contraindications to SLT (history of uveitis, unable to sit at slit-lamp, poor view of trabecular meshwork); patients unable to use eye drops; patients who had a symptomatic cataract; patients who were under active treatment for another ophthalmic condition
(c) Groups: eye drops group, SLT group
(d) Primary endpoint: health-related quality of life measured using the EuroQol EQ-5D 5 levels utility scores
(e) Secondary endpoint(s): glaucoma-specific treatment related quality of life assessed with the Glaucoma Utility Index (GUI); patient-reported disease and treatment-related symptoms assessed using the Glaucoma Symptom Scale (GSS); patient-reported visual function assessed using the Glaucoma Quality of Life-15 questionnaire (GQL-15); clinical effectiveness (proportion of visits at target IOP, number of treatment escalations); visual function (VA, VF); safety
(f) Follow up: 36 months
Results: 652 patients
(a) Primary endpoint: no significant difference in EQ-5D scores at 36 months
(b) Secondary endpoints: mean GUI score, mean GQL-15 and mean GSS scores were similar between the 2 groups at 36 months; 2 groups had similar endpoint VA, IOP, and VF loss MD; 74.2% of eyes in the SLT group remained drop free at 36 months; SLT was more cost effective; 11 eyes (1.8%) required trabeculectomy in the eye drops group compared with none in the SLT group
Conclusions of study: SLT should be offered as first line treatment for OAG and OHT

- Discuss the benefits and risks of stopping treatment with people with OHT who have a low risk of developing visual impairment within their lifetime **and** an acceptable IOP. If a person decides to stop treatment after this discussion, offer to assess their IOP in 1 month

to 4 months with further reassessment if clinically indicated
- Follow up:
  - If conversion to COAG is not detected or uncertain and IOP is not controlled, review management plan and reassess between 1 month and 4 months
  - If uncertain conversion to COAG and IOP is controlled, reassess between 6 months and 12 months
  - If no conversion to COAG detected and IOP is controlled, reassess between 18 months and 24 months
  - If conversion to COAG is detected, follow up according to COAG recommendations as stated below

People with suspected COAG:
- Do not offer treatment to people with suspected COAG and IOP less than 24 mmHg unless they are at risk of visual impairment within their lifetime.
- Follow up:
  - If conversion to COAG not detected or uncertain and IOP is not controlled, review management plan and reassess between 1 month and 4 months
  - If uncertain conversion to COAG and IOP is controlled, reassess between 6 months and 12 months
  - If no conversion to COAG is detected and IOP is controlled, reassess between 12 months and 18 months
  - If conversion to COAG is detected, follow up according to COAG recommendations as stated below

People with COAG:
- Offer 360° SLT to people with newly diagnosed COAG (excluding cases associated with PDS). For advanced COAG, offer glaucoma surgery with pharmacological augmentation (Mitomycin C). Offer people who present with advanced COAG and who are listed for glaucoma surgery, interim treatment with a generic PGA
- Consider a second 360° SLT for people with COAG if the effect of an initial successful SLT has subsequently reduced over time
- Offer a generic PGA if:
  - Patient chooses not to have SLT **or**
  - 360° SLT is not suitable (e.g. they have PDS) **or**
  - They are waiting for an 360° SLT and need an interim treatment **or**
  - They have previously had 360° SLT but need additional treatment to reduce IOP sufficiently to prevent the risk of visual impairment
- Encourage people to continue with the same pharmacological treatment unless:
  - Their IOP cannot be reduced sufficiently to prevent the risk of progression to sight loss
  - There is progression of optic nerve head damage
  - There is progression of visual field defect
  - They cannot tolerate the medicine
- Offer one of the following to people with satisfactory adherence to treatment and eye drop instillation technique whose IOP has not been reduced sufficiently to prevent the risk of progression to sight loss:
  - A medicine from another therapeutic class (a beta-blocker, carbonic anhydrase inhibitor or sympathomimetic); topical medications from different therapeutic classes may be needed at the same time to control IOP **or**
  - 360° SLT **or**
  - Glaucoma surgery with pharmacological augmentation (Mitomycin C)
- Consider 360° SLT or glaucoma surgery with pharmacological augmentation (Mitomycin C) as indicated for people with COAG who are at risk of progressing to sight loss despite treatment with medicines from 2 therapeutic classes
- Consider one of the following for people with COAG who cannot tolerate a pharmacological treatment:
  - A medicine from another therapeutic class (a beta-blocker, carbonic anhydrase inhibitor or sympathomimetic) **or**
  - Preservative-free eye drops if there is evidence that the person is allergic to the preservative or has clinically significant and symptomatic ocular surface disease
  - After treatment with medicines from 2 therapeutic classes, consider 360° SLT or glaucoma surgery with pharmacological augmentation (Mitomycin C)

- Offer one of the following to people with COAG whose IOP has not been reduced sufficiently to prevent the risk of progression to sight loss after glaucoma surgery:
  - Pharmacological treatment; topical medicines from different therapeutic classes may be needed at the same time to control IOP **or**
  - Further glaucoma surgery **or**
  - 360° SLT **or**
  - Cyclodiode laser treatment
- Offer one of the following to people with COAG (including advanced COAG) who prefer not to have glaucoma surgery or for whom glaucoma surgery is not suitable:
  - Pharmacological treatment; topical medicines from different therapeutic classes may be needed at the same time to control IOP **or**
  - 360° SLT **or**
  - Cyclodiode laser treatment
- Follow up:
  - If progression of COAG is not detected and IOP is not controlled, review treatment plan and reassess between 1 month and 4 months
  - If progression or uncertain progression of COAG and IOP is not controlled, review treatment plan and reassess between 1 month and 2 months
  - If no progression of COAG and low clinical risk and IOP is controlled, reassess between 12 months and 18 months
  - If no progression of COAG and high clinical risk and IOP is controlled, reassess between 6 months and 12 months
  - If progression or uncertain progression of COAG and IOP is controlled, review treatment plan and reassess between 2 months and 6 months

NICE Guidance [TA1009] [85]:

Latanoprost-netarsudil (Roclanda) is recommended as an option for reducing IOP in adults with COAG or OHT when a prostaglandin analogue alone has not reduced IOP enough, only if:

- They have then tried a fixed-dose combination treatment and it has not reduced IOP enough, ***or***
- A fixed-dose combination treatment containing beta-blockers is unsuitable

3.21 Aqueous Misdirection

3.21.1 Definition

- Posterior misdirection of aqueous into the vitreous causing anterior displacement of vitreous, ciliary processes, and lens/IOL with secondary angle closure

3.21.2 Risk Factors

- Short axial length
- Nanophthalmos
- Uveal effusion syndrome
- History of angle closure: previous acute angle closure, chronic angle closure
- Post procedures: trabeculectomy, GDI, cataract extraction, surgical iridectomy, Yag PI

3.21.3 History

- Ask about history of angle closure
- Ask about previous ocular surgeries including trabeculectomy, GDI, cataract extraction, surgical iridectomy, Yag PI

3.21.4 Examination

- Raised IOP
- Shallow/flat central (see Fig. 3.38) and peripheral AC—significant myopic shift

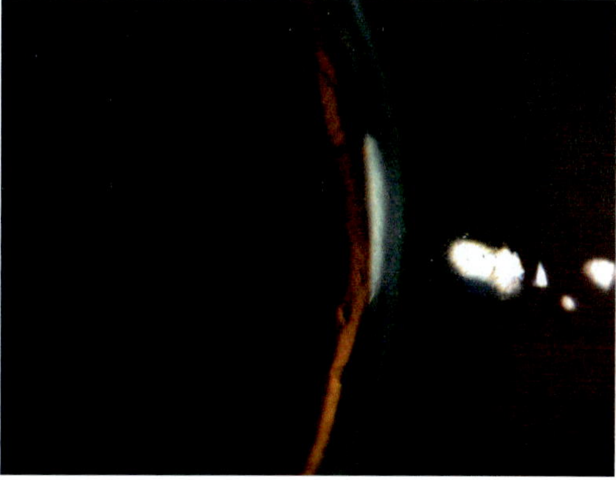

Fig. 3.38 Anterior segment image of a patient with aqueous misdirection showing a shallow central AC

- Patent PI—no iris bombe
- No suprachoroidal haemorrhage or detachments on fundus examination

3.21.5 Treatment

- Ensure patent PI before commencing treatment
- Medical:
  - Atropine
  - Reduction of IOP with systemic and topical medications
- Laser:
  - Yag laser disruption of posterior capsule (if pseudophakic) + anterior vitreous face
  - Trans-scleral cyclodiode photocoagulation of the ciliary body in 1 quadrant
- Surgical:
  - If pseudophakic: pars plana vitrectomy + posterior capsulotomy
  - If phakic: cataract extraction + posterior capsulotomy + pars plana vitrectomy

3.22 Vernal Keratoconjunctivitis (VKC) (Table 3.32)

3.22.1 Associated Diseases

- HSV keratitis
- Keratoconus
- Anterior capsular cataract

3.22.2 History

- History of atopy: eczema, hayfever, asthma

Table 3.32 Key facts about VKC

Atopic disease in which an allergic response is mounted to common environmental allergens, dust, or pollen
Usually develops in the first decade of life (82% by age 10 years with a mean age of 7 years)
More common in males
Seasonal propensity

3.22.3 Examination

- Skin of the lids may be eczematous with excoriation at the canthi +/− reactive ptosis
- Palpebral VKC: giant papillae (>1 mm diameter) giving a cobblestone appearance (see Fig. 3.39) +/− mucus accumulation between the papillae
- Limbal VKC: white Horner-Trantas dots (aggregates of degenerated eosinophils and epithelial cells) on the apices of papillae at the limbus
- Cornea:
  - Punctate epithelial erosions on the superior and central cornea with adherent mucus
  - Macroerosion: confluent area of epithelium breakdown
  - Vernal plaque (shield ulcer): deposition of calcium and mucus deposited on Bowman's layer—prevent re-epithelialisation

3.22.4 Treatment

- Inflammation:
  (a) Topical mast cell stabilisers (e.g. cromolyn sodium)/topical anti-histamines (e.g. emedastine)/topical mast cell stabilisers + anti-histamines (e.g. olopatadine, lodoxamide)
  (b) Topical corticosteroids: risk of glaucoma, ocular herpetic infection, cataract

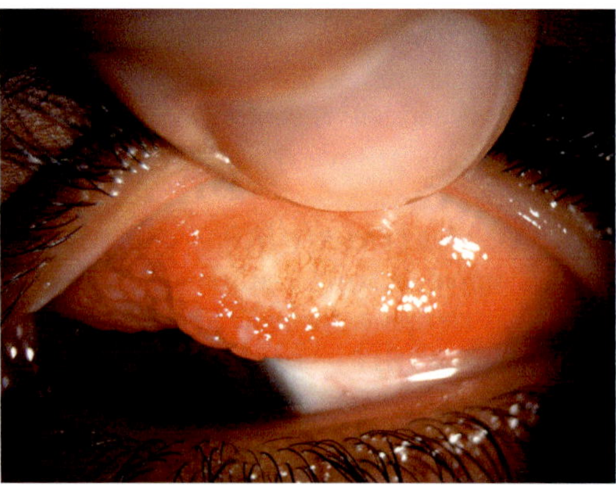

Fig. 3.39 Anterior segment image of a patient with VKC showing giant papillae

Table 3.33 Key facts of AKC

Bilateral, chronic inflammation of the conjunctiva and lids associated with atopic dermatitis
Onset of disease usually in the second through fifth decade
Male:Female ratio as 2.4:1
Consists of type I and type IV hypersensitivity reactions

(c) Topical acetylcysteine: reduces mucus adherence to the cornea during exacerbations
(d) Steroid (e.g. triamcinolone 40 mg/ml) injected into the supratarsal space after lid eversion: reserved for severe disease not responding to topical treatment or given following surgery for a vernal plaque
(e) Topical cyclosporin A: alternative to topical corticosteroid
(f) Oral steroid: reserved for severe unremitting disease with corneal complications

- Vernal plaque:
  (a) Debridement of plaque
  (b) Superficial keratectomy after the local allergic inflammatory disease has been medically controlled

3.23 Atopic Keratoconjunctivitis (AKC) (Table 3.33)

3.23.1 History

- Periocular itching associated with dermatitis
- Hx of seasonal or exposure-related exacerbations is usually present
- FHx of atopic disease in 1 or both parents
- Hx of atopy: asthma, eczema, hayfever
- Hx of CL wear: lack of CL wear aids in differentiating AKC from GPC

3.23.2 Examination

- Periocular and lid dermatitis—scaling, flaking skin with reddened base
- Loss of cilia, meibomianitis, keratinization, and punctal ectropion.
- The conjunctiva of the tarsal surfaces has a papillary reaction and possibly a pale white oedema +/− subepithelial fibrosis
- Inferior fornix shortening with symblepharon
- Perilimbal gelatinous hypertrophy +/− Horner-Trantas dots
- Punctate epithelial keratopathy, persistent epithelial defects, scarring, microbial ulceration, and neovascularisation
- Anterior or posterior subcapsular cataract.
- Signs of KC (see Sect. 8.21)

3.23.3 Investigations

- Skin testing to determine nature of the irritants
- Corneal topography if clinical signs of KC is present

3.23.4 Treatment

- Environmental control: removal of environmental irritants in both the home and the employment or school setting
- Correction of trichiasis or lid position abnormalities if contributing in any way to corneal compromise, correction of blepharitis, lubricants for dry eye
- Topical medications: anti-histamines, topical steroids (for 7–10 days)—potential for cataract or glaucoma, mast-cell stabilisers—for recommended for patients with perennial symptoms, mast cell stabilisers + antihistamines (olopatadine, azelastine, epinastine, ketotifen), ciclosporin A, tacrolimus
- Systemic medications: oral prednisolone in cases of uncontrolled dermatitis with vision threatening complications

3.23.5 Other Diagnoses to Consider

- Vernal keratoconjunctivitis (VKC)—AKC patients are usually older and have major lid involvement compared to patients with VKC

- Giant papillary conjunctivitis (GPC)—hx of CL wear
- Seasonal allergic conjunctivitis (SAC)—no or markedly diminished symptoms out of their season and show no evidence of chronic inflammation in the conjunctiva
- Perennial allergic conjunctivitis

3.24 Bacterial Keratitis

3.24.1 Risk Factors

- Ocular
  - Contact lens wear (gram negative pseudomonas is the most common cause of bacterial keratitis in CL wearers)
  - Trauma causing a corneal abrasion or epithelial defect: chemical and thermal injuries, foreign bodies, local irradiation
  - Corneal surgery: LASIK, RK, PK +/− loose sutures
  - Ocular surface disease: dry eye, bullous keratopathy, chronic keratitis (e.g. HSV), neurotrophic keratitis (e.g. HSV, HZV, tumours of the cerebellopontine angle with CN VII palsy), OCP, SJS, atopic keratoconjunctivitis
  - Lid abnormalities: entropion, lagophthalmos, trichiasis
- Systemic
  - Immunosuppression: diabetes, drugs
  - Vitamin A deficiency
- Other
  - Male sex

3.24.2 History

- Ask about risk factors for bacterial keratitis (see Sect. 3.24.1)
- For contact lens wearers, enquire about the following:
  - Type of contact lens worn
  - Duration of contact lens wear
  - Hygiene of contact lenses
  - Does the patient sleep, swim or shower with contact lens in their eyes?
  - Lifestyle: wearing of contact lenses for sports or at work
  - Purchasing of contact lenses: over the internet, from opticians

3.24.3 Examination

- Features suggestive of bacterial keratitis:
  - Suppurative stromal infiltrate (particularly those greater than 1 mm in size) with indistinct edges, oedema, and white cell infiltration in surrounding stroma
  - Epithelial defect is typically present
  - An AC reaction is often seen +/− hypopyon (see Fig. 3.40)
- Pseudomonas: stromal necrosis exhibiting a shaggy surface and adherent mucopurulent exudate

3.24.4 Investigation

- Corneal scrapes:
  - Stain: gram stain, giemsa stain, Ziehl-Neelson stain
  - Culture: blood agar, chocolate agar, Lowenstein-Jensen
- If patient wears CL—send lenses, solutions, cases for culture

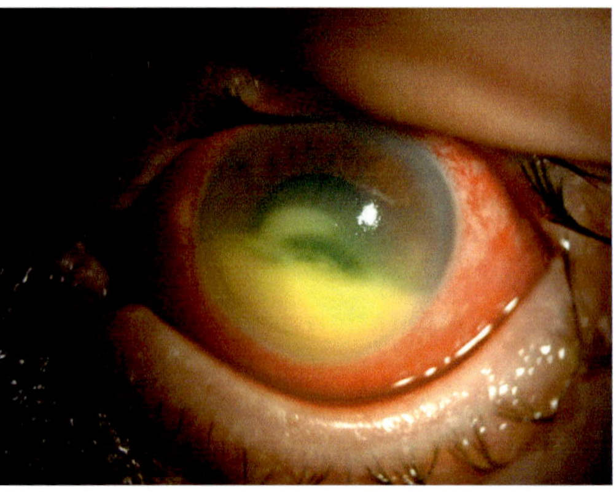

Fig. 3.40 Anterior segment image of a patient with a bacterial keratitis

3.24.5 Treatment

- Admit and daily review if:
  - Severe infection: >1.5 mm diameter infiltrate, central corneal ulcer, hypopyon
  - Poor compliance likely: either with administering drops or returning for daily review
  - Only eye
  - Failing to improve
- Stop CL wear if patient wears CL
- Medications:
  - Intensive topical broad-spectrum antibiotics
  - Cycloplegia
  - Topical corticosteroids: no difference in BCVA at 3 months [98] but corticosteroid use was associated with a mean 1-line improvement in BCVA at 12 months among patients with non-Nocardia ulcers [99]
- If an initial scrape result in no growth and current regimen proves clinically ineffective, consider withholding treatment for 12 to 24 hours before rescraping or performing a formal corneal biopsy
- Surgery:
  - Cyanoacrylate tissue adhesive: progressive corneal thinning, corneal perforation
  - Therapeutic PK: impending or overt perforation
  - Optical PK: can be used after complete resolution of the corneal infection to remove corneal scarring and to rehabilitate vision
  - Conjunctival flap: non-healing corneal ulcer

3.25 Herpes Simplex Virus (HSV) Keratitis

3.25.1 History

- History of cold sores
- History of previous attacks of HSV keratitis

3.25.2 Examination

- Epithelial keratitis (see Fig. 3.41 and Fig. 3.42)
  - Dendritic ulcer: branching linear lesion with terminal bulbs (stain with fluorescein) and raised swollen epithelial borders (negative staining with fluorescein + stain with rose bengal), lesion extends through basement membrane (true ulcer) –pseudodendrites are raised rather than ulcerated and do not stain with fluorescein
  - Geographic ulcer: non-linear enlarged dendritic ulcer, scalloped borders of swollen epithelial cells
  - Marginal ulcer: anterior stromal infiltrate with overlying ED, limbal injection with neovascularisation of the infiltrate, progresses centrally
  - Corneal vesicles: small raised clear vesicles in the epithelium
- Stromal keratitis (see Fig. 3.43)
  - Necrotising stromal keratitis: stromal infiltration with overlying epithelial defect

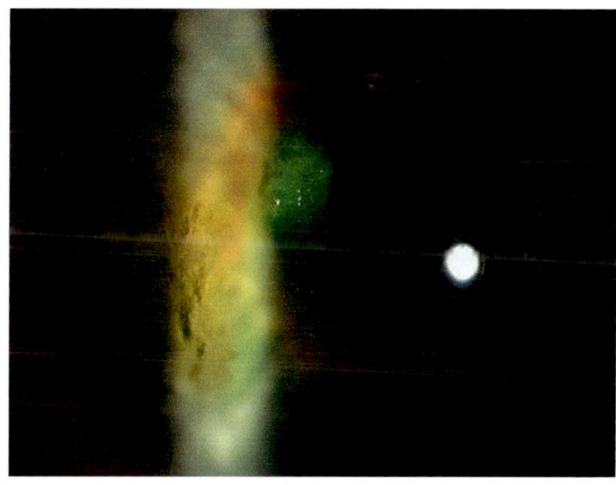

Fig. 3.41 Anterior segment image of a patient with a dendritic ulcer

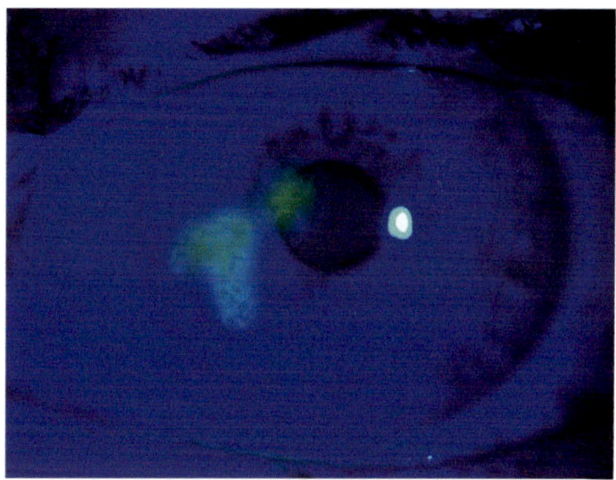

Fig. 3.42 Anterior segment image of the same patient in Fig. 3.41 showing fluorescein staining of the dendritic lesion

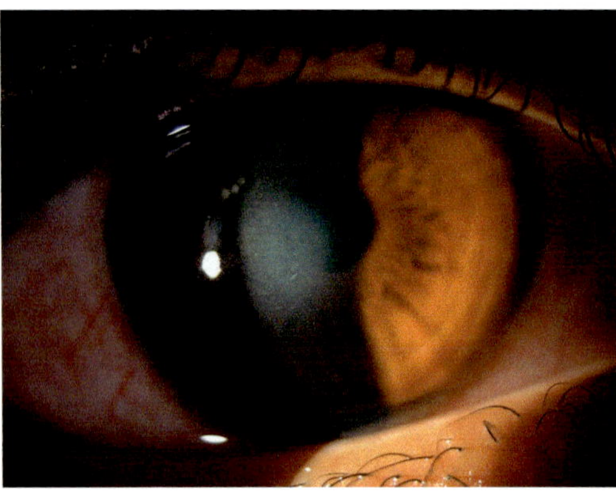

Fig. 3.43 Anterior segment image of a patient with HSV stromal keratitis

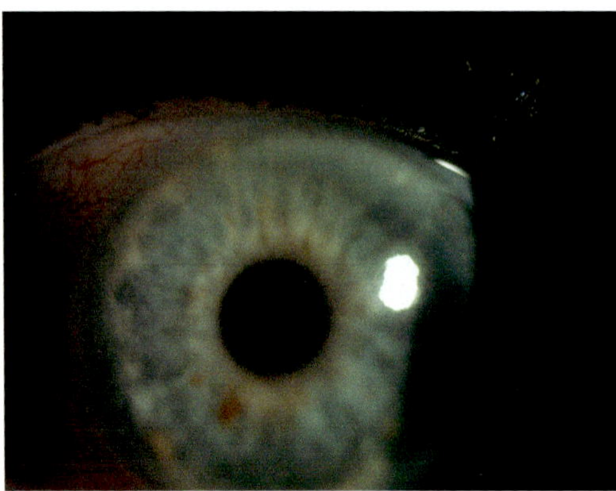

Fig. 3.44 Anterior segment image of a patient with HSV endotheliitis

  - Interstitial keratitis: stromal infiltration with intact overlying epithelium, stromal oedema, stromal neovascularisation +/− ghost vessels +/− lipid exudation
- Endotheliitis (see Fig. 3.44)
  - Disciform endotheliitis: round area of stromal +/− epithelial oedema without stromal infiltrate overlying KP's, iritis
  - Diffuse endotheliitis: diffuse stromal oedema with diffusely scattered KP's
  - Linear endotheliitis: line of KP's accompanied by stromal + epithelial oedema between the KP's and the limbus
- Iridocyclitis
  - Sectoral iris atrophy
  - Raised IOP

3.25.3 Treatment

- Epithelial keratitis
  - Topical aciclovir 3% 5x/day for 10–14 days
  - Cycloplegia
- Stromal keratitis
  - Topical corticosteroids (defer possible until epithelium intact)
  - Topical aciclovir 3% 5x/day to prevent outbreak of epithelial keratitis
  - Cycloplegia
  - Monitor IOP and treat if necessary
- Endotheliitis
  - Topical corticosteroids (defer where possible until epithelium intact)
  - Topical aciclovir 3% 5x/day to prevent outbreak of epithelial keratitis
  - Oral aciclovir 400 mg 5x/day for 7 days then 400 mg BD
  - Cycloplegia
  - Monitor IOP and treat if necessary
- Iridocyclitis
  - Topical corticosteroids
  - Oral aciclovir 400 mg 5x/day for 7 days
  - Cycloplegia
  - Monitor IOP and treat if necessary

3.25.4 Herpetic Eye Disease Study (HEDS)

- A set of multicentre RCT's designed to address 6 HSV-associated clinical questions:
  (1) Topical corticosteroids in treating stromal keratitis already on a topical antiviral [127]
    - Time to failure (new focal stromal inflammation, increase in area of inflammed cornea) comparison was highly in favour of the treatment group at 10 weeks (73% vs 26%)
    - Delaying steroid initiation does not affect visual outcome at 6 months
  (2) Oral aciclovir in treating stromal keratitis already on a topical steroid and antiviral [2]
    - Time to treatment failure at 16 weeks was not delayed significantly in the treatment group

- No benefit of adding oral aciclovir (400 mg 5X/day) in patient on topical antiviral and topical corticosteroids

(3) Oral aciclovir in treating iridocyclitis already on topical steroid [113]
- The rate ratio for the protective effect of aciclovir on time to failure at 10 weeks bordered on significant

(4) Oral aciclovir in preventing recurrence of epithelial and stromal keratitis [114]
- Aciclovir prophylaxis (400 mg BD) reduced recurrence of ocular HSV from 32% (placebo group) to 19% (aciclovir group) at 12 months
- Effect applied to both epithelial (14% to 9%) and stromal keratitis (28% to 14%)—greatest for stromal keratitis patients with at least one prior episode

(5) Demographic and disease-specific predictors of recurrent HSV keratitis [46]
- History of epithelial keratitis was not a risk factor for recurrent epithelial keratitis
- The more prior episodes of stromal keratitis, the higher the likelihood of recurrence

(6) Risk factors for recurrence of ocular HSV [45]
- Stress, systemic infection, sunlight exposure, menstruation, CL wear, and eye injury were not deemed significant

3.26 Acanthamoeba Keratitis

3.26.1 Risk Factors

- Contact lens wear: poor CL hygiene (e.g. rinsing in tap water), extended wear CL (soft—90% or rigid CL), swimming with CL insitu (ponds, hot tubs, swimming pools)
- Trauma: agricultural or rural setting

3.26.2 History

- Disproportionate incapacitating ocular pain to clinical findings
- Ask about risk factors (see Sect. 3.26.1)

3.26.3 Examination

- Radial keratoneuritis (see Fig. 3.45): represents amoebic migration along the corneal nerves (can also be seen in pseudomonas keratitis)
- Epitheliitis (flat diffuse microcystic form with perilimbal sparing) +/− epithelial ridges +/− pseudodendrites
- Anterior stromal infiltrate +/− overlying ED that progresses circumferentially to form a stromal ring infiltrate with subsequent stromal scarring
- Scleritis
- Uveitis

3.26.4 Investigations

- Corneal scrape:
  - Culture on non-nutrient agar with E. coli overlay
  - Stain with Calcofluor white (stains cysts visualised under UV light) or gram stain (stains organisms)
  - DNA detection using PCR
- If patient wears CL—send lenses, solutions, cases for culture
- Invivo confocal microscopy (IVCM):
  - Direct visualisation of cysts (high contrast round bodies—see Fig. 3.46)
- Corneal biopsy for culture if other tests negative but there is a strong suspicion of acanthamoeba keratitis

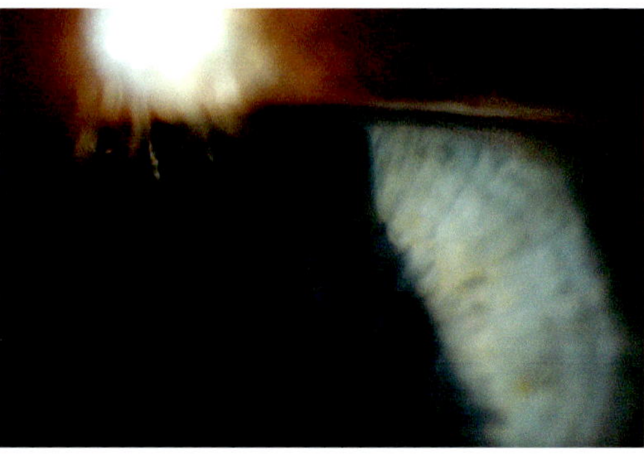

Fig. 3.45 Anterior segment image of a patient with acanthamoeba keratitis showing radial keratoneuritis

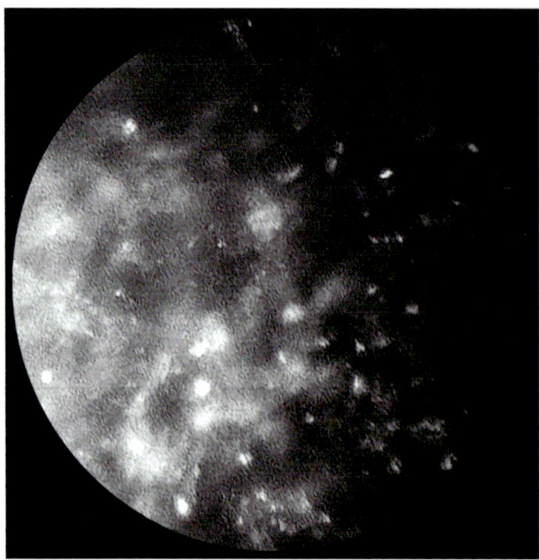

Fig. 3.46 IVCM of a patient with acanthamoeba keratitis showing high contrast round bodies suggestive of acanthamoeba cysts

3.26.5 Treatment

- Admit and daily review
- Stop CL wear if patient wears CL
- Educate patient about CL wear and hygiene
- Medical:
- Intensive topical anti-amoebic agents:
  (a) Biguanides: PHMB 0.02% or chlorhexidine 0.02%
  (b) Diamidine: propamidine 0.1% or hexamidine 0.1%
- Cyclopentolate
- Scleritis: systemic steroids +/− steroid sparing agent
- Surgical:
- Severe stromal scarring: PK an option once free of infection—3 months after discontinuation of anti-acanthamoebal medications
- Extensive stromal necrosis and impending or overt perforation: emergency PK—high risk of persistent or recurrent disease in grafted tissue
- Severe intractable pain: enucleation

3.27 Fungal Keratitis

3.27.1 Risk Factors

- Trauma involving plant matter
- Contact lens wear
- Immunosuppression: topical corticosteroids, alcoholism, diabetes, HIV positive, systemic immunosuppression
- Corneal surgery: PK, LASIK, RK
- Chronic keratitis: neurotrophic cornea (HSV, HZV, topical anaesthetic abuse), dry eye

3.27.2 History

- Ask about risk factors (see Sect. 3.27.1)

3.27.3 Examination

- Non-specific: conjunctival injection, epithelial defect, stromal infiltration, AC reaction or hypopyon
- Filamentous fungi: stromal infiltrates with irregular feathery margins, elevated edges, dry rough texture, satellite lesions (see Fig. 3.47)

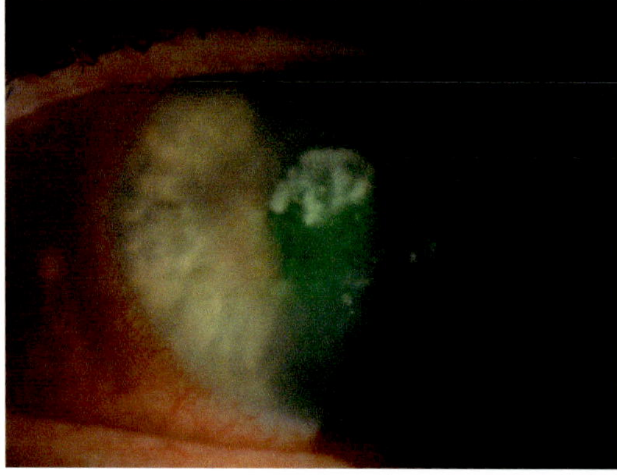

Fig. 3.47 Anterior segment image of a patient with a fungal keratitis

- Yeast: localised with "button" appearance, expanding stromal infiltrate, relatively small epithelial ulceration
- It is not always possible to differentiate clinically between bacterial and fungal keratitis, especially in cases where yeasts are the infecting fungi

3.27.4 Investigations

- Corneal scrapes
- Stains: gram stain, giemsa stain, Grocott's methenamine silver (GMS) stain
- Culture: Sabouraud's dextrose agar (for most fungi), sheep blood agar (for fusarium)
- In vivo confocal microscopy (IVCM): look for filaments (see Fig. 3.48)
- Corneal biopsy if corneal scrapings for culture are negative and there is a strong suspicion of fungal keratitis

3.27.5 Treatment

- Admit and daily review, stop CL wear if patient wears CL
- Medical treatment:
  - Topical:

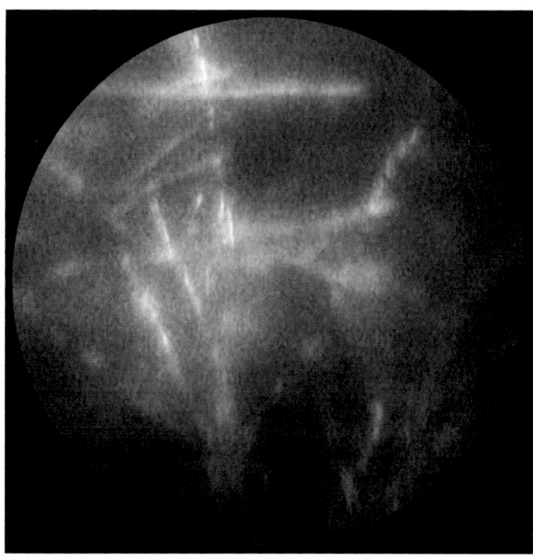

Fig. 3.48 IVCM of a patient with a fungal keratitis secondary to a filamentous fungus

    (a) Intensive topical broad spectrum antifungal agents: natamycin 5% (fusarium infection), voriconazole 1% (candidal infection), amphotericin 0.15% (candida, aspergillus): natamycin treatment is associated with significantly better clinical and microbiological outcomes than voriconazole treatment for filamentous fungal keratitis [88]
    (b) Cyclopentolate
  - Systemic:
    (a) Oral fluconazole (candida and aspergillus)
    (b) Oral voriconazole
- Visual rehabilitation after a treated fungal infection begins with spectacle correction and hard contact lenses. If these modalities fail to improve vision sufficiently—surgery
- Surgical treatment: PK in a quiet but visually compromised eye or therapeutic PK or for impending or overt perforation, conjunctival flap for a non-healing ulcer

3.28 Ectopia Lentis

3.28.1 Differential Diagnosis

- Systemic
  - Marfan syndrome (AD—fibrillin gene on chromosome 15, clinical diagnosis):
    (a) Ocular: bilateral superotemporal lens subluxation, accommodation intact, RD, glaucoma, keratoconus, high myopia, blue sclera
    (b) Musculoskeletal: arachnodactyly, disproportionately long limbed, joint laxity, high-arched palate
    (c) Cardiovascular: mitral valve prolapse, aortic dilatation, aortic regurgitation, aortic dissection
  - Weill-Marchesani syndrome (AR):
    (a) Ocular: bilateral inferonasal lens subluxation, microspherophakia, RD, high myopia
    (b) Musculoskeletal: brachydacytyly, short stature
    (c) Neurological: reduced IQ
  - Homocystinuria (AR):

(a) Ocular: bilateral inferonasal lens subluxation, myopia, glaucoma
(b) Musculoskeletal: marfanoid habitus
(c) Haematological: thromboses, especially associated with GA
(d) Neurological: reduced IQ3.28.2
- Hyperlysemia (AR)
- Sulfite oxidase deficiency (AR)
- Ehlers-Danlos syndrome (AR)

- Ocular
  - Trauma
  - PXF
  - High myopia
  - Hypermature cataract
  - Buphthalmos
  - Ciliary body tumour
  - Aniridia
  - Hereditary ectopia lentis
  - Ectopia lentis et pupillae: lens subluxation with pupil displacement in opposite direction

3.28.2 History

- History of trauma
- Positive FHx
- Cardiovascular or musculoskeletal abnormalities in patient or family

3.28.3 Examination

- Ectopia lentis (see Fig. 3.49) +/– uveitis +/– corneal decompensation +/– pupil block
- Check IOP
- Perform gonioscopy to look for angle closure
- Perform a dilated fundus examination to look for RD, signs of glaucoma
- Systemic examination

3.28.4 Investigations

- Refraction
- Cardiac evaluation (echocardiography) in Marfan's syndrome

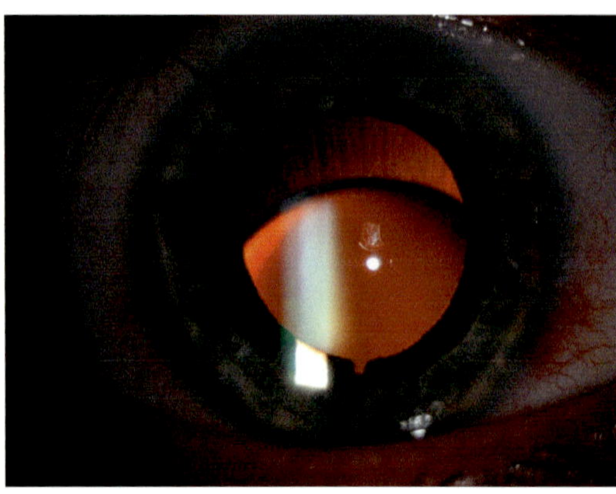

Fig. 3.49 Anterior segment image of a patient with ectopic lentis

- Plasma homocysteine level in homocystinaemia

3.28.5 Treatment

- Genetic counselling
- Vision
  (a) Correction of refractive error: spectacles, CL
  (b) Surgical: Lensectomy +/– vitrectomy with post-op aphakia correction or secondary artisan IOL, or scleral sutured PCIOL
- Ectopia lentis
  (a) Migration of lens into AC: mydriatics + lie pt on their back to permit posterior migration of lens behind the iris
  (b) Pupil block glaucoma: Yag PI and topical medications to reduce IOP
  (c) Lensectomy +/– vitrectomy +/– artisan IOL +/– scleral sutured PCIOL:
  Indications:
  - Lens induced glaucoma/uveitis
  - Lens in AC with corneal decompensation
  - Lens opacity is mature or hypermature
  - Inadequate VA not correctable by refraction
  - RD

3.29 High Myopia and Cataract Surgery

3.29.1 Preoperative Considerations

- Assess visual potential: myopic degeneration, macular holes, myopic foveoschisis, previous RD repair with silicone oil
- Discuss refractive outcome: anisometropia—less need for second eye operation if patient already wears CL
- Biometry
  - Use of IOL master rather than A-scan to measure the axial length (AL) of the eye (posterior staphyloma can generate an erroneously long axial length when measured with the A scan giving rise to a postoperative hypermetropic refractive surprise)
  - Convert speed of sound through vitreous to 987 metres/second on IOL master to measure true AL in a silicone oil (viscosity 1000 centistokes) filled eye / true AL of a silicone oil filled (viscosity 1300 centistokes) eye can be estimated from the measured AL (MAL) obtained on A/B scan US by multiplying MAL by a conversion factor of 0.71
  - Formula choice: SRK/T if axial length > 26.5 (NICE Guidance [NG77] [76])
  - IOL power choice: A constant increases as IOL power is lower, which leads to selection of a higher dioptric power implant to lessen the odds of a postoperative hyperopic surprise—select a power of IOL which leaves some residual of postoperative myopia
  - IOL material selection: avoid silicone lenses

3.29.2 Intraoperative Considerations

- Anaesthesia: retrobulbar and peribulbar anaesthesia carry the risk of perforation of the globe in a long, myopic eye
- Deeper AC: break reverse pupillary block by using the chopper to slightly tent up the iris at the pupillary margin to establish a channel for anterior-posterior fluid flow (equalise anterior and posterior chamber pressures), decrease infusion pressure by lowering bottle height (increased risk of surge)
- Increased risk of post-op RD (0.9–3.8% risk if AL > 26.0 mm): prevent collapse of the AC when removing the phaco probe or I&A probe from the eye to avoid traction or tension on the vitreous during surgery (once AC collapses, the vitreous has a tendency to move anteriorly)—inject viscoelastic via the paracentesis prior to removing the phaco probe or IA probe from the eye
- Zonular weakness: minimise nuclear manipulation to protect damaged zonules from a previously vitrectomised eye

3.29.3 Postoperative Considerations

- Floppy large bag: postop refraction can take time to stabilise due to the variation in effective lens position as the capsular bag shrinks and wraps around the IOL
- Repeat fundus exam to search for retinal breaks that may have been created during the surgery
- Timely surgery on the fellow eye (within 6 weeks) will minimise the imbalance caused by the large degree of anisometropia

3.30 Pseudoexfoliation and Cataract Surgery

3.30.1 Preoperative Considerations

- Risk of wipe out (progression of VF) to a vulnerable nerve
- Control of high IOP: risk for suprachoroidal haemorrhage
- Phacodonesis: when there is severe zonular instability, the surgeon may consider pars plana lensectomy with an ACIOL or sutured PCIOL

- Zonular dialysis: quantified by the number of clock hours involved—a capsular tension ring (CTR) can be used if 4 clock hours or less of zonule loss
- AC depth: AC depth < 2.5 mm centrally may indicate anterior displacement of the lens-iris diaphragm from zonular weakness
- Poor mydriasis: look for iris atrophy and transillumination defects

3.30.2 Intraoperative Considerations

- Pupil size: ensure adequate pupil dilation by use of intracameral injection of phenylephrine, iris stretching or iris hooks
- Avoid overinflating AC with viscoelastic causing posterior pressure on the lens can further weakening the zonules
- Capsulorrhexis: large capsulorrhexis (risk of post-op anterior capsular phimosis), provide counter traction via the non-dominant hand using a second instrument via the paracentesis (if wrinkling of the anterior capsule when piercing the anterior capsule)
- Hydrodissection: avoid overfilling of the AC causing excessive zonular stress
- Nucleus removal: for soft nuclei consider prolapsing the nucleus anteriorly, for denser nuclei consider chopping techniques
- Cortex removal: lower flow rate and maximum vacuum settings, perform circumferential removal of cortex rather than radial stripping (less stress on zonules)
- Consider insertion of CTR if up to 4 clock hours of zonular dehiscence present
- IOL insertion: IOL placed in the capsular bag—orientation of haptics towards the area of zonular loss to bolster support at the equator / IOL placed in the ciliary sulcus—orientation of haptics 90° away from the area of zonular loss

3.30.3 Postoperative Considerations

- IOP spike: acetazolamide (diamox) tablets for 3/7 postoperatively

3.31 Intraoperative Floppy Iris Syndrome (IFIS)

3.31.1 Features

- Syndrome characterised by a triad of occurrences
  - Fluttering and billowing of the iris stroma in response to normal irrigation currents
  - A propensity for the floppy iris stroma to prolapse towards the phaco and side incisions
  - Progressive pupillary constriction that occurs during the surgical procedure

3.31.2 Preoperative Considerations

- Past or present use of α1-antagonists (tamsulosin, alfuzosin, doxazosin) in the treatment of BPH and HTN

3.31.3 Intraoperative Considerations

- Pupil size: intracameral injection of phenylephrine (0.25 ml 2.5% phenylephrine mixed with 1 ml BSS—1:200 solution), iris hooks / pupil expansion devices
- Wound construction: longer incision within the clear cornea and move incisions more anteriorly into the cornea to help with flow dynamics and iris prolapse

3.32 Endothelium in Cataract Surgery

3.32.1 Endothelial Cell Counts

- 4000 cells/mm^2 at birth
- 2500 cells/mm^2 in middle age
- 2000 cells/mm^2 in old age

3.32.2 Ophthalmic Viscosurgical Devices (OVDs)

- OVDs are solutions of long chain polymers
- Dispersive OVDs:

- Lower viscosity + cause less IOP spikes (more difficult to remove from the eye)
- Uses: isolate part of surgical field e.g. protect cornea or keeping the iris or vitreous out of the way
- Examples: Viscoat (sodium chondroitin sulfate + sodium hyaluronate with molecular weight of 100-500 kDa)

- Cohesive OVDs:
  - Higher viscosity + cause higher IOP spikes (easier to remove from the eye)
  - Uses: deep AC creation, opening the bag prior to IOL implantation
  - Examples: Healon (sodium hyaluronate with molecular weight of 1000-2000 kDa), Provisc (sodium hyaluronate with molecular weight of 1000-2000 kDa), Healon GV (sodium hyaluronate with molecular weight of 4000-8000 kDa)
- Viscoadaptive OVDs:
  - Has components of both cohesive and dispersive OVDs
  - At high flow rates (e.g. phacoemulsification) it acts like a dispersive OVD and stays within the eye to protect the corneal endothelium
  - At low flow rates (e.g. I/A) it acts like a cohesive OVD for easier removal
  - Example: Healon 5 (sodium hyaluronate with molecular weight of 4000-8000 kDa)

3.32.3 Soft-Shell Technique

- Dispersive OVD to protect the corneal endothelium
- Cohesive OVD to maintain the AC space

3.32.4 Ultimate Soft-Shell Technique

- Viscoadaptive OVD + Basic Salt Solution

3.32.5 Irrigating Solutions

- Basic Salt Solution
  - Composition per 1 ml: sodium and potassium chloride, calcium chloride dehydrate, magnesium chloride hexahydrate, sodium acetate trihydrate, sodium citrate dehydrate, sodium hydroxide, hydrochloric acid
- Basic Salt Solution Plus
  - Has been shown to minimise endothelial pleomorphism and polymegathism though Invivo studies
  - Part I: 480 ml solution in a 500 ml single dose bag to which the part II concentrate is added. Each ml of part I contains (5 salts and a buffer): sodium and potassium chloride, dibasic sodium phosphate, sodium bicarbonate, hydrochloric acid, sodium hydroxide
  - Part II: sterile concentrate in a 20 ml single dose vial for addition to part I. Each ml of part II contains: calcium chloride dehydrate, magnesium chloride hexahydrate, dextrose (energy source), glutathione disulfide (antioxidant)

3.33 Endophthalmitis (Table 3.34)

3.33.1 Other Diagnoses to Consider

- Toxic anterior segment syndrome (TASS)
  - Acute post-operative non-infectious inflammatory reaction due to inadvertent entry of toxic substances in the AC
  - Rapid onset: 12–24 hours post-surgery
  - Mild/moderate or no pain
  - Corneal oedema (limbus to limbus) with moderate-to-severe AC inflammation +/− fibrin/hypopyon, raised IOP

Table 3.34 Key facts about endophthalmitis

National rate of post cataract surgery endophthalmitis was 0.14% in the BOSU study [53] and 0.055% in the Bolton study [54]
Acute post-operative endophthalmitis: usually 3–5 days after ocular surgery
Chronic post-operative endophthalmitis: usually 6 weeks after ocular surgery
White plaque on posterior capsule suggest Propionobacterium acnes infection
Current advice is to continue with the local arrangements for preventative treatment of endophthalmitis if audited figures reveal a rate similar to the Bolton study. If figures are higher, the use of intracameral cefuroxime should be considered

  - Vitritis is rare
  - Highly sensitive to topical steroids
- Occult retention of lens cortex or nucleus
- Hypopyon uveitis (e.g. Behcet's)
- Inflammatory reaction to intravitreal drug

3.33.2 Investigations

- B-scan
  - Indication: significant media opacification prevents adequate view of the fundus
  - Findings: dispersed vitreous opacities with vitritis, chorioretinal thickening
  - Rule out RD or choroidals, dislocated lens material, retained foreign bodies

3.33.3 Treatment of Acute Endophthalmitis

- Admit
- If VA hand motion (HM) or better
  - Perform a vitreous needle tap (27G needle attached to a TB syringe) +/− AC tap (30G needle attached to a TB syringe) with simultaneous injection of intravitreal antibiotics (vancomycin 1 mg/0.1 mL + amikacin 0.4 mg/0.1 mL or ceftazidime 1 mg/0.1 mL)
  - Oral ciprofloxacin 750 mg BD: no evidence of clinical benefit
  - Corticosteroids: topical (e.g dexamethasone 0.1% hourly), systemic (e.g. oral prednisolone 1 mg/kg OD rapidly reducing to zero over 7–10 days): no evidence it improves VA and should be avoided in fungal infections
  - If failure to respond at 48–72 hours consider repeating needle vitreous tap +/− AC tap with simultaneous injection of intravitreal antibiotics (repeat intravitreal antibiotics may increase the risk of retinal toxicity)
- If VA light perception (LP) or worse
  - Pars plana vitrectomy (PPV) with intravitreal injection of antibiotics:
    In the Endopthalmitis Vitrectomy Study [28]), patients with postop endophthalmitis within 6 weeks of cataract surgery who presented with LP only VA has a significant threefold improved chance of obtaining 6/12 vision after immediate vitrectomy compared to tap and inject
  - Oral ciprofloxacin 750 mg BD: no evidence of clinical benefit. Potential resistance from pseudomonas and gram-positive cocci organisms
  - Corticosteroids: topical (e.g dexamethasone 0.1% hourly), systemic (e.g. oral prednisolone 1 mg/kg OD rapidly reducing to zero over 7–10 days): no evidence it improves VA and should be avoided in fungal infections
  - If failure to respond at 48–72 hours consider repeating needle vitreous tap +/− AC tap with simultaneous injection of intravitreal antibiotics (repeat intravitreal antibiotics may increase the risk of retinal toxicity)

3.33.4 Prevention

- Pre-operative
  - Identification and treatment of blepharitis, conjunctivitis, mucocele or chronic dacryocystitis before elective surgery is performed
  - Avoidance of intraocular procedures in patients with significant active non-ocular infections
- Intra-operative
  - Skin and conjunctival preparation with 5% povidone iodine 5 minutes before op
  - Eyelid speculum and careful draping to eliminate eyelashes from surgical field
  - Suturing of any leaking wounds at the completion of the operation
  - Avoidance of serious intraoperative complications such as PCR and vitreous loss and avoidance of overly prolonged surgery
  - Intracameral cefuroxime (1 mg in 0.1 ml) at the completion of cataract surgery:
    ESCRS study [29]: five-fold decrease in incidence of postoperative endophthalmitis with intracameral cefuroxime compared with topical levofloxacin

NICE Guidance [NG77] [76]: recommends use of intracameral cefuroxime during cataract surgery to prevent endophthalmitis
- Post-operative
  - Topical antibiotics

3.33.5 Prognosis

- Prognosis depends on organism (e.g. poor prognosis with pseudomonas, staphylococcus aureus and streptococcus pneumoniae), patient factors (e.g. diabetes, advanced age, post complicated cataract surgery), time to intravitreal injection

3.34 The RCOphth Ophthalmic Services Guidance on Managing an Outbreak of Post-operative Endophthalmitis 2016 [122]

3.34.1 Outbreak Definition

- More than 1 case in a short time frame e.g. days to weeks

3.34.2 Determine if there is an Outbreak

- Incident report all cases
- Review cases for risk and causes with particular concern if:
  - Analysis of the cases demonstrate a common organism especially an unusual organism
  - Analysis of the cases demonstrates the same apparent underlying cause of concern
  - Analysis of the cases demonstrates the cases related clearly to only one team member, one surgeon, one theatre/site, one session in the week, a particular instrument or consumables batch number
  - 2 or more cases have arisen during the same theatre list
  - Cluster occurring over a very short time frame e.g. days to weeks
- Regularly assess incidence
- Use agreed system as cut off for action

3.34.3 Notification

- Notify/involve colleagues: ophthalmology, risk team, microbiology, infection control, management (clinical and medical director)
- Make patients aware of symptoms and provide easy emergency postop access
- Consider resuming early follow up

3.34.4 Immediate Measures

- Consider cessation of all surgery/procedures
- Cease bilateral simultaneous cataract surgery if performed
- Ensure all know and follow current prophylaxis regime

3.34.5 Investigation

- Review cases and check all aspects for risks and common factors:
  - Patient factors—blepharitis, diabetes, concurrent systemic illness, vitreous loss, postop wound leak, duration of surgery, non-compliance with prescribed drops
  - Surgeon factors: surgical and draping technique
- Check theatre environment, cleanliness, airflow/ventilation system
- Microbiological sampling of intraocular tap samples (looking for a common organism or subtype), equipment, theatre, drugs, irrigating and viscoelastic solutions
- Review and obey theatre discipline and correct operating practices
- Ensure equipment/devices up to date, used properly, maintained well
- Check instrument cleaning and sterilisation procedures

- Keep detailed records of investigations and actions
- Eliminate specific cause if found
- If specific cause not found:
  - Revise and improve current prophylaxis protocol
  - Introduce intracameral antibiotics
  - Consider external review from other unit or College

3.35 Idiopathic Intracranial Hypertension (IIH) (Table 3.35)

3.35.1 Differential Diagnosis of Disc Swelling

- Pseudopapilloedema
  - Features:
    No disc hyperaemia, no dilation of surface microvasculature, no blurring of retinal vessels at the disc margin
  - Causes:
    Optic disc drusen
    Myelinated peripapillary nerve fibers: dense white opacity
    Tilted discs
    Hypermetropic discs
    Myopic discs
- Papilloedema
  - Features:
    Patients retain good visual function (VA, VF, colour vision) until late in disease course regardless of how swollen the nerve appears
    Bilateral disc swelling
  - Causes:
    Raised intracranial pressure (ICP)

Table 3.35 Key facts about IIH

The syndrome of increased ICP without ventriculomegaly or mass lesion, and with normal CSF composition
Diagnosis of exclusion
Obesity is the major risk factor

- Local disc swelling
  - Causes:
    Inflammatory: optic neuritis, uveitis, scleritis
    Vascular: AION, CRVO, diabetic papillitis
    Granulomatous: TB, sarcoid
    Infiltrative: leukaemia, lymphoma
    Trauma causing hypotony
    Tumours of optic nerve: optic nerve sheath meningioma, glioma
    Hereditary: LHON
    Iatrogenic: surgery causing hypotony

3.35.2 Causes of Raised ICP

- Mass effect: tumours, haemorrhage, trauma—oedema, haematoma
- Increased CSF production: choroid plexus tumour
- Reduced CSF drainage: IIH
- Drugs ("I LOVE PTC"): isotretinoin, lithium, OCP, vitamin A derivatives, endocrine (synthetic growth hormone), prednisolone withdrawal, tetracyclines, cyclophosphamide
- Haematological: cerebral venous sinus thrombosis
- Endocrine: Addison's disease, hypoparathyroidism, obesity

3.35.3 Terminology

- Primary pseudotumor cerebri
  - IIH: includes patients with obesity, recent weight gain, polycystic ovarian syndrome, and thin children
- Secondary pseudotumor cerebri
  - Cerebral venous abnormalities:
    Cerebral venous sinus thrombosis
    Bilateral jugular vein thrombosis or surgical ligation
    Middle ear or mastoid infection
    Increased right heart pressure
    Superior vena cava syndrome
    Arteriovenous fistula

Decreased CSF absorption from previous intracranial infection or subarachnoid hemorrhage
Hypercoagulable states
- Medications and exposures
Antibiotics: tetracycline, minocycline, doxycycline, nalidixic acid, sulfa drugs
Vitamin A and retinoids: hypervitaminosis A, isotretinoin, all-trans retinoic acid for promyelocytic leukaemia, excessive liver ingestion
Hormones: human growth hormone, thyroxine (in children), leuprorelin acetate, levonorgestrel, anabolic steroids
Withdrawal from chronic corticosteroids
Lithium
Chlordecone
- Medical conditions
Endocrine disorders: Addison disease, Hypoparathyroidism
Hypercapnia: sleep apnoea, Pickwickian syndrome
Anaemia
Renal failure
Turner syndrome
Down syndrome

3.35.4 Criteria for Diagnosis of IIH

- Revised diagnostic criteria for the pseudotumor cerebri syndrome in adults and children [35]
  1. Required for diagnosis of pseudotumor cerebri syndrome:
     - A diagnosis of pseudotumor cerebri syndrome is definite if the patient fulfils criteria A-E. The diagnosis is considered probable if criteria A-D are met but the measure CSF pressure is lower than specified for a definite diagnosis
       A. Papilledema
       B. Normal neurologic examination except for cranial nerve abnormalities
       C. Neuroimaging: normal brain parenchyma without evidence of hydrocephalus, mass, or structural lesion and no abnormal meningeal enhancement on MRI, with or without gadolinium, for typical patients (female and obese), and MRI, with and without gadolinium, and magnetic resonance venography for others; if MRI is unavailable or contraindicated, contrast-enhanced CT may be used
       D. Normal CSF composition
       E. Elevated lumbar puncture opening pressure (at least 250 mm CSF in adults and at least 280 mm CSF in children [250 mm CSF if the child is not sedated and not obese]) in a properly performed lumbar puncture
  2. Diagnosis of pseudotumour cerebri without papilledema:
     - In the absence of papilledema, a diagnosis of pseudotumor cerebri syndrome can be made if B-E from above are satisfied, and in addition the patient has a unilateral or bilateral sixth nerve palsy
     - In the absence of papilledema or sixth nerve palsy, a diagnosis of pseudotumor cerebri syndrome can be suggested but not made if B-E from above are satisfied, and in addition at least 3 of the following neuroimaging criteria are satisfied:
       I. Empty sella
       II. Flattening of the posterior aspect of the globe
       III. Distension of the perioptic subarachnoid space with or without a tortuous optic nerve
       IV. Transverse venous sinus stenosis
- IIH: consensus guidelines on management [64]
  A. Papilloedema
  B. Normal neurological examination (except CN VI palsy)
  C. Neuroimaging: normal brain parenchyma (no hydrocephalus, mass, structural lesion or meningeal enhancement). Venous thrombosis excluded in all
  D. Normal CSF constituents

  - Topiramate and furosemide can be considered if patients are intolerant to acetazolamide or if acetazolamide is ineffective
- Surgical:
  - Optic nerve sheath fenestration: for progressive visual loss despite maximally tolerated medical therapy
  - CSF diversion procedure (lumboperitoneal or ventriculoperitoneal shunt): for intractable headache despite maximally tolerated medical therapy

3.36 Septo-Optic Dysplasia (De Morsier Syndrome)

3.36.1 Risk Factors for Optic Nerve Hypoplasia

- Young maternal age
- Maternal drug (LSD) and alcohol abuse (fetal alcohol syndrome) during pregnancy
- Exposure to sodium valproate or phenytoin during pregnancy
- Maternal diabetes: superior segmental optic nerve hypoplasia (topless disc syndrome—superior entrance of central retinal vessels, superior disc pallor)

3.36.2 Examination

- Optic nerve hypoplasia (subnormal number of optic nerve axons with normal mesodermal elements and glial supporting tissue): small optic nerves with crowded vessels and a pale ring around the nerve (double ring sign—inner ring is the abnormal extension of the retina and RPE over the outer portion of the lamina cribrosa, outer ring is the consists of the normal junction between sclera and lamina cribrosa—see Fig. 3.51)

3.36.3 Investigations

- Bloods: hypopituitarism (GH, TSH, ACTH, ADH deficiency)

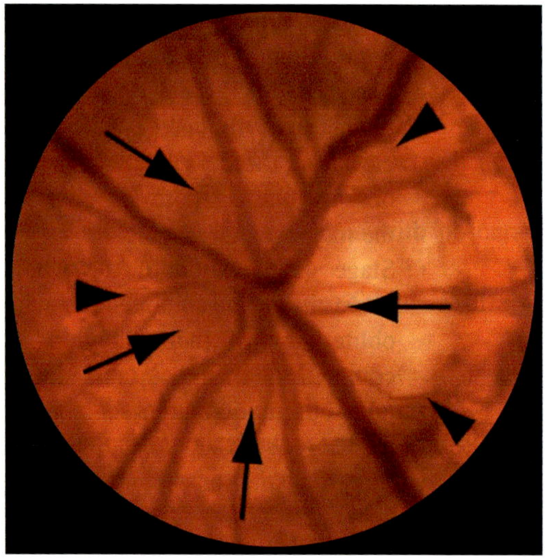

Fig. 3.51 Colour fundus image of a patient with optic nerve hypoplasia showing the double ring sign. Black arrows show the inner ring and the black arrowheads show the outer ring

- MRI head and orbit: midline abnormalities—absent septum pellucidum and agenesis or thinning of corpus callosum

3.36.4 Treatment

- Refer to endocrinologists for hormonal supplementation
- Visual impairment registration

3.37 Tobacco-Alcohol Amblyopia

3.37.1 Pathophysiology

- Both smoking and alcohol can cause B12 deficiency. B12 and B9 (folate) deficiencies lead to increased formic acid production, which impairs the electron transport chain (mitochondrial oxidative phosphorylation). This leads to ATP deficiency, thus causing optic neuropathy
- Abuse of tobacco can lead to increased levels of cyanide in the body, which can impair the electron transport chain similarly to that of formic acid. Tobacco can also be toxic by

causing disturbances in the metabolism of the vitamin B complex and by impairing vitamin B12 absorption

- Tobacco and alcohol act synergistically to cause optic nerve damage via a disease referred to as "tobacco-alcohol amblyopia". The theoretical mechanism of this disease is based on the decreased consumption of vitamin B12 from alcohol abuse combined with the decreased absorption of B12 from tobacco use leading to severely low levels of this vitamin in the body

3.37.2 Differential Diagnosis

- Toxic optic neuropathy
  - Drugs: vigabatrin, ethambutol, amiodarone, isoniazid, lead, methanol
- Inflammatory optic neuropathy
  - Typical / atypical optic neuritis
  - Sarcoidosis
  - Vasculitis e.g. SLE, PAN
- Inherited
  - LHON: VA typically 6/60—HM
  - Kjer syndrome
  - Behr syndrome
  - Wolfram syndrome (DIDMOAD)
- Compressive/infiltrate optic neuropathy

3.37.3 History

- Symptoms:
  - Subacute, painless, bilateral progressive central vision loss
  - Colour desaturation (red desaturation)
  - Isolated numbness or paraesthesia
  - Gait abnormalities
  - Psychiatric or cognitive symptoms
- Alcohol abuse with malnourishment—caloric needs from alcohol. Which is lacking in the vitamin B complex—chronic alcohol abuse leads to systemic deficiencies in B1, B9, and B12
- Smoking
- FHx: inherited optic atrophy
- DHx: toxic optic neuropathy

3.37.4 Examination

- Bilateral decreased VA (typically 6/9–6/60) due to preferential damage to the papillomacular bundle
- Reduced colour vision
- Sluggish pupil reactions; however, there may be no RAPD VF demonstrate bilateral central or cecocentral scotomas
- Optic discs may look normal initially or slight hyperaemic, progressing to temporal pallor over time
- Rule out any signs of intraocular inflammation

3.37.5 Investigations

- Bloods: vitamin B1 (thiamine), B2 (riboflavin), B3 (niacin or nicotinamide), B6 (pyridoxine), folate (B9), B12 (cobalamin)

3.37.6 Treatment

- Abstain from alcohol
- Abstain from tobacco
- Supplement deficient vitamins, specifically B12 (IM injections) and folate (oral)
- Pabrinex:
  - Indication: prophylaxis and treatment (to prevent irreversible Korsakoff's syndrome—reduced ability to acquire new memories) of Wernicke's encephalopathy (thiamine deficiency with triad of confusion, ataxia with wide spaced gait, ophthalmoplegia or nystagmus)
  - Contents: vitamins B and C (B1, B2, B3, B6, ascorbic acid)

3.38 Optic Atrophy in Infancy and Childhood

3.38.1 Causes

- Unilateral (other eye clinically normal with normal ERG/VEPs)

  - Tumour compression anterior to chiasm: optic nerve glioma—fusiform enlargement of optic nerve on MRI scan
  - Tumour infiltration anterior to chiasm: leukaemia
  - Trauma
  - Leber's hereditary optic neuropathy (LHON) before other eye affected (other eye usually affected within 2 months)
  - Glaucoma
- Bilateral +/− nystagmus
  - Severe hypoxia
  - Hereditary optic neuropathies (LHON, ADOA—Kjer syndrome, AROA—Behr syndrome, Wolfram syndrome [AR]—DIDMOAD)
  - Tumour: glioma of the optic chiasm, craniopharyngioma
  - Increased ICP: congenital hydrocephalus, IIH
  - Optic neuritis
  - Toxic or nutritional optic neuropathy: drugs, avitaminosis
  - Neurometabolic

3.38.2 History

- History of birth (prematurity with IVH) or perinatal problems (whether child had to be in an incubator, have added oxygen, be ventilated, or had any difficulty in breathing, episodes of bradycardia or apnoea, resuscitation): perinatal asphyxia
- FHx of poor vision: hereditary optic neuropathy (LHON, ADOA, optic nerve gliomas in NF-1) or retinal dystrophies
- History of diabetes and hearing loss
- Headaches, vomiting: raised ICP
- History of trauma: traumatic optic neuropathy
- Sudden visual loss:
  - With pain: optic neuritis, infiltrations (leukaemia)
  - Without pain: LHON—peripapillary telangiectasia, NMO
- History of toxic drugs (anti-TB agents e.g. ethambutol, systemic antibiotics e.g. linezolid, immunomodulatory agents e.g. infliximab), malnutrition (anorexia nervosa): toxic / nutritional optic neuropathy
- History of seizures: hereditary degenerative diseases
- History of other systemic disorders: syndromic optic neuropathy
- Any photophobia, blepharospasm, buphthalmos: congenital glaucoma

3.38.3 Examination

- Optic nerve function: VA, RAPD, colour vision (blue-yellow tritanopia of ADOA)
- Check for proptosis (axial for optic nerve glioma)
- Check IOP and measure the horizontal corneal diameter: glaucoma
- Examine parents and siblings: hereditary optic neuropathy (LHON, ADOA)
- Full systemic examination including dermatological (NF-1) and neurological

3.38.4 Investigations

- VF (age ≥ 5 years old): central or cecocentral scotomas for LHON or toxic/nutritional optic neuropathies
- MRI head/orbits: exclude tumours
- ERG: exclude a primary retinal disease (even if the retina appears normal)
- VEP: delayed with abnormal amplitude and waveform in the acute stage of optic neuritis
- Bloods: glucose, vitamin B1 (thiamine), B2 (riboflavin), B6 (pyridoxine), B12, folic acid levels
- Raised ICP: LP
- LHON: Mitochondrial DNA analysis for mutations (11,778, 14,484, 3460)

3.38.5 Treatment

- Treat the underlying cause
  - Nutritional optic neuropathy: Oral vitamin supplementation
  - Toxic optic neuropathy: stop drugs
  - Optic nerve glioma:
    - (a) Observation: isolated optic nerve involvement distant from the chiasm, good vision, non-disfiguring proptosis
    - (b) Surgical excision: reduced vision, pain, severe proptosis, posterior spread threatening the chiasm
    - (c) Chemotherapy / radiotherapy: chiasmal or midbrain involvement
- Visual impairment registration

3.39 Giant Cell Arteritis (GCA)

3.39.1 History

- Symptoms: abrupt onset headaches (usually unilateral in the temporal area), scalp tenderness/hyperaesthesia, jaw or tongue claudication, visual symptoms (diplopia, reduced colour vision, reduced VA—transient or permanent), constitutional symptoms (fever, weight loss, loss of appetite), vascular claudication of the limbs, pain and stiffness of the shoulder and hip girdles
- History of comorbidities and medications that might predispose to glucocorticoid-related adverse events: infection, hypertension, diabetes, osteoporosis, low-trauma fracture, dyslipidaemia, peptic ulcer, psychiatric adverse events
- Features that may suggest alternative diagnosis e.g. neurological deficits, very severe constitutional symptoms or localised ear, nose and throat signs

3.39.2 Examinations

- Abnormal superficial temporal artery: tenderness, nodularity or reduced/absent pulsation
- RAPD suggesting AION or CRAO
- CN III, IV, VI palsy

3.39.3 Investigations

- Bloods [60]:
  - Laboratory markers of inflammation (measures of activity of GCA): FBC (anaemia, thrombocytosis), raised CRP, raised ESR
  - Baseline laboratory tests of major organ system function: plasma glucose, renal and liver function tests, calcium and alkaline phosphatase
- Consider serum protein electrophoresis and urine Bence-Jones protein/serum free light chains if ESR elevated out of proportion to CRP [60]
- Screening tests for risk of serious infection (may include urine dipstick, CXR, tests for latent TB according to local or national protocol)
- Screening tests for osteoporosis risk (may include TSH, vitamin D, bone density test [DXA])
- Temporal artery duplex US: hypoechoic halo due to vessel wall oedema in temporal arteries, positive for over 2 weeks post-steroid initiation
- Temporal artery biopsy: samples should be at least 1 cm in length [60], aim for within 1 week but sample can remain positive for 2–6 weeks after the commencement of treatment
  - Consent: risks—visible scarring, haematoma, wound infection, scalp or skin necrosis, facial nerve injury, cerebral infarction
  - Procedure:
    Map the artery by palpation or US doppler (mark skin overlying the artery)
    Hair removal for good surgical exposure
    Clean the skin and inject local anaesthetic
    Skin incision
    Blunt dissection to artery—artery lies superficially in the superficial temporalis fascia
    Tie the proximal and distal end of the artery with 4/0 silk or Vicryl before cutting
    Close subcutaneous tissue with 5/0 interrupted Vicryl and skin closure with a running 6/0 Vicryl subcuticular suture
    Compression bandage for 24 hours

- High resolution 3 T MRI of the cranial arteries: can be used if neither vascular ultrasound nor biopsy is possible
- CXR: every 2 years in patients with large vessel GCA

3.39.4 Interpretation of Investigations

- Bloods
  - ESR (upper limit in women: age+10/2, upper limit in men: age/2): can be raised in patients with anaemia
- TAB
  - Length of specimen biopsied should be documented and known in order to be able to interpret findings correctly
  - TAB may be negative in some patients. Patients should be regarded as having GCA if there is a typical clinical picture and response to glucocorticosteroids. If features considered atypical or alternative explanations are available and TAB is negative, rapid glucocorticosteroid tapering (within 2 weeks).

3.39.5 Treatment

British Society for Rheumatology Guideline [60]

- Glucocorticoid therapy:
  - High dose glucocorticosteroid therapy should be initiated immediately when clinical suspicion of GCA is raised
  - Starting dosages:

    GCA in the absence of ischaemic visual manifestations: 40–60 mg oral prednisolone per day—vast majority of patients with GCA respond symptomatically within 1–7 days to a 40–60 mg daily dose of prednisolone, apart from irreversible sequelae such as established visual loss, stroke or tissue necrosis

    GCA in the presence of ischaemic visual manifestations (acute or intermittent visual loss): 500 mg to 1 g of IV methylprednisolone for 3 consecutive days before commencing oral prednisolone therapy. If IV therapy is not immediately possible, this should not delay initiation of oral prednisolone. If IV glucocorticoid therapy is not possible, 60–100 mg oral prednisolone may be given for up to 3 consecutive days
  - Tapering regime:

    Glucocorticoid dose should be tapered to zero over 12–18 months, providing there is no return of GCA symptoms, signs or laboratory markers of inflammation. A more rapid dose reduction is appropriate for patients at high risk of glucocorticoid toxicity and/or those receiving concomitant glucocorticoid-sparing therapy

    Initial dose of prednisolone continued until symptoms and laboratory abnormalities resolve (usually 3–4 weeks)

    Reduce dose by 10 mg every 2 weeks to 20 mg

    Reduce dose by 2.5 mg every 2–4 weeks to 10 mg

    Reduce dose by 1 mg every 2–3 months providing there is no relapse

    One week after any change in dose, review the person to exclude any relapse of symptoms (it may be possible to do this by telephone)
  - Proton pump inhibitors
  - Recommended for GI protection (risk of GI bleed from corticosteroids and aspirin)
  - Osteoporosis prophylaxis
  - Follow up:

    Weeks 0, 1, 3, 6, then months 3, 6, 9, 12 in the first year

    Arrange routine reviews a week after any change in dose

    After the first year, the person should be seen every 3–6 months (with extra visits for relapses or adverse events)
  - Low dose aspirin if there are no contraindications:

    People with GCA are at risk of developing ischaemic cranial complications (vision loss, CVA). Evidence indicates that low-dose aspirin may protect against these events

- Methotrexate:
  - Methotrexate might be considered for GCA, in combination with a glucocorticoid taper, in patients at high risk of glucocorticoid toxicity or who relapse
- Tocilizumab:
  - Giant-Cell Arteritis Actemra (GiACTA) trial [101]: tocilizumab with a tapering course of glucocorticosteroids was more effective than glucocorticosteroids alone at increasing the proportion of patients sustaining remission and time to first flare up at 52 weeks
  - NICE Guidance [TA518] [77]: when used with a tapering course of glucocorticosteroids (and when used alone after glucocorticosteroids), is recommended as an option for treating GCA in adults only if:
    They have relapsing or refractory disease
    They have not already had tocilizumab
    Tocilizumab is stopped after 1 year of uninterrupted treatment at most

3.39.6 Complications

- Second eye involvement is 10% if treated and 95% if untreated
- Vascular: thoracic aortic aneurysms, TIA/CVA, MI
- Death

3.40 Comitant Esotropia (ET)

3.40.1 Other Diagnoses to Consider

- Type 1 Duane's syndrome: limitation of abduction, globe retraction in adduction
- Congenital CN VI palsy: limitation of abduction
- Convergence spasm: intermittent spasm of convergence, of miosis, and of accommodation, high myopia on dry retinoscopy accompanying the failure of abduction—treatment options include cycloplegia and bifocals

3.40.2 Classification of Comitant ET

- Primary ET
  (a) Accommodative ET:
    - Refractive fully accommodative ET
    - Refractive partially accommodative ET
    - Non-refractive convergence excess ET with high AC/A ratio
  (b) Non-accommodative ET:
    - Constant:
      Starting <6 months: infantile ET
      Starting >6 months: basic ET—muscle surgery
    - Variable with distance:
      Distance fixation only: distance ET (divergence insufficiency)—orthoptic exercises initially
      Near fixation only: non-accommodative convergence excess—muscle surgery
- Secondary sensory ET
- Consecutive ET

3.40.3 Infantile ET

Definition:
- Infantile esotropia is a constant non-accommodative ET with onset before 6 months of age in a neurologically normal child

Examination:
- The angle is >30PD with mild or no amblyopia (alternate fixation) and mild hyperopia
- Full extraocular motility: can elicit by monocular occlusion or performing a doll's head manoeuvre
- Dissociated vertical deviation (DVD): eye elevates and extorts and is not associated with a corresponding downwards movement of the other eye when fixation is resumed—can occur spontaneously or when the eye is occluded
- Inferior oblique overaction (IOOA): visible in adduction only and is associated with fundus

excyclotorsion, if the eye elevates in adduction and there is a corresponding hypodeviation in the opposite eye the deviation is due to IOOA
- Latent nystagmus: horizontal jerk nystagmus that occurs on monocular occlusion, fast phase toward the uncovered eye (fixing eye), nystagmus lessened in adduction and worsened in abduction
- Optokinetic asymmetry: greater sensitivity to objects moving from temporal to nasal than from nasal to temporal
- Normal anterior/posterior segment examination

Investigations
- Cycloplegic refraction

Treatment
- Full hypermetropic correction if hyperopia ≥2.5D
- Treat any amblyopia present: atropine penalisation or patching
- Muscle surgery (before age 2—better stereopsis outcomes): bilateral MR recession, unilateral MR recession and LR resection, IO recession or myectomy for IOOA

3.40.4 Accomodative ET

Definition:
- Accommodative ET describes an ET caused in whole, or in part, by the use of accommodation to clear vision in the presence of uncorrected hypermetropia

Classification
- Refractive fully accommodative ET
  - Equal distance and near deviation
  - ET resolves with full hypermetropic correction
- Refractive partially accommodative ET
  - Equal distance and near deviation
  - ET partially resolves with full hypermetropic correction
- Non-refractive accommodative convergence excess ET
  - Near ET
  - Little or no ET at distance
  - Deviation at least 10PD more at near than at distance

Examination
- Full extraocular motility +/− IOOA
- Normal anterior/posterior segment examination
- Determine AC/A ratio based on near-distance discrepancy (≥10PD)

Investigations
- Cycloplegic refraction: hypermetropia ≥2.5D

Treatment
- Refractive error correction
  - Full hypermetropic correction
  - Myopic correction if > −3.0D
  - Executive bifocals (+3.00 near add) + full hypermetropic correction for non-refractive accommodative convergence excess ET
- Miotics: phospholine iodide—non-refractive accommodative convergence excess ET
- Treat any amblyopia present: atropine penalisation or patching
- Muscle surgery (for potential BSV or cosmesis when eyes not aligned adequately with glasses): bilateral MR recession

3.41 Comitant Exotropia (XT)

3.41.1 Other Diagnoses to Consider

- Sensory XT: abnormal anterior/posterior segment
- Type 2 Duane's syndrome: limitation of adduction, globe retraction in adduction
- Convergence insufficiency: near point of convergence greater than age for normal, no manifest deviation but may be exophoric for near—treatment options include full myopic correction, convergence exercises (e.g. pencil push ups), prisms, Botox, surgery

3.41.2 Classification of Comitant XT

- Primary XT:
  (a) Constant:
    - Starting <6 months: Infantile XT
    - Starting >6 months: Basic XT
  (b) Intermittent:
    - Distance fixation only:
      True divergence excess XT (normal AC/A ratio)
      Simulated divergence excess XT (high AC/A ratio)
    - Near fixation only: Near XT
- Secondary sensory XT
- Consecutive XT

3.41.3 Intermittent XT

Definition
- Intermittent XT is a strabismus condition with outward drifting of either eye interspersed with periods of good alignment or orthotropia
- Onset usually before 18 months of age
- XT at distance fixation with eyes remaining aligned for near fixation

Classification
- True divergence excess XT
  - Deviation ≥10 PD larger when measured at distance fixation than at near
- Simulated divergence excess XT
  - Initial deviation ≥10PD larger when measured at distance fixation than at near
  - Misalignment at near fixation increases to less than10 PD of the angle at distance following disruption of near binocular vision by 1 hour of monocular occlusion or with +3.0D lenses or pharmacological cycloplegia

Newcastle control score (NCS) for intermittent XT
- A scoring system for grading the severity of intermittent distance XT [41]. The components of the NCS are
  - Home control (subjective criteria):
    Score 0: XT or monocular eye closure never noticed
    Score 1: XT or monocular eye closure seen <50% of time child observed for distance fixation
    Score 2: XT or monocular eye closure seen >50% of time child observed for distance fixation
    Score 3: XT or monocular eye closure seen for distance and near fixation
  - Clinic control near (objective criteria):
    Score 0: Manifest only after cover test (CT) and resumes fusion without need for blink or refixation
    Score 1: Blink or refixate to control after CT
    Score 2: Manifest spontaneously or with any form of fusion disruption without recovery
  - Clinic control distance (objective criteria):
    Score 0: Manifest only after cover test (CT) and resumes fusion without need for blink or refixation
    Score 1: Blink or refixate to control after CT
    Score 2: Manifest spontaneously or with any form of fusion disruption without recovery
- Total score 0–7
- Surgical intervention indicated for NCS ≥ 3 to achieve a cure (NCS 0 or 1)

Examination
- Full extraocular motility: can elicit by monocular occlusion or performing a doll's head manoeuvre
- Normal anterior/posterior segment examination

Investigations
- Cycloplegic refraction

Treatment
- Refractive error correction:
  - Full myopic correction in children
  - Hypermetropia correction if greater than +4.00D
- Muscle surgery (NCS ≥ 3):
  - Simulated distance XT: unilateral MR resection and LR recession
  - True distance XT: bilateral LR recession

3.42 Amblyopia Management (Table 3.36)

3.42.1 Classification

- Strabismic amblyopia
- Refractive amblyopia
- Stimulus deprivation amblyopia

3.42.2 Methods of Detection

- Reduced BCVA in the absence of an organic cause
- Crowding phenomenon: scores better with single optotypes
- Tolerance of a neutral density filter: classically in amblyopia VA is reduced less by the addition of neutral density filters than in other causes of reduced VA

3.42.3 Methods of Treatment

- Refractive error correction alone first—spectacle adaptation phase of 18 weeks:
  - Correct anisometropia >1.00D and correct astigmatism >1.50D
  - Full myopic correction in children >3.5 years old if VA < 6/9 and myopia > −0.75D
- Occlusion therapy (if reduced VA remains after 18 weeks of refractive error correction):
  - Moderate amblyopia (6/12 to 6/24): 2 hours per day of total occlusion is as effective as 6 hours per day of total occlusion for improving visual acuity in children aged 3–7 years [117]
  - Severe amblyopia (6/30 to 6/120): 6 hours per day of total occlusion is as effective as all-day full-time occlusion for improving visual acuity in children aged 3 to less than 7 years of age [118]
  - Teenagers (13–17 years old) who have never before received amblyopia treatment may improve visual acuity from a trial of occlusion therapy for 2 to 6 hours per day [87]
- Penalisation therapy:
  - Moderate amblyopia (6/12 to 6/24): atropine is as effective as 6 hours per day of total occlusion for improving visual acuity in children aged 3 to less than 7 years [116]

Table 3.36 Key facts about amblyopia

Amblyopia is the decrease of best corrected visual acuity (BCVA) by 1 line or more caused by pattern vision deprivation or abnormal binocular interaction for which no causes can be detected by the physical examination of the eye
Development of amblyopia occurs during the critical period of visual development (the first 7–8 years of life)

3.43 Retinopathy of Prematurity (ROP)

3.43.1 Classification of ROP

International Classification of ROP (International Classification of Retinopathy of Prematurity Third Edition [17]):

- Plus disease
  - Retinal arterial tortuosity +/− venous dilatation in the posterior pole in at least 2 quadrants
  - Pre-plus disease is the presence of retinal arterial tortuosity +/− venous dilatation in the posterior pole in 1 quadrant only
- Zones
  - Concentric retinal zones are centered on the disc and extend to the ora serrata. The location of the most posterior retinal vascularisation or ROP lesion denotes the zone for the eye)
  - Zone I:

    Area in a circle twice the radius of the distance from the optic disc to the foveola

    Approximate temporal extent of Zone I can be determined by using a 25- or 28-D lens:
    - Place nasal edge of optic disc at one edge of the field of view
    - Limit of Zone I is at the temporal field of view

- Zone II:
  Area in a circle centered on the optic disc with a radius of the distance from the optic disc to the nasal ora serrata
- Posterior Zone II:
  Begins at the margin of zone I and zone II and extends into zone II for 2 disc diameters
- Zone III:
  Includes remainder of the fundus outside zones I and II
- Notch:
  The term notch is used to describe an incursion by the ROP lesion of 1–2 clock hours into a more posterior zone. The ROP zone for such eyes should be noted by the most posterior zone of retinal vascularisation with the qualifier "notch" (e.g. 'zone I secondary to notch")

• Staging
  - Stage 1 (see Fig. 3.52):
    Flat demarcation line separating vascular and avascular retina
  - Stage 2 (see Fig. 3.53):
    Border thickens and appears elevated (ridge); small tufts of vessels may be present at border
  - Stage 3 (see Fig. 3.54):
    Presence of a ridge with extraretinal fibrovascular proliferations
    Blood vessels grow through the ILM of the retina at the ridge into the vitreous
  - Stage 4:
    A. Macula on partial tractional RD
    B. Macula off partial tractional RD
  - Stage 5 (CDE labelling is incorrect - it has to be ABC as it correlates to stage 5A, 5B and 5C):
    A. Open funnel total tractional RD (optic disc visible by ophthalmoscopy)
    B. Closed funnel total tractional RD (optic disc not visible by ophthalmoscopy)
    C. Stage 5B accompanied by anterior segment changes (e.g marked anterior chamber shallowing, iridocorneolenticular adhesions, corneal opacification)

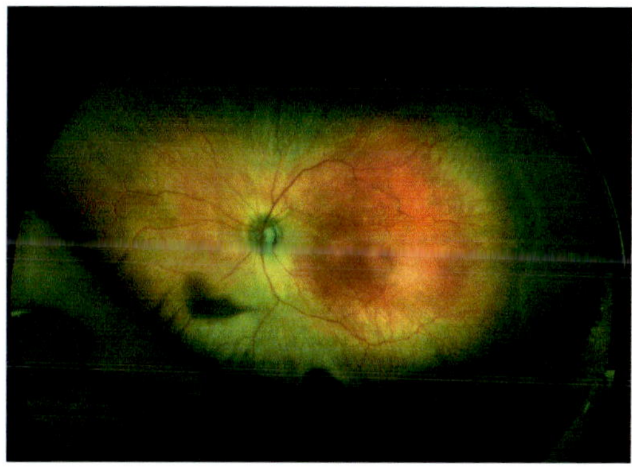

Fig. 3.52 Optos pseudocolour ultra-widefield fundus image of a patient with stage I ROP with no plus disease

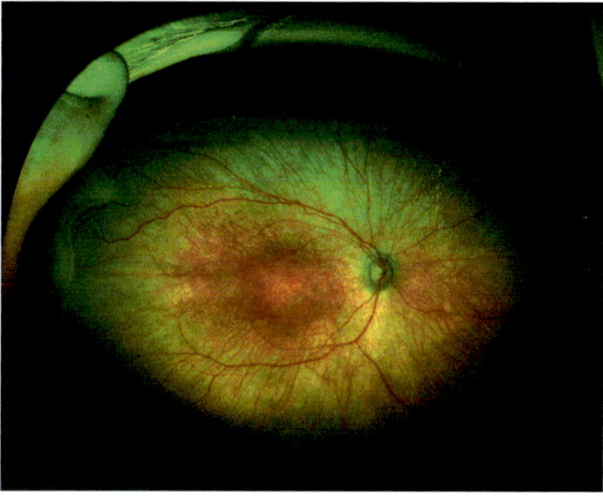

Fig. 3.53 Optos pseudocolour ultra-widefield fundus image of a patient with stage II ROP with pre-plus disease

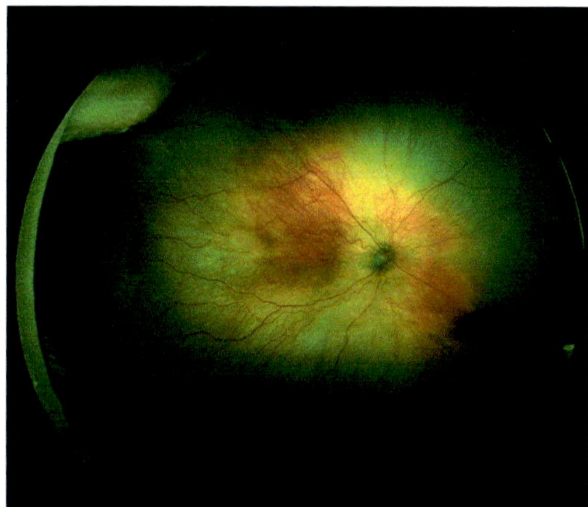

Fig. 3.54 Optos pseudocolour ultra-widefield fundus image of a patient with stage III ROP with plus disease

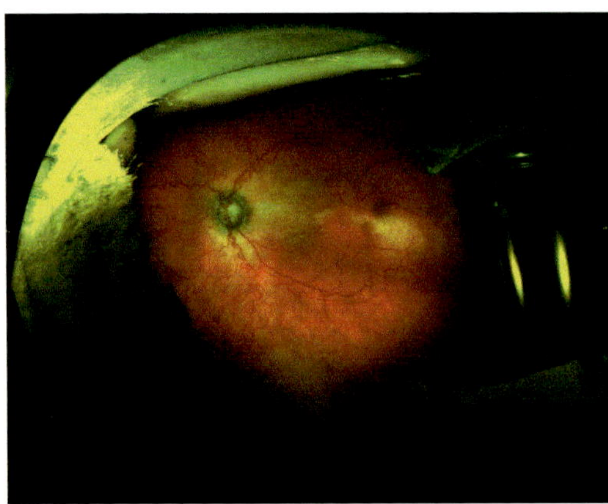

Fig. 3.55 Optos pseudocolour ultra-widefield fundus image of a patient with aggressive ROP

– Aggressive ROP (see Fig. 3.55):
  Replaced the term aggressive-posterior ROP which was previously used to describe a severe, rapidly progressive form of ROP located in posterior zones I or II.

3.43.2 UK Screening of ROP Guideline 2022 [91] and the RCOphth Clinical Guideline on Treating ROP in the UK 2022 [124]

3.43.2.1 Screening Inclusion Criteria

- Must be screened: birth weight < 1501 g &/or gestational age < 31 weeks (up to and including 30 weeks and 6 days) (UK screening of ROP guideline 2022 [91])
- Should be considered for screening: infants born between 31 + 0 and 31 + 6 weeks gestational age (UK screening of ROP guideline 2022 [91])

3.43.2.2 First Screening Examination

- For infants born before 31 + 0 weeks gestational age, the first ROP screening examination should be performed between 31 + 0 and 31 + 6 weeks post-menstrual age, or at 4 completed weeks postnatal age (28–34 days), whichever is later (UK screening of ROP guideline 2022) [91]
- For infants born from 31 + 0 weeks gestational age (irrespective of birthweight), the first ROP screening examination should be performed between 36 + 0 and 36 + 6 weeks post-menstrual age or at 4 completed weeks postnatal age (28–34 days), whichever is sooner (UK screening of ROP guideline 2022) [91]

3.43.2.3 Frequency of Screening

- After the first ROP screening, if treatment is not required, re-examine at least weekly when (1) the vessels end in zone I or posterior Zone II with or without any stage of ROP; ***OR*** (2) there is any plus or pre-plus disease; ***OR*** (3) there is stage 3 ROP in Zone II or III, until the criteria for treatment or 2 weekly examination or termination of screening have been reached (UK screening of ROP guideline 2022 [91])
- After the first ROP screening, if treatment is not required and criteria for weekly examinations are not present, re-examine at least every 2 weeks when (1) the vessels end in mid or anterior zone II or in Zone III; ***AND*** (2) there is no plus or pre-plus disease; ***AND*** (3) there is no ROP or stage 1 or 2 ROP, until the criteria for treatment or weekly examination or termination of screening have been reached (UK screening of ROP guideline 2022 [91])

3.43.2.4 Termination of Screening

- For infants with any stage of ROP, consider discontinuing screening examinations when any of the following characteristics of regression are detected on at least 2 consecutive examinations (UK screening of ROP guideline 2022 [91]):
  – Partial resolution progressing towards complete resolution
  – Change in colour of the ridge from salmon-pink to white
  – Growth of vessels through the demarcation line
- For infants without ROP, continue examination until vascularisation has extended into Zone III (UK screening of ROP guideline 2022 [91])

3.43.2.5 Treatment Criteria

- Treat infants in whom a screening examination has detected (The RCOphth Clinical Guideline on Treating ROP in the UK 2022 [124]):
  - Zone I any stage ROP with plus disease
  - Zone I stage 3 ROP without plus disease
  - Zone II stage 2 or 3 with plus disease
  - Aggressive ROP

3.43.2.6 Timing of Treatment

- Aggressive ROP or Zone I stage 3 ROP with plus disease should be treated ASAP and within 48 hours (The RCOphth Guideline on treating ROP in the UK 2022 [124])
- All other ROP requiring treatment (Zone I stage 1 or 2 ROP with plus disease, Zone I stage 3 ROP without plus disease, Zone II stage 2 or 3 ROP with plus disease) should be treated within 48–72 hours (The RCOphth Clinical Guideline on Treating ROP in the UK 2022 [124])

3.43.2.7 Treatment Technique

- Anti-VEGF:
  - Intravenous injection of an anti-VEGF agent should be used for infants with aggressive ROP and ROP in Zone I (The RCOphth Clinical Guideline on Treating ROP in the UK 2022 [124])
  - Posterior Zone II (2-disc diameters anterior to the junction of Zone 1 and Zone II) or any "notch" of ROP that encroaches backwards into Zone I, may behave in a similar way to Zone I and may be treated accordingly (The RCOphth Clinical Guideline on Treating ROP in the UK 2022 [124])
  - Anti-VEGF agents must not be administered if there are any signs of periocular infection
  - Injection should be performed 1.00–1.50 mm from the limbus and the 30 g needle should be directed in a vertically backward manner to avoid damaging the crystalline lens (The RCOphth Clinical Guideline on Treating ROP in the UK 2022 [124])
- Transpupillary laser:
  - Treatment-requiring ROP in zone II (except posterior Zone II) should be treated with transpupillary diode laser, to produce near confluent ablation of the entire avascular retina (The RCOphth Clinical Guideline on Treating ROP in the UK 2022 [124])

3.43.2.8 Post-treatment Follow-Up

- Anti-VEGF:
  - First examination should take place 1–2 days and 5–7 days after treatment to detect any adverse effects of treatment (The RCOphth Clinical Guideline on Treating ROP in the UK 2022 [124])
  - Following partial or complete disease regression, regular examinations must be maintained to detect disease reactivation: weekly for 4 weeks, 2 weekly for a further 12 weeks and then 4 weekly for a further 8 weeks (total of 24 weeks) and up to 32 weeks in eyes treated for aggressive ROP with bevacizumab after treatment (The RCOphth Clinical Guideline on Treating ROP in the UK 2022 [124])
  - Subsequent examinations at 1 year, 18 months, 2 years, 3 years, 4 years and 5 years. Discharge to community services at 5 years if stable (The RCOphth Clinical Guideline on Treating ROP in the UK 2022 [124])
- Transpupillary laser:
  - First examination at one week post treatment. The second examination at 2 weeks, preferably with wide angle photography, is used to observe disease regression and determine whether "top up" treatment for untreated "skip" areas within 10 days of baseline (The RCOphth Clinical Guideline on Treating ROP in the UK 2022 [124])
  - Subsequent examinations at 3–4 weeks, 3 months, 6 months, 1 year, 18 months, 2 years, 3 years, 4 years and 5 years. Discharge to community services at 5 years if stable (The RCOphth Clinical Guideline on Treating ROP in the UK 2022 [124])

3.43.2.9 Retreatment / Rescue Treatment

- Anti-VEGF:
  - Disease reactivation (plus disease and/or extraretinal new vessels) should be treated with transpupillary laser, to produce near-confluent ablation of the entire avascular retina (The RCOphth Clinical Guideline on Treating ROP in the UK 2022 [124])
  - Following initial anti-VEGF treatment consider EUA / examination under sedation with possible transpupillary laser to produce near-confluent ablation of the entire avascular retina if the retina has not fully vascularised or this is uncertain (The RCOphth Clinical Guideline on Treating ROP in the UK 2022 [124]) ***AND***:
    1. Regular follow-up is becoming unsustainable for social and/or geographic reasons
    2. The growing child's limited cooperation precludes adequate examination of the peripheral retina
    3. There is uncertainty about the presence of signs of disease reactivation
  - ***OR***:
    1. During longer term follow-up a significant area of persistent avascular retina is seen or suspected
- Transpupillary laser:
  - Failure of disease regression after 2 weeks in the presence of optimal laser cover of anterior retina should prompt consideration of rescue treatment with an anti-VEGF agent
  - Anti-VEGF rescue treatment following primary laser treatment requires initial follow-up as for primary anti-VEGF treatment

3.44 Penetrating Eye Injury

3.44.1 History

- Mechanism of injury
- Tetanus status

3.44.2 Examination

- IOP: may be reduced
- Lids: lid lacerations with or without involvement of the lid margin or canaliculus
- Conjunctiva: conjunctival lacerations, subconjunctival haemorrhage
- Cornea: penetrating corneal injury—perform a seidel test
- Sclera: penetrating scleral injury
- AC: formed or flat, hypopyon, hyphaema
- Iris: iris hole (transillumination), peaked pupil
- Perform gonioscopy to look for angle recession and occult intraocular foreign body (IOFB) in angle
- Lens: traumatic cataract (focal) +/− disruption of anterior/posterior lens capsule +/− zonular dehiscence +/− subluxation/dislocation, IOFB
- Fundus: vitreous/retinal haemorrhage, retinal tear(s), RD, commotio retinae, choroidal rupture, IOFB (see Fig. 3.56)

3.44.3 Investigations

- B-scan (if poor view of fundus): IOFB (highly reflective mobile appearing opacity), RD or choroidal haemorrhage
- CT orbit with 2 mm slices: orbital fractures, IOFB
- Full field ERG: siderosis causes a progressive reduction in the B-wave with eventual total extinguishing

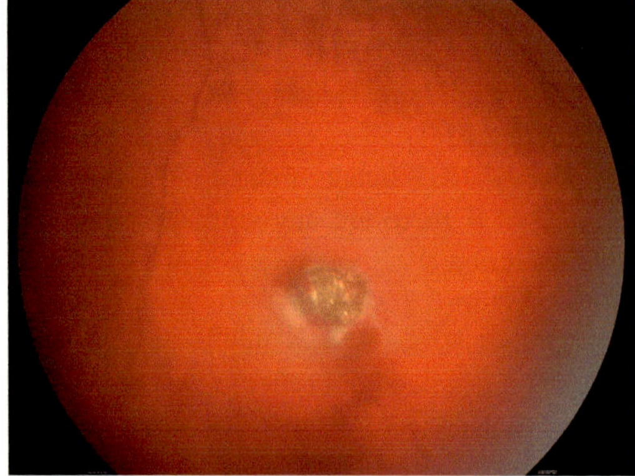

Fig. 3.56 Colour fundus image of a patient with a metallic IOFB dislodged in the retina

3.44.4 Treatment

- Pre-operative
  (a) Admit and prepare for GA (NBM, determine last meal/drink, liaise with anaesthetist, ECG/bloods if indicated)
  (b) Protect globe with clear plastic shield
  (c) Systemic antibiotics e.g. ciprofloxacin 750 mg BD +/− topical antibiotics
  (d) Administer tetanus vaccine / toxoid if indicated
- Intraoperative
  (a) Primary globe repair:
    – Limbus is repaired first typically with 9/0 nylon sutures
    – Any corneal laceration is then repaired typically with 10/0 nylon sutures (longer compression suture throws are used in the peripheral cornea and shorter suture throws used in the central cornea)—rotate sutures to bury knots; return exposed viable iris tissue through perforation; abscise exposed tissue if non-viable
    – Any scleral laceration is then repaired (following a conjunctival peritomy) in an anterior to posterior direction with 8/0 nylon sutures; return exposed viable uveal tissue through perforation; cut prolapsed vitreous flush to wound taking care not to induce vitreous traction
  (b) IOFB removal
    – AC IOFB: corneal approach, removal with fine forceps
    – Angle IOFB: scleral trapdoor approach
    – Lenticular IOFB: consider leaving insitu or remove with lens at cautious cataract surgery
    – Posterior segment IOFB: intraocular magnet or vitrectomy forceps
  (c) Lid laceration repair
  (d) Secondary procedures
    – Traditionally performed 4–10 days after initial injury, in part, to allow for the formation of a PVD
    – PPV + tamponade (C3F8 or silicone oil) +/− membrane dissection (if PVR) +/− encircling buckle (if breaks) +/− lensectomy (if cataract; IOL commonly deferred) +/− intravitreal antibiotics (if endophthalmitis)

3.44.5 Tetanus Prophylaxis

- Tetanus vaccine treatment (3 doses of 0.5 mL IM Td/IPD, separated by 4 weeks, with a booster after 10 years) if
  (a) Patient non-immune and wound is clean or tetanus prone
  (b) Patient is uncertain of vaccination status and wound is clean or tetanus prone
- Tetanus immunoglobulin treatment if
  (a) Patient non-immune and wound is tetanus prone
  (b) Patient is uncertain of vaccination status and wound is tetanus prone

3.45 Atypical Optic Neuritis (Table 3.37)

3.45.1 Features of Typical Optic Neuritis (Acute Demyelinating Optic Neuritis)

- Age 20–50
- Unilateral
- Worsens over hours / days
- Recovery starts within 2 weeks
- Retrobulbar pain (may be worse on eye movements)—present in 92% of cases

Table 3.37 Key facts about atypical optic neuritis

Atypical optic neuritis is a heterogenous collection of disorders whose presenting features suggest inflammation of the optic nerve
Inflammation of the optic nerve may be divided into papillitis (disc is swollen), retrobulbar neuritis (disc is spared), and neuroretinitis (retinal involvement, macular star)
If an acute optic neuropathy does not fulfil the criteria for typical optic neuritis (see Sect. 3.45.1) then it must be investigated further as an atypical optic neuritis to exclude a compressive lesion or other serious pathology

- Reduced colour vision
- RAPD—disc swelling only present in 1/3 of cases

3.45.2 Features of Atypical Optic Neuritis

- Absence of pain
- Grossly swollen optic disc with peripapillary haemorrhages
- Bilateral
- Severe loss of vision over several weeks
- Recurrence on cessation of steroids

3.45.3 Causes of Atypical Optic Neuritis

- Infection: syphilis, TB, lyme, HIV
- Lymphoproliferative (directly or indirectly related to the haematological disease): lymphoma, leukaemia, neurotoxic treatments post bone-marrow transplant
- Systemic immune mediated disorders: neurosarcoidosis, IBD, systemic vasculitis, connective tissue disease
- Antibody mediated neurological illness: NMO spectrum disorder (NMOSD), MOG antibody mediated demyelinating disease

3.45.4 History

- Course of optic nerve dysfunction both current and in the past: persistent visual loss, negligible spontaneous improvement
- Presence of paraesthesia, weakness of limbs—clumsiness with dropping things frequently, bowel and bladder incontinence—NMOSD
- Any recent infections or vaccinations—vaccinations induced optic neuritis
- History of lymphoproliferative diseases, IBD, connective tissue disorders
- History of autoimmunity (e.g. MG, hypothyroidism): NMOSD frequently associated with systemic autoimmune disorders
- Concurrent or recent treatments e.g. bone marrow transplant, new biologic agents such as monoclonals

3.45.5 Examination

- Optic nerve function: VA, RAPD, colour vision, confrontational VF
- Cranial nerve: CN VII involvement in Sarcoidosis—Heerfordt's syndrome (CN VII palsy, uveitis, parotid/submandibular gland enlargement)
- Uveitis (anterior, intermediate or posterior): sarcoidosis, infective causes, lymphoproliferative causes
- Skin: erythema nodosum (red tender elevated lesions on the shins)

3.45.6 Investigations

- HVF
- MRI brain with gadolinium contrast +/− spinal cord (transverse myelitis—lesion extending continuously over ≥3 vertebral segments)
- Bloods:
  - VDRL: syphilis
  - FBC, ESR: lymphoproliferative
  - ACE: sarcoidosis
  - Aquaporin-4 antibodies: NMOSD
  - Myelin oligodendrocyte glycoprotein (MOG) antibodies
- CXR: sarcoidosis (hilar lymphadenopathy, pulmonary fibrosis), TB

3.45.7 Treatment

- High dose oral/IV corticosteroids, followed by a reducing dose oral steroid programme
- Refer to respiratory team for bronchoscopy
- Refer to neurologists for full neurological examination

3.46 Carotid Artery Dissection (Table 3.38)

3.46.1 History

- Symptoms: headache, ocular pain, neck pain, Horner's syndrome (caused by compression of the ascending sympathetic supply within the carotid sheath), symptoms of TIA/CVA (Over 50% of patients with a spontaneous ICA dissection present initially as a stroke or TIA with hemiplegia, dysarthria, dysphagia, or amaurosis fugax)
- History of neck trauma (e.g from car accident with seat belt injury to neck)
- History of hereditary connective tissue disorders

3.46.2 Examination

- Horner's syndrome
- Deviation of tongue to affected side: compression of hypoglossal nerve (CN XII)
- Neurological examination

3.46.3 Investigation

- CTA or MRA

Table 3.38 Key facts about carotid artery dissection

Dissection occurs when a tear forms within the inner wall of an artery
Bloods enters tunica media of the vessel and forms an intramural haematoma along plane of the vessel wall—may cause vessel wall to bulge toward the lumen, leading to stenosis, or it may cause outward pseudoaneurysmal bulging of the vessel wall
Cervical artery dissection accounts for only 1–2% of all ischaemic strokes, but in young and middle-aged people it accounts for 10–25% of strokes [22]
May occur spontaneously or secondary to trauma, hereditary connective tissue disorders (Marfan syndrome, Ehlers-Danlos syndrome, osteogenesis imperfecta)

3.46.4 Treatment

- Patients are treated empirically with either antiplatelet (aspirin, clopidogrel, dipyridamole) or anticoagulation (warfarin, heparin) therapy to prevent formation of a thrombus at the site of dissection and subsequent embolisation. However, there is no difference in efficacy of antiplatelet and anticoagulant drugs at preventing stroke and death in patients with symptomatic carotid and vertebral artery dissection [62, 109]

3.46.5 Prognosis

- The risk of stroke is zero for patients who present with anything other than an initial stroke [109]
- For patients who present initially with symptoms of a stroke, only 2% will have a stroke recurrence [109]
- All stroke events occur in the first 10 days [109]

3.47 Transient Ischaemic Attack (TIA) and Stroke: NICE Guidance [NG128] [78]

3.47.1 Prompt Recognition of Symptoms of Stroke and TIA

- FAST (Face Arm Speech Test):
  - Validated tool used outside of hospital to screen for a diagnosis of stroke or TIA in people with sudden onset of neurological symptoms:
    Face: ask the person to smile
    Arm: ask the person to raise both arms
    Speech: ask the person to repeat a simple phrase
- Exclude hypoglycaemia in people with sudden onset of neurological symptoms as the cause of these symptoms

- For people who are admitted to the emergency department with a suspected stroke or TIA, establish the diagnosis rapidly using a validated tool, such as ROSIER (Recognition of Stroke in the Emergency Room)

3.47.2 Initial Management of Suspected and Confirmed TIA

- Offer aspirin 300 mg daily, unless contraindicated, to people who have had a suspected TIA, to be started immediately
- Refer immediately people who have had a suspected TIA for specialist assessment and investigation, to be seen within 24 hours of onset of symptoms
- Do not use scoring systems, such as the $ABCD^2$ score, to assess risk of subsequent stroke or to inform urgency of referral for people who have had a suspected or confirmed TIA
- Offer secondary prevention, in addition to aspirin, as soon as possible after the diagnosis of TIA is confirmed

3.47.3 Imaging for People Who Have Had a Suspected TIA or Acute Non-disabling Stroke

- Do not offer CT brain scanning to people with a suspected TIA unless there is clinical suspicion of an alternative diagnosis that CT could detect
- After specialist assessment in the TIA clinic, consider MRI (including diffusion-weighted and blood-sensitive sequences) to determine the territory of ischaemia, or to detect haemorrhage or alternative pathologies. If MRI is done, perform it on the same day as the assessment
- Everyone with a TIA who after specialist assessment is considered as a candidate for carotid endarterectomy should have urgent carotid imaging. Ensure that carotid imaging reports clearly state which criteria (ECST [30] or NASCET [33]) were used when measuring the extent of carotid stenosis
- Perform brain imaging immediately with a non-enhanced CT for people with suspected acute stroke if any of the following apply:
  - Indications for thrombolysis or thrombectomy
  - On anticoagulant treatment
  - A known bleeding tendency
  - A depressed level of consciousness (Glasgow Coma Score below 13)
  - Unexplained progressive or fluctuating symptoms
  - Papilloedema, neck stiffness or fever
  - Severe headache at onset of stroke symptoms
- If thrombectomy might be indicated, perform imaging with CT contrast angiography following initial non-enhanced CT. Add CT perfusion imaging (or MR equivalent) if thrombectomy might be indicated beyond 6 hours of symptom onset
- Perform scanning as soon as possible and within 24 hours of symptom onset in everyone with suspected acute stroke without indications for immediate brain imaging

3.47.4 Urgent Carotid Endarterectomy and Carotid Stenting

- People with stable neurological symptoms from acute non-disabling stroke or TIA who have symptomatic carotid stenosis of 50–99% according to the North American Symptomatic Carotid Endarterectomy (NASCET) Trial criteria [33], or 70–99% according to the European Carotid Surgery Trial (ECST) criteria [30] should:
  - Be assessed and referred urgently for carotid endarterectomy to a service following current national standards

  - Receive best medical treatment (control of BP, antiplatelet agents, cholesterol lowering through diet and drugs, lifestyle advice)
- People with stable neurological symptoms from acute non-disabling stroke or TIA who have symptomatic carotid stenosis of less than 50% according to the NASCET criteria, or less than 70% according to the ECST criteria should:
  - Not undergo surgery
  - Receive best medical treatment (control of BP, antiplatelet agents, cholesterol lowering through diet and drugs, lifestyle advice)

3.47.5 Pharmacological Treatments and Thrombectomy for People with Acute Stroke

- Thrombolysis with alteplase:
  - Recommended for treating acute ischaemic stroke in adults if:

    Treatment is started as early as possible within 4.5 hours of onset of stroke symptoms **and**

    Intracranial haemorrhage has been excluded by appropriate imaging techniques
- Thrombectomy:
  - Offer thrombectomy as soon as possible and within 6 hours of symptom onset, together with intravenous thrombolysis (if not contraindicated and within the licensed time window), to people who have:

    Acute ischaemic stroke **and**

    Confirmed occlusion of the proximal anterior circulation demonstrated by CTA or MRA
  - Offer thrombectomy as soon as possible to people who were last known to be well between 6 hours and 24 hours previously (including wake-up strokes):

    Who have acute ischaemic stroke and confirmed occlusion of the proximal anterior circulation demonstrated by CTA or MRA **and**

    If there is the potential to salvage brain tissue, as shown by imaging such as CT perfusion or diffusion-weighted MRI sequences showing limited infarct core volume
  - Consider thrombectomy together with intravenous thrombolysis (where not contraindicated and within the licensed time window) as soon as possible for people last known to be well up to 24 hours previously (including wake-up strokes):

    Who have acute ischaemic stroke and confirmed occlusion of the proximal posterior circulation (that is, basilar or posterior cerebral artery) demonstrated by CTA or MRA **and**

    If there is potential to salvage brain tissue, as shown by imaging such as CT perfusion or diffusion-weighted MRI sequences showing limited infarct core volume
- Aspirin and anticoagulant treatment
  - People with acute ischaemic stroke:

    All people presenting with acute ischaemic stroke who have had a diagnosis of primary intracerebral haemorrhage excluded by brain imaging should, as soon as possible but certainly within 24 hours, be given:

    - Aspirin 300 mg PO if they are not dysphagic
    - Aspirin 300 mg PR or by enteral tube if they are dysphagic

    Thereafter aspirin should be continued until 2 weeks after the onset of stroke symptoms, at which time definitive long-term antithrombotic treatment should be initiated

    Offer a protein pump inhibitor, in addition to aspirin, to anyone with acute ischaemic stroke for whom previous dyspepsia associated with aspirin is reported

    Offer an alternative antiplatelet agent to anyone with acute ischaemic stroke who is allergic to or genuinely intolerant of aspirin

– People with stroke associated with acute arterial dissection:
  Treat with either anticoagulants or antiplatelet agents
– People with acute venous stroke:
  People diagnosed with cerebral venous sinus thrombosis should be given full-dose anticoagulant treatment (initially full dose heparin and then warfarin INR 2–3) unless there are comorbidities that preclude its use

3.48 Amaurosis Fugax (Table 3.39)

3.48.1 Causes

- Embolic
  - Carotid artery disease:
    Atherosclerosis
    Dissection
    Aneurysms
  - Cardiac disease:
    Valvular heart disease
    Mural thrombi e.g. lesions associated with AF or MI
    Intracardiac tumour e.g. atrial myxoma
  - Drug abuse:
    Talc retinopathy
- Haemodynamic
  - Inflammatory arteritis:
    Takayasu's disease
  - Hypoperfusion:
    Heart failure
    Acute hypovolaemia
- Ocular
  - AION
  - CRAO / BRAO
  - CRVO
- Neurologic
  - Optic neuritis, optic nerve or chiasm compression
  - Papilloedema
  - MS
  - Migraine
- Idiopathic

Table 3.39 Key facts about amaurosis fugax

Defined as transient monocular visual loss attributed to ischaemia or vascular insufficiency
Typically, patients describe diminished or absent vision in one eye that progresses over a few seconds and lasts for seconds to a few minutes followed by complete recovery

3.48.2 History

- Ask about symptoms of GCA: headache, jaw claudication, scalp tenderness, weight loss, fever
- Ask about cardiovascular risk factors: HTN, DM, hypercholesterolaemia, smoking
- Ask about use of recreational drug use: talc
- Ask about symptoms of migraine: unilateral headache, photophobia/phonophobia, nausea/vomiting, aura that usually precedes the headache (visual—starts paracentrally and expands temporally with advancing edge forms a positive scotoma, motor—hemiparesis, speech—dysphasia, somatosensory—hemianaesthesia/paraesthesia)
- Ask about symptoms of MS
  - Ocular symptoms: pain on eye movements, rapid decrease of vision over hours/days with recovery starting at 2 weeks
  - Systemic symptoms: limb weakness, paraesthesia, urine retention, incontinence

3.48.3 Examination

- Ophthalmic examination to exclude
  - Retinal vascular diseases
  - Optic neuropathy

3.48.4 Investigations

- Bloods: FBC, CRP, ESR
- TAB
- Carotid doppler
- Cardiac echocardiography
- MRI head

3.48.5 Treatment

- Treat underlying cause
- Refer to TIA clinic

3.49 Juvenile Idiopathic Arthritis (JIA) (Table 3.40)

3.49.1 International League of Associations for Rheumatology (ILAR) Classification

- Systemic disease
- Polyarticular rheumatoid factor positive: 5 or more joints affected during the first 6 months of disease
- Polyarticular rheumatoid factor negative: 5 or more joints affected during the first 6 months of disease
- Oligoarticular persistent: 1–4 joints affected throughout the first 6 months of disease
- Oligoarticular extended: 1–4 joints affected throughout and after the first 6 months of disease
- Psoriatic arthritis
- Enthesitis-related arthritis
- Undifferentiated arthritis

Table 3.40 Key facts about JIA

Chronic rheumatic disease of childhood characterised by chronic inflammatory arthritis (swelling within a joint or limitation in range of movement with joint pain or tenderness which persists for a minimum of 6 weeks)
Onset prior to age 16 years old
More common in girls but boys get higher rates of visual loss and complications
Annual incidence in the UK is 1:10,000 with a prevalence of 1:1000 [8]
Type of arthritis and the age at onset dictates the risk of developing uveitis
Uveitis in JIA is asymptomatic until visual complications arise and therefore screening by slit-lamp is essential for diagnosis
Visual impairment arises mainly from complications of the uveitis including cataract, glaucoma, macular oedema, hypotony

3.49.2 Risk Factors for Developing Uveitis in JIA

- Oligoarticular group
- ANA positive
- Female
- < 7 years old at age of onset

3.49.3 Examination

- Articular
- Ocular
  - Chronic recurrent anterior uveitis with a white eye, usually bilateral
  - Complications of uveitis:
    Band keratopathy
    Macular oedema
    Cataract
    Glaucoma
    Hypotony that may lead to phthisis bulbi

3.49.4 Investigations

- Bloods: ANA
- OCT: macular oedema

3.49.5 Treatment

- Arthritis
  - Physiotherapy
  - Occupational therapy
  - Joint inflammation:
    (a) NSAIDs
    (b) Oral corticosteroids
    (c) Immunosuppresants
    (d) Biologics: adalimumab, etanercept, tocilizumab are recommended for treating polyarticular and extended oligoarticular JIA (NICE guidance)
- Anterior uveitis and macular oedema
  - Topical steroids + mydriatics
  - Subtenon injection of steroids / orbital floor injections
  - Oral corticosteroids

- Immunosuppresants: methotrexate (MTX)
- Biologics: infliximab, adalimumab

- Complications of ocular inflammation
  - Glaucoma:
    Topical medications
    Trabeculectomy
    GDI
  - Cataract:
    Cataract extraction once uveitis quiescent for at least 3 months
    Preoperative considerations:
    - Determine visual potential
    - Concurrent surgery: co-existing ERM, vitreous opacity
    - Frequent topical +/− oral steroid 1–2 week before surgery

    Intraoperative considerations:
    - Maximise pupil size: synechialysis, intracameral phenylephrine, iris hooks
    - Large capsulorrhexis to prevent post-operative capsular phimosis
    - Meticulous removal of all nuclear matter and cortical matter

    Postoperative considerations:
    - Frequent topical +/− oral steroids (if started preoperatively) that are tapered slowly to zero or maintenance dose
    - Close follow up: 1 day post-op, 1/52 post-op, 6 weeks post-op
  - Band keratopathy:
    Chelation with ETDA
    PTK

3.49.6 The British Society of Paediatric and Adolescent Rheumatology (BSPAR) and the RCOphth Guidelines for Screening for Uveitis in JIA 2006 [8]

3.49.6.1 Principles

- Initial screening examination within 6 weeks of referral
- Symptomatic patients or patient suspected of cataracts or synechiae should be seen within 1 week of referral
- EUA should be considered if the patient is uncooperative at initial screening or for an urgent symptomatic examination in a young child
- Screening should restart at 2 monthly intervals after stopping MTX or any other immunosuppressant therapy during the period of maximum risk for 6 months before reverting to the previous screening arrangements

3.49.6.2 Specific Screening Schedules

- First screening within 6 weeks of referral
- 2 monthly intervals from onset of arthritis for 6 months, then 3–4 monthly screening for time outlined below:
  (a) Oligoarticular JIA, Psoriatic arthritis onset and Enthesitis related arthritis irrespective of ANA status onset under 11 years:
    - <3 years old at onset: screen for 8 years
    - 3–4 years old at onset: screen for 6 years
    - 5–8 years old at onset: screen for 3 years
    - 9–10 years old at onset: screen for 1 year

  (b) Polyarticular ANA+ JIA onset under 10 years:
    - <6 years old at onset: screen for 5 years
    - 6–9 years old at onset: screen for 2 years

  (c) Polyarticular ANA- JIA onset under 7 years:
    - All children need 5 years of screening
- Alternative method is to screen all these groups until age 11–12 years
- Older patients presenting for the first time after the age of 11 should undergo 1 year of screening

3.50 Paediatric Cataract

3.50.1 History

- Any FHx of childhood cataracts (parents, siblings)
- Exposure to corticosteroid or radiation therapy

- Ocular trauma: accidental or non-accidental
- Co-morbidities suggesting systemic disease:
  - Galactosaemia: failure to thrive
  - Lowe syndrome: hypotonia, problems with weight gain, delayed milestones, feeding difficulties
  - Dysmorphic features suggestive of a syndrome
- Intrauterine infections (TORCH): associated with severe intraocular disease
- Age child was first noted to squint or have leukocoria
- If bilateral cataracts, ask parents when they first noted abnormal visual behaviour or nystagmus

3.50.2 Examination

- Vision testing
  - Fix and following a target (CSM method: Central—location of corneal light reflex under monocular conditions, Steady—steadiness of fixation as light is held motionless and slowly moved around under monocular conditions, Maintained—binocular conditions): 3 months onwards
  - Forced choice preferential looking tests (e.g Teller acuity card): 0–1 year
  - Cardiff cards: 0–2 years
  - 3 m logMAR uncrowded Kay pictures: 18 months to 3 years
  - 3 m logMAR crowded Kay pictures: 2–4 years
  - 3 m logMAR crowded letters: Above 3 years
- Pupillary reflexes for an RAPD: suggests poor visual potential
- Look for nystagmus: suggests severe visual impairment and poor visual potential
- Slit lam exam
  - Evaluate cornea
  - Evaluate iris
  - Evaluate morphology of cataract:

    Anterior polar: AD inheritance, minimal visual deprivation, non-progressive

    Anterior subcapsular: atopic dermatitis

    Posterior subcapsular: radiation

    Lamellar: rubella, diabetes, galactosaemia

    Sutural: Fabry's disease, mannosidosis

    Posterior cortical with lenticonus: Alport's syndrome

    Nuclear: rubella, galactosaemia ("oil droplet" cataract)
- Dilated fundus examination
  - Optic nerve
  - Retina
- Examine parents and siblings: presence of asymptomatic cataracts may establish the heredity

3.50.3 Investigations

- B-scan: if density of cataract precludes an adequate view of the fundus
- Unilateral cataracts: no tests required as most are isolated ocular problems
- Bilateral cataracts
  - No tests required if +ve FHx and child has no other medical problems
  - If no FHx—investigate for systemic associations:

    Paediatric systemic evaluation

    Galactosaemia: urinalysis for reducing substances, galactokinase levels

    Lowe syndrome: urine amino acids, serum electrolytes, enzyme assay on cultured skin fibroblasts, OCRL gene testing

    TORCH screen: serology for toxoplasma, syphilis, rubella, CMV, HSV

    Karyotyping and geneticist involvement if dysmorphic features are present in child

3.50.4 Treatment

- Non-surgical
  - Observation: cataracts that are not in the visual axis, <3 mm in diameter, partial density
  - Dilation
- Surgical
  - Indications: visually significant cataracts: cataracts that are dense, central/axial, posterior, >3 mm in diameter

22. Debette S, Leys D. Cervical artery dissections: predisposing factors, diagnosis, and outcome. Lancet Neurol. 2009;8:668–78.
23. De Bustros S. Vitrectomy for prevention of macular holes. Results of a randomised multicenter clinical trial. Vitrectomy for Prevention of Macular Hole Study Group. Ophthalmology. 1994;101:1055–9.
24. Diabetes Control and Complications Trial Research Group. Progression of retinopathy with intensive versus conventional treatment in the diabetes control and complications trial. Ophthalmology. 1995;102:647–61.
25. Duker JS, Kaiser PK, Binder S, de Smet MD, Gaudric A, Reichel E, Sadda SR, Sebag J, Spaide RF, Stalmans P. The International Vitreomacular Traction Study Group classification of vitreomacular adhesion, traction, and macular hole. Ophthalmology. 2013;120:2611–9.
26. Early Treatment Diabetic Retinopathy Study Research Group. Early photocoagulation for diabetic retinopathy. ETDRS report number 9. Early Treatment Diabetic Retinopathy Study Research Group. Ophthalmology. 1991;98:766–85.
27. Early Treatment Diabetic Retinopathy Study Research Group. Fundus photographic risk factors for progression of diabetic retinopathy. ETDRS report number 12. Ophthalmology. 1991;98:823–33.
28. Endophthalmitis Vitrectomy Study Group. Results of the Endophthalmitis Vitrectomy Study. A randomised trial of immediate vitrectomy and of intravenous antibiotics for the treatment of postoperative bacterial endophthalmitis. Arch Ophthalmol. 1995;113:1479–96.
29. ESCRS Endophthalmitis Study Group. Prophylaxis of postoperative endophthalmitis following cataract surgery: results of the ESCRS multicenter study and identification of risk factors. J Cataract Refract Surg. 2007;33:978–88.
30. European Carotid Surgery Trialists Collaborative Group. MRC European Carotid Surgery Trial: interim results for symptomatic patients with severe (70-99%) or with mild (0-29%) carotid stenosis. Lancet. 1991;337:1235–43.
31. Ezra E, Wells JA, Gray RH, Kinsella FM, Orr GM, Grego J, Arden GB, Gregor ZJ. Incidence of idiopathic full-thickness macular holes in fellow eyes. A 5-year prospective natural history study. Ophthalmology. 1998;105:353–9.
32. Ezra E. Idiopathic full thickness macular hole: natural history and pathogenesis. Br J Ophthalmol. 2001;85:102–8.
33. Ferguson GG, Eliasziw M, Barr HWK, Clagett P, Barnes RW, Wallace MC, Taylor DW, Haynes RB, Finan JW, Hachinski VC, Barnett HJM. The North American symptomatic carotid endarterectomy trial. Stroke. 1999;30:1751–8.
34. Freeman WR, Azen SP, Kim JW, el-Haig W, Mishell DR III, Bailey I. Vitrectomy for the treatment of full-thickness stage 3 or 4 macular holes. Results of a multicentered randomised clinical trial. The Vitrectomy for Treatment of Macular Hole Study Group. Arch Ophthalmol. 1997;115:11–21.
35. Friedman DI, Liu GT, Digre KB. Revised diagnostic criteria for the pseudotumor cerebri syndrome in adults and children. Neurology. 2013;81:1159–65.
36. Frisen L. Swelling of the optic nerve head: a staging scheme. J Neurol Neurosurg Psychiatry. 1982;45:13–8.
37. Garcia GH, Harris GJ. Criteria for nonsurgical management of subperiosteal abscess of the orbit: analysis of outcomes 1988-1998. Ophthalmology. 2000;107:1454–6.
38. Gillies MC, Lim LL, Campain A, Quin GJ, Salem W, Li J, Goodwin S, Aroney C, McAllister IL, Fraser-Bell S. A randomised clinical trial of intravitreal bevacizumab versus intravitreal dexamethasone for diabetic macular edema: the BEVORDEX study. Ophthalmology. 2014;121:2473–81.
39. Guillaubey A, Malvitte L, Lafontaine PO, Hubert I, Bron A, Berrod JP, Creuzot-Garcher C. Incidence of retinal detachment after macular surgery. Br J Ophthalmol. 2007;91:1327–30.
40. Guzzard G, Konstantakopoulou E, Garway-Heath D, Garg A, Vickerstaff V, Hunter R, Ambler G, Bunce C, Wormald R, Nathwani N, Barton K, Rubin G, Buszewicz M. Selective laser trabeculoplasty versus eye drops for first-line treatment of ocular hypertension and glaucoma (LiGHT): a multicentre randomised controlled trial. Lancet. 2019;393:1505–16.
41. Haggerty H, Richardson S, Hrisos S, Strong NP, Clarke MP. The Newcastle Control Score: a new method of grading the severity of intermittent distance exotropia. Br J Ophthalmol. 2004;88:233–5.
42. Haller JA, Bandello F, Belfort R, Blumenkranz MS, Gillie M, Heier J, Loewenstein A, Yoon YH, Jacques ML, Jiao J, Li XY, Whitcup SM. Randomised, sham-controlled trial of dexamethasone intravitreal implant in patients with macular edema due to retinal vein occlusion. Ophthalmology. 2010;117:1134–46.
43. He M, Jiang Y, Huang S, Chang DS, Munoz B, Aung T, Foster PJ, Friedman DS. Laser peripheral iridotomy for the prevention of angle closure: a single-centre, randomised controlled trial. Lancet. 2019;393:1609–18.
44. Heijl A, Leske C, Bengtsson B, Hyman L, Bengtsson B, Hussein M. Reduction of intraocular pressure and glaucoma progression. Results from the early manifest glaucoma trial. Arch Ophthalmol. 2002;120:1268–79.
45. Herpetic Eye Disease Study Group. Psychological stress and other potential triggers for recurrences of herpes simplex virus eye infections. Arch Ophthalmol. 2000;118:1617–25.
46. Herpetic Eye Disease Study Group. Predictors of recurrent herpes simplex virus keratitis. Cornea. 2001;20:123–8.
47. Hillier RJ, Felfeli T, Berger AR, Wong DT, Altomare F, Dai D, Giavedoni LR, Kertes PJ, Kohly RP, Muni RH. The pneumatic retinopexy versus vitrectomy for the management of primary rhegmatogenous retinal

detachment outcomes randomized trial (PIVOT). Ophthalmology. 2019;126:531–9.

48. Holz FG, Roider J, Ogura Y, Korobelnik JF, Simader C, Groetzbach G, Vitti R, Berliner AJ, Hiemeyer F, Beckmann K, Zeitz O, Sandbrink R. VEGF trap-eye for macular oedema secondary to central retinal vein occlusion: 6-month results of the phase III GALILEO study. Br J Ophthalmol. 2013;97:278–84.
49. Hubschman JP, Govetto A, Spaide RF, Schumann R, Steel D, Figueroa MS, Sebag J, Gaudric A, Staurenghi G, Haritoglou C, Kadonosono K, Thompson JT, Chang S, Bottoni F, Tadayoni R. Optical coherence tomography-based consensus definition for lamellar macular hole. Br J Ophthalmol. 2020;104:1741–7.
50. Infant Aphakia Treatment Study Group, Lambert SR, Buckley EG, Drews-Botsch C, DuBois L, Hartmann EE, Lynn MJ, Plager DA, Wilson ME. A randomised clinical trial comparing contact lens with intraocular lens correction of monocular aphakia during infancy: grating acuity and adverse events at age 1 year. Arch Ophthalmol. 2010;128:810–8.
51. Infant Aphakia Treatment Study Group, Lambert SR, Lynn MJ, Hartmann EE, DuBois L, Drews-Botsch C, Freedman SF, Plager DA, Buckley EG, Wilson ME. Comparison of contact lens and intraocular lens correction of monocular aphakia during infancy: a randomised clinical trial of HOTV optotype acuity at age 4.5 years and clinical findings at age 5 years. JAMA Ophthalmol. 2014;132:676–82.
52. Ip MS, Baker BJ, Duker JS, Reichel E, Baumal CR, Gangnon R, Puliafito CA. Anatomic outcomes of surgery for idiopathic macular hole as determined by optical coherence tomography. Arch Ophthalmol. 2002;120:29–35.
53. Kamalarajah S, Silvestri G, Sharma N, Khan A, Foot B, Ling R, Cran G, Best R. Surveillance of endophthalmitis following cataract surgery in the UK. Eye (Lond). 2004;18:580–7.
54. Kelly SP, Mathews D, Mathews J, Vail A. Reflective consideration of postoperative endophthalmitis as a quality marker. Eye (Lond). 2007;21:1419–26.
55. Klein R, Klein BE, Moss SE, Davis MD, DeMets DL. The Wisconsin Epidemiologic Study of Diabetic Retinopathy. II. Prevalence and risk of diabetic retinopathy when age at diagnosis is less than 30 years. Arch Ophthalmol. 1984;102:520–6.
56. Leaute-Labreze C, Hoeger P, Mazereeuw-Hautier J, Guiband L, Baselga E, Posiunas G, Phillips RK, Caceres H, Gutierrez JCL, Ballona R, Friedlander SF, Powell J, Perek D, Metz B, Barbarot S, Maruani A, Szalai ZZ, Krol A, Boccara O, Foelster-Holst R, Bosch MI, Su J, Buckova H, Torrelo A, Cambazard F, Grantzow R, Wargon O, Wyrzykowski D, Roessler J, Bernabeu-Wittel J, Valencia AM, Przewratil P, Glick S, Pope E, Birchall N, Benjamin L, Mancini AJ, Vabres P, Souteyrand P, Frieden IJ, Berul CI, Mehta CR, Pray S, Boralevi F, Morgan CC, Heritier S, Delarue A, Voisard JJ. A randomised, controlled trial of oral propranolol in infantile haemangioma. N Engl J Med. 2015;372:735–46.
57. Lichter PR, Musch DC, Gillespie BW, Guire KE, Janz NK, Wren PA, Mills RP. Interim clinical outcomes in the collaborative initial glaucoma treatment study comparing initial treatment randomised to medications or surgery. Ophthalmology. 2001;108:1943–53.
58. Lincoff H, Gieser R. Finding the retinal hole. Arch Ophthalmol. 1971;85:565–9.
59. MacEwan CJ, Young JD. The fluorescein disappearance test (FDT): an evaluation of its use in infants. J Pediatr Ophthalmol Strabismus. 1991;28:302–5.
60. Mackie SL, Dejaco C, Appenzeller S, Camellino D, Duftner C, Gonzalez-Chiappe S, Mahr A, Mukhtyar C, Reynolds G, de Souza AWS, Brouwer E, Bukhari M, Buttgereit F, Bryne D, Cid MC, Cimmino M, Direskeneli H, Gilbert K, Kermani TA, Khan A, Lanyon P, Luqmani R, Mallen C, Mason JC, Matteson EL, Merkel PA, Mollan S, Neill L, O'Sullivan E, Sandovici M, Schmidt WA, Watts R, Whitlock M, Yacyshyn E, Ytterberg S, Dasgupta B. British Society of Rheumatology guideline on diagnosis and treatment of giant cell arteritis: executive summary. Rheumatology. 2020;59:487–94.
61. McCannel CA, Ensminger JL, Diehl NN, Hodge DN. Population-based incidence of macular holes. Ophthalmology. 2009;116:1366–9.
62. Markus HS, Levi C, King A, Madigan K, Norris J. Antiplatelet therapy vs anticoagulation therapy in cervical artery dissection: the cervical artery dissection in stroke study (CADISS) randomized clinical trial final results. JAMA Neurol. 2019;76:657–64.
63. Mitchell P, Bandello F, Schmidt-Erfurth U, Lang GE, Massin P, Schlingemann RO, Sutter F, Simader C, Burian G, Gerstner O, Weichselberger A. The RESTORE study. Ranibuzumab monotherapy or combined with laser versus laser monotherapy for diabetic macular edema. Ophthalmology. 2011;118:615–25.
64. Mollan SP, Davies B, Silver NC, Shaw S, Mallucci CL, Wakerley BR, Krishnan A, Chavda SV, Ramalingam S, Edwards J, Hemmings K, Williamson M, Burdon MA, Hassan-Smith G, Digre K, Liu GT, Jensen RH, Sinclair AJ. Idiopathic intracranial hypertension: consensus guidelines on management. J Neurol Neurosurg Psychiatry. 2018;89:1088–100.
65. Mourits MP, Prummel MF, Wiersinga WM, Koornneef L. Clinical activity score as a guide in the management of patients with Graves ophthalmopathy. Clin Endocrinol. 1997;47:9–14.
66. National Institute for Health and Care Excellence. Dexamethasone intravitreal implant for the treatment of macular oedema secondary to retinal vein occlusion [TA229]. [Online]. London: NICE; 2011 [Accessed 11th December 2019]. Available at https://www.nice.org.uk/guidance/ta229.
67. National Institute for Health and Care Excellence. Ranibizumab for treating diabetic macular oedema [TA274]. [Online]. London: NICE; 2013 [Accessed 11th December 2019]. Available at https://www.nice.org.uk/guidance/ta274.

68. National Institute for Health and Care Excellence. Ranibizumab for treating visual impairment caused by macular oedema secondary to retinal vein occlusion [TA283]. [Online]. London: NICE; 2013 [Accessed 11th December 2019]. Available at https://www.nice.org.uk/guidance/ta283.
69. National Institute for Health and Care Excellence. Fluocinolone acetonide intravitreal implant for treating chronic diabetic macular oedema after an inadequate response to prior therapy [TA301]. [Online]. London: NICE; 2013 [Accessed 11th December 2019]. Available at https://www.nice.org.uk/guidance/ta301.
70. National Institute for Health and Care Excellence. Aflibercept for treating visual impairment caused by macular oedema secondary to central retinal vein occlusion [TA305]. [Online]. London: NICE; 2014 [Accessed 11th December 2019]. Available at https://www.nice.org.uk/guidance/ta305.
71. National Institute for Health and Care Excellence. Aflibercept for treating diabetic macular oedema [TA346]. [Online]. London: NICE; 2015 [Accessed 11th December 2019]. Available at https://www.nice.org.uk/guidance/ta346
72. National Institute for Health and Care Excellence. Diabetes in pregnancy: management from preconception to the postnatal period [NG3]. [Online]. London: NICE; 2015 [Accessed 11th December 2019]. Available at https://www.nice.org.uk/guidance/ng3.
73. National Institute for Health and Care Excellence. Dexamethasone intravitreal implant for treating diabetic macular oedema [TA349]. [Online]. London: NICE; 2015 [Accessed 11th December 2019]. Available at https://www.nice.org.uk/guidance/ta349
74. National Institute for Health and Care Excellence. Aflibercept for treating visual impairment caused by macular oedema after branch retinal vein occlusion [TA409]. [Online]. London: NICE; 2016 [Accessed 11th December 2019]. Available at https://www.nice.org.uk/guidance/ta409.
75. National Institute for Health and Care Excellence. Glaucoma: diagnosis and management [NG81]. [Online]. London: NICE; 2017 [Accessed 10th December 2024]. Available at https://www.nice.org.uk/guidance/ng81.
76. National Institute for Health and Care Excellence. Cataracts in adults: management [NG77]. [Online]. London: NICE; 2017 [Accessed 30th November 2019]. Available at https://www.nice.org.uk/guidance/ng77.
77. National Institute for Health and Care Excellence. Tocilizumab for treating giant cell arteritis [TA518]. [Online]. London: NICE; 2018 [Accessed 11th December 2019]. Available at https://www.nice.org.uk/guidance/ta518.
78. National Institute for Health and Care Excellence. Stroke and transient ischaemic attack in over 16s: diagnosis and initial management [NG128]. [Online]. London: NICE; 2019 [Accessed 17th December 2024]. Available at https://www.nice.org.uk/guidance/ng128.
79. National Institute for Health and Care Excellence. Diabetic retinopathy: management and monitoring [NG242]. [Online]. London: NICE; 2024 [Accessed 6th November 2024]. Available at http://www.nice.org.uk/guidance/ta242.
80. National Institute for Health and Care Excellence. Hypertension in adults diagnosis and management [NG136]. [Online]. London: NICE; 2019 [Accessed 6th November 2024]. Available at http://www.nice.org.uk/guidance/ta136.
81. National Institute for Health and Care Excellence. Faricimab for treating diabetic macular oedema [TA799]. [Online]. London: NICE; 2022 [Accessed 6th November 2024]. Available at http://www.nice.org.uk/guidance/ta799.
82. National Institute for Health and Care Excellence. Brolucizumab for treating diabetic macular oedema [TA820]. [Online]. London: NICE; 2022 [Accessed 6th November 2024]. Available at http://www.nice.org.uk/guidance/ta820.
83. National Institute for Health and Care Excellence. Type 2 diabetes in adults: management [NG28]. [Online]. London: NICE; 2015 [Accessed 7th November 2024]. Available at http://www.nice.org.uk/guidance/ng28.
84. National Institute for Health and Care Excellence. Faricimab for treating visual impairment caused by macular oedema after retinal vein occlusion [TA1004]. [Online]. London: NICE; 2024 [Accessed 7th November 2024]. Available at http://www.nice.org.uk/guidance/TA1004.
85. National Institute for Health and Care Excellence. Latanoprost-netarsudil for previously treated primary open-angle glaucoma or ocular hypertension [TA1009]. [Online]. London: NICE; 2024 [Accessed 22nd December 2024]. Available at http://www.nice.org.uk/guidance/TA1009.
86. Nguyen QD, Brown DM, Marcus DM, Boyer DS, Patel S, Feiner L, Gibson A, Sy J, Rundle AC, Hopkins J, Rubio RG, Ehrlich JS. Ranibizumab for diabetic macular edema. Results from 2 phase III randomised trials: RISE and RIDE. Ophthalmology. 2012;119:789–801.
87. Pediatric Eye Disease Investigator Group. Randomised trial of treatment of amblyopia in children aged 7 to 17 years. Arch Ophthalmol. 2005;123:437–47.
88. Prajna NV, Krishnan T, Mascarenhas MD, Rajaraman R, Prajna L, Srinivasan M, Raghavan A, Oldenburg CE, Ray KJ, Zegans ME, McLeod SD, Porco TC, Acharya NR. The mycotic ulcer treatment trial. A randomised trial comparing natamycin vs voriconazole. JAMA Ophthalmol. 2013;131:422–9.
89. Public Health England. NHS Diabetic Eye Screening Programme. Grading definitions for referable disease. Public Health England leads the NHS Screening Programmes. [Online]. London: Public Health England; 2017 [Accessed 11th December

2019]. Available at https://assets.publishing.service.gov.uk/government/uploads/system/uploads/attachment_data/file/582710/Grading_definitions_for_referrable_disease_2017_new_110117.pdf.

90. Risk factors for central retinal vein occlusion. The eye disease case-control study group. Arch Ophthalmol. 1996;114:545–54.
91. Royal College of Paediatrics and Child Health, Royal College of Ophthalmologists, British Association of Perinatal Medicine. UK screening of retinopathy of prematurity guideline 2022. [Online]. London: Royal College of Paediatrics and Child Health. London: Royal College of Ophthalmologists. London: British Association of Perinatal Medicine [Accessed 22nd December 2024]. Available at https://www.rcpch.ac.uk/sites/default/files/2024-10/rop-screening-guideline-full-2022_updated-2024.pdf.
92. Ruby AJ, Williams DF, Grand MG, Thomas MA, Meredith TA, Boniuk I, Olk RJ. Pars plana vitrectomy for treatment of stage 2 macular holes. Arch Ophthalmol. 1994;112:359–64.
93. Saidkasimova S, Mitry D, Singh J, Yorston D, Charteris DG. Retinal detachment in Scotland is associated with affluence. Br J Ophthalmol. 2009;93:1591–4.
94. Scott CJ, Kardon RH, Lee AG, Frisen L, Wall M. Diagnosis and grading of papilledema in patients with raised intracranial pressure using optical coherence tomography vs clinical expert assessment using a clinical staging scale. Arch Ophthalmol. 2010;128:705–11.
95. Sharma MC, Regillo CD, Shuler MF, Borrillo JL, Benson WE. Determination of the incidence and clinical characteristics of subsequent retinal tears following treatment of the acute posterior vitreous detachment-related initial retinal tears. Am J Ophthalmol. 2004;138:280–4.
96. Smiddy WE, Michels RG, Glaser BM, de Bustros S. Vitrectomy for impending idiopathic macular holes. Am J Ophthalmol. 1988;105:371–6.
97. Solebo AL, Cumberland P, Rahi JS. 5-year outcomes after primary intraocular lens implantation in children aged 2 years or younger with congenital or infantile cataract: findings from the IoLunder2 prospective inception cohort study. Lancet Child Adolesc Health. 2018;2:863–71.
98. Srinivasan M, Mascarenhas J, Rajaraman R, Ravindran M, Lalitha P, Glidden DV, Ray KJ, Hong KC, Oldenburg CE, Lee SM, Zegans ME, Mcleod SD, Lietman TM, Acharya NR. Corticosteroids for bacterial keratitis. The steroids for corneal ulcers trial (SCUT). Arch Ophthalmol. 2012;130:143–50.
99. Srinivasan M, Mascarenhas J, Rajaraman R, Ravindran M, Lalitha P, O'Brien KS, Glidden DV, Ray KJ, Oldenburg CE, Zegans ME, Whitcher JP, Mcleod SD, Porco TC, Lietman TM, Acharya NR. The steroids for corneal ulcers trial (SCUT): secondary 12-month clinical outcomes of a randomised controlled trial. Am J Ophthalmol. 2014;157:327–33.
100. Steel DH, Donachie PHJ, Awlward GW, Laidlaw DA, Williamson TH, Yorston D. Factors affecting anatomical and visual outcome after macular hole surgery: findings from a large prospective UK cohort. Eye (Lond). 2021;35:316–25.
101. Stone JH, Tuckwell K, Dimonaco S, Klearman M, Aringer M, Blockmans D, Brouwer E, Cid MC, Dasgupta B, Rech J, Salvarani C, Schott G, Schulze-Koops H, Spiera R, Unizony SH, Collinson N. Trial of Tocilizumab in Giant-cell arteritis. N Engl J Med. 2017;377:317–28.
102. Tadayoni R, Paris LP, Danzig CJ, Abreu F, Khanani AM, Brittain C, Lai TYY, Haskova Z, SakamotoT KA, Schlottmann PG, Liu Y, Seres A, Retiere A, Willis JR, Yoon YH. Efficacy and safety of faricimab for macular edema due to retinal vein occlusion: 24-week results from the BALATON and COMINO trials. Ophthalmology. 2024;131:950–60.
103. Tanner V, Williamson TH. Watzke-Allen slit beam test in macular holes confirmed by optical coherence tomography. Arch Ophthalmol. 2000;118:1059–63.
104. The ACCORD Study Group and ACCORD Eye Study Group. Effects of medical therapies on retinopathy progression in type 2 diabetes. N Engl J Med. 2010;363:233–44.
105. The AGIS Investigators. The advanced glaucoma intervention study (AGIS): 4. Comparison of treatment outcomes within race. Ophthalmology. 1998;105:1146–64.
106. The AGIS Investigators. The advanced glaucoma intervention study (AGIS): 9. Comparison of glaucoma outcomes in black and white patients within treatment groups. Am J Ophthalmol. 2001;132:311–20.
107. The Branch Vein Occlusion Study Group. Argon laser photocoagulation for macular edema in branch vein occlusion. Am J Ophthalmol. 1984;98:271–82.
108. The Branch Vein Occlusion Study Group. Prevention of neovascularisation and vitreous hemorrhage in branch vein occlusion. Arch Ophthalmol. 1986;104:34–41.
109. The CADISS trial investigators. Antiplatelet treatment compared with anticoagulation treatment for cervical artery dissection (CADISS): a randomised trial. Lancet Neurol. 2015;14:361–7.
110. The Central Vein Occlusion Study Group. Natural history and clinical management of central retinal vein occlusion. Arch Ophthalmol. 1997;115:486–91.
111. The Diabetic Retinopathy Vitrectomy Study Research Group. Early vitrectomy for severe proliferative diabetic retinopathy in eyes with useful vision. Results of a randomised trial—diabetic retinopathy vitrectomy study report 3. Ophthalmology. 1988;95:1307–20.
112. The Diabetic Retinopathy Study Research Group. Photocoagulation treatment of proliferative diabetic retinopathy. Clinical application of diabetic retinopathy study (DRS) findings, DRS report number 8. Ophthalmology. 1981;88:583–600.

113. The Herpetic Eye Disease Study Group. A controlled trial of oral acyclovir for iridocyclitis caused by herpes simplex virus. Arch Ophthalmol. 1996;114:1065–72.
114. The Herpetic Eye Disease Study Group. Acyclovir for the prevention of recurrent herpes simplex virus eye disease. N Engl J Med. 1998;339:300–6.
115. The NORDIC idiopathic intracranial hypertension study group writing committee. Effect of acetazolamide on visual function in patients with idiopathic intracranial hypertension and mild visual loss: the idiopathic intracranial hypertension treatment trial. JAMA. 2014;311:1641–51.
116. The Pediatric Eye Disease Investigator Group. A randomized trial of atropine vs patching for treatment of moderate amblyopia in children. Arch Ophthalmol. 2002;120:268–78.
117. The Pediatric Eye Disease Investigator Group. A randomised trial of patching regimens for treatment of moderate amblyopia in children. Arch Ophthalmol. 2003;121:603–11.
118. The Pediatric Eye Disease Investigator Group. A randomised trial of prescribed patching regimens for treatment of severe amblyopia in children. Ophthalmology. 2003;110:2075–87.
119. The Royal College of Ophthalmologists. Diabetic Retinopathy Guidelines 2012. [Online]. London: The Royal College of Ophthalmologists. [Accessed 11th December 2019]. Available at https://www.rcophth.ac.uk/wp-content/uploads/2014/12/2013-SCI-301-FINAL-DR-GUIDELINES-DEC-2012-updated-July-2013.pdf.
120. The Royal College of Ophthalmologists. Retinal Vein Occlusion (RVO) Guidelines 2022. [Online]. London: The Royal College of Ophthalmologists. [Accessed 6th November 2024]. Available at https://www.rcophth.ac.uk/wp-content/uploads/2015/07/Retinal-Vein-Occlusion-Guidelines-2022.pdf.
121. The Royal College of Ophthalmologists. Ophthalmic Services Guidance for the Management of Acute Retinal Detachment 2010. [Online]. London: The Royal College of Ophthalmologists. [Accessed 11th December 2019]. Available at https://www.rcophth.ac.uk/wp-content/uploads/2014/12/2010_PROF_064_OSG-Retinal-Detachment-June-2010.pdf.
122. The Royal College of Ophthalmologists. Ophthalmic Services Guidance for Managing an outbreak of postoperative endophthalmitis 2016. [Online]. London: The Royal College of Ophthalmologists. [Accessed 11th December 2019]. Available at https://www.rcophth.ac.uk/wp-content/uploads/2016/07/Managing-an-outbreak-of-postoperative-endophthalmitis.pdf.
123. The Royal College of Ophthalmologists. The Management of Angle Closure Glaucoma Clinical Guidelines 2021. [Online]. London: The Royal College of Ophthalmologists. [Accessed 4th June 2024]. Available at https://www.rcophth.ac.uk/wp-content/uploads/2021/10/The-Management-of-Angle-Closure-Glaucoma-Clinical-Guidelines.pdf.
124. The Royal College of Ophthalmologists. Treating Retinopathy of Prematurity in the UK. Clinical Guidelines 2022. [Online]. London: The Royal College of Ophthalmologists. [Accessed 22nd December 2024]. Available at: https://www.rcophth.ac.uk/resources-listing/uk-retinopathy-of-prematurity-guideline/.
125. The Royal College of Ophthalmologists. Idiopathic Full Thickness Macular Holes. Clinical Guidelines 2025. [Online]. London: The Royal College of Ophthalmologists. [Accessed 23rd February 2025]. Available at: https://www.rcophth.ac.uk/wp-content/uploads/2025/02/Macular-Holes-Guidelines-final-version-jan-2025.pdf.
126. UK Prospective Diabetes Study (UKPDS) Group. Intensive blood-glucose control with sulphonylureas or insulin compared with conventional treatment and risk of complications in patients with type 2 diabetes (UKPDS 33). Lancet. 1998;352:837–53.
127. Wilhelmus KR, Gee L, Hauck WW, Kurinij N, Dawson CR, Jones DB, Barron BA, Kaufman HE, Sugar J, Hyndiuk RA, Laibson PR, Stulting RD, Asbell PA. Herpetic Eye Disease Study. A controlled trial of topical corticosteroids for herpes simplex stromal keratitis. Ophthalmology. 1994;101:1883–96.
128. Wilkinson CP, Ferris FL 3rd, Klein RE, Lee PP, Agardh CD, Davis M, Dills D, Kampik A, Pararajasegaram R, Verdaguer JT, Global Diabetic Retinopathy Project Group. Proposed international clinical diabetic retinopathy and diabetic macular edema disease severity scales. Ophthalmology. 2003;110:1677–82.
129. Writing committee for the diabetic retinopathy clinical research network, Fong DS, Strauber SF, Aiello LP, Beck RW, Callanan DG, Danis RP, Davis MD, Feman SS, Ferris F, Friedman SM, Garcia CA, Glassman AR, Han DP, Le D, Kollman C, Lauer AK, Recchia FM, Solomon SD. Comparison of the modified early treatment diabetic retinopathy study and mild macular grid laser photocoagulation strategies for diabetic macular edema. Arch Ophthalmol. 2007;125:469–80.
130. Wycoff CC, Abreu F, Adamis AP, Basu K, Eichenbaum DA, Haskova Z, Lin H, Loewenstein A, Mohan S, Pearce IA, Sakamoto T, Schlottmann PG, Silverman D, Sun JK, Wells JA, Willis JR, Tadayoni R. Efficacy, durability, and safety of intravitreal faricimab with extended dosing up to every 16 weeks in patients with diabetic macular oedema (YOSEMITE and RHINE): two randomised, double-masked, phase 3 trials. Lancet. 2022;399:741–55.
131. Yamashita T, Uemara A, Uchino E, Doi N, Ohba N. Spontaneous closure of traumatic macular hole. Am J Ophthalmol. 2002;133:230-235.

4 Attitudes, Ethics and Responsibilities in Clinical Practice

Timothy H. M. Fung and Winfried M. K. Amoaku

Abstract

Staying informed about the guidelines from various organisations is essential for ensuring high standards of practice and patient care. This chapter summarises key guidelines from the General Medical Council, the Royal College of Ophthalmologists, and the UK government.

4.1 GMC Guidance—Doctors Use of Social Media 2013 [1]

4.1.1 Facebook: Patient Asking to Add You as a Friend on Facebook

- It is important that doctors maintain a professional boundary between themselves and their patients, however minimal the professional contact may be. This professional boundary is important to maintain trust
- If the boundary is breached, whether the breach is deliberate or accidental, this can undermine a patient's trust in their doctor, and society's trust in the medical profession more widely
- Using social media also creates risks, particularly where social and professional boundaries become unclear
- If a patient contacts you about their care or other professional matters, through your private profile, you should indicate that you cant mix social and professional relationships and, where appropriate, direct them to your professional profile
- You must consider the potential risks involved in using social media and the impact that inappropriate use could have on your patients trust in you and society's trust in the medical profession.
- Social media can blur the boundaries between a doctor's personal and professional lives and may change the nature of the relationship between a doctor and a patient

4.1.2 Facebook: Posting Messages on a Groups Facebook Page

- Doctors must be careful not to share identifiable information about patients
- Although individual pieces of information may not breach confidentiality on their own, the sum of published information online could be enough to identify a patient or someone close to them. This would be in breach of the

T. H. M. Fung (✉)
University Hospitals of Derby & Burton NHS Foundation Trust, Royal Derby Hospital, Derby, UK
e-mail: timothy.fung@nhs.net

W. M. K. Amoaku
Eye, Ear, Nose and Throat Centre, Queens Medical Center, Nottingham University Hospitals NHS Trust, Nottingham, UK

T. H. M. Fung, W. M. K. Amoaku (eds.), *Viva and OSCE Exams in Ophthalmology*,
https://doi.org/10.1007/978-3-031-97401-4_4

GMC's guidance on Confidentiality, Social Media and Good Medical Practice

- Doctors must also ensure that their tone online is in keeping with professional practice and that their comments don't risk damaging public trust in the profession
- The standards expected of doctors do not change because they are communicating through social media rather than face to face or through other traditional media
- You must make sure that your conduct justifies your patient's trust in you and the publics trust in the profession
- When communicating publicly, including speaking to or writing in the media, you must maintain patient confidentiality
- You should remember when using social media that communications intended for friends or family may become more widely available
- You must not use publicly accessible social media to discuss individual patients or their care, with those patients or anyone else
- Many doctors use professional social media sites that are not accessible to the public. However, you must still be careful not to share identifiable information about your patients. Although individual pieces of information may not breach confidentiality on their own, the sum of published information online could be enough to identify a patient or someone close to them.

4.1.3 Twitter: Doctor Tweeting Messages on Twitter

- You must make sure that your conduct justifies your patient's trust in you and the publics trust in the profession
- When communicating publicly, including speaking to or writing in the media, you must maintain patient confidentiality
- You should remember when using social media that communications intended for friends or family may become more widely available
- Using of social media has blurred the boundaries between public and private life, and online information can be easily accessed by others.
- You should be aware of the limitations of privacy online and you should regularly review the privacy settings for each of your social media profiles. This is for the following reasons:
  (a) Social media sites cannot guarantee confidentiality whatever privacy settings are in place
  (b) Patients, your employer and potential employers, or any other organisation that you have a relationship with, may be able to access your personal information
  (c) Information about your location may be embedded within photographs and other content and available for others to see
  (d) Once information is published online it can be difficult to remove as other users may distribute it further or comment on it
- Using social media also creates risks, particularly where social and professional boundaries become unclear.
- You must not use publicly accessible social media to discuss individual patients or their care, with those patients or anyone else
- You must consider the potential risks involved in using social media and the impact that inappropriate use could have on your patients trust in you and society's trust in the medical profession.
- Social media can blur the boundaries between a doctor's personal and professional lives and may change the nature of the relationship between a doctor and a patient
- If doctors are using social media to comment on health or healthcare issues, it is good practice for them to say who they are.

4.2 GMC Guidance—Consent: Patients and Doctors Making Decisions Together 2008 [2]

- Assess capacity for patient to consent to investigation or treatment, starting from the presumption that the patient has capacity
- You must work on the presumption that every adult patient has the capacity to make decisions about their care, and to decide whether to agree to, or refuse, an examination, investigation or treatment.
- You must assess a patient's capacity to make a particular decision at the time it needs to

be made. You must not assume that because a patient lacks capacity to make a decision on a particular occasion, they lack capacity to make a decision at all, or will not be able to make similar decisions in the future

- You must give patients the information they want or need to know in a way they can understand. You should make sure that arrangements are made, wherever possible, to meet patient's language and communication needs.
- How you discuss a patient's diagnosis, prognosis and treatment options is often as important as the information itself. You should share information in a way that the patient can understand and, whenever possible, in a place and at a time when they are best able to understand and retain it
- You should check whether the patient needs any additional support to understand the information, to communicate their wishes, or to make a decision. You must make sure, wherever practical, that arrangements are made to give the patient any necessary support. This might include, for example: using an advocate or interpreter; asking those close to the patient about the patient's communication needs; or giving the patient a written or audio record of the discussion and any decisions that were made
- Ask the patient if there is anything that would help them remember information, or make it easier to make a decision; such as bringing a relative, partner, friend, carer or advovate to consultations, or having written or audio information about their condition or the proposed investigation or treatment
- If a patient is likely to have difficulty retaining information, you should offer them a written record of your discussions, detailing what decisions were made and why.
- You must only regard a patient as lacking capacity once it is clear that, having been given all appropriate help and support, they cannot understand, retain, use or weigh up the information needed to make that decision, or communicate their wishes by whatever means possible.
- If your assessment leaves you in doubt about the patients capacity to make a decision, you should seek advice from:
  (a) Nursing staff or others involved in the patients care, or those close to the patient, who may be aware of the patients usual ability to make decisions and their particular communication needs
  (b) Colleagues with relevant specialist experience, such as psychiatrists, neurologists, or speech and language therapists
- If you are still unsure about the patients capacity to make a decision, you must seek legal advice with a view to asking a court to determine capacity

4.2.1 Patients Who Lacks Capacity to Consent

- In England and Wales (under the Mental Capacity Act 2005) and in Northern Ireland (under the common law), decisions must be made in a patient's best interest
- Best interest can be assessed by evidence of patients previously expressed preferences (e.g. advance directive) and by consulting those who are familiar with the patient e.g. relatives or carers
- Independent mental capacity advocates (IMCA) must be instructed in relation to individuals who lack capacity and who have no family or friends whom it is appropriate to consult when:
  (a) An NHS body is proposing to provide, withhold or withdraw "serious medical treatment"; or
  (b) An NHS body or local authority is proposing to arrange accomodation, or a change in accomodation, in a hospital or care home, and the stay in hospital will be more than 28 days, or the stay in the care home more than 8 weeks

  The IMCA cannot make decisions, but represents the patient by bringing to the attention of decision makers the important factors that need to be considered, such as the patient's beliefs, feelings, and values

- In making decisions about the treatment and care of patients who lack capacity, you must:
  (a) Make the care of your patient your first concern
  (b) Treat patients as individuals and respect their dignity
  (c) Support and encourage patients to be involved, as far as they want to and are able, in decisions about their treatment and care
  (d) Treat patients with respect and not discriminate against them
- You must also consider:
  (a) Whether the patients lack of capacity is temporary or permanent
  (b) Which options for treatment would provide overall clinical benefit for the patient
  (c) Which option, including the option not to treat, would be least restrictive of the patient's future choices
  (d) Any evidence of patient's previously expressed preferences, such as an advance statement or decision (advance directive)
  (e) The views of anyone the patient asks you to consult, or who has legal authority to make a decision on their behalf, or has been appointed to represent them (lasting powers of attorney)
  (f) The views of people close to the patient on the patient's preferences, feelings, beliefs and values, and whether they consider the proposed treatment to be in the patients best interest
  (g) What you and the rest of the healthcare team know about the patients wishes, feelings, beliefs and values
- Unless the patient has signed an advance directive, the management decisions will rest with the doctor. Legally, relatives and others only have an advisory role.

4.2.2 Delegating Consent

- Clinical, legal and professional responsibility for ensuring that valid consent has been obtained before treatment is provided rests with the person carrying out the procedure
- The GMC's guidance states:
  (a) If you are the doctor undertaking an investigation or providing treatment, it is your responsibility to discuss it with the patient. If this is not practical, you can delegate the responsibility to someone else, provided you make sure that the person you delegate to:
    1. is suitably trained and qualified
    2. has sufficient knowledge of the proposed investigation or treatment, and understands the risk involved
    3. understands, and agrees to act in accordance with the GMC's guidance
  (b) If you delegate, you are still responsible for making sure that the patient has been given enough time and information to make an informed decision, and has given their consent, before you start any investigation or treatment

4.2.3 Capacity in Children

- All children aged 16 or above can be assumed to have the capacity to make decisions about their care, and to decide whether to agree to, or refuse, an examination, investigation or treatment (i.e. essentially they can be treated in exactly the same way as an adult)
- Children under the age of 16 can give consent to an examination, investigation or treatment if they are deemed to be Gillick competent
- A child is deemed Gillick competent if they can understand, retain, use and weigh the information given and their understanding of benefits, risks and consequences.
- Even if a child is competent enough to make a decision to consent to a given procedure or treatment, you should make every effort to encourage the child to involve their parents. Whatever their involvement, parents cannot override consent given by a competent child

4.2.4 Children Refusing Treatment

- Parents cannot override the competent consent of a young person to treatment that you consider is in their best interests. You can rely on parental consent when a child lacks the capacity to consent.
- In Scotland, children can refuse treatment and the child's decision cannot be overridden by the parents
- In England, Wales and Northern Island, the law on parents overriding young people's competent refusal is complex. You should involve other members of the multi-disciplinary team, an independent advocate, or a named or designated doctor for child protection or seek legal advice if you think treatment is in the best interests of a competent young person who refuses.

4.3 GMC Guidance—Confidentiality: Good Practice in Handling Patient Information 2017 [3]

- Not leaving computers with patient records unattended
- Not leaving patient details showing on screen where they can be viewed by others
- Not letting patient notes lie around and not taking notes home with you unless they have been anonymised
- Not leaving handover sheets where they can be seen by patients and their families
- Ensuring you check the identity of patients, particularly if you are discussing matters over the phone
- If the patient comes accompanied, asking the patient if they are comfortable with a third person sitting in on the consultation
- Not using the public as translators, even if they offer. There are a number of commercial interpreters available via telephone (e.g. LanguageLine)
- If an adult who has capacity to make the decision refuses to consent to information being disclosed that you consider necessary for their protection, you should explore their reasons for this. It may be appropriate to encourage the patient to consent to the disclosure and to warn them of the risks of refusing to consent.
- You should, however, usually abide by the patients refusal to consent to disclosure, even if their decision leaves them (but no one else) at risk of death or serious harm.
- You should do your best to give the patient the information and support they need to make decisions in their own interests e.g. by arranging contact with agencies to support people who experience domestic violence

4.3.1 Breaching Patient Confidentiality

- There are various legal requirements (e.g. court order) to disclose information about adults who are known or considered to be at risk or, or to have suffered, abuse or neglect. You must disclose information if it is required by law. You should:
  (a) Satisfy yourself that the disclosure is required by law
  (b) Only disclose information that is relevant to the request, and only in the way required by the law
  (c) Tell patients about such disclosures whenever practicable, unless it would undermine the purpose of the disclosure to do so
- You must not disclose personal information to a third party such as a solicitor, police officer or officer of a court without the patients explicit consent, unless it is required by law or can be justified in the public interest. You may disclose information without consent to your own legal advisors.
- In very exceptional circumstances, disclosure without consent may be justified in the public interest to prevent a serious crime such as murder, manslaughter or serious assault even where no other than the patient is at risk. This is only likely to be justifiable where there is clear evidence of an imminent risk of serious harm to the individual, and where there are no

alternative (and less intrusive) methods of preventing that harm
- Disclosing information about serious communicable diseases:
    (a) You may disclose information to a known sexual contact of a patient with a sexually transmitted serious communicable disease if you have reason to think that they are at risk of infection and that the patient has not informed them and cannot be persuaded to do so. This guidance applies, even if the sexual contact is not a patient
    (b) In such circumstances, you should tell the patient before you make the disclosure (and should consider any reason the patient gives for refusing to consent), if it is practicable and safe to do so.
    (c) You must be prepared to justify a decision to disclose personal information without consent

4.4 GMC Guidance—Financial and Commercial Arrangements and Conflicts of Interest 2013 [4]

- You must be honest in financial and commercial dealings with patients, employers, insurers and other organisations or individuals
- You must not allow any interests you have to affect the way you prescribe for, treat, refer or commission services for patients
- If you are faced with a conflict of interest, you must be open about the conflict, declaring your interest formally, and you should be prepared to exclude yourself from decision making
- You must not ask for or accept—from patients, colleagues or others—any inducement, gift or hospitality that may affect or be seen to affect the way you prescribe for, treat or refer patients or commission services for patients. You must not offer these inducements
- You should use your professional judgement to identify when conflicts of interest arise
- Avoid conflicts of interest wherever possible
- Declare any conflicts of interest to anyone affected, formally and as early as possible, in line with the policies of your employer or the organisation contracting your services
- Get advice about the implications of any potential conflict of interest
- Make sure that the conflict does not affect your decisions about patient care

4.5 GMC Guidance—Revalidation [5]

- The process by which all licensed doctors are required to demonstrate on a regular basis that they are up to date and fit to practice in their chosen field and able to provide a good level of care. This means that holding a licence to practice is becoming an indicator that the doctor continues to meet the professional standards set by the GMC
- All doctors who wish to retain their licenses to practice are now legally required to be revalidated every 5 years to prove they are up to date and fit to practice.
- Revalidation aims to protect patients from poorly performing doctors, promote good medical practice, and increase public confidence in doctors.
- Revalidation is based on annual whole practice appraisals usually carried out by someone from your workplace.
- Need to collect evidence and examples of your work throughout the year. At your appraisal you can reflect on these and identify your strengths and any areas for development.
- There are three ways to get revalidated:
    1. Responsible officer:
        - For the vast majority of doctors, this decision is based on a recommendation from a senior doctor in your organisation called a responsible officer
        - Your responsible officer bases their recommendation on your appraisals and any relevant evidence such as clinical governance information
    2. Suitable person:

- If you are a small number of doctors who don't have a responsible officer, you will need another senior doctor to take on their duties, known as a suitable person

3. Annual return.
   - If you don't have a responsible officer or a suitable person you will need to send the GMC an annual return showing that you are having annual appraisals and that there are no outstanding concerns about your practice
   - In this case, the GMC may ask you to sit a written knowledge test

4.6 GMC Guidance—Appraisal

- A constructive discussion with a senior colleague during which doctors reflect on their performance over the last 12 months and consider their future development needs (PDP, CME, CPD)
- There are three stages in the appraisal process:
  1. Inputs to appraisal, including a record of the doctors scope and nature of work and relevant supporting information
  2. The confidential appraisal discussion
  3. Outputs of appraisal, including the doctors PDP and a summary of the appraiser discussion and the appraiser's statements

4.7 UK Government Guidance—Parental Rights and Responsibilities [6]

- Defined as "all the rights, duties, powers, responsibilities and authority which by law a parent of a child has in relation to the child and his property"
- This can include:
  (a) Consenting to a child's operation or certain medical treatment
  (b) Accessing a child's medical records
- Mothers automatically have parental responsibility and will not lose it if divorced
- Married fathers automatically have parental responsibility and will not lose it if divorced
- Unmarried fathers do not automatically have parental responsibility:
  - If an unmarried father has a child after 1st December 2003 and he is registered on the birth certificate, he will have parental responsibility
  - If a child's birth was registered before 1st December 2003 and the father was not named on the birth certificate, the birth can be re-registered to include the father's name—the father will then have parental responsibility
  - If a child's birth was registered before 1st December 2003 and includes the name of the unmarried father, the father will not have parental responsibility (unless obtained by other means)
- Step fathers and step mothers do not automatically have parental responsibility
- Grandparents do not automatically have parental responsibility

4.8 UK Government Guidance—Driving Eyesight Rules [7]

- Group 1 drivers (car and light vehicles):
  - Vision requirements:
    - BCVA of at least 6/12 with both eyes open (or in the only eye if monocular) AND
    - Read a standard number plate at 20 meters
  - Visual field requirements (Esterman programme on the Humphrey analyser—maximum of 20% false positives is allowed):
    - At least 120 degrees on the horizontal, with at least 50 degrees left and right AND
    - No significant defect on the binocular field encroaching within 20 degrees of fixation above or below the horizontal meridian

    - Significant defect:
        - A cluster of 4 adjoining points that is either wholly or partly within the central 20 degrees
        - Loss consisting of both a single cluster of 3 adjoining missed points up to and including 20 degree from fixation AND any additional separate missed point within the central 20 degree area
        - Any central loss that is an extension of hemianopia or quadrantanopia of size greater than 3 missed points
    - Where a driver has fully adapted to a static long-standing defect, the DVLA may consider them as an exceptional case and perform a practical driving assessment
- Group 2 drivers (large goods vehicles and passenger-carrying vehicles)
    - Vision requirements:
        - BCVA of at least 6/7.5 in the better eye AND
        - BCVA of at least 6/60 in the worst eye AND
        - Glasses, if required, should be up to +8D in strength
    - Visual field requirements (Esterman programme on the Humphrey analyser—maximum of 20% false positives is allowed):
        - At least 160 degrees on the horizontal, with at least 70 degrees left and right and 30 degrees above and below AND
        - No defects in the central 30 degrees
- Monocularity:
    - Group 1 drivers: do not need to tell DVLA if the other eye satisfies the usual vision and visual field requirements and may drive when clinically advised that they have adapted to the disability
    - Group 2 drivers: must not drive and must inform the DVLA
- Diplopia:
    - Group 1 drivers: must inform the DVLA, driving may be resumed if diplopia controlled—patching is acceptable (must not drive if diplopia uncontrolled)
    - Group 2 drivers: must not drive and must inform the DVLA, patching not acceptable
- Blepharospasm:
    - Patients with severe blepharospasm must not drive. Patients with mild treated blepharospasm may drive subject to consultant approval
    - Group 1 drivers: must inform DVLA
    - Group 2 drivers: must inform DVLA
- TIA:
    - Group 1 drivers: must not drive for 1 month and only restart when the doctor tells the patient they are safe to resume driving, do not need to inform DVLA if patient had a TIA and have recovered
    - Group 2 drivers: must inform the DVLA and must not drive for 1 year following a TIA and can only restart when the doctor tells the patient they are safe to resume driving
- Glaucoma:
    - Group 1 drivers: do not need to inform DVLA if glaucoma affects only one eye and your other eye has normal vision and visual field
    - Group 2 drivers: must inform DVLA if glaucoma affects one eye or both eyes
- Diabetic retinopathy:
    - Group 1 drivers: must inform DVLA only when both eyes affected
    - Group 2 drivers: must inform DVLA if one or both eyes affected

4.9 UK Government Guidance—Registering Vision Impairment as a Disability [8]

- Sight impaired:
    - VA 3/60 to 6/60 with full field
    - VA 6/60 to 6/24 with moderate constriction of field (superior or patchy loss), media opacities or aphakia
    - VA 6/18 or better with marked field defect (e.g. homonymous hemianopia advanced glaucoma, RP)
- Severely sight impaired:

- Legally defined as "so blind that they cannot do any work for which eyesight is essential"
- VA worse than 3/60
- VA 3/60 or better but worse than 6/60 with contraction of their visual field
- VA 6/60 or better with a clinically significant contracted visual field which is functionally impairing the person (e.g. loss of inferior field or homonymous or bitemporal hemianopia)
- Homonymous or bitemporal hemianopia is specifically excluded unless VA worse than 6/18

4.10 UK Government Guidance—Data Protection Act 2018 [9]

- Data protection is the fair and proper use of information about people (ensuring people can trust you to use their data fairly and responsibly)
- If you collect information about individuals for any reason other than your own personal, family or household purposes (e.g. personal social media activity, private letters and emails, or use of your own household gadgets), you need to comply
- The data protection act 2018 is the UK's implementation of the European General Data Protection Regulation (GDPR forms part of the UK law)
- The information commissioners office (ICO) regulates data protection in the UK
- Everyone responsible for using personal data has to follow strict rules called Caldicott principles or "data protection principles":
  1. Personal data processed lawfully, fairly and in a transparent manner
  2. Purpose limitation:
     - Data collected for specified, explicit and legitimate purposes and not further processed in a manner that is incompatible with those purposes
  3. Data minimization:
     - Adequate, relevant and limited to what is necessary in relation to the purposes for which they are processed
  4. Accuracy:
     - Inaccurate data should be erased or rectified without delay
  5. Storage limitation:
     - Kept in a form which permits identification of data subjects for no longer than is necessary or the purposes for which the personal data are processed
  6. Integrity and confidentiality (security):
     - Appropriate security of the personal data, including protection against unauthorized or unlawful processing and against accidental loss, destruction or damage, using appropriate technical or organizational measures
  7. Accountability
- The data protection officer (Caldicott guardian) is responsible for providing advice, monitoring compliance, and is the first point of contact in the organisation for data protection matters

4.11 UK Government Guidance—Safeguarding Policy: Protecting Vulnerable Adults and Children [10]

- Safeguarding is about protecting an adult's or child's right to live in safety, free from abuse and neglect
- Vulnerable adult: person aged 18 or over who is or may be in need of community care services by reason of mental or other disability, age or illness; and who is or may be unable to take care of him or herself, or unable to protect him or herself against significant harm or exploitation
- Neglect: persistent failure to meet a person's basic physical or psychological needs to a level that is likely to result in serious impairment of the persons health or development
- Alert the adults safeguarding team for vulnerable adults—contact the named nurse

for adult safeguarding and named doctor who lead on issues related to adult safeguarding
- Alert the child protection team for vulnerable children—contact the named nurse and named doctor who lead on issues related to child protection

4.12 Never Events

NHS Improvement Never Events policy and framework 2018 [11]:

- Never events are defined as serious incidents that are wholly preventable because guidance or safety recommendations that provide strong systemic protective barriers are available at a national level and should have been implemented and followed by all healthcare providers
- Never events list applicable to Ophthalmology include:
  - Wrong site surgery
  - Wrong implant/prosthesis: an error in IOL choice after the time out WHO check is a never event. An error in IOL choice up to the time out WHO check is a serious incident (The RCOphth Ophthalmic Service Guidance for Correct IOL implantation in cataract surgery 2018)
  - Retained foreign objects post procedure
- Never events require full investigation (completed within 60 days) under the Serious Incident Framework:
  - Describes the process and procedures to help ensure serious incidents are identified correctly, investigated thoroughly and, most importantly, learned from to prevent the likelihood of similar incidents happening again
  - Incident report required within 2 days on Strategic Executive Information System (StEIS) and National Reporting and Learning System (NRLS)
  - Disclose information to patients as soon as possible
  - Organisational leaders must undertake with the whole multidisciplinary team a root-cause analysis to determine the reasons for the incident
  - Leaders must then establish strategies and implementation tools to stop it from happening again

4.13 Non-accidental Injury (NAI)

- When to suspect a NAI:
  - Frequent attendance or unusual pattern of presentation to healthcare services most commonly due to injuries
  - There is a delay between injury and seeking medical advice. If there is a delay, there is no satisfactory explanation
  - History is not consistent with the injury. Parents have given different accounts at different times
  - On examination, the child has unexplained injuries and there are patterns of injury typical of abuse (e.g. multiple facial bruises, scalds, cigarette burns, any unexplained injuries in non-ambulant babies, bites, hand or implement marks, head injuries with intracranial haemorrhages in babies, multi-layered retinal haemorrhages, unexplained abdominal or genital injuries or long bone fractures especially in babies)
  - The child's behaviour and interaction with parents/carers is not appropriate
  - Unusual or marked change in the child's behaviour or emotional state, different from what is expected for their age and developmental stage, and not explained by a medical condition, neurodevelopment disorder or stressful situation
  - Any children who present with unexplained injuries or a history that is inconsistent with the injury should be referred to the Named Doctor and Named Nurse for child protection
  - If a child is thought to be in immediate danger, refer immediately to Children's Social Care and/or the police
- Standards of ophthalmology assessment (The RCOphth Clinical Guideline on Abusive Head Trauma and the Eye 2024 [12]

- Ophthalmology assessment must be carried out by an ophthalmologist using a standardised clinical proforma designed for documentation
- Visual acuity: rarely possible in a very sick child and the reason should be recorded such as due to sedation or intubated
- The periocular area, eyelids, conjunctiva, anterior segments, pupillary reactions and ocular movements (or dolls head manoeuvre if necessary) of both eyes should be examined and the findings recorded
- Posterior segment examination with an indirect ophthalmoscope and condensing lens (dilate with short acting mydriatics such as phenylephrine 2.5%, tropicamide 0.5%). The following should be recorded:
  1. The presence or absence of retinal haemorrhages unilaterally or bilaterally
  2. Details of the layer of retinal involvement (preretinal, intraretinal, subretinal)
  3. Location in the retina (posterior pole/periphery)
  4. Severity of the retinal haemorrhages in terms of number (few, many, too numerous to count) and size
  5. The presence or absence of additional features such as retinal folds, haemorrhagic retinoschisis, presence of large macular or vitreous haemorrhages
- The use of the RetCam (see Fig. 4.1) or Optos for retinal imaging and the use of a handheld OCT can help to record findings if available
- It is recommended that ophthalmology assessment by the on-call ophthalmology team should ideally be undertaken within 24–48 hours of the initial paediatric assessment. If any findings need to be reviewed by a paediatric ophthalmologist this should be undertaken preferably within 72 hours of the initial paediatric referral

• Communication with parents
  - It is important that parents are kept informed about the child's medical care throughout any investigations
  - Parents prefer honest, clear, and early communication on what a child protection enquiry means; what referral to social services or the police means; whether emergency proceedings are taking place; what the child protection medical examination involves; how long the child has to stay in the hospital; what different tests involve; whether further tests are needed and how long it will take to receive test results
  - Sensitively explaining to parents that there is a protocol that the professional has to follow and clearly outlining the process may help parents to accept and understand. For example, "Examination findings are consistent with a non-accidental injury and it was the procedure in those cases therefore to inform social services and also to do a full skeletal x-ray and dilated fundus examination in those cases".

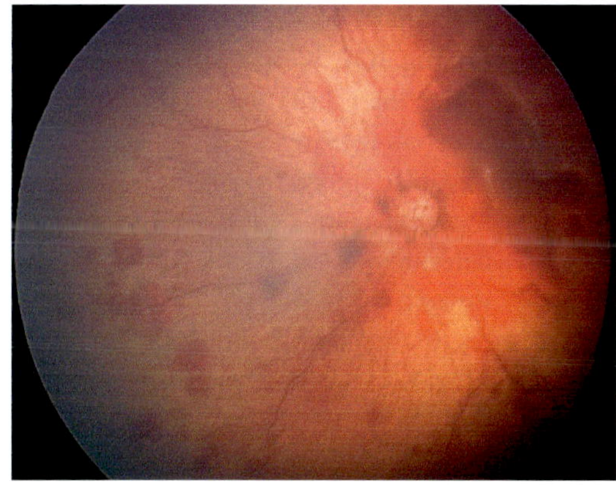

Fig. 4.1 Colour fundus photo of a patient with multi-layered retinal haemorrhages from NAI

4.14 Approach to Patient with Refractive Surprise

4.14.1 Verify the Problem

• RCOphth guidelines [13]: achieve 85% within 1 diopter of intended refractive outcome
• What is the postop refraction (have it checked by a clinician experienced at refraction)?
  - Causes of a myopic surprise:
    (a) Previous hyperopic refractive surprise

(b) Error in A constant calculations (e.g. placing IOL with A constant of 118 rather than 113) leading to a higher lens power than required
(c) Capsular block syndrome (capsular hyperextension, IOL displacement anteriorly, AC shallowing, postop myopic shift)
– Causes of a hyperopic surprise:
(a) Previous unrecognized myopic refractive surgery
(b) Unrecognised staphyloma at most posterior portion of the globe (anatomic axial length may not correspond with the center of the macula i.e. refractive axial length)

4.14.2 Case Note Review

- Was the correct IOL selected intraoperatively?
- Was the preoperative biometry/ lens selection valid?
  - Check biometry used does indeed belong to your patient
  - Look for intraocular consistency in axial length and K values
  - Look for interocular consistency in axial length and K values
- Check appropriate formula used
- Had they had previous refractive surgery?

4.14.3 Clinical Examination

- Has there been a change in the corneal curvature (K) reading since the operation?
  - Wounds: poorly constructed wounds or use of LRI's (hypermetropic effect)
  - Corneal oedema
  - Other corneal pathology previously unrecognised e.g. keratoconus, previous refractive laser surgery, CL use
- Is the IOL correctly positioned?
  - Check IOL centered and completely in the bag
  - Is their retention of Healon within the bag?
  - Is early capsule healing/phimosis affecting IOL position?

4.14.4 Investigations

- Repeat biometry +/− B scan to confirm axial length (on pseudophakic mode)
- Repeat keratometry +/− corneal topography

4.14.5 Treatment

- Small errors
  (a) Observation: post-op changes in corneal curvature may improve as oedema settles and wound heals
  (b) No treatment: a small myopic refractive surprise in a non-dominant eye may be useful for reading
  (c) Trial of spectacles
  (d) Intervention for specific problem: surgical repositioning of poorly placed IOL, YAG laser for capsular phimosis
- Large errors
  (a) CL
  (b) Secondary piggyback IOL: IOL power based on postop refraction
  (c) Laser refractive surgery for residual errors
  (d) IOL exchange: least preferable as carries a greater surgical risk and offers less predictability

4.15 Consenting for Cataract Surgery

- Explain what a cataract is ("clear lens in your eye has become cloudy") and what the operation does ("operation replaces the cloudy lens with a new clear plastic lens")
- General risks
  - Intraoperative risks:
    - PC rupture +/− vitreous loss
    - Dropped nucleus with need for a second operation
  - Postoperative risks:
    - Endophthalmitis

    - Retinal detachment/tear
    - Choroidal haemorrhage
    - Posterior capsular opacification with need for laser treatment
- Specific risks
  - Technical difficulties e.g. patient positioning
  - Guarded visual prognosis e.g. amblyopia, corneal opacity, macular disease, vitreous opacities, optic nerve disease
  - Increased risk of sight-threatening complications in certain conditions:
    - High myopia: RD
    - Endothelial dystrophy (e.g. FED): corneal decompensation
    - PXF: zonular dehiscence
    - Posterior polar cataract (see Fig. 4.2): PC rupture
    - IFIS: iris trauma
- Anaesthetic options
  - Topical anaesthetic
  - Subtenon anaesthetic
    - Globe rupture (0.006–0.1%)
    - Oculocardiac reflex (0.03%)
  - General anaesthetic
- Desired refractive outcome
  - Emmetropia: require no/weak glasses for distance but will definitely require reading glasses
  - High ametropia:
    - Aim for emmetropia and perform second eye operation within 6 weeks
    - Aim to leave ametropic but up to 2D nearer emmetropia than the other eye
    - Aim for emmetropia and use a CL on the second eye until surgery is indicated
- IOL choice
  - Monofocal IOL
  - Toric IOL
  - Multifocal IOL

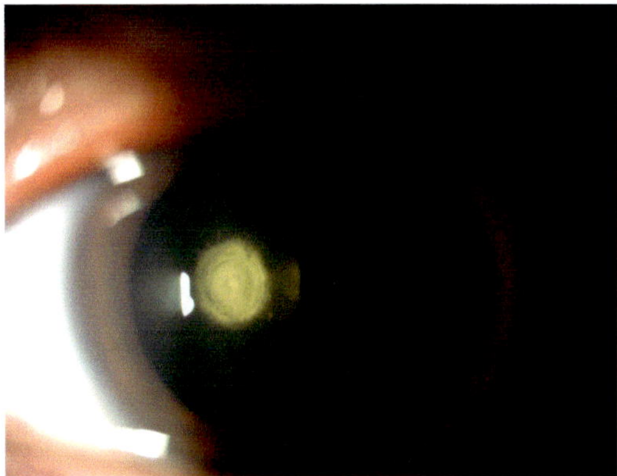

Fig. 4.2 Anterior segment image of a patient with a polar cataract

4.16 Cataract Surgery in Patients Living with Dementia

The RCOphth Concise Practice Points on Cataract surgery in patients living with dementia 2023:

- Preoperative considerations:
  - Risk vs benefit assessment—a patient with a known diagnosis of dementia who has a clinical frailty score ≥8 is unlikely to benefit from surgery
  - Preassessment and biometry on the same day, if possible, to allow refractive aim plan
  - Mild myopia (-1D) should be considered in people with severe dementia who may be housebound, as near tasks without spectacles such as feeding are of importance
  - Offer cataract surgery as early as possible to patients with a known diagnosis of dementia with the option of general anaesthesia available if the patient is deemed suitable. Try for topical or local anaesthesia if possible. Where general anaesthesia is deemed the most suitable option for the patient, consider immediate sequential bilateral cataract surgery
  - Assess mental capacity for decision making using the Mental Capacity Act. Where they lack mental capacity to decide/refuse cataract surgery, consult with their advocate (can be a friend). Clearly establish whether their advocate holds Lasting Power of Attorney for health (i.e. has the legal right to make the decision on their behalf, or is acting as a next of kin in a best interest decision). Where someone lacks

mental capacity and has no advocate, decision making requires referral to an Independent Mental Capacity Advocate (IMCA). You cannot perform surgery without an IMCA for those with no advocate

- Perioperative considerations:
  - Avoid early morning theatre slots
  - Experienced surgeon, preferably known to the patient
  - Theatre briefing for all staff including comfort (e.g. hand-holding, blanket) and minimise distraction for patient
  - For a designated person familiar with the patient (e.g. next of kin) to be prepared to be present in the theatre to accompany the patient, if this helps the individual
  - Intracameral dexamethasone has been successfully used to reduce the postoperative burden of drops in this patient group and should be considered in medium to high-risk cases
- Postoperative considerations:
  - Consider optometrist-led local follow-up

4.17 Clinical Supervision of Trainees in Difficulty

- Seek information (what is the issue, is there actually a problem, is this a one-off situation or is there a pattern)
  - Collate information from consultant colleagues who have worked with trainee
  - Initial conversation with the trainee to inform them of the concerns that have been raised and the action that is being taken and also to get their perspective
  - Encourage trainee to commit their comments to paper
  - Training environment issues:
    - Mismatches between trainee and trainer
    - Alleged bullying or harassment
    - Wrong levels of expertise expected of trainee
    - Supervision not congruent with level of expertise expected
  - Personal issues:
    - Partner/spouse relationship
    - Bereavement
    - Critical family illness
    - VISA problems
  - Clinical performance issues:
    - Clinical or surgical skill issues
  - Generic professional development issues:
    - Communication issues with patients &/ or staff
    - Motivation, maturity, a lack of insight
    - Time management and basic organisational skills
  - Professional behaviour issues:
    - Integrity
    - Probity
    - Substance abuse
- Patient safety (is patient care compromised)
  - Training environment issues:
  - Personal issues:
  - Clinical performance issues:
  - Generic professional development issues:
  - Professional behaviour issues:
    - Substance abuse: suspension from clinical duties pending full investigation
- Initiative (can you do anything yourself before you escalate the situation)
  - Training environment issues:
  - Personal issues:
    - Encourage trainees to access counselling and support services of their deanery through human resources (HR) and occupational health (OH) departments
  - Clinical performance issues:
    - Increased supervision of trainee
    - SMART (specific, measurable, achievable, relevant, time bound) objectives
  - Generic professional development issues:
  - Professional behaviour issues:
- Escalate (involve other colleagues as needed, who will you go to, who is the most appropriate person)
  - Training environment issues:
    - Discussion with educational supervisor
    - Discussion with training programme director (TPD)
  - Personal issues:
    - Discussion with educational supervisor
    - Discussion with TPD

  - Clinical performance issues:
    - Discussion with educational supervisor
    - Discussion with TPD
  - Generic professional development issues:
    - Discussion with educational supervisor
    - Discussion with TPD
    - Discussion with postgraduate dean
  - Professional behaviour issues:
    - Probity—inform GMC
    - Substance abuse—inform local HR department, medical director, GMC
- Support (can you support the individual or team)
  - Training environment issues:
    - Relocation to a more appropriate training environment
  - Personal issues:
    - Arrangements of future placements closer to trainees home or support network
    - Out of programme career break (OOPC)
  - Clinical performance issues:
    - Use of simulator/wet-lab facilities
    - Targeted or repeat training with clear educational objectives and yardsticks of success (SMART objectives)
  - Generic professional development issues:
    - Behavioural or psychometric assessment through psychologists identified through deanery or NCAS (national clinical assessment service)
  - Professional behaviour issues:
    - Behavioural or psychometric assessment through psychologists identified through Deanery or NCAS
    - Stress counselling service

4.18 The RCOphth Ophthalmology Service Guidance on Theatre Procedures 2018 [14]

- Consent
  - Discuss the options of no surgery and of other or lesser interventions
  - Best practice to consent before the day of surgery in all but emergency or minor operation situations
  - On the day of surgery, the consent should be rechecked with the patient and resigned by a consenter
  - Consent must be obtained in the full knowledge of risks relevant to both the operation and anaesthesia. It is the responsibility of the individual administering the anaesthetic to discuss possible complications of the anaesthetic. A separate consent for the anaesthetic per se is not required, although it is advisable to record the discussion in the patient records
- Pre-operative assessment
  - Purpose: identify abnormalities or issues that might interfere with the safe performance and outcome of the operation and confirm the decisions made at the decision to admit were appropriate and still apply
  - Undertaken normally by trained specialist nurses or other trained ophthalmic healthcare professionals with medical anaesthetic input as required
  - General medical records should be available. If the relevant information is not available, planned surgery should be deferred
  - Should take place before the day of surgery and occur within 3–4 months of the surgery. A telephone call to confirm nothing has changed may be done in the week preceding the surgery if there is a long gap between assessment and procedure
  - Telephone pre-assessment may be appropriate when a second procedure is planned in healthy patients (e.g. second eye for cataract surgery) within 3–4 months of the first operation
  - Some patients may need help (e.g. friend, relative, carer) to accompany them to surgery and at discharge, or support from the community nursing team at home
  - Specific checks to ensure suitability for day case surgery if planned; living alone is not a contraindication but it needs to be confirmed that the aftercare, particularly instilling the eyedrops effectively at the right times, is possible
  - Specific checks to highlight any concerns about mental capacity, ability to lie flat and

still for the whole duration of the operation, and communication difficulties
  - Results should be recorded on a checklist
  - Following examinations should be undertaken:
    - BP
    - HR and rhythm
    - Hearing, comprehension, co-operation
    - Tremor and abnormal body movements
    - Infection control screening (e.g. MRSA swabs)
  - Following examinations are performed if indicated:
    - If there is respiratory distress or SOB present, measure the RR, O2 sats, and the patient review by or discussed with a doctor or an anaesthetist
    - Practice patients ability to lie flat and still in the appropriate position for the duration of the operation
    - Examination for non-ocular sepsis
    - Slit lamp examination e.g. blepharitis
  - Tests routinely indicated for the following situations:
    - Clotting profile for those on anticoagulants (e.g. warfarin)
    - Electrolytes for patients on dialysis
    - Blood glucose measurement and HBA_1C for those with diabetes
- On admission
  - Nurses, or HCA's under the supervision of nurses, will perform the pre-operative patient preparation on wards or day case areas. Results of the preoperative assessment should be available and, together with the following, be recorded on a checklist:
    - Patients identity should be confirmed and a name badge should be attached to the patient's wrist
    - Ensure the next of kin details are documented/updated in the patient's medical records
    - Confirm that the patient has been well since the pre-operative assessment visit and does not have any acute illness e.g. URTI
    - Confirm whether the patient has taken his/her medication
    - Confirm allergy status as this may affect the order of the list e.g. type I latex allergy
    - Ensure the patient has provision for a safe return home
    - BP, HR, temperature and O2 saturation should be checked
    - Check that the consent form has been signed and rechecked on the day of surgery
    - Check the marking side forms and biometry/IOL data are present
    - Ensure that the pre-operative medications including eye drops or inserts are administered
  - Any change in the patient's condition or therapy since pre-operative assessment, or other concerns from these assessments, should be brought to the attention of the surgeon and, where relevant, the anaesthetist
  - The findings of the preoperative assessment and checks should be reviewed by the ophthalmologist, and where appropriate, the anaesthetist
  - The eye/adnexae should be checked to exclude acute inflammation or infection and rechecked for other factors that may affect safe local anaesthesia or surgery
  - Preop marking:
    - Mandatory to mark procedure site shortly before the procedure but not in the anaesthetic room or the theatre
    - Marking must be performed by the surgeon or a nominated deputy, who will be present during the procedure. It is the surgeon's responsibility to check that he/she is operating on the correct eye/side
    - Mark the eye or side/site to be operated on with a clear, indelible mark. This mark should remain visible after surgical cleaning, and after draping if at all possible

- Handover to procedure teams:
  - There must be a formal handover process from the ward or admission team to a member of the theatre team receiving the patient
  - The handover should include a check of:
    - Patient identification (name, DOB, active confirmation), checked against identity band
    - Allergies
    - Procedure, and site or side
    - Site marking
    - Whether patient has any plates, pins, or any metal implants if monopolar diathermy is going to be used
    - Fasting status
    - Relevant clinical features e.g. blood sugar for diabetic patients, INR for warfarin
    - An appropriate patient records
    - A properly completed consent form
    - A biometry sheet if relevant
- In theatre
  - Staffing levels:
    - For most LA ophthalmic lists, the following staff are the minimum acceptable theatre team:
      - 2 scrub nurses or practitioners: 1 for the current case and the other preparing the instruments for the next case
      - Runner (can be a HCA): role is to supply the scrub practitioner with the necessary equipment and consumables, set up the phaco equipment etc., help position the patient and microscope, adjust the lights and other essential duties.
  - Patient monitoring:
    - For LA patients:
      - Patients should be continuously monitored—clinical observation, communication and pulse oximetry as a minimum, from before the administration of the LA to the end of the operation
      - ECG and BP should be monitored in sedated patients and those who are at risk of cardiovascular complications (e.g. hypertensives, patients with pacemaker, diabetics) and higher risk situations such as strabismus surgery, intraoperative use of ocular sympathomimetics (such as phenylephrine and mydricaine)
      - In stable patients the non-invasive BP measurements should be kept to a minimum to avoid discomfort and undue disturbance during surgery
      - A suitably trained individual must have responsibility for monitoring the patient throughout. This task may be carried out by an anaesthetist, a nurse, an ODP, an ODA, an anaesthetic nurse or, in some cases, a suitably trained HCA as long as they are trained in basic life support (BLS)
      - The ultimate responsibility for the patient rests with the operating surgeon and, when present, the anaesthetist
  - Anaesthetics and resuscitation:
    - GA and sedation requires the assistance of a trained anaesthetic technician/or anaesthetic nurse as well as an anaesthetist. In addition there should be trained recovery staff
    - An anaesthetist is not essential when topical, subconjunctival or sub-tenon's techniques without sedation are used
    - Ideally, an anaesthetist should be available in the theatre complex, particularly when sharp needle blocks such as peribulbar, retrobulbar are used, and when complex or long cases are being performed
    - For any operation, all theatre staff must be regularly trained and able to perform BLS, understand local resuscitation arrangements, and there should be a resuscitation trolley easily and quickly available
    - Where there is backup from a formal cardiac arrest/medical emergency team, there should be at least 1 person available with immediate life support (ILS),

who should be supported by staff with the knowledge and skills to assist in resuscitation
- Where the unit is free-standing and there is no immediate access to a formal cardiac arrest team there should be at least 1 person with advanced life support (ALS)
- If an anaesthetist is not immediately available, the operating ophthalmologist is directly responsible for the management of any untoward event and should have the appropriate skills to safely manage resuscitation, or to have these skills within the theatre team

– Five steps to safer surgery:
  - Team brief:
    – Performed before the first patient arrives in the theatre area
    – Any team member may lead the safety briefing
    – As many members of the surgical team as possible should attend the briefing, but it must include the surgeon and anaesthetist who have seen and consented the patients
  - Sign in (first part of the WHO checklist):
    – Performed when patient arrives at the procedure area
    – For cataract surgery a specific cataract or ophthalmic checklist is recommended. For other ocular surgery the standard WHO checklist or an ophthalmic specific checklist can be used
    – Must be performed by at least 2 people involved in the procedure. For procedures involving an anaesthetist, these should include the anaesthetist or anaesthetic assistant
    – Any omissions, discrepancies or uncertainties identified during the sign in should be resolved before the time out is performed or any procedure starts
    – Immediately before the insertion of a block anaesthetic, the anaesthetist and anaesthetic assistant must simultaneously check the surgical site marking and the site and side of the block
  - Time out (second part of the WHO checklist):
    – Must be performed immediately before the start of the procedure
    – Any member of the procedure team may lead the time out
    – All team members involved in the procedure should be present at the time out. This will usually require that they stop all other tasks and face the time out lead
    – The team member leading the time out should verify that all team members are participating
    – Any omissions, discrepancies or uncertainties identified during the time out should be resolved before the procedure starts
  - Sign out (third part of the WHO checklist):
    – Performed at end of procedure before patient is awoken from GA or before the patient leaves theatre
    – Any member of the procedure team may lead the sign out
    – All team members involved in the procedure should be present at the sign out. This will usually require that they stop all other tasks and face the sign out lead
    – The team member leading the sign out should verify that all team members are participating
  - Team debrief:
    – Performed at the end of all lists
    – Every member of the procedural team should take part in the debriefing
    – Any team member may lead the debriefing, but the surgeon and anaesthetist (if an anaesthetist has been involved) must be present
    – If any team member, and especially the senior surgeon, scrub practitioner

or anaesthetist, has to leave before the debriefing is conducted, they should have the opportunity to feedback any issues they wish to see addressed during the debriefing

- Postoperatively
  - Pain should be assessed and managed
  - After the operation, and before discharge, the patient should feel well and have stable key signs
  - For patients who have undergone GA, ensure patient has passed urine before discharge
  - Before discharge the safety arrangements for the patient's return to home, and the level of support available, should be confirmed.
  - Information (including written) should be provided about post-operative recovery (postop instructions, medication dispensing and advice, advice on post-op appointments, what to expect during recovery)
  - Written instructions should be given to the patient about what to do and whom to contact in the event of problems or concerns, especially signs of postop infections such as endophthalmitis
- Organising theatre lists
  - There should be unambiguous use of language in all communications relating to the scheduling and listing of procedures. Laterality must always be written in full i.e. 'left' or 'right'
  - The information to schedule a procedure should include when relevant:
    - Source of patient e.g. ward or day case area
    - Significant comorbidities
    - Allergies e.g. latex or iodine
    - Unusual infection risk including prion disease
    - Any non-standard equipment requirements or non-stock prostheses
    - Unusual BMI or extreme obesity where normal hospital equipment may have difficulty safely accommodating the patients weight e.g. theatre trolley, mobile patient hoist
  - The clinical team performing the procedures is responsible for deciding the order of procedures within a list of cases. In determining the order of a list, priority should be given to clinical criteria e.g. urgency, extremes of age, allergies such as latex allergy, and medical conditions e.g. diabetes
  - Late list changes should be avoided if possible. Any list changes made after the deadline for the publication of a final version of the list must be agreed with identified key members of the procedure team, and should be discussed by all members of the procedure team at the safety briefing

4.19 Needle Stick Injury

4.19.1 Transmission Rates

- Needle stick transmission rates from infected patients are estimated at around 0.3% for HIV (The RCOphth Ophthalmic Services Guidance on Prevention of transmission of blood-borne viruses in ophthalmic surgery 2010 [15]), up to 10% for Hepatitis C (The RCOphth Ophthalmic Services Guidance on Prevention of transmission of blood-borne viruses in ophthalmic surgery 2010 [15]), and up to 30% for Hepatitis B (The RCOphth Ophthalmic Services Guidance on Prevention of transmission of blood-borne viruses in ophthalmic surgery 2010 [15])

4.19.2 Management

- Immediate
  - Encourage the injury to bleed
  - Wash under running water
  - If body fluids splashed onto eyes, irrigate them copiously
  - Incident report
  - Inform patient and take patient details (name, unit number, contact details)
  - Inform head of department

- Within 1 hour
  - Report to the occupational health department (or A&E department if out of hours). If high risk (exposure to blood or high-risk body fluid from patient with known or suspected HIV) of HIV transmission, start post-exposure prophylaxis (e.g. TRUVADA once a day)—this should be started within 1 hour by the occupational health/A&E physician:
    - If donor is HIV positive (already known or discovered on testing):
      - Continue post-exposure prophylaxis for 4 weeks
      - Test recipient for HIV seroconversion at 6 weeks, 3 months, 6 months
      - Follow up with occupational health
    - If donor is HIV negative:
      - Discontinue post-exposure prophylaxis
      - Test recipient for HIV seroconversion at 3 months and 6 months
      - Follow up with occupational health
  - Store blood from the donor and the recipient:
    - Screening for Hepatitis B and HIV (HIV antibody AND p24 antigen simultaneously), where appropriate, is generally arranged by the occupational health physician
    - The donors blood sample should not be taken by the recipient
    - The donor must be counseled before taking blood samples/testing for HIV (no written consent required but the benefits of testing to the individual and the details of how the result will be given [face to face provision of test result] must be discussed)

4.20 Ophthalmia Neonatorum

4.20.1 Definition

- Defined as conjunctivitis (inflammatory or infection) occurring within the first month of life

4.20.2 Causes

- Chemical neonatal conjunctivitis
  - Post-instillation of 2% silver nitrate (agglutinates and inactivates gonococci) into the conjunctival fornix immediately after birth
  - Typically appears within 1–2/7 after the administration of a topical agent
  - Withdrawal of the offending agent results in resolution of symptoms within 2/7
  - Ocular features: conjunctival injection, tearing
- Bacterial neonatal conjunctivitis

  (a) Gonococcal neonatal conjunctivitis:
    - Typically appears 2–5 days after birth
    - Ocular features: hyperpurulent discharge, severe conjunctival injection +/− pseudomembrane, chemosis, eyelid oedema, corneal ulcer +/− perforation (gonococcus can invade the cornea through intact corneal epithelium)
    - Systemic features: meningitis, endocarditis
    - Investigations: prewet swab or conjunctival scrapings for gram stain (gram negative diplococci) and Gonococcal culture using modified Thayer-Martin medium. Giemsa stain and chlamydial culture should also be performed in view of frequent maternal co-infection with chlamydia

  - Treatment: single dose of IV or IM cefotaxime or ceftriaxone by paediatricians, frequent saline lavage of the purulent discharge, topical antibiotics are unnecessary
  - Referral of mother (with partner) to GUM clinic

(b) Chlamydial neonatal conjunctivitis:
  - Typically appears 5–14 days after birth
  - Ocular features: mucopurulent discharge, conjunctivitis +/− pseudomembrane, keratitis +/− corneal scarring
  - Systemic features: otitis media, pneumonia, rhinitis
  - Investigations: prewet swab or conjunctival scrapings for Giemsa stain or PCR
  - Treatment: oral erythromycin (50 mg/kg/day divided into four daily doses) for 14 days (risk of infantile hypertrophic pyloric stenosis)—for infants with conjunctivitis but no pneumonia, systemic erythromycin can be delayed while awaiting confirmatory diagnostic tests for Chlamydia
  - Referral of mother (with partner) to GUM clinic (single dose of azithromycin 1 g PO)

- HSV neonatal conjunctivitis:
  - Typically occur 5–14 days after exposure
  - Ocular features: eyelid vesicles and erythema, conjunctivitis, keratitis, ant uveitis
  - Systemic features: pneumonitis, hepatitis, meningoencephalitis
  - Investigations: viral swabs or conjunctival, corneal epithelium or skin vesicle scrapings for HSV culture +/− PCR, LFT's, CSF analysis
  - Treatment: IV aciclovir (60 mg/kg/day TDS) for 14 days, or for 21 days in the presence of disseminated or CNS disease + topical anti-viral (aciclovir ointment 5×/day for 7 days) +/− topical steroids (for corneal stromal and endothelial disease or ant uveitis)

4.20.3 Chlamydia/Gonorrhoea

- Symptoms:
  - Females—vaginal discharge, dysuria, lower abdominal pain
  - Males—urethral discharge, dysuria, genital ulcers, testicular pain and swelling
- Treatment:
  (a) Antibiotics
  (b) Educate and counsel
  (c) Promote condom use and provide condoms
  (d) Manage and treat partner
  (e) Offer HIV counseling and testing

References

1. General Medical Council (GMC). Doctors use of social media. [Online]. London: GMC; 2013. Available at: https://www.gmc-uk.org/-/media/documents/doctors-use-of-social-media_pdf-58833100.pdf?la=en&hash=61BDC9EAA79FE4F877797D8C76515EA39BC8D516. Accessed 12 Dec 2019
2. General Medical Council (GMC). Consent: patients and doctors making decisions together. [Online]. London: GMC; 2008. Available at: https://www.gmc-uk.org/-/media/documents/consent%2D%2Denglish-0617_pdf-48903482.pdf?la=en&hash=C77983ADC0B63D655CC6BCFA89209B9C1A3D86A2. Accessed 12 Dec 2019.
3. General Medical Council (GMC). Confidentiality: good practice in handling patient information. [Online]. London: GMC; 2017. Available at: https://www.gmc-uk.org/-/media/documents/confidentiality-good-practice-in-handling-patient-information%2D%2D-english-0417_pdf-70080105.pdf?la=en&hash=2F39E0A8258FE82F573040DBB14617D5DB9E84C1. Accessed 12 Dec 2019.
4. General Medical Council (GMC). Financial and commercial arrangements and conflicts of interest. [Online]. London: GMC; 2013. Available at: https://www.gmc-uk.org/-/media/documents/financial-and-commercial-arrangements-and-conflicts-of-interest_pdf-58833167.pdf?la=en&hash=4C9B2012B935EEA94E26AAF0C121AF3A3269BB1A. Accessed 12 Dec 2019
5. General Medical Council (GMC). Revalidation. [Online]. London: GMC. Available at: https://www.gmc-uk.org/registration-and-licensing/managing-your-registration/revalidation#doctors-with-no-connection. Accessed 12 Dec 2019.

6. UK Government Guidance. Parental rights and responsibilities. [Online]. Available at: https://www.gov.uk/parental-rights-responsibilities. Accessed 12 Dec 2019.
7. UK Government Guidance. Driving Eyesight Rules. [Online]. Available at: https://www.gov.uk/driving-eyesight-rules. Accessed 12 Dec 2019.
8. UK Government Guidance. Registering vision impairment as a disability. [Online]. Available at: https://www.gov.uk/government/publications/guidance-published-on-registering-a-vision-impairment-as-a-disability. Accessed 12 Dec 2019.
9. UK Government Guidance. Data Protection Act 2018. [Online]. Available at: https://www.gov.uk/government/collections/data-protection-act-2018. Accessed 12 Dec 2019.
10. UK Government Guidance. Safeguarding policy: protecting vulnerable adults. [Online]. Available at: https://www.gov.uk/government/publications/safeguarding-policy-protecting-vulnerable-adults. Accessed 12 Dec 2019.
11. NHS Improvement. Never events policy and framework 2018. [Online]. London: NHS Improvement. Available at: https://improvement.nhs.uk/documents/2265/Revised_Never_Events_policy_and_framework_FINAL.pdf. Accessed 12 Dec 2019.
12. The Royal College of Ophthalmologists. Abusive head trauma and the eye in infancy guideline 2024. [Online]. London: The Royal College of Ophthalmologists. Available at: https://www.rcophth.ac.uk/wp-content/uploads/2021/08/Abusive-Head-Trauma-and-the-Eye.pdf. Accessed 9 Jan 2025.
13. The Royal College of Ophthalmologists. Ophthalmic service guidance for correct IOL implantation in cataract surgery 2018. [Online]. London: The Royal College of Ophthalmologists. Available at https://www.rcophth.ac.uk/wp-content/uploads/2018/03/Correct-IOL-implantation-in-cataract-surgery-quality-standard.pdf. Accessed 30 Nov 2019.
14. The Royal College of Ophthalmologists. Ophthalmic service guidance for theatre procedures 2018. [Online]. London: The Royal College of Ophthalmologists. Available at: https://www.rcophth.ac.uk/wp-content/uploads/2018/02/Theatre-procedures.pdf. Accessed 12 Dec 2019.
15. The Royal College of Ophthalmologists. Ophthalmic services guidance on prevention of transmission of blood-borne viruses in ophthalmic surgery 2010. [Online]. London: The Royal College of Ophthalmologists. Available at: https://www.rcophth.ac.uk/wpcontent/uploads/2014/12/2010_PROF_053_Blood_Borne_Viruses.pdf. Accessed 12 Dec 2019.

5 Health Promotion, Audit, Research & Evidence-Based Medicine

Timothy H. M. Fung and Winfried M. K. Amoaku

Abstract

Evidence-based medicine focuses on using high-quality research, such as randomised clinical trials, to inform clinical decisions. This chapter highlights several key clinical trials that have significantly influenced practice and improved health outcomes in eyecare. Additionally, it discusses the principles of screening and how these principles are applied in various eyecare programs.

5.1 Steroids

- Mechanisms of action
  - Reduction of inflammation by corticosteroids is via inhibition of phospholipase A2, thereby blocking the production of prostaglandins and leukotrienes
  - Corticosteroids have an immunosuppressive role via inhibition of NF-kB transcription factor signaling, thereby blocking the production of IL-2 and other pro-inflammatory cytokines
- Clinical applications of intravitreal corticosteroids
  - Ozurdex (Dexamethasone 700 micrograms intravitreal implant):
    - NICE Guidance [TA349] [33]: option for treatment of DMO if eye is pseudophakic and CSMO does not respond to non-corticosteroid treatment or such treatment is unsuitable
    - NICE Guidance [TA229] [31]: recommend as an option for treatment of macular oedema due to a CRVO or a BRVO when treatment with laser photocoagulation has not been beneficial or treatment with laser photocoagulation is not considered suitable because of the extent of retinal haemorrhages
    - NICE Guidance [TA460] [34]: recommended as an option for treating non-infectious uveitis in the posterior segment of the eye in adults only if there is active disease (current inflammation in the eye) and worsening vision with a risk of blindness
    - Clinical trials:
      - **MEAD** study [5]: diabetic macular oedema
      - **GENEVA** study [21]: retinal vein occlusion (BRVO/CRVO)

T. H. M. Fung (✉)
University Hospitals of Derby & Burton NHS Foundation Trust, Royal Derby Hospital, Derby, UK
e-mail: timothy.fung@nhs.net

W. M. K. Amoaku
Eye, Ear, Nose and Throat Centre, Queens Medical Centre, Nottingham University Hospitals NHS Trust, Nottingham, UK

T. H. M. Fung, W. M. K. Amoaku (eds.), *Viva and OSCE Exams in Ophthalmology*,
https://doi.org/10.1007/978-3-031-97401-4_5

- **HURON** study [27]: non-infectious posterior uveitis
- Iluvien (Flucinolone Acetonide 170 μg):
  - NICE Guidance [TA301] [32]: option for the treatment of chronic diabetic macular oedema that is insufficiently responsive to available therapies if an eye is pseudophakic
  - NICE Guidance [TA590] [36]: option for preventing relapse in recurrent non-infectious uveitis affecting the posterior segment of the eye
  - Clinical trials:
    - **FAME** study [11]: diabetic macular oedema
    - **PSV-FAI-001** Study (NICE Guidance [TA590] [36]): non-infectious posterior uveitis
- Monitoring
  - Pre-treatment:
    - BP, glucose, weight
    - CXR if there is any possibility of TB
  - During treatment:
    - BP, glucose, weight every 3 months
    - Lipids every year
    - Bone density (DXA scan) if steroid course ≥3 months
- Side-effects of corticosteroids
  - Ocular:
    - Glaucoma
    - Cataracts—posterior subcapsular cataracts
    - Microbial keratitis
  - Systemic:
    - Endocrine:
      - Cushing' syndrome
      - Adrenal suppression—risk of Addisonian crisis with withdrawal
      - Weight gain
    - GI:
      - Peptic ulcer
      - Pancreatitis
    - Musculoskeletal:
      - Osteoporosis
      - Osteopenia
    - Skin:
      - Hirsutism
    - Haematological:
      - Immunosuppression
    - Psychiatric:
      - Insomnia
      - Psychosis
    - Neurological:
      - Raised ICP +/− papilloedema
- Prophylaxis of corticosteroid-induced osteoporosis:
  - Risk assessment (NICE Guidance [CG146] [35]):
    - Consider assessment of fracture risk:
      - In all women aged ≥65 years and all men ≥75 years
      - In women aged under 65 years and men aged under 75 years in the presence of risk factors e.g. current use or frequent recent use of oral or systemic glucocorticoids, previous fragility fracture, smoking, history of falls, family history of hip fracture, alcohol intake of more than 14 units per week, BMI <18.5 kg/m^2
    - Tools for risk assessment (see Table 5.1):
      - Use either FRAX (without a bone mineral density [BMD] value if DXA scan has not previously been undertaken) or QFracture, within their

Table 5.1 Measurement tools used to assess fragility fracture risk

FRAX
Based on individual patient models that integrate the risks associated with clinical risk factors as well as BMD
Output is a 10-year probability of hip fracture and the 10-year probability of a major osteoporotic fracture (clinical spine, forearm, hip or shoulder fracture)
QFracture
Uses a series of questions to identify individuals at risk of developing a fracture of the hip, wrist or spine
Offers a 10-year risk prediction for osteoporotic fractures
DXA scan
Compares the BMD of the femoral neck or lumbar spine against normal (i.e. healthy Caucasian adults aged 20–29 years). The difference is calculated in SD to give the T score:
T score 0 to −1 SD = normal
T score −1 to −2.5 SD = osteopenia
T score ≤−2.5 SD = osteoporosis
Z score is used to determine whether the BMD is less than the age-related bone loss (i.e. no. of SD the measurement is above or below the age matched mean BMD)

allowed age ranges, to estimate 10-year predicted absolute fracture risk when assessing risk of fracture. Above the upper age limits defined by the tools, consider people to be at high risk.
- FRAX can be used for people aged between 40 and 90 years, either with or without BMD values, as specified. QFracture can be used for people aged between 30 and 84 years. BMD values cannot be incorporated into the risk algorithm
- Following risk assessment with FRAX (without a BMD value) or QFracture, consider measuring BMD with DXA in people whose fracture risk is in the region of an intervention threshold for a proposed treatment, and recalculate absolute risk using FRAX with the BMD value
- Do not routinely measure BMD with DXA to assess fracture risk without prior assessment using FRAX (without a BMD value) or QFracture
- Measure BMD with DXA to assess fracture risk in people aged under 40 years who have a major risk factor such as history of multiple fragility fractures, major osteoporotic fracture, or current or recent use of high-dose oral or high-dose systemic glucocorticoids (more than 7.5 mg prednisolone or equivalent per day for 3 months of longer)

- Treatment [10]:
  - Women and men age ≥70 years with a previous fragility fracture, or taking high doses of glucocorticoids (≥7.5 mg/day prednisolone) should be considered for bone protective therapy
  - In other individuals fracture probability should be estimated using FRAX with adjustment for glucocorticoid dose. FRAX assumes an average dose of prednisolone (2.5–7.5 mg/day or its equivalent) and may overestimate fracture risk in those taking lower doses and underestimate fracture risk in patients taking higher risks
  - Bone-protective treatment should be started at the onset of glucocorticoid therapy in individuals at high risk of fracture.
  - Adequate calcium intake should be achieved through dietary intake, if possible, with the use of supplementation if required. An adequate vitamin D status should be maintained, using supplements if required.
  - Alendronate (see Table 5.2) and risedronate are first line treatment options. Where these are not tolerated, zoledronic acid, teriparatide or denosumab are alternative options
  - If glucocorticoid therapy is stopped, withdrawal of bone protective therapy may be considered, but if glucocorticoids are continued long term, bone protection should be maintained in the majority of cases
  - Bone protective therapy may be appropriate in some premenopausal women and younger man, particularly in individuals with a previous history of fracture or receiving high doses of glucocorticoids
- Prophylaxis of GI side effects:
  - Higher doses of corticosteroids
  - History of GI disease
  - Co-administration of NSAIDs (avoid if possible)
- Withdrawal of corticosteroids:

Table 5.2 Key facts about alendronate

Mechanism of action: Bisphosphonate that induces apoptosis of osteoclasts
10 mg OD or 70 mg once weekly by mouth for up to 5 years. Treatment review should be performed after 5 years.
Side effects include upper GI symptoms, bowel disturbance, musculoskeletal pains and headaches
Should be taken after an overnight fast and at least 30 min before the first food or drink (other than water) of the day or any other oral medicinal products or supplementation
Tablets should be swallowed whole with a glass of plain water (200 ml) while the patient is sitting or standing in an upright position (to prevent reflux). Patients should not lie down for 30 min after taking the tablet (to prevent reflux)

- Tapering of corticosteroids is required if there is a risk of adrenal suppression:
  - Daily dose has been >40 mg/d prednisolone (or equivalent)
  - Duration has been >3 weeks
  - Frequency has been >1x/d
  - There have been other courses recently, or long-term steroid administration within the last year
- 5 mg prednisolone is equivalent to: Dexamethasone 750 µg, Betamethasone 750 µg, Methylprednisolone 4 mg, Triamcinolone 4 mg, Hydrocortisone 20 mg

5.2 Trials in Glaucoma Involving Trabeculectomy

5.2.1 Collaborative Initial Glaucoma Treatment Study [26]

- Primary outcome: A RCT to determine whether patients with newly diagnosed OAG are best treated by initial treatment with topical medications or by immediate trabeculectomy
- Methods
  - Inclusion criteria: newly diagnosed open angle glaucoma (POAG, PXF glaucoma, pigmentary glaucoma); one of three combinations of qualifying IOP (IOP ≥20 mmHg), VF changes, and optic disc findings; BCVA of 20/40 or better in both eyes; age 25–75 years; no prior ocular surgery (laser, refractive, conjunctival, intraocular); little (≤14 cumulative days of topical therapy) or no prior treatment of glaucoma
  - Exclusion criteria: use of glaucoma medication >14 cumulative days; CIGST VF score >16 in either eye; ocular disease that might affect measurement of IOP, VA, or VF; undergone ophthalmic laser, refractive, conjunctival, or intraocular surgery in either eye; PDR, DMO, or NPDR with >10 MA's by clinical count; current or expected chronic use of corticosteroids; likely require cataract surgery within 1 year of randomisation
  - Groups: topical medication group—escalating drops, if further treatment was required start with ALT, then trabeculectomy+/– 5-FU, drops, then trabeculectomy + anti-fibrotic agent, then medication / trabeculectomy group—trabeculectomy +/– 5-FU, if further treatment was required start with ALT, then escalating drops, then repeat trabeculectomy + anti-fibrotic agent, then medication
  - Primary endpoint: increasing CIGST VF score (0–20) reflecting increased VF loss
  - Secondary endpoints: change in VA, change in IOP, occurrence of cataract extraction, QOL (questionnaire)
  - Follow up: 5 years (initial report)
- Results: 607 patients
  - Primary endpoint: no significant difference in VF scores at 5 years in both groups
  - Secondary endpoints: initial decrease in VA in the trabeculectomy group that was not observed in the topical medication group and resulted in lower mean VA in the trabeculectomy group, that persisted through 3.5 years after surgery. After that time, mean VA levels were comparable in the 2 treatment groups up to 5 years of follow up (VA less in trabeculectomy group compared to topical medications group); there were no significant differences in the QOL between the 2 groups; both groups had significantly decreased mean IOP after treatment initiation (3 mmHg better reduction with trabeculectomy) although the amount of decrease was greater in the trabeculectomy group (48% in trabeculectomy group vs 35% in the topical medication group), and the difference was maintained over 5 years of observation; the trabeculectomy group had a higher cataract extraction probability over time compared to the topical medications group
  - Risk factors for VF progression: older age, non-white race, DM, development of cataract, maximal IOP, IOP fluctuation between visits
- Conclusion of study: CIGTS clinical outcomes do not suggest a change in the way ophthalmologists currently manage their patients with newly diagnosed OAG

5.2.2 Advanced Glaucoma Intervention Study [48, 49]

- Primary outcome: A RCT that assessed the effects of two surgical intervention sequences in patients with advanced POAG after the failure of medical therapy.
- Methods
  - Inclusion criteria: eyes with either advanced (defined as glaucoma that can no longer be controlled adequately despite maximum tolerated medical therapy in the presence of some glaucomatous VF defect) POAG without previous surgery or advanced POAG in a phakic eye 4 weeks or more after PI, phakic VA better than 20/80 [6/24]), age 35–80 years old, reproducible glaucomatous VF defects in at least one eye, a table of specific combinations of elevated IOP and VF defect (range of very mild to severe) was used to define uncontrolled glaucoma and was used to determine if a second or third operation was required
  - Exclusion criteria: secondary glaucoma or congenital angle anomalies, other active eye diseases particularly those that cause field of loss or previous surgery (except PI or localised retinopexy)
  - Groups: A-T-T group: ALT followed if necessary, by trabeculectomy, followed if necessary, by repeat trabeculectomy/T-A-T group: trabeculectomy followed if necessary, by ALT, followed if necessary, by repeat trabeculectomy
  - Primary endpoints: VA and/or VF (score 0 normal to-20 blind)
  - Follow up: 7 years (initial report)
- Results: 332 black patients, 249 white patients, 10 patients of other races
  - Low post intervention IOP is associated with reduced progression of VF defect
    - (a) Predictive analysis (IOP averaged over the first three 6-month visits—designed to assess whether IOP during early follow up is predictive of subsequent change from baseline in VF defect score): Initial mean IOP <14 mmHg over the first 18 months after surgery had a mean VF score deterioration of less than 1 point from baseline and those with an initial IOP ≥18 mmHg had a mean score deterioration of 3 points over 7 years
    - (b) Associative analysis (% of visits over the first 6 years of follow up for which an eye presented with IOP <18 mmHg): IOP <18 mmHg on 100% of follow up visits over 6 years resulted in a mean score deterioration of close to zero, but those achieving IOP <18 mmHg on <100% of visits had a mean deterioration of 2–3 points
  - After 7 years of follow-up, overall (in both black and white patients) the mean decrease in IOP from baseline is greater in eyes assigned to T-A-T than in those assigned to A-T-T
  - In white patients, VF was better preserved by T-A-T only after the first year of follow-up and thereafter favour the A-T-T sequence, and acuity was better preserved by A-T-T throughout follow up.
  - For black patients, the VF and acuity loss was less for eyes in the A-T-T sequence
  - Complications of trabeculectomy: relative risk of cataract in the 5 years after trabeculectomy was 1.78 compared to those participants who avoided trabeculectomy. Youth and high IOP were key risk factors for failure of either ALT or trabeculectomy. DM or persistent postop inflammation were also significant risk factors for trabeculectomy failure
- Conclusion of study: Low IOP reduces risk of VF progression. Data supports the use of the A-T-T sequence for all black patients. For white patients the data supports the use of the T-A-T sequence

5.2.3 Tube Versus Trabeculectomy (TVT) Study [19]

- Primary outcome: A RCT designed to prospectively compare the safety and efficacy of tube shunt surgery and trabeculectomy with mitomycin C (MMC 0.4 mg/ml) in eyes with prior ocular surgery (cataract extraction with IOL implantation or failed trabeculectomy) with uncontrolled glaucoma

- Methods
  - Inclusion criteria: age 18–85 years; previous trabeculectomy and/or cataract extraction with IOL implantation; IOP ≥18 mmHg and ≤40 mmHg on maximum tolerated medical therapy
  - Exclusion criteria: NPL vision; pregnant or nursing women; active NVI or proliferative retinopathy; ICE syndrome; aphakia; epithelial or fibrous downgrowth; vitreous in the AC for which a vitrectomy was anticipated; chronic or recurrent uveitis; severe posterior blepharitis; previous cyclodestructive procedure; prior scleral buckling procedure; presence of silicone oil; conjunctival scarring precluding a superior trabeculectomy; unwillingness to discontinue contact lens use after surgery
  - Groups: 350mm^2 Baerveldt glaucoma implant group / trabeculectomy + MMC group
  - Endpoints: IOP, VA, use of supplemental medical therapy, surgical complications, visual fields, failure (IOP >21 mmHg or less than 20% reduction below baseline on 2 consecutive follow up visits after 3 months, IOP ≤5 mmHg on 2 consecutive follow up visits after 3 months, reoperation for glaucoma—additional glaucoma surgery requiring a return to the OR, loss of light perception vision)
  - Follow up: 5 years
- Results: 212 eyes of 212 patients
  - IOP reduction: mean IOP was similar between the 2 treatment groups at 5 years (14.3 mmHg in the tube group vs 13.6 mmHg in the trabeculectomy group)
  - Use of supplemental medical therapy: no significant difference in the mean number of supplemental medications between treatment groups at 5 years
  - Failure rate: a significantly higher failure rate was seen in the trabeculectomy group than the tube group at 5 years (33% in the tube group vs 50% in the trabeculectomy group)
  - Reoperation for glaucoma: a significantly higher rate of reoperation for glaucoma was observed in the trabeculectomy group compared with the tube group at 5 years (9% in the tube group vs 29% in the trabeculectomy group)
- Conclusion of study: Tube shunt surgery had a higher success rate compared to trabeculectomy with MMC at 5 years. Both procedures were associated with similar IOP reductions and use of supplemental medical therapy at 5 years. Additional glaucoma surgery was needed more frequently after trabeculectomy with MMC than tube shunt surgery

5.2.4 Primary Tube Versus Trabeculectomy (PTVT) Study [20]

- Primary outcome: A RCT designed to prospectively compare the safety and efficacy of tube shunt surgery and trabeculectomy with mitomycin C (MMC 0.4 mg/ml) in eyes with no prior incisional ocular surgery with uncontrolled glaucoma
- Methods
  - Inclusion criteria: age 18–85 years; previous trabeculectomy and/or cataract extraction with IOL implantation; IOP ≥18 mmHg and ≤40 mmHg on maximum tolerated medical therapy
  - Exclusion criteria: NPL vision; pregnant or nursing women; active NVI or proliferative retinopathy; ICE syndrome; aphakia; epithelial or fibrous downgrowth; vitreous in the AC for which a vitrectomy was anticipated; chronic or recurrent uveitis; severe posterior blepharitis; previous cyclodestructive procedure; prior scleral buckling procedure; presence of silicone oil; conjunctival scarring precluding a superior trabeculectomy; unwillingness to discontinue contact lens use after surgery

- Groups: 350mm^2 Baerveldt glaucoma implant group/trabeculectomy + MMC group
- Endpoints: IOP, VA, use of supplemental medical therapy, surgical complications, visual fields, failure (IOP >21 mmHg or less than 20% reduction below baseline on 2 consecutive follow up visits after 3 months, IOP ≤5 mmHg on 2 consecutive follow up visits after 3 months, reoperation for glaucoma—additional glaucoma surgery requiring a return to the OR, loss of light perception vision)
- Follow up: 1 year

- Results: 242 eyes of 242 patients
  - IOP reduction: mean IOP was significantly lower in the trabeculectomy group at 1 year (13.8 mmHg in the tube group vs 12.4 mmHg in the trabeculectomy group)
  - Use of supplemental medical therapy: a significantly lower mean number of supplemental glaucoma medications was used in the trabeculectomy group at 1 year (2.1 in the tube group vs 0.9 in the trabeculectomy group)
  - Failure rate: a significantly higher failure rate was seen in the tube group than the trabeculectomy group at 1 year (17.3% in the tube group vs 7.9% in the trabeculectomy group)
  - Reoperation for glaucoma: a significantly higher rate of reoperation for glaucoma was observed in the trabeculectomy group compared with the tube group at 1 year (1% in the tube group vs 7% in the trabeculectomy group)
- Conclusion of study: Trabeculectomy + MMC had a higher surgical success rate than tube shunt surgery at 1 year. Lower IOP with use of fewer glaucoma medications was achieved after trabeculectomy + MMC compared with tube shunt surgery at 1 year. Additional glaucoma surgery was needed more frequently after trabeculectomy with MMC than tube shunt surgery

5.3 The RCOphth Guideline on Standards for the Retrieval of Human Ocular Tissue Used in Transplantation, Research and Training 2008 [55]

- Eyebanks
  - 4 in the UK: Moorfields, East Grinstead, Manchester, Bristol
  - 2 Corneal Transplant Service: Bristol, Manchester
- Consent
  - If a person has expressed a wish to be an eye donor, for example through the National Organ Donor Register or in a will, that consent is paramount and cannot be overridden by relatives
  - In the absence of prior consent given by a potential donor, consent may be given by a nominated representative of the donor or by a person in a qualifying relationship/nearest relative
  - Inform relatives that not every cornea will be suitable for transplantation, but that suitability cannot be determined before the eyes have been collected
  - Consent should also be obtained for a sample of the donor's blood to be taken for the testing of viral and other microbiological markers of transmissible disease
  - Relatives should also be asked for their permission to seek further information about a donor's medical history and behavioural background from the donor's medical records, GP and other relevant healthcare professionals
  - Research consent using a separate consent/authorisation form
  - Strongly recommended good practice that consent is recorded by a specially trained healthcare professional, such as a transplant or tissue coordinator, using the NHSBT Consent/Authorisation forms and Management Process Document or their equivalent

- Donor age
  - Upper age:
    - Currently no need to set an upper age limit for eye donation
    - Corneal endothelium is to be carefully examined by microscopy before transplantation to exclude those corneas with low endothelial cell densities endothelial damage, or other abnormalities
  - Lower age:
    - There will be very little demand for corneas from donors under 3 years old
- Post-mortem time
  - Enucleation can be performed up to 24 h post-mortem time after a donors death
  - Blood sample must be taken within 24 h of a donors death
- Medical and behavioural history
  - Sources of information about donors:
    - Hospital medical records
    - Consultant/Senior Nursing Staff with clinical responsibility for the deceased
    - Family/most relevant life partner
    - GP
    - Post-mortem examination request form
  - NHSBT assessment form used to record the family/partner interview
  - NHSBT GP form used to obtain information from the donors GP
  - Check for medical contraindications for donation and transplantation of ocular tissue
- Eye retrieval
  - Eye retrievers:
    - Must be carried out by a person who is competent in enucleation
    - Check:
      - Consent/authorization has been obtained
      - All relevant sources of medical information has been checked
  - NHS Blood Transport (NHSBT) Human Tissue Transport box:
    - Contains:
      - A set of sterile, single-use instruments with a paper wrapper for use as a drape
      - Blood sample tube
      - Alcohol swabs for cleaning the skin around the eyes and the eyelids
      - Sterile saline for irrigating eyes
      - Sterile pots, 25G needles, eye stands, cotton balls and saline for creating moist chambers
      - Eye caps and cotton balls for restoring the donor's appearance
      - Enucleation protocol, list of medical contraindications, NHSBT Ocular Tissue Donor Information and Retrieval Site Risk Assessment forms
    - Additional required items not included in the transport box:
      - At least 1 kg of ice is needed to keep the contents of the transport box below 5 °C for up to 24 h during transportation to the eye bank
      - 10 ml syringe and 19G needle for taking the blood sample
      - Sterile gloves and appropriate protective clothing
  - Retrieval site risk assessment:
    - A requirement that a risk assessment is carried out to ensure that the retrieval site is suitable and appropriate for the removal of tissue from a deceased donor
  - Donor identification:
    - In hospitals and hospices, the donor should be identified by the wrist or ankle tag using name, DOB, hospital number and any other available identifiers
    - Strongly recommended good practice for identification of the donor to be confirmed by the eye retriever and another person
  - Physical examination of the donor:
    - Examine those parts of a donor's body that are readily accessible, noting the areas examined and findings such as tattoos, piercings and scars on the body map provided on the NHSBT Ocular Tissue Donor information form
  - Blood sample:
    - If the mandatory blood tests for transmissible disease are not carried out

    locally, a sample of the donor's blood must be sent to the eye bank with the donor's eyes
    - If an ante-mortem blood sample taken not more than 7 days before death is not available, a blood sample should be taken from the deceased as soon after death as possible and not more than 24 h after death
  - Enucleation:
    - A standard enucleation protocol, such as that provided in the NHSBT Human Tissue Transport Box should be followed
    - Carefully transfer the eye to a plastic eye stand, passing the stump of the optic nerve through the hole in the base of the stand. Secure the eye on the stand by placing a sterile 25G hypodermic needle through the side of the optic nerve. Place the eye stand and eye (cornea uppermost) on top of a cotton wool ball moistened with saline in a sterile pot (moist chamber). The eye must not be immersed in any liquid in the moist chamber
  - Restoring the donor's appearance:
    - Orbits should be packed with cotton wool and the lids closed over plastic eye caps to restore the original profile of the lids
  - Packaging, labeling and transport to a Corneal Transplant Service (CTS) eye bank:
    - Labelling:
      - Essential that the moist chambers and the blood sample tube are clearly and correctly labelled with the date, donor's name, DOB and at least one other identifier (e.g. hospital name)
    - Packaging:
      - Eyes must be packed in an NHSBT Human Tissue Transport Box with the blood sample, NHSBT Retrieval Site Risk Assessment form, an NHSBT Ocular Tissue Donor form completed to the best of the eye retrievers knowledge, and any other information that may be available at the time such as a consent form, a medical history check list, or an NHSBT GP form
      - Box must be packed according to the instructions provided, including at least 1 kg of ice to ensure correct maintenance of temperature during transport
    - Transport:
      - Box should be closed using the supplied tamper-evident security tag
      - Eye retriever should contact UK Transplant (UKT) when the eyes are ready for collection, providing specific details of the location and reporting the security tag number
      - UKT will specify the eye bank address, which should then be clearly written on the label provided and attached to the side of the box
      - The eyes must be kept at a secure location until they are collected
- Contraindications to ocular tissue transplantation
  - Infections:
    - HIV/AIDS
    - Viral hepatitis (A-C)
    - TB
    - HTLV
    - Syphilis
    - Septicaemia
    - Congenital rubella
    - Rabies
    - Behaviour leading to risk of contracting HIV, hepatitis or HTLV
    - Tattoos and body piercing within the 6 months before death
    - Acupuncture within the 6 months before death
    - Imprisonment within the 12 months before death
  - Previous surgery/medical treatment:
    - Immunosuppression
    - Receipt of an organ transplant
    - Receipt of dura mater or brain/spinal surgery before August 1992
    - Receipt of human pituitary hormones

    - Receipt of a cornea, sclera or other human tissue allograft
  - Unknown aetiology and CNS disorders:
    - Death from unknown cause
    - CJD, Alzheimer's disease, Parkinson's disease, MS, motor neurone disease
  - Malignancies:
    - Leukaemia
    - Lymphoma
    - Myeloma
    - Polycythaemia Ruba Vera
    - Myelodysplastic syndrome
  - Intrinsic eye disease:
    - Active ocular inflammation/uveitis
    - Any congenital or acquired disorders of the eye, or previous ocular surgery (including corneal laser surgery), that would preclude successful graft outcome
    - Retinoblastoma
    - Malignant tumours of the anterior segment

5.4 Recent Pivotal Age-Related Macular Degeneration Clinical Trials

5.4.1 ANCHOR Study [6]

- Primary outcome: To compare ranibizumab with photodynamic therapy with verteporfin (vPDT) in the treatment of predominantly classic neovascular AMD
- Methods
  - Groups—0.3 mg ranibizumab + sham vPDT group, 0.5 mg ranibizumab + sham vPDT group, sham injections + active vPDT group. Injections were administered monthly and vPDT (sham or active) was administered at day 0 and then if needed on the basis of investigator's evaluation of angiography at 3, 6, 9 and 12 months
  - Primary endpoint—proportion of patients losing fewer than 15 letters from baseline VA at 12 months
  - Secondary endpoints—structural outcomes on fluorescein angiography
  - Follow up—12 months
- Results—423 patients
  - Primary endpoint
    - 94.3% of patients in the 0.3 mg ranibizumab group and 96.4% in the 0.5 mg ranibizumab group lost fewer than 15 letters from baseline VA, as compared with 64.3% in the vPDT group
    - The proportion of patients whose VA improved from baseline by 15 or more letters was significantly greater among those receiving ranibizumab treatment (35.7% in the 0.3 mg ranibizumab group and 40.3% in the 0.5 mg ranibizumab group, as compared with 5.6% in the vPDT group)
    - Significantly greater proportions of ranibizumab-treated patients than patients in the vPDT group had VA of 20/40 or better and smaller proportions had VA of 20/200 or worse
    - A severe loss of vision (defined as decrease of 30 letters or more) did not occur in any patient in the ranibizumab groups but occurred in 13.3% of patients in the vPDT group
    - At 12 months, 7.1% of patients in the 0.3 mg ranibizumab group and 6.4% of patients in the 0.5 mg ranibizumab group had VA of 20/20 or better, as compared with 0.7% of patients in the vPDT group
  - Secondary endpoints
    - At 12 months, the area occupied by classic CNV decreased by a mean of 0.52 optic disc area in the 0.3 mg ranibizumab group and 0.67 optic disc area in the 0.5 mg ranibizumab group, as compared with a mean increase of 0.54 optic disc area in the vPDT group
    - The area of leakage from CNV plus intense, progressive staining of the RPE at 12 months decreased by a mean of 2.05 optic disc area in the 0.5 mg ranibizumab group and 1.80 optic disc area in the 0.3 mg ranibizumab group, as compared with a mean increase of 0.32 optic disc area in the vPDT group

- Conclusion of study: Ranibizumab was superior to vPDT as treatment of predominantly classic neovascular AMD

5.4.2 MARINA Study [43]

- Primary outcome: To evaluate ranibizumab for the treatment of minimally classic or occult with no classic CNV associated with AMD
- Methods
  - Groups—0.3 mg ranibizumab group, 0.5 mg ranibizumab group, sham injection. Injections were administered monthly for 2 years
  - Primary endpoint—proportion of patients who had lost fewer than 15 letters from baseline VA
  - Secondary endpoint—structural outcomes on fluorescein angiography
  - Follow up—2 years
- Results—716 patients
  - Primary endpoints
    - At 12 months, 94.5% of the patients receiving 0.3 mg ranibizumab and 94.6% of the patients receiving 0.5 mg ranibizumab had lost fewer than 15 letters from baseline VA, as compared with 62.2% in the sham-injection group
    - At 24 months, 92% of the patients receiving 0.3 mg ranibizumab and 90% of the patients receiving 0.5 mg ranibizumab had lost fewer than 15 letters from baseline VA, as compared with 52.9% in the sham-injection group
    - At 12 and 24 months, approximately 25% of patients treated with 0.3 mg ranibizumab and 33% of patients treated with 0.5 mg ranibizumab had gained 15 or more letters in VA, as compared with 5% or less of those in the sham-injection group
    - At 12 months, mean increases in VA were 6.5 letters in the 0.3 mg ranibizumab group and 7.2 letters in the 0.5 mg ranibizumab group, as compared with a decrease of 10.4 letters in the sham-injection group. The benefit in VA was maintained at 24 months
    - At 12 months, approximately 40% of patients receiving ranibizumab had 20/40 vision or better, as compared with 11.3% in the sham-injection group. At 24 months, of the patients receiving ranibizumab, 34.5% of those in the 0.3 mg ranibizumab group and 42.1% in the 0.5 mg ranibizumab group had at least 20/40 vision, whereas the proportion in the sham injection group had dropped to 5.9%
    - Among patients receiving ranibizumab, 3.8% in the 0.3 mg ranibizumab group and 7.9% in the 0.5 mg ranibizumab group had 20/20 vision or better at 24 months. In the sham injection group, 0.8% of patients had 20/20 vision or better at 12 months and 0.4% of patients had 20/20 vision or better at 24 months
  - Secondary endpoints
    - Ranibizumab treatment was associated with arrested growth of and leakage from CNV
- Conclusion of study: Intravitreal administration of ranibizumab for 2 years prevented vision loss and improved mean VA in patients with minimally classic or occult with no classic CNV secondary to AMD

5.4.3 PrONTO Study [18]

- Primary outcome: To evaluate an OCT-guided, variable-dosing regimen with intravitreal ranibizumab for the treatment of patients with neovascular AMD (eligibility—BCVA 20/40 to 20/400 in the study eye and OCT central retinal thickness ≥300 μm)
- Methods
  - Groups—all patients received intravitreal injections of ranibizumab at baseline, month 1, and month 2. Additional reinjections were given if: [1] VA loss of at least 5 letters with OCT evidence of fluid in the macula, [2] an increase in OCT central retinal thickness ≥100 μm, [3] new macular haemorrhage, [4] new area of classic CNV, or [5] evidence of persistent fluid on OCT

at least one month after the previous injection
  - Primary endpoints—change in VA and OCT measurements from baseline
  - Secondary endpoints—number of consecutive monthly injections required from baseline to achieve a fluid-free macula as determined by OCT
  - Follow up—12 months
- Results—40 patients
  - Primary endpoints:
    - At 12 months, the mean and median VA scores improved compared with baseline by 9.3 letters and 11 letters, respectively
    - At 12 months, the mean and median central retinal thickness measurements decreased by 177.8 μm and 185.5 μm, respectively
  - Secondary endpoints
    - The mean number of injections for the first year were 5.6 (SD 2.3) and 5.0 (range, 3–13), respectively, of a possible 13 injections from day 0 through month 12
    - A total of 39 eyes eventually became fluid-free; 37 of these eyes eventually developed some recurrent fluid during the first year. Of the 37 eyes that developed some recurrent fluid, 32 received a retreatment during the first 12 months
    - After the first 3 injections, 7 patients never needed another injection. One eye never became fluid-free and received a total of 13 injections
    - Of the 39 eyes that eventually achieved a fluid-free macula, the mean and median number of monthly consecutive injections from baseline that were required to achieve a fluid-free macula were 1.5 (SD 1.1) and 1.0 (range, 1–6), respectively
- Conclusion of study: OCT-guided, variable-dosing regimen with ranibizumab resulted in VA outcomes similar to the phase III clinical trials MARINA and ANCHOR. OCT appears useful for determining when retreatment with ranibizumab is necessary

5.4.4 PIER Study [42]

- Primary outcome: To evaluate the efficacy and safety of ranibizumab administered monthly for 3 months and then quarterly in patients with subfoveal CNV secondary to AMD
- Methods
  (a) Groups—0.3 mg ranibizumab group, 0.5 mg ranibizumab group, sham treatment group. Injections were administered monthly, for the first 3 doses, followed by three-monthly intervals. Verteporfin photodynamic therapy (vPDT) was permitted at the investigator's discretion
  (b) Primary endpoint—mean change from baseline to 12 months in VA score
  (c) Secondary endpoint—proportion of subjects losing 15 letters or less from baseline; proportion gaining ≥15 letters from baseline; proportion with a Snellen equivalent of 20/200 or worse; mean change from baseline in the near activities, distance activities, and vision-specific dependency NEI VFQ-25 subscales; and mean change from baseline in total area of CNV and total area of leakage from CNV
  (d) Follow up—12 months
- Results—184 patients
  (a) Primary endpoints
    - At 12 months, sham-treated eyes had lost a mean of 16.3 letters, whereas ranibizumab-treated subjects had lost a mean of 1.6 letters (0.3 mg ranibizumab group) or 0.2 letters (0.5 mg ranibizumab group)
    - On average, there was a 4.5 letter decline in VA between month 3 and month 12 for both ranibizumab dose groups, reflecting the effect of quarterly dosing; these declines were statistically significant
  (b) Secondary endpoints
    - Significantly greater proportions of the ranibizumab groups than the sham

group had lost fewer than 15 letters from baseline VA: 83.3% and 90.2% of the 0.3 mg and 0.5 mg ranibizumab groups, respectively, compared with 49.2% of the sham group
  - The 3 treatment groups did not differ significantly in the proportions gaining at least 15 letters: 9.5% in the sham group, 11.7% in the 0.3 mg ranibizumab group, and 13.1% in the 0.5 mg ranibizumab group
  - Significant smaller proportions of the ranibizumab groups than the sham group had VA of 20/200 of worse snellen equivalent at month 12: 23.3% and 24.6% of the 0.3 mg and 0.5 mg ranibizumab groups, respectively, compared with 52.4% of the sham group
  - There was no statistically significant difference between either ranibizumab dose group and the sham control for any of the 3 NEI VFQ-25 subscales that were prespecified as secondary endpoints
  - Ranibizumab reduced the total area of leakage of CNV plus intense progressive RPE staining on average, whereas the sham group exhibited an increase trend
- Conclusion of study: Ranibizumab administered monthly for 3 months and then quarterly provided significant VA benefits to patients with AMD-related subfoveal CNV

5.4.5 The Comparison of Age-Related Macular Degeneration Treatment Trial [50]

- Primary outcome—A RCT to assess the relative efficacy and safety of ranibizumab (0.5 mg) and bevacizumab (1.25 mg) and to determine whether an as-needed regimen would compromise long term VA, as compared to a monthly regimen
- Methods
  - Groups—ranibizumab monthly group, bevacizumab monthly group, ranibizumab as needed group, bevacizumab as needed group
  - Primary endpoint—mean change in VA between baseline and 1 year
  - Secondary endpoints—proportion of patients with a change in VA of 15 letters or more, the number of injections, the change in fluid and foveal thickness on OCT, change in lesion size on FA, the incidence of ocular and systemic adverse effects
  - Follow up—1 year
- Results—1208 patients
  - Primary endpoint
    - Bevacizumab monthly (+8.0 letter) was equivalent to ranibizumab monthly (+8.5 letters)
    - Bevacizumab as needed (+5.9 letters) was equivalent to ranibizumab monthly (+6.8 letters)
    - Ranibizumab as needed was equivalent to monthly ranibizumab
    - Comparison of bevacizumab as needed and bevacizumab monthly was inconclusive
  - Secondary endpoints
    - The proportion of patients who did not have a decrease in VA of 15 letters or more from baseline was 94.4% in the ranibizumab monthly group, 94.0% in the bevacizumab monthly group, 95.4% in the ranibizumab as needed group, and 91.5% in the bevacizumab as needed group
    - The proportion of patients who gained at least 15 letters did not differ significantly among the groups, ranging from 24.9% in the group that received ranibizumab as needed to 34.2% in the group that received ranibizumab as needed
    - The proportion of patients with arteriothrombotic events (CVA, MI, death from vascular causes) were similar among the groups
    - The proportion of patients with serious systemic adverse events (hospitalisation

from infections e.g. pneumonia, UTI, GI disorders e.g. haemorrhage, nausea and vomiting) was higher with bevacizumab (24.1%) than with ranibizumab (19.0%)

- Conclusion of study
  - At 1 year, effect on visual acuity of bevacizumab were non-inferior to that ranibizumab when administered according to the same schedule. Ranibizumab given as needed with monthly evaluation had effects on vision that were similar to those of ranibizumab administered monthly.
  - At 2 years [28], bevacizumab and ranibizumab had similar effects on visual acuity. Treatment as needed resulted in less gain in VA, whether instituted at enrolment or after 1 year of monthly treatment
  - Non-inferiority was not shown between as required bevacizumab and monthly ranibizumab or monthly bevacizumab
  - As required ranibizumab was non-inferior to monthly ranibizumab
  - In order to achieve similar effects, prn bevacizumab needs to be administered more often than prn ranibizumab
  - There was a higher incidence of adverse events associated with bevacizumab compared to ranibizumab

5.4.6 VIEW 1 and VIEW 2 Studies [22]

- Primary outcome: To compare intravitreal aflibercept, monthly or every 2 months, with monthly ranibizumab in treatment of nAMD
- Methods
  - Groups—0.5 mg aflibercept every 4 weeks group, 2 mg aflibercept every 4 weeks group, 2 mg aflibercept every 8 weeks after 3 injections at week 0, 4 and 8 group, 0.5 mg ranibizumab every 4 weeks group
  - Primary endpoint—noninferiority (margin of 10%) of the intravitreal aflibercept regimens to ranibizumab in the proportions of patients maintaining vision at week 52 (losing less than 15 ETDRS letters)
  - Secondary endpoint—compare baseline and 52-week data regarding mean change in BCVA; gaining 15 or more letters; change in total National Eye Institute 25-Item Visual Function Questionnaire (NEI VFG-25) score; change in CNV area on fluorescein angiography
  - Follow up—12 months
- Results—2419 patients
  - Primary endpoints
    - All aflibercept groups achieved statistical noninferiority compared with monthly ranibizumab in the treatment of CNV secondary to AMD
  - Secondary endpoints
    - Similar VA scores across the entire 52-week study for all treatment groups
    - On the basis of the hierarchical testing sequence, only the 2 mg aflibercept every 4 weeks group was statistically superior to ranibizumab, and only in VIEW 1, with a gain of +10.9 versus +8.1 letters
    - In both studies, the proportion of patients gaining 15 or more ETDRS letters from baseline to week 52 was similar in all treatment groups
    - Vision-related quality of life, assessed by the change of total score of the NEI VFQ-25, improved in all groups in both studies
    - All groups demonstrated a comparable decrease in area of active CNV
    - All aflibercept groups in both studies had reductions in central retinal thickness similar to those for monthly ranibizumab as assessed by OCT, with a large and rapid reduction evident by week 4 that was maintained to week 52
- Conclusion of study: Intravitreal aflibercept dosed monthly or every 2 months after 3 initial monthly doses produced similar efficacy and safety outcomes as monthly ranibizumab in the treatment of nAMD

5.4.7 Inhibition of VEGF in Age-Related Choroidal Neovascularisation (IVAN) Trial [7]

- Primary outcome—A RCT to compare the efficacy and safety of ranibizumab (0.5 mg) and bevacizumab (1.25 mg) to treat neovascular age-related macular degeneration
- Methods
  - Groups—ranibizumab continuous group, bevacizumab continuous group, ranibizumab discontinuous group, bevacizumab discontinuous group
  - Primary endpoint—BCVA at 2 years
  - Secondary endpoints—near VA, reading index, contrast sensitivity, lesion morphology and metrics from FA and OCTs, adverse events
  - Follow up—2 years
- Results—525 patients reached the visit at 2 years
  - Primary endpoint
    - BCVA was similar between ranibizumab and bevacizumab groups and continuous and discontinuous treatment groups.
    - Bevacizumab was neither inferior or non-inferior to ranibizumab
    - Discontinuous regimen was neither inferior or non-inferior to the continuous regimen
  - Secondary endpoints
    - Near VA, reading index, and contrast sensitivity did not differ significantly between drug groups
    - Near VA and contrast sensitivity were significantly worse with the discontinuous regimen
    - Mortality was higher at 2 years with discontinuous treatment than continuous treatment
- Conclusion of study: ranibizumab and bevacizumab have similar efficacy. Reduction in the frequency of retreatment resulted in a small loss of efficacy irrespective of drug. Safety was worse when treatment was administered discontinuously.

5.4.8 HAWK and HARRIER Trials [14]

- Primary outcome –To demonstrate that brolucizumab is noninferior to fixed-dose aflibercept with respect to the change in best corrected visual acuity (BCVA) from baseline to week 48 in patients with neovascular AMD
- Methods
  - Groups—HAWK: brolucizumab 3 mg group, brolucizumab 6 mg group, or aflibercept 2 mg group; HARRIER: brolucizumab 6 mg group or aflibercept 2 mg group. For both trials, all treatment arms had 3 loading injections at weeks 0, 4, and 8 followed by 8 weeks before the next possible treatment. Brolucizumab was injected every 12 weeks (q12w) unless disease activity was identified, resulting in permanent adjustment to 8 weekly injections (q8w). Aflibercept was injected every 8 weeks (q8w)
  - Primary endpoint—mean BCVA change from baseline to week 48
  - Secondary endpoints—BCVA change from baseline averaged over the period of week 36 through week 48 (to account for differences in timing of treatment), q12w treatment status at week 48 (brolucizumab groups only), q12w treatment status at week 48 among eyes with no q8w need during the first q12w cycle (to evaluate the predictive value of the first q12w cycle; brolucizumab groups only), anatomic retinal fluid outcomes
  - Follow up—48 weeks
- Results—total of 1817 patients (HAWK + HARRIER)
  - Primary endpoint
    - In both trials, each brolucizumab arm demonstrated noninferiority versus aflibercept in least squares (LS) mean BCVA change from baseline to week 48

5.5 The Optic Neuritis Treatment Trial (ONTT)

- The ONTT was a randomised trial that evaluated the use of corticosteroids in the treatment of acute optic neuritis
- Methods—3 treatment regimens
  - 250 mg of IV methylprednisolone every 6 h for 3 days followed by 1 mg of oral prednisolone per kg of body weight per day for 11 days (IV-methylprednisolone group)
  - 1 mg of oral prednisolone per kg per day for 14 days (oral prednisolone group)
  - Oral placebo for 14 days (placebo group)
- Results
  - A 3-day course of pulsed IV treatment with methylprednisolone (250 mg QDS) followed by an 11-day course of oral prednisolone (1 mg/kg) accelerated visual recovery but did not significantly improve visual outcome at 6 months [2]. However, this regimen temporarily reduced the rate of new demyelinating events over a 6–24 month follow up period [3]
  - A regimen of oral prednisolone alone (1 mg/kg for 14 days) did not improve visual outcome at 6 months and was associated with an increased rate of new attacks of optic neuritis [2]
  - At 10 years, the probability of developing MS was 22% for patients with no white matter lesions on MRI and 56% for patients with one or more white matter lesions on MRI [39]
  - The aggregate cumulative probability of developing MS by the 15-year examination was 50% and was strongly related to the presence of lesions on the baseline MRI [53]
  - At 15 years, the probability of developing MS was 25% for patients with no white matter lesions on MRI and 72% for patients with one or more white matter lesions on MRI [53]
  - Among patients without MS at the 10-year examination, the probability of developing MS by the 15-year examination was 32% when 1 or more baseline lesions were present vs 2% when there were no baseline lesions [53]

5.6 Zoster Eye Disease Study (ZEDS)

- Primary objective [8]: to evaluate whether one year of suppressive valacyclovir 1000 mg daily in patients with herpes zoster ophthalmicus (HZO) reduces specific eye disease manifestations including new or worsening episode of dendriform epithelial keratitis, stromal keratitis, endothelial keratitis, and/or iritis and/or postherpetic neuralgia (PHN) compared to placebo
- Secondary objectives [8]:
  - To evaluate the effect of treatment on the primary endpoint at 18 months (6 months after the completion of study drug treatment) by:
    1. Comparing the rates of new or worsening dendriform epithelial keratitis, stromal keratitis, endothelial keratitis, and/or iritis in study participants randomized to valacyclovir versus placebo
    2. Comparing time to development of the primary endpoint over the 18-month period from randomization and
    3. Comparing the occurrence of the primary endpoint during the 6-month post treatment period
  - To test the hypothesis that suppressive treatment for 12 months with oral valacyclovir 1000 mg daily reduces the incidence, severity and duration of PHN compared to placebo at 12 and 18 months in study participants with HZO
- Methods [8]:
  - Inclusion criteria: 18 years and older, immunocompetent, have a history of a typical rash at disease onset, and have had a record of active epithelial or stromal keratitis or iritis within 1 year before enrollment
  - Exclusion criteria: estimated glomerular filtration rate less than 45 or pregnancy
  - Groups: participants were randomly assigned to valacyclovir or placebo in 4 groups: age of *onset* of HZO: younger <60 years vs older ≥60 years; time of onset of HZO at *enrollment*: recent <6 months vs chronic ≥6 months

  - Primary endpoint: time to first occurrence of new or worsening dendriform epithelial keratitis, stromal keratitis without or with ulceration, endothelial keratitis, or iritis due to HZO during 12 months of study treatment, requiring prespecified treatment changes. The primary endpoint is compared for participants randomized to study medication or placebo
  - Secondary endpoints: to find out whether there is persistent treatment benefit at 18 months, 6 months after cessation of treatment, and whether development of PHN (defined by trial as zoster brief pain inventory score of worst pain in last 24 hours of 3/10 or more occurring 3 or more months after HZO onset) varies by treatment group; the effect of valacyclovir treatment on medication usage for pain was also analysed
  - Follow-up: March 2020—June 2024
- Results [9, 61]—490 participants completed 12 months of treatment and 460 completed 18 months:
  - Primary endpoint: no significant treatment benefit in reducing new/worsening keratitis or iritis at 12 months of treatment
  - Secondary endpoints: significant treatment benefit in reducing new/worsening keratitis or iritis at 18 months; participants randomised to valacyclovir had a significantly lower likelihood of experiencing subsequent disease flare-ups compared to those on placebo at 12 and 18 months; participants <60 years at HZO onset on valacyclovir had a significantly lower prevalence of PHN at 18 months; participants in the <60 years onset, chronic stratum on valacyclovir had significantly lower pain scores at 12 and 18 months; among all participants there was a significant decrease in pain duration for those on valacyclovir compared to placebo at 18 months; there was a statistically significant reduction in the dose of neuropathic medications at 12 and 18 months for participants on valacyclovir
- Conclusions [9, 61]:
  - Evidence supports suppressive valacyclovir treatment 1000 mg daily for one year to reduce new or worsening keratitis or iritis in immunocompetent, non-pregnant adults with good renal function
  - Evidence supports suppressive valacyclovir treatment to reduce multiple episodes of keratitis or iritis
  - Recommend one year of suppressive valacyclovir to significantly decrease pain duration at 18 months (overall) and significantly lower pain scores (if HZO onset <60 years and in chronic stratum) at 12 and 18 months
  - Recommend one year of suppressive valacyclovir to significantly reduce dose of neuropathic pain medications at 12 and 18 months

5.7 Principles of Screening Applied to the NHS Diabetic Eye Screening Programme

- Screening is the presumptive identification of unrecognised disease or defect by the application of tests, examinations, or other procedures which can be applied rapidly [63]
- World Health Organisation (WHO) Criteria for screening [63]
  - **Condition**:
    - The condition should be an important health problem:
      - Sight threatening DR is an important public health problem
      - In 1990–1991 DR was the leading cause of people registered blind among people of working age in England and Wales [17]
    - There should be a recognisable latent or early symptomatic stage:
      - Sight threatening DR has a recognisable latent or early symptomatic

stage in both type 1 and 2 diabetes [15]
- The natural history of the condition, including development from latent to declared disease, should be adequately understood
  - The natural history of sight-threatening diabetic retinopathy is well understood [25]

- **Test**:
  - There should be a suitable test or examination:
    - Two field mydriatic digital photography with a sensitivity of 87.8%, specificity of 86.1%, and poor image quality rate of 3.7% [44, 45]
  - The test should be acceptable to the population
    - Two field mydriatic digital photography [45]
  - Facilities for diagnosis and treatment should be available
    - Hospital Eye Service (HES)
- **Treatment**:
  - There should be an acceptable treatment for patients with recognised disease:
    - PRP is of benefit in preventing severe visual loss in eyes with PDR [51]
    - Focal photocoagulation of CSMO is of benefit in reducing moderate visual loss [15]
  - There should be an agreed policy on whom to treat as patients
    - All patients with PDR and CSMO require treatment [15, 51]
- **Cost**:
  - The cost of case finding (including diagnosis and treatment of patients diagnosed) should be economically balanced in relation to possible expenditure on medical care as a whole:
    - The costs of screening and effective treatment of sight threatening DR are balanced economically in relation to total expenditure on health care including the consequences of leave the disease untreated [46]
- **Process**:
  - Case finding should be a continuing process and not a "once and for all" project
    - Annual eye examination for DR is offered to all people with diabetes over the age of 12

5.8 Public Health England NHS Diabetic Eye Screening Programme (DESP) (Table 5.3)

5.8.1 NHS DESP Grading Definitions for Diabetic Retinopathy [41]

- R0: no retinopathy
- R1 (background DR/mild NPDR):
  - Venous loop
  - Microaneurysms
  - Retinal haemorrhage
  - Any exudate or cotton wool spot in presence of other non-referable DR features
- R2 (pre-proliferative DR/moderate NPDR):
  - Venous beading
  - Venous reduplication
  - Multiple blot haemorrhages (if uncertain, refer only in the presence of IRMA that are definitely seen)
    - Blot haemorrhages (located in OPL and INL) are larger than the width of the smallest of the 4 branches of the central retinal vein as it crosses the edge of the disc
  - IRMA (check that they can still be seen on the colour image as well as the red-free image that has not been enlarged)

Table 5.3 Key facts about the NHS DESP

Key facts
Aim is to reduce the risk of sight loss amongst people with diabetes by the prompt identification and effective treatment if necessary, of sight-threatening DR, at the appropriate stage during the disease process
Two 45-degree field mydriatic digital photographic screening
All people with diabetes aged 12 or above are offered annual screening eye examinations for DR

- R3 (proliferative DR):
  - R3A (active PDR):
    - NVD
    - NVE
    - Pre-retinal or vitreous haemorrhage
    - Pre-retinal fibrosis +/− tractional RD
  - R3S (stable treated PDR):
    - Evidence of peripheral laser retinal treatment AND
    - Stable retina with respect to reference images taken at or shortly after discharge from the hospital eye service (HES)

5.8.2 NHS DESP Grading Definitions for Diabetic Maculopathy [41]

- Macula is defined as that part of the retina which lies within a circle centered on the centre of the fovea whose radius is the distance between the centre of the fovea and the temporal margin of the disc
- M0
  - No maculopathy
- M1:
  - Exudate within 1-disc diameter of the centre of the fovea
  - Circinate or group of exudates within the macula:
    - A group of exudates is an area of exudates that is greater than or equal to half the disc area and this area is all within the macular area
    - To work out the area, the outer points of the exudates are joined and compared to half the area of the optic disc
  - Any microaneurysm or haemorrhage within 1-disc diameter of the centre of the fovea only if associated with a best VA of 6/12 or worse

5.8.3 NHS DESP Referral Criteria to Hospital Eye Service (HES) [41]

- Retinopathy
  - R0: screen annually
  - R1: screen annually
  - R2: Referral to HES—seen ≤13 weeks
  - R3A: Urgent referral to HES—seen ≤2 weeks
  - R3S: screen annually
- Maculopathy
  - M0: screen annually
  - M1: Referral to HES—seen ≤13 weeks

5.8.4 Treatment Time at HES

- PRP for PDR within 2 weeks
- Focal/grid laser for maculopathy within 10 weeks

5.9 Diabetic Retinopathy Clinical Research Network (DRCR.net) Protocols

- PDR
  - Protocol S [13]:
    - Purpose
      - Prompt PRP vs 0.5 mg ranibizumab +/− deferred PRP
    - Results
      - Treatment with ranibizumab resulted in VA that was non-inferior to PRP treatment at 2 years
- DMO
  - Protocol B [12]:
    - Purpose
      - Intravitreal triamcinolone vs focal/grid laser for DMO
    - Results
      - At 2 years, focal/grid laser is more effective and has fewer side effects than intravitreal triamcinolone
      - For center-involving DMO, focal/grid laser produces gradual VA improvement of ≥2 lines in approximately one-third of eyes with VA of ≤20/40 at 2 years
      - For center-involving DMO, approximately 20% of laser treated eyes worsen by ≥2 lines at 2 years

- Protocol I [16]:
  - Purpose
    - Sham injection + prompt focal/grid laser (within 3–10 days after injection) vs Intravitreal 0.5 mg ranibizumab + prompt (within 3–10 days after injection) focal/grid laser vs Intravitreal 4 mg triamcinolone + prompt (within 3–10 days after injection) focal/grid laser vs Intravitreal ranibizumab + deferred (≥24 weeks) focal/grid laser
  - Results
    - Intravitreal ranibizumab with prompt or deferred focal/grid laser resulted in superior VA and OCT outcomes compared with prompt focal/grid laser alone for the treatment of DMO involving the central macula at 1 year
    - In pseudophakic eyes, intravitreal triamcinolone with prompt focal/grid laser resulted in superior VA and OCT outcomes than focal/grid laser alone and the VA and OCT outcomes were comparable to intravitreal ranibizumab with prompt or deferred focal/grid laser for the treatment of DMO involving the central macula at 1 year
- Protocol T [52, 62]:
  - Purpose
    - Aflibercept (2 mg), bevacizumab (1.25 mg) and ranibizumab (0.3 mg) comparison for center-involved DMO
  - Results
    - If initial VA letter score was 78–69 (20/32 to 20/40), there was no significant difference in mean improvement in VA letter score from baseline at 1 year between the 3 anti-VEGF drugs
    - If initial VA score was <69 (<20/40), the mean improvement in VA letter score from baseline at 1 year was significantly greater with aflibercept than with bevacizumab or ranibizumab
    - If initial VA letter score was 78–69 (20/32 to 20/40), there was no significant difference in mean improvement in VA letter score from baseline at 2 years between the 3 anti-VEGF drugs
    - If initial VA score was (<20/40), the mean improvement in VA letter score from baseline at 2 years was significantly greater with aflibercept than bevacizumab but not with ranibizumab

5.10 Hydroxychloroquine & Chloroquine Retinopathy

5.10.1 Pathogenesis

- Hydroxychloroquine and chloroquine can cause toxic retinopathy due to their binding of melanin in the RPE as well as direct toxicity to retinal ganglion cells

5.10.2 History

- Symptoms: asymptomatic, reduced vision, reduced colour vision, paracentral scotomas, reduced night vision, photopsias, glare, metamorphopsia
- Ask about risk factors
  - Concomitant tamoxifen use
  - Impaired renal function with eGFR less than 60
  - >5-year duration of hydroxychloroquine use and >5 mg/kg/day dose of hydroxychloroquine

5.10.3 Examination

- Mottling of the RPE (early sign)
- Blunted foveal reflex (early sign)
- Bull's eye maculopathy (late sign): ring of depigmentation surrounding the fovea
- Geographic atrophy
- Optic atrophy

5.10.4 Investigation

- OCT: loss of IS/OS junction in early toxicity, parafoveal thinning of the ONL in moderate toxicity, widespread RPE atrophy and retinal thinning in severe cases, "flying saucer" sign—ovoid appearance of central fovea created by preservation of central foveal outer retinal structures surrounded by perifoveal loss of IS/OS junction and perifoveal outer retinal thinning
- Fundus autofluorescence (FAF): ring of increased autofluorescence initially with parafoveal hypofluorescence in severe cases
- HVF: Paracentral scotomas

5.10.5 The RCOphth Clinical Guidelines on Hydroxychloroquine and Chloroquine Retinopathy 2020: Recommendations on Monitoring [59]

- Monitoring criteria
  - Annual monitoring for individuals who have taken hydroxychloroquine for more than 5 years
  - Annual monitoring for individuals who have taken chloroquine for more than 1 year
  - All individuals taking hydroxychloroquine who have additional risk factors for retinal toxicity (concomitant tamoxifen use, impaired renal function with eGFR <60 ml/min/1.75 m^2, dose of hydroxychloroquine >5 mg/kg/day) may be monitored annually after the initiation of therapy
  - It is the responsibility of the prescribing physician to refer patients eligible for screening to the local HES
- Monitoring Protocol: Tests
  - All patients should undergo both SD-OCT and FAF, widefield if available
  - Patients with abnormalities on either SD-OCT or FAF imaging should undergo automated visual fields testing using either a 10–2 or 30–2 protocol depending on the location of the structural abnormality
  - Patients with confirmed structural abnormalities on SD-OCT or FAF who do not demonstrate an anatomically consistent visual defect on repeated testing should undergo multifocal ERG
- Interpretation of Monitoring: Results
  - No toxicity: no abnormalities suggestive of toxicity detected on OCT or FAF
  - Possible toxicity: OCT or FAF result typical of hydroxychloroquine retinopathy, but neither visual fields of multifocal ERG abnormal
  - Definite toxicity: two tests with corresponding abnormalities consistent with hydroxychloroquine retinopathy. This definition can be satisfied in the following scenarios:
    1. OCT ***and*** FAF typical of hydroxychloroquine retinopathy
    2. Either OCT ***or*** FAF typical of hydroxychloroquine retinopathy, supported by either visual field testing or multifocal ERG findings corresponding to the anatomical defect
- Management of patients with Possible Retinopathy
  - Continue drug treatment
  - Patients with one abnormal test result on retinal imaging (SD-OCT or widefield FAF) but normal visual fields on repeat testing should be referred for multifocal ERG. Treatment should continue until the outcome of mfERG is known.
- Management of patients with Definite Toxicity
  - Recommendation to stop hydroxychloroquine should be made to the prescribing physician
  - Inappropriate for ophthalmologists to stop hydroxychloroquine treatment
  - Patients should be referred for appropriate support at the point of detection of hydroxychloroquine retinopathy e.g. low vision or eye clinic liaison officer (ECLO) services, certification of visual impairment, and referral to local and/or national charities

  - Patients who are drivers should inform the DVLA and be advised not to drive until an Estermann VF test confirms it is legal to do so
  - Some description by the ophthalmologist of disease severity (mild, moderate or severe) may be helpful to facilitate discussion between patient and prescribing physician
- Termination of Monitoring
  - Screening discontinued if patients stop taking hydroxychloroquine

5.11 The RCOphth Review of the Ocular Side Effects of Topiramate 2010 [57]

5.11.1 Indications

- Monotherapy or adjunct in the control of partial and primary generalised epilepsy in adults and children above the age of 2
- Migraine prophylaxis
- Trigeminal neuralgia
- Bipolar disorder, depression, eating disorders
- IIH

5.11.2 Ocular Side-Effects

- Secondary acute angle closure glaucoma
  - Occurs within 2 weeks of initiation of treatment
  - Suprachoroidal or cilio-choroidal detachments and ciliary body oedema: causes a forward rotation of the ciliary body which displaces the iris-lens plane anteriorly to close the AC angle
  - Treatment:
    - Withdrawal of topiramate
    - Topical atropine
    - Topical ocular hypotensive agents
    - Cautious use of oral acetazolamide—may worsen ciliary body oedema
- Acute myopia on its own or with angle closure
  - Suprachoroidal or cilio-choroidal detachments and ciliary body oedema—causes a forward rotation of the ciliary body which displaces the iris-lens plane anteriorly
  - Myopia on its own resolves following discontinuation of the drug
- Diplopia and nystagmus
- Posterior scleritis

5.11.3 Recommendations

- Screening patient on topiramate for asymptomatic disease is not useful
- In case of visual blurring or ocular pain, initial advice from their local optometrist should be encouraged
- Patients referred to Ophthalmologists with acute myopia should consider drug replacement following advice from a neurologist
- Acute angle closure should be managed with:
  - Withdrawal or replacement of topiramate with an alternative drug
  - Topical atropine drops + topical ocular hypotensive agents

5.12 The Ocular Side-Effects of Vigabatrin (Sabril) Information and Guidance for Screening [54]

5.12.1 Indications for Vigabatrin

- Anti-epileptic drug (selective irreversible inhibitor of GABA-transaminase) licensed for first line treatment of infantile spasms and for the treatment of partial epilepsy +/− secondary generalization which is not satisfactorily controlled by other drugs
- Vigabatrin is not recommended for patients with pre-existing visual field defects
- No relationship between the daily or cumulative dose of vigabatrin and the risk of visual field constriction

5.12.2 History

- Symptoms: normal VA, asymptomatic absolute field loss
- Risk factors: male (two-fold higher chance of developing VF constriction compared with females—effect independent of any differences in dose duration or cumulative dose of vigabatrin)

5.12.3 Examination

- Absolute field loss can occur in the absence of any demonstratable fundal pathology observed clinically
- Optic nerve pallor
- RNFL atrophy

5.12.4 Investigations

- ERG: reduced or absent oscillatory potentials
- HVF: bilateral concentric predominantly peripheral and nasal constriction of the VF with temporal and macular sparing (spares the central field)

5.12.5 Prognosis

- VF constriction does not reverse on cessation of the drug
- Progression of VF constriction after stopping vigabatrin has not been reported to date

5.12.6 Screening

- Baseline VF (Humphrey 120/Octopus 07 or Goldmann kinetic perimetry—less sensitive compared to Humphrey) should be obtained before starting treatment (age ≥9 years). Threshold testing is not recommended
- VF testing after baseline should be repeated every 6 months for 5 years. Test interval can then be extended to annually in patients who have no defect detected.
- If VF constriction is detected it is advisable, if possible, to conduct a confirmatory field test within 1 month before considering cessation of vigabatrin
- If the drug is discontinued VF should be repeated at a future date to monitor the field loss

5.13 Uveitis

5.13.1 Classification of Uveitis

- International Uveitis Study Group Anatomical Classification [4]
  - Anterior uveitis: anterior chamber
  - Intermediate uveitis: vitreous
  - Posterior uveitis: retina or choroid
  - Panuveitis: anterior chamber, vitreous, and retina or choroid
- The Standardisation of Uveitis Nomenclature (SUN) Working Group 2005 Descriptors of Uveitis Descriptors of Uveitis [60]
  - Onset:
    - Sudden
    - Insidious
  - Course:
    - Acute: episode with sudden onset and limited duration
    - Chronic: persistent uveitis with relapse in <3 months after discontinuing treatment
    - Recurrent: repeated episodes separated by periods of inactivity without treatment >3 months duration
  - Duration:
    - Limited <3 months
    - Persistent >3 months

5.13.2 The SUN Working Group Grading Scheme of Anterior Chamber Cells [60]

- Field size of 1 × 1 mm slit beam:
  - 0: no cells
  - 0.5+: 1–5 cells
  - 1+: 6–15 cells

- 2+: 16–25 cells
- 3+ 26–50 cells
- 4+: >50 cells

5.13.3 The SUN Working Group Grading Scheme for Anterior Chamber Flare [60]

- 0: none
- 1+: faint
- 2+: moderate—iris and lens details clear
- 3+: severe—iris and lens details hazy
- 4+: intense—fibrin or plastic aqueous

5.13.4 Nussenblatt Scale for Vitreous Haze 1985 [38]

- Performed with an indirect ophthalmoscope and 20-diopter lens by visually comparing the degree of haze on examination to a colour fundus photograph printout of the 6-step ordinal scale
  - 0: no evident vitreal haze at all
  - Trace (0.5+): slight blurring of optic disc margin, no visualisation of the normal striations and reflex of the nerve fiber layer
  - 1+: permits better definition of both the optic nerve head and the retinal vessels
  - 2+: permits better visualisation of the retinal vessels
  - 3+: optic nerve head is visible to the observer but its borders are blurry
  - 4+: optic nerve head is obscured

5.13.5 The SUN Working Group Activity of Uveitis Terminology 2005 [60]

- Inactive: grade 0 cells
- Worsening activity: 2-step increase in level of inflammation (AC cells or vitreous haze) or increase from grade 3+ to 4+
- Improved activity: 2-step decrease in level of inflammation (AC cells or vitreous haze) or decrease to grade 0
- Remission: inactive disease for >3 months after discontinuing all treatments for eye disease

5.13.6 NICE Guidance [TA460] on Adalimumab [34]

- Based on evidence from the **VISUAL I** [24] and **VISUAL II** [29] trials
- Recommended as an option for treating of non-infectious uveitis in the posterior segment of the eye in adults with inadequate response to corticosteroids, only if there is:
  - Active disease (current inflammation in the eye) AND
  - Inadequate response or intolerance to immunosuppresants AND
  - Systemic disease or both eyes are affected (or 1 eye is affected if the second eye has poor visual acuity) AND
  - Worsening vision with a high risk of blindness
- Stop adalimumab for non-infectious uveitis in the posterior segment of the eye in adults with inadequate response to corticosteroids if there is 1 of the following:
  - New active inflammatory chorioretinal or inflammatory retinal vascular lesions, or both or
  - A 2 step increase in vitreous haze or AC cell grade or
  - Worsening of BCVA by 3 or more lines or 15 letters

5.13.7 NICE Guidance [TA460] on Ozurdex [34]

- Based on evidence from the HURON study [27]
- Dexamethasone intravitreal implant is recommended as an option for treating non-

infectious uveitis in the posterior segment of the eye in adults, only if there is:
  - Active disease (that is, current inflammation in the eye) AND
  - Worsening vision with a risk of blindness

5.13.8 NICE Guidance [TA590] on Fluocinolone Acetonide Intravitreal Implant [36]

- Based on evidence from the PSV-FAI-001 trial [40]
- Flucinolone acetonide intravitreal implant is recommended as an option for preventing relapse in recurrent non-infectious uveitis affecting the posterior segment of the eye

5.14 Creutzfeldt-Jakob Disease (CJD)

- CJD is a progressive, fatal neurological disease that belongs to a wider group of neurodegenerative disorders known as transmissible spongiform encephalopathies (TSE) or prion diseases
- A novel form of human prion disease, variant CJD (vCJD) is believed to result from consumption of food derived from cattle infected with bovine spongiform encephalopathy (BSE)—ingestion of contaminated beef
- The prion protein is a normal cellular protein that is widely expressed in almost all human tissues, with the highest levels seen in nerve cells. Prions are infectious particles composed of abnormally folded forms of the prion protein.
- Transmission (NICE Guidance [IPG196] [30])
  - Iatrogenic:
    - Recipient of human cadaveric derived pituitary hormones
    - Antecedent neurosurgery with dura mater transplantation
    - Blood transfusion
    - Contaminated surgical instruments:
      - High risk procedures for transmission of CJD:
        - Posterior eye procedures that involve the retina or optic nerve:
          - Excision of eye e.g. evisceration + orbital implant
          - Operations on the optic nerve e.g. optic nerve decompression
          - Operations of vitreous body ONLY if they come into contact with the posterior hyaloid face e.g. PPV + membrane peel
          - Scleral buckling with drainage of SRF
          - Photocoagulation of retina for detachment (only when the retina is handled directly)
          - Destruction of lesion of retina
          - Operations on the retina and RPE
      - Medium risk procedures for transmission of CJD:
        - Anterior eye procedures
  - Familial
  - Variant (see Table 5.4): contaminated foods of bovine origin
  - Sporadic (see Table 5.4): de novo spontaneous generation of self-replicating protein
- Decontamination practices to reduce transmission (NICE Guidance [IGG196])
  - Keep instruments wet immediately after use until they are cleaned
  - Eliminate instrument migration between sets (keep instrument sets together)
  - Single use instruments for patients who have previously undergone high-risk procedures with incineration of instrument post usage
  - Decontamination of re-useable instruments: immerse in sodium hypochlorite for 1 h, rinse in water and subject to routine sterilisation
  - Decontamination of work surfaces: disinfection by flooding, for 1 h, with sodium hypochlorite, followed by water rinses

Table 5.4 Comparison of sporadic and variant CJD

Characteristic	Sporadic CJD	Variant CJD (vCJD)
Median age at death	68 years	28 years
Median duration of illness	4–5 months	13–14 months
Clinical signs and symptoms	Progressive dementia; early neurologic signs (myoclonus, visual or cerebellar signs, pyramidal/extrapyramidal signs)	Prominent psychiatric symptoms (depression, anxiety, delusions, apathy); painful dysaesthesia; delayed neurologic signs
Periodic sharp waves (generalised triphasic periodic complexes) on EEG	Often present	Often absent
"Pulvinar sign" on MRI (hyperintensities in the posterior thalamus FLAIR sequences on brain MRI)	Not reported. High signal in caudate/putamen on MRI brain or at least 2 cortical regions (parietal, temporal, occipital)	Present in >75% of cases
Presence of "florid plaques" on neuropathology	Rare or absent	Present in large numbers
Immunohistochemical analysis of brain tissue	Variable accumulation of protease-resistance prion protein, spongiform change	Marked accumulation of protease-resistance prion protein, spongiform change
Presence of agent in lymphoid tissue	Not readily detected	Readily detected
Increased glycoform ratio on immunoblot analysis of protease-resistance prion protein	Not reported	Marked accumulation of protease-resistance prion protein

5.15 The RCOphth Ophthalmic Services Guidance on Ophthalmic Instrument Decontamination 2016 [58]

- Decontamination is the term used to describe a combination of processes (cleaning, disinfection and/or sterilisation) used to make re-usable items safe for further use
- Cleaning
  - Most important stage in the decontamination process
  - Removes dust, dirt, excretions, secretions, organic matter and all contamination including harmful and undesirable substances as well as a large proportion of micro-organisms which may be present
  - Mechanical/automated cleaning is the most effective and reproducible method
- Disinfection
  - Process that removes or destroys potentially harmful micro-organisms (apart from spores) to a level non-harmful to health
  - Achieved by use of liquid chemicals or by moist heat
  - Moist heat is the first-choice method except for devices unable to withstand high temperatures
- Sterilisation
  - Process that removes or destroys all micro-organisms and spores
  - Preferred method for instruments is autoclaving which achieves sterilisation by applying steam under pressure at the highest temperature compatible with the instruments being processed
- All patients undergoing elective or emergency surgery must be asked, "Have you ever been notified that you are at increased risk of CJD or vCJD for public health purposes?"—consult local infection control team if there is a positive response
- For high risk procedures, a further set of questions should be asked about FHx of CJD, growth hormone treatment, brain or spinal cord surgery, blood transfusions
- Guidance for use of instruments in the ophthalmic clinic
  - For patients with known or potential CJD (e.g. dementia of unknown cause or unexplained neurodegenerative condition):

    - Single use devices or non-contact devices where possible
    - For reusable contact devices, either the device must be under strict quarantine and only reused on that patient or be disposed of
  - For the majority of patients:
    - Use of non-contact or disposable devices where possible
    - For reusable contact devices use disposable covers if possible and after usage:
      - Do not allow the device to dry
      - Rinse immediately for at least 30 seconds in water for irrigation
      - Clean with liquid soap or detergent for at least 20 s
      - Rinse again with water for 30 s
      - Immerse in freshly prepared hypochlorite 10,000 ppm of chlorine (1%) for at least 10 min
      - Rinse in 3 changes of sterile water or saline for at least 10 min
      - Shake, dry with tissue and store dry
- Guidance for use of surgical instruments
  - For patients with no extra risk of carrying CJD prion protein:
    - Low risk surgery: no extra precautions
    - High risk surgery:
      - Ensure reusable instruments do not migrate between sets and that they should be fully trackable
      - Single use supplementary instruments
  - For patients with extra risk of carrying CJD or who have CJD:
    - Low risk surgery:
      - Minimise instrument migration and instruments should be trackable
    - High risk surgery:
      - Consider whether procedure is required at all or whether deferral might allow the diagnosis of CJD to be excluded if not certain
      - Perform procedure with minimal number of staff in theatre and at the end of the list
      - Use single instruments and incinerate at the end of the procedure
      - Reusable instruments should be kept quarantined and for reuse solely on that individual patient

5.16 The RCOphth Ophthalmic Services Guidance on the Prevention of Transmission of Blood-Borne Viruses in Ophthalmic Surgery [56]

- Standard precautions
  - General measures:
    - Hand-washing
    - Barrier protection: wearing of intact gloves, surgical face masks, protective clothing
  - Avoiding sharps usage wherever possible, and exercising care in their handling and disposal:
    - Sharps should not be recapped
    - Sharps should not be handed from one person to another
    - Avoid manipulation of sharps by hands or fingers
    - Surgeons should announce the movement of sharps
    - Magnetic pads should be used for keeping discarded needles
  - Exclude theatre personnel with open skin wounds on their hands or arms
- Non-exposure prone procedures
  - Hands and fingers of the surgeon are completely visible at all times during the procedure
  - Pose no risk for transmission of a blood borne virus from an infected healthcare worker to a patient
- Exposure prone procedures (EPPs)
  - Hands or fingers of the surgeon are inside a wound or body cavity and not completely visible at all times during the procedure
  - Orbital surgery and some operations in oculoplastic and lacrimal surgery
- Surgeons who are HIV, hepatitis B (HBV) or Hepatitis C (HCV) positive should inform

their occupational health department. An infected practitioner does not need to disclose to prospective patients of his/her infective status
- Preventing doctor to patient transmission of HIV
  - After a single needle stick injury the risk of seroconversion is approximately 0.3%
  - No risk of transmission when blood is in contact with intact skin
  - There is a less than 1 in 1000 risk for exposure to intact mucous membranes
  - EPPs should not be performed by HIV positive surgeons
  - There are no restrictions on performing non-exposure prone procedures
  - Not all patients who have undergone an EPP by an HIV positive surgeon need to be notified and tested
- Preventing doctor to patient transmission of HBV
  - After a single needle stick injury from an e-antigen (high infectivity) positive source to a non-immunised recipient the risk of seroconversion is up to 30% (the presence of hepatitis B surface antigen—HbsAg—indicates infection)
  - If the injured party is fully up to date with their immunisation and has shown a good antibody response to the vaccine (immunity is recognised by anti-hepatitis B surface antibodies: anti-Hbs), they are protected against infection with HBV
  - Hepatitis B surface antigen positive and e-antigen positive surgeons should not perform EPP's
- Preventing doctor to patient transmission of HCV
  - Risk of seroconversion in a healthcare worker following a single percutaneous injury from a HCV positive source is probably between 1.2% and 3%
  - Surgeons who are hepatitis C RNA positive should not perform EPPs
  - Hepatitis C infected surgeons who have responded successfully to treatment with antiviral therapy may resume EPPs.
- General principles of management of needlestick injury
  - Gently squeezing the wound to encourage bleeding
  - Washing the wound with plain soap and copious water and then covering it with a waterproof dressing
  - Injury reported to a line manager
  - Healthcare practitioner designated to manage exposure should conduct a risk assessment
  - Blood from the source, taken with their consent, should be tested for blood borne virus status—when the source lacks capacity for consent, their tissue can only be tested if held to be in their best interests in accordance with the Mental Capacity Act 2005
- HIV post-exposure prophylaxis (PEP)
  - Estimated risk of HIV transmission from a known HIV positive source after a needlestick injury is estimated at 0.3%
  - Testing of the source is performed (with consent and after pre-test counselling, and not by the direct health professional involved) ideally within 8 h and not more than 24 h after source blood is taken in order to minimise unnecessary use of PEP
  - PEP is typically given as a 3-drug combination for the duration of 4 weeks. It should be commenced within 72 h after exposure
  - Post exposure HIV antibody testing should be performed at least 12 weeks after exposure or completion of PEP

5.17 Audit

- Systematic examination of current practice to assess how well an institution or a practitioner is performing against set standards. Essentially it is a method for systematically reflection on, reviewing and improving practice.
- Audit cycle
  - Identify a problem or issue
  - Identify standards
  - Collect data on current practice

- Data analysis with comparison to the standard
- Identify changes required and implement change
- Re-audit to monitor effect of change

5.18 Laser Safety in Hospitals

- Designated laser protection advisor (medical engineer who is responsible for ensuring that the safety and use of lasers is in accordance with the health and safety law and regulations) is present in every hospital in the UK
- There are 2 designated laser safety officers (responsible for ensuring that all staff are trained to safely use lasers and that all laser procedures and clinics are in keeping with the health and safety requirements) at the local departmental level
- Safety measures for lasering patients:
  - Laser personnel:
    - Ensure that any member of staff who is to perform a laser treatment on a patient has attended an up-to-date training session on the fundamentals of laser safety
  - Prior to laser treatment of a patient:
    - Ensure laser machines are working correctly
    - Ensure any windows or reflective surfaces are covered
    - Ensure you have the correct patient
    - Lock the laser room door before you commence the laser treatment
    - Switch the "laser in use" sign on
  - During laser treatment of a patient:
    - Ensure the correct protective eyewear for the correct laser machine is worn by any relatives or members of staff who will be in the laser room during the laser treatment

References

1. Age-Related Eye Disease Study Research Group. A randomised, placebo-controlled, clinical trial of high-dose supplementation with vitamins C and E, Beta carotene, and zinc for age-related macular degeneration and vision loss: AREDS Report No.8. Arch Ophthalmol. 2001;119:1417–36.
2. Beck RW, Cleary PA, Anderson MM, Keltner JL, Shults WT, Kaufman DI, Buckley EG, Corbett JJ, Kupersmith MJ, Miller NR, Savino PJ, Guy JR, Trobe JD, McCrary JA, Smith CH, Chrousos GA, Thomson S, Katz BJ, Brodsky MC, Goodwin JA, Atwell CW. A randomised, controlled trial of corticosteroids in the treatment of acute optic neuritis. N Engl J Med. 1992;326:581–8.
3. Beck RW, Cleary PA, Trobe JD, Kaufman DI, Kuppersmith MJ, Paty DW, Brown CH. The effect of corticosteroids for acute optic neuritis on the subsequent development of multiple sclerosis. N Engl J Med. 1993;329:1764–9.
4. Bloch-Michel E, Nussenblatt RB. International Uveitis Study Group recommendations for the evaluation of intraocular inflammatory disease. Am J Ophthalmol. 1987;103:234–5.
5. Boyer DS, Yoon YH, Belfort R, Bandello F, Maturi RK, Augustin AJ, Li XY, Cui H, Hashad Y, Whitcup SM. Three-year, randomised, sham-controlled trial of dexamethasone intravitreal implant in patients with diabetic macular edema. Ophthalmology. 2014;121:1904–14.
6. Brown DM, Kaiser PK, Michels M, Soubrane G, Heier JS, Kim RY, Sy JP, Schneider S. Ranibizumab versus verteporfin for neovascular age-related macular degeneration. N Engl J Med. 2006;355:1432–44.
7. Chakravarthy U, Harding SP, Rogers CA, Downes SM, Lotery AJ, Culliford LA, Reeves BC. Alternative treatments to inhibit VEGF in age-related choroidal neovascularisation: 2-year findings of the IVAN randomised controlled trial. Lancet. 2013;382:1258–67.
8. Cohen EJ, Hochman JS, Troxel AB, Colby KA, Jeng BH. Zoster eye disease study: rationale and design. Cornea. 2022;41:562–71.
9. Cohen EL, Jeng B, Troxel A, Hochman J. Zoster eye disease study results [PowerPoint Presentation]. 2024. Available at: https://med.nyu.edu/departments--institutes/ophthalmology/sites/default/files/zoster-eye-disease-study-results.pdf. Accessed 4 Feb 2025.
10. Compston J, Cooper A, Cooper C, Gittoes N, Gregson C, Harvey N, Hope S, Kanis JA, McCloskey EV, Poole KES, Reid DM, Selby P, Thompson F, Thurston A, Vine N. UK clinical guideline for the prevention and treatment of osteoporosis. Arch Osteoporos. 2017;12:43.
11. Cunha-Vaz J, Ashton P, Iezzi R, Campochiaro P, Dugel PU, Holz FG, Weber M, Danis RP, Kuppermann BD, Bailey C, Billman K, Kapik B, Kane F, Green K. Sustained delivery fluocinolone acetonide vitreous implants. Long term benefits in patients with chronic diabetic macular oedema. Ophthalmology. 2014;121:1892–903.
12. Diabetic Retinopathy Clinical Research Network. A randomised trial comparing intravitreal triamcinolone acetonide and focal/grid photocoagulation for diabetic macular edema. Ophthalmology. 2008;115:1447–59.

13. Diabetic Retinopathy Clinical Research Network. Panretinal photocoagulation vs intravitreous ranibizumab for proliferative diabetic retinopathy. A randomised clinical trial. JAMA. 2015;314:2137–46.
14. Dugel PU, Koh A, Ogura Y, Jaffe GJ, Schmidt-Erfurth U, Brown DM, Gomes AV, Warburton J, Weichselberger A, Holz FG. HAWK and HARRIER: phase 3, multicenter, randomized, double-masked trials of brolucizumab for neovascular age-related macular degeneration. Ophthalmology. 2020;127:72–84.
15. Early Treatment Diabetic Retinopathy Study Research Group. Fundus photographic risk factors for progression of diabetic retinopathy. ETDRS report number 12. Ophthalmology. 1991;98:823–33.
16. Elman MJ, Aiello LP, Beck RW, Bressler NM, Bressler SB, Edwards AR, Ferris FL III, Friedman SM, Glassman AR, Miller KM, Scott IU, Stockdale CR, Sun JK. Randomized trial evaluating ranibizumab plus prompt or deferred laser or triamcinolone plus prompt laser for diabetic macular edema. Ophthalmology. 2010;117:1064–77.
17. Facey K, Cummins E, Macpherson K, Morris A, Reay L, Slattery J. Organisation of services for diabetic retinopathy screening. Glasgow: Health Technology Board for Scotland; 2002. p. 1–224.
18. Fung AE, Lalwani GA, Rosenfeld PJ, Dubovy SR, Michels S, Feuer WJ, Puliafito CA, Davis JL, Flynn HW, Esquiabro M. An optical coherence tomography-guided, variable dosing regimen with intravitreal ranibizumab (Lucentis) for neovascular age-related macular degeneration. Am J Ophthalmol. 2007;143:566–83.
19. Gedde SJ, Schiffman JC, Feuer WJ, Herndon LW, Brandt JD, Budenz DL. Treatment outcomes in the tube versus trabeculectomy (TVT) study after five years of follow-up. Am J Ophthalmol. 2012;153:789–803.
20. Gedde SJ, Feuer WJ, Shi W, Lim KS, Barton K, Goyal S, Ahmed IIK, Brandt J. Treatment outcomes in the primary tube versus trabeculectomy study after 1 year of follow up. Ophthalmology. 2018;125:650–63.
21. Haller JA, Bandello F, Belfort R, Blumenkranz MS, Gillie M, Heier J, Loewenstein A, Yoon YH, Jacques ML, Jiao J, Li XY, Whitcup SM. Randomised, sham-controlled trial of dexamethasone intravitreal implant in patients with macular edema due to retinal vein occlusion. Ophthalmology. 2010;117:1134–46.
22. Heier JS, Brown DM, Chong V, Korobelnik JF, Kaiser PK, Nguyen QD, Kirchhof B, Ho A, Ogura Y, Yancopoulos GD, Stahl N, Vitti R, Berliner AJ, Soo Y, Anderesi M, Groetzbach G, Sommerauer B, Sandbrink R, Simader C, Schmidt-Erfurth U. Intraviteal aflibercept (VEGF trap-eye) in wet age-related macular degeneration. Ophthalmology. 2012;119:2537–48.
23. Heier JS, Khanani AM, Ruiz CQ, Basu K, Ferrone PJ, Brittain C, Figueroa MS, Lin H, Holz FG, Patel V, Lai TYY, Silverman D, Regillo C, Swaminathan B, Viola F, Cheung CMG, Wong TY. Efficacy, durability, and safety of intravitreal faricimab up to every 16 weeks for neovascular age-related macular degeneration (TENAYA and LUCERNE): two randomised, double-masked, phase 3, non-inferiority trials. Lancet. 2022;399:729–40.
24. Jaffe GJ, Dick AD, Brezin AP, Nguyen QD, Thorne JE, Kestelyn P, Barisani-Asenbauer T, Franco P, Heiligenhaus A, Scales D, Chu DS, Camez A, Kwatra NV, Song AP, Kron M, Tari S, Suhler EB. Adalimumab in patients with active non-infectious uveitis. N Engl J Med. 2016;375:932–43.
25. Kohner EM. The natural history of proliferative diabetic retinopathy. Eye. 1991;5:222–5.
26. Lichter PR, Musch DC, Gillespie BW, Guire KE, Janz NK, Wren PA, Mills RP. Interim clinical outcomes in the collaborative initial glaucoma treatment study comparing initial treatment randomised to medications or surgery. Ophthalmology. 2001;108:1943–53.
27. Lowder C, Belfort R Jr, Lightman S, Foster CS, Robinson MR, Schiffman RM, Li XY, Cui H, Whitcup SM. Dexamethasone intravitreal implant for noninfectious intermediate or posterior uveitis. Arch Ophthalmol. 2011;129:545–53.
28. Martin DF, Maguire MG, Fine SL, Ying GS, Jaffe GJ, Grunwald JE, Toth C, Redford M, Ferris FL. Ranibizumab and bevacizumab for treatment of neovascular agerelated macular degeneration. Two-year results. Ophthalmology. 2012;119:1388–98.
29. Nguyen QD, Merrill PT, Jaffe GJ, Dick AD, Kurup SK, Sheppard J, Schlaen A, Pavesio C, Cimino L, Van Calster J, Camez AA, Kwatra NV, Song AP, Kron M, Tari S, Brezin AP. Adalimumab for prevention of uveitic flare in patients with inactive non-infectious uveitis controlled by corticosteroids (VISUAL II): a multicenter, double-masked, randomised, placebo-controlled phase 3 trial. Lancet. 2016;388:1183–92.
30. National Institute for Health and Care Excellence. Patient safety and reduction of risk of transmission of Creutzfeldt-Jakob disease (CJD) via interventional procedures [IPG196]. [Online]. London: NICE; 2006. Available at https://www.nice.org.uk/guidance/ipg196. Accessed 13 Dec 2019.
31. National Institute for Health and Care Excellence. Dexamethasone intravitreal implant for the treatment of macular oedema secondary to retinal vein occlusion [TA229]. [Online]. London: NICE; 2011. Available at https://www.nice.org.uk/guidance/ta229. Accessed 11 Dec 2019.
32. National Institute for Health and Care Excellence. Fluocinolone acetonide intravitreal implant for treating chronic diabetic macular oedema after an inadequate response to prior therapy [TA301]. [Online]. London: NICE; 2013. Available at https://www.nice.org.uk/guidance/ta301. Accessed 11 December 2019.
33. National Institute for Health and Care Excellence. Dexamethasone intravitreal implant for treating diabetic macular oedema [TA349]. [Online]. London: NICE; 2015. Available at https://www.nice.org.uk/guidance/ta349. Accessed 11 Dec 2019.
34. National Institute for Health and Care Excellence. Adalimumab and dexamethasone for treating non-infectious uveitis [TA460]. [Online]. London: NICE;

2017a. Available at https://www.nice.org.uk/guidance/ta460. Accessed 13 Dec 2019.
35. National Institute for Health and Care Excellence. Osteoporosis: assessing the risk of fragility fracture [CG146]. [Online]. London: NICE; 2017b. Available at https://www.nice.org.uk/guidance/cg146. Accessed 13 Dec 2019.
36. National Institute for Health and Care Excellence. Fluocinolone acetonide intravitreal implant for treating recurrent non-infectious uveitis [TA590]. [Online]. London: NICE; 2019. Available at https://www.nice.org.uk/guidance/ta590. Accessed 13 Dec 2019.
37. National Institute for Health and Care Excellence. Bevacizumab gamma for treating wet age-related macular degeneration [TA1022]. [Online]. London: NICE; 2024. Available at https://www.nice.org.uk/guidance/ta1022. Accessed 22 Dec 2024.
38. Nussenblatt RB, Palestine AG, Chan CC, Roberge F. Standardization of vitreal inflammatory activity in intermediate and posterior uveitis. Ophthalmology. 1985;92:467–71.
39. Optic Neuritis Study Group. High- and low-risk profiles for the development of multiple sclerosis within 10 years after optic neuritis. Experience of the optic neuritis treatment trial. Arch Ophthalmol. 2003;121:944–9.
40. Pouwels XGLV, Petersohn S, Carrera VH, Denniston AK, Chalker A, Raatz H, Armstrong N, Shah D, Witlox W, Worthy G, Noake C, Riemsma R, Kleijnen J, Joore MA. Fluocinolone acetonide intravitreal implant for treating recurrent non-infectious uveitis: an evidence review group perspective of a NICE single technology appraisal. PharmacoEconomics. 2020;38:431–41.
41. Public Health England. NHS diabetic eye screening Programme. Grading definitions for referable disease. Public Health England leads the NHS screening programmes. [Online]. London: Public Health England; 2017. Available at https://assets.publishing.service.gov.uk/government/uploads/system/uploads/attachment_data/file/582710/Grading_definitions_for_referrable_disease_2017_new_110117.pdf. Accessed 11 Dec 2019.
42. Regillo CD, Brown DM, Abraham P, Yue H, Ianchulev T, Schneider S, Shams N. Randomised, double-masked, sham-controlled trial of ranibizumab for neovascular age-related macular degeneration: PIER study year 1. Am J Ophthalmol. 2008;145:239–48.
43. Rosenfeld PJ, Brown DM, Heier JS, Boyer DS, Kaiser PK, Chung CY, Kim RY. Ranibizumab for neovascular age-related macular degeneration. N Engl J Med. 2006;355:1419–31.
44. Scanlon PH, Malhotra R, Thomas G, Foy C, Kirkpatrick JN, Lewis-Barned N, Harney B, Aldington SJ. The effectiveness of screening for diabetic retinopathy by digital imaging photography and technician ophthalmoscopy. Diabet Med. 2003a;20:467–74.
45. Scanlon PH, Malhotra R, Greenwood RH, Aldington SJ, Foy C, Flatman M, Downes S. Comparison of two reference standards in validating two field mydriatic digital photography as a method of screening for diabetic retinopathy. Br J Ophthalmol. 2003b;87:1258–63.
46. Scanlon PH. The English national screening programme for sight threatening diabetic retinopathy. J Med Screen. 2008;15:1–4.
47. The Age-Related Eye Disease Study 2 (AREDS2) Research Group. Lutein + zeaxanthin and omega-3 fatty acids for age-related macular degeneration: the age-related eye disease study 2 (AREDS2) randomized clinical trial. JAMA. 2013;309:2005–15.
48. The AGIS Investigators. The advanced glaucoma intervention study (AGIS): 4. Comparison of treatment outcomes within race. Ophthalmology. 1998;105:1146–64.
49. The AGIS Investigators. The advanced glaucoma intervention study (AGIS): 9. Comparison of glaucoma outcomes in black and white patients within treatment groups. Am J Ophthalmol. 2001;132:311–20.
50. The CATT Research Group. Ranibizumab and Bevacizumab for neovascular age-related macular degeneration. N Engl J Med. 2011;364:1897–908.
51. The Diabetic Retinopathy Study Research Group. Photocoagulation treatment of proliferative diabetic retinopathy. Clinical application of diabetic retinopathy study (DRS) findings, DRS report number 8. Ophthalmology. 1981;88:583–600.
52. The Diabetic Retinopathy Clinical Research Network. Aflibercept, Bevacizumab, or Ranibizumab for Diabetic Macular Edema. N Engl J Med. 2015;372:1193–203.
53. The Optic Neuritis Study Group. Multiple sclerosis risk after optic neuritis. Final optic neuritis treatment trial follow-up. Arch Neurol. 2008;65:727–32.
54. The Royal College of Ophthalmologists. The Ocular Side-Effects of Vigabatrin (Sabril) Information and Guidance for Screening 2008a. [Online]. London: The Royal College of Ophthalmologists. Available at: https://www.rcophth.ac.uk/wp-content/uploads/2015/01/2008-SCI-020-The-Ocular-Side-Effects-of-Vigabatrin-Sabril.pdf. Accessed 12 Dec 2019.
55. The Royal College of Ophthalmologists. Standards for the retrieval of human ocular tissue used in transplantation, research and training 2008b. [Online]. London: The Royal College of Ophthalmologists. Available at http://bmec.swbh.nhs.uk/wp-content/uploads/2013/03/RETRIEVAL-OF-HUMAN-OCULAR-TISSUE.pdf. Accessed 12 Dec 2019.
56. The Royal College of Ophthalmologists. Ophthalmic Services Guidance. Prevention of transmission of blood-borne viruses in ophthalmic surgery 2008c. [Online]. London: The Royal College of Ophthalmologists. Available at https://www.rcophth.ac.uk/wpcontent/uploads/2014/12/2010_PROF_053_Blood_Borne_Viruses.pdf.Accessed 12 Dec 2019.

57. The Royal College of Ophthalmologists. A Review of the Ocular side effects of Topiramate 2010. [Online]. London: The Royal College of Ophthalmologists. Available at https://www.rcophth.ac.uk/wp-content/uploads/2014/12/2010_PROF_122_Review_of_Ocular_side_effects_of_Topiramate-2.pdf. Accessed 12 Dec 2019.
58. The Royal College of Ophthalmologists. Ophthalmic Services Guidance. Ophthalmic Instrument Decontamination 2016. [Online]. London: The Royal College of Ophthalmologists. Available at https://www.rcophth.ac.uk/wp-content/uploads/2014/12/Ophthalmic-Instrument-Decontamination.pdf. Accessed 12 Dec 2019.
59. The Royal College of Ophthalmologists. Hydroxychloroquine and chloroquine retinopathy: Recommendations on Screening 2020. [Online]. London: The Royal College of Ophthalmologists. Available at https://www.rcophth.ac.uk/wp-content/uploads/2020/12/Hydroxychloroquine-and-Chloroquine-Retinopathy-Monitoring-Guideline.pdf. Accessed 04 Jan 2025.
60. The Standardisation of Uveitis Nomenclature (SUN) Working Group. Standardization of uveitis nomenclature for reporting clinical data. Results of the first international workshop. Am J Ophthalmol. 2005;140:509–16.
61. Warner DB, Jeng BH, Kim J, Liu M, Troxel AB, Hochman JS, Baratz KH, Mian SI, Choulakian MY, Meyer JJ, Lu Y, Twi-Yeboah A, Lee TF, Lopez-Jimenez C, Laury SC, Cohen EJ. Low-dose valacyclovir for postherpetic neuralgia in the zoster eye disease study—a randomized clinical trial. JAMA Ophthalmol Published online. 2025;143:277. https://doi.org/10.1001/jamaophthalmol.2024.6113.
62. Wells JA, Glassman AR, Ayala AR, Jampol LM, Bressler NM, Bressler SB, Brucker AJ, Ferris FL, Hampton GR, Jhaveri C, Melia M, Beck RW. Aflibercept, bevacizumab, or ranibizumab for diabetic macular edema. Two-year results from a comparative effectiveness randomized clinical trial. Ophthalmology. 2016;123:1351–9.
63. Wilson JMG, Jungner G, World Health Organisation. Principles and practice of screening for disease. World Health Organization Geneva 1968. [Online]. Available at https://apps.who.int/iris/bitstream/handle/10665/37650/WHO_PHP_34.pdf?sequence=17.

Communication Skill Scenarios 6

Timothy H. M. Fung, Delicia Jayakumar, and Winfried M. K. Amoaku

Abstract

Effective communication skills are essential for all doctors. In an exam setting, these skills can be evaluated through simulated doctor-patient encounters. This chapter presents examples of common communication scenarios that candidates may encounter during an exam. These include breaking bad news, explaining a diagnosis and management plan, discussing surgical complications and errors, obtaining consent for treatment, encouraging adherence to treatment, managing interactions with an angry patient, and addressing issues of confidentiality.

6.1 Explaining a Diagnosis to Patients/Parents

6.1.1 Scenario 1

Re: Mr. Steven Shaw, aged 55 years

Mr. Shaw has primary open angle glaucoma in both his eyes. He has raised intraocular pressure in both eyes and cupped optic discs with correlating visual field defects.

Your task is to explain the diagnosis, addressing his concerns

6.1.1.1 Approach

- Introduce yourself and confirm the patient's identity
- Take any relevant history from the patient that has not been provided:
  - Driving status
  - Occupation
  - Family history of glaucoma
- Clarify the task in your mind. Begin discussing the diagnosis:
  - *"Your examination and test results show that you have glaucoma"*
- Establish what the patient already knows about the diagnosis:
  - *"Have you heard of the condition glaucoma before?"*

T. H. M. Fung (✉)
University Hospitals of Derby & Burton NHS Foundation Trust, Royal Derby Hospital, Derby, UK
e-mail: timothy.fung@nhs.net

D. Jayakumar
Kingsmill Hospital, Mansfield, UK

W. M. K. Amoaku
Eye, Ear, Nose and Throat Centre, Queens Medical Centre, Nottingham University Hospitals NHS Trust, Nottingham, UK

T. H. M. Fung, W. M. K. Amoaku (eds.), *Viva and OSCE Exams in Ophthalmology*,
https://doi.org/10.1007/978-3-031-97401-4_6

- *"I wonder if you know anything about this condition before we start?"*
- Tell the patient that you are going to start giving them some information (*"I am going to tell you some information now, so please feel free to stop me at any point if there is anything you don't understand"*)
- Order the explanation—possible discussion points include:
  - What is glaucoma (*"a disease of the optic nerve, which is a long cable at the back of the eye"*)
  - Why glaucoma occurs (*"multiple reasons why it can occur including genetic factors and the presence of high pressures in the eye"*)
  - Likely history of glaucoma with and without treatment (*"if the pressures in the eyes remain persistently high then you will lose vision permanently over time. With treatment to lower the pressures in your eyes, you can slow the progression of the condition"*)
  - Treatment options (*"the aim of treatment is to lower the eye pressure. Initial options include drops or laser"*)
  - Follow-up (*"we will need to see you again in clinic in ….."*)
  - Driving regulations (*"you will need to inform the DVLA as you have glaucoma in both your eyes"*)
- Check that the patient is following your explanation and encourage patient feedback and questions:
  - *"Are you happy with everything I have said so far?"*
  - *"Do you have any questions so far?"*
  - *"I appreciate that I have given you a lot of information. Would you like me to go over anything again or do you have any questions that you would like to ask me?"*
- Provide a summary of the main points of the discussion to provide the patient with any key take home messages (*"To summarise our discussion….."*)
- Provide the patient with a point of contact should he have any questions or concerns
- General points:
  - Keep your explanations clear without using any complex medical jargon. Ensure you use language that the patient will understand (without being patronising!)
  - Throughout your explanation, take into account any ideas, concerns or expectations you elicit from the patient
  - Be prepared to admit uncertainty if the patient asks you something you don't know (assure the patient that you will find the answer and let them know)

6.1.2 Scenario 2

Re: Master Simon Baines, aged 2 years

A GP has referred a 2-year-old child with a white pupillary reflex. You have seen the child in your clinic and have seen a large white, round retinal mass on clinical examination. Ultrasonography shows intralesional calcification with high internal reflectivity, confirming a diagnosis of retinoblastoma. The mother of the child is present.

Your task is to explain the diagnosis to his mother, possible prognosis, and propose referral to a specialist retinoblastoma treatment centre

6.1.2.1 Approach

- Introduce yourself and confirm the patient's and mother's identity
- Take any relevant history from the mother that has not been provided
  - Other children in family
  - Health status of other children in family
  - Any medical problems that run in the family
  - Identify mother's support system (family/friends) (*"who is at home with you?"*)
- Establish what the patient's mother already knows (*"Do you know why your son was referred by your GP to the hospital?"*)
- Give a warning shot to the mother (*"I am afraid that I have some bad news"*). Give the

mother time to digest the warning shot. They may signal that more information is wanted or that they want some time before further information is wanted.

- Be open, honest and informative to the mother (*"the examination and ultrasound result show that your son has a type of eye cancer called a retinoblastoma"*)
- Acknowledge distress and support ventilation of feelings from the mother (*"I understand that this is very hard and its normal to be upset"*)—offer tissues if the mother becomes teary
- Check if mother has had previous experience/know relatives or friends with the same condition (*"do you know anyone else with the same condition to your son?"*)
- Establish what the mother wants to know (*"before I provide you with further information, I just wanted to know whether you are you the type of person who likes to know everything about your sons condition?*)
- Prioritise and identify any concerns from the mother before providing the mother with information (*"what are the particular things you are thinking about?"*)
- Provide information—possible discussion points (depending on the mother's earlier responses) include
  - Causes (*"40% of cases is caused by a faulty gene. The faulty gene may be inherited from a parent or a change to the gene occurred at an early stage of the child's development in the womb. Unknown what causes the remaining 60% of cases"*)
  - Incidence (*"about 45 children per year are diagnosed with retinoblastoma in the UK"*)
  - Referral (*"Your child will need to be referred to a specialist retinoblastoma team at either The Royal London Hospital or Birmingham Children's hospital. Do you any preference?"*)
  - Treatment (*"depends on the stage of the cancer. Further details will be provided by the specialist retinoblastoma team you will be referring the child too"*)
  - Prognosis (*"over 90% cure rate with appropriate treatment if the cancer has not spread beyond the eyeball"*)
- Check that you have provided the mother with all her information needs (*"do you have anything else you want to ask me about?"*)
- Provide contact details so that the mother can contact you if she or her relatives/friends have any questions. Make clear to the mother that she can be seen any time if she wishes to discuss any issues or concerns
- Offer to provide contact details about the Childhood Eye Cancer Trust that can give the mother further information about retinoblastoma
- Provide a summary of the main points of the discussion to provide the patient with any key take home messages (*"To summarise our discussion....."*)

6.2 Discussing Management with Patients/Parents

6.2.1 Scenario 1

Re: Mrs. Anna Smith, aged 56 years

Mrs. Smith has been referred by the GP for possible cataract surgery as the patient has noticed a reduction in her vision in her right eye. She had a breast mastectomy for breast cancer 5 years ago. On examination you see a visually insignificant cataract but have found an elevated mass at her right macula.

Your task is to explain your findings to the patient, possible diagnoses and your proposed management plan

6.2.1.1 Approach

- Introduce yourself and confirm the patient's identity
- Take any relevant history from the patient that has not been provided
  - Ask if she was given the all clear from her breast cancer since her mastectomy and whether she has been discharged from oncology
- Establish what the patient already knows (*"can you tell me what you understand about the problem with your eye?"*)
- Give a warning shot (*"I am afraid that it is not a cataract that is causing the reduction in your vision"*). Give the patient time to digest the warning shot. They may signal that more information is required
- Be open, honest and informative to the patient (*"there is a lump in the back of your eye that is causing a reduction in your vision"*)
- Outline the possibilities (*"There are several causes for a lump to appear in the back of the eye. Some are serious and others are not so serious. At this stage I am not certain of the cause of your lump. However, given your previous history of breast cancer, there is a possibility that the lump in the back of the eye is cancerous"*)
- Acknowledge distress and support ventilation of feelings from the patient (*"I understand that this is very hard and its normal to be upset"*)—offer tissues if the patient becomes teary
- Explain to the patient that you will be urgently referring her to a specialist centre (*"I will be urgently referring you to a specialist center to investigate the cause of the lump in the back of your eye. This will be at Liverpool, Sheffield or London. Do you have a preference?"*)
- Check that the patient is following your explanation and encourage patient feedback and questions (*"I appreciate that I have given you a lot of information. Would you like me to go over anything again or do you have any questions that you would like to ask me?"*)
- Provide contact details so that the patient can contact you if she or her relatives/friends have any questions. Make clear to the patient that she can be seen any time if she wishes to discuss any issues or concerns
- Identify patient support systems (*"who do you live at home with?"*)
- Provide a summary of the main points of the discussion to provide the patient with any key take home messages (*"To summarise our discussion….."*)

6.2.2 Scenario 2

Re: Miss Tina Carter, aged 30 years

You are seeing Mrs. Carter in the outpatient's clinic. She was seen in eye casualty 6 weeks ago with pain on eye movements and loss of vision in her left eye (VA HM). Her right eye was unaffected. She presents to you today in clinic with the vision in her left eye remaining poor at 6/60 and her vision in her right eye has now dropped to 6/36. On examination both optic nerves are pale.

Your task is to address her questions and to talk about management

6.2.2.1 Approach

- Introduce yourself and confirm the patient's identity
- Take any relevant history from the patient that has not been provided
  - Presence of paraesthesia, weakness of limbs, bowel and bladder incontinence
  - Any recent infections or vaccinations
  - Past medical history (autoimmune disorders, lymphoproliferative diseases, connective tissue disorders)
  - Concurrent or recent treatments
  - Driving status

  - Occupation
- Establish what the patient already knows (*"can you tell me what you understand about the problem with your eyes?"/"have you thought about any possibilities for the cause of your symptoms?"*)
- Prioritise and identify any concerns from the patient before providing the patient with information (*"what are the particular things you are thinking about?"*)
- Provide information (be open and honest)—possible discussion points (depending on the patient's earlier responses)
  - Reason for the patient's symptoms (*"In the back of each eye there is a bright long yellow cable called the optic nerve, which contains lots of wires that enable us to see well with our eyes. In your eyes your optic nerves are pale, which is why your vision is reduced in both of your eyes. At this point I am not sure what has caused this"*)
  - Outline the possible causes (*"There are several different causes of pale optic nerves which requires investigations with tests. Would you like to know all the possibilities?"*)
  - Outline the tests you want (*"I would advise blood tests, a chest x-ray, and an MRI scan of the brain to investigate possible causes for your pale disc"*)
  - Follow-up (*"we will see you in clinic again in …."*)
  - Driving (*"your current level of vision does not meet the legal requirements for driving and you must inform the DVLA"*)
- Check that the patient is following your explanation and encourage patient feedback and questions (*"I appreciate that I have given you a lot of information. Would you like me to go over anything again or do you have any questions that you would like to ask me?"*)
- Provide contact details so that the patient can contact you if she or her relatives/friends have any questions. Make clear to the patient that she can be seen any time if she wishes to discuss any issues or concerns
- Offer to provide contact details about support groups such as the macular society and the RNIB
- Provide a summary of the main points of the discussion to provide the patient with any key take home messages (*"To summarise our discussion….."*)

6.2.3 Scenario 3

Re: Master Robert Gale, aged 5 years

Robert is a 5-year-old boy who you have been seeing regularly in clinic. He is currently under treatment with patching for amblyopia secondary to a squint. His mother is insisting on squint surgery.

Your tasks are to explore her reasons for wanting squint surgery, addressing her concerns

6.2.3.1 Approach

- Introduce yourself and confirm the patient's and mother's identity
- Establish what the mother already knows (*"can you tell me what you understand about the problem with the eyes of your son?"*)
- Explore the reasons for why the mother wants squint surgery (*"you have expressed that you are keen for your son to have squint surgery. What are your reasons for this?"*)
- Counter any misunderstandings (*"squint surgery will not improve the vision in your child's eyes. It will only improve the cosmetic appearance. The patching is necessary to try to maximise the vision in your child's eyes"*)
- Explore whether compliance with patching is an issue (*"how are you finding the patching regimen for your son?"*). If patching compliance is an issue then advise on possible solu-

tions (e.g. possible reward for son by letting him put a sticker on a calendar for each day they wear the patch)

- Check that the mother is following your explanation and encourage feedback and questions from the mother ("*I appreciate that I have given you a lot of information. Would you like me to go over anything again or do you have any questions that you would like to ask me?*")
- Agree a way forward ("*at present we need to try to maximise the vision in your child's eyes with patching. Once we have achieved this then squint surgery can be an option in the future if the cosmetic appearance becomes an issue*") and ensure appropriate follow up arrangements are in place
- Provide a summary of the main points of the discussion to provide the mother with any key take home messages (*"To summarise our discussion….."*)
- Provide the mother with a point of contact should she have any questions or concerns

6.2.4 Scenario 4

Re: Mr. Jackson Francis, aged 72 years

Mr. Francis was referred by his optician for possible diagnosis of age-related macular degeneration (AMD). On clinical examination he has a dry disciform macular scar in both eyes with a visual acuity of CF in his right eye and 6/60 in his left eye.

Your task is to consult and advise on appropriate management, addressing his concerns

6.2.5.1 Approach

- Introduce yourself and confirm the patient's identity
- Take any relevant history from the patient that has not been provided
  - Smoking history
  - Past medical history: hypertension
  - Family history of AMD
  - Driving status
  - Identify patients support system ("*Who is at home with you*")
- Establish what the patient already knows ("*can you tell me what you understand about the problem with your eyes?*")
- Clarify the task in your mind. Begin discussing the diagnosis:
  - *"Your examination shows that you have age-related macular degeneration"*
- Establish what the patient already knows about the diagnosis:
  - *"Have you heard of the condition age-related macular degeneration before?"*
  - *"I wonder if you know anything about this condition before we start?"*
- Prioritise and identify any concerns from the patient before providing the patient with information ("*what are the particular things you are thinking about?*")
- Order the explanation (be open, honest and informative)—possible discussion points (depending on the patient's earlier responses)
  - What is AMD ("*age-related macular degeneration is a common condition that affects the middle part of your vision*")
  - What is the cause of AMD ("*the exact cause is unknown. It has been linked to smoking, high blood pressure and genetic factors*")
  - Types of AMD ("*there are 2 forms of age-related macular degeneration: a dry form and a wet form*")
  - Treatment options ("*unfortunately you have the dry form of AMD. This form of*

AMD has no treatment to help improve your vision")
  - Support for the patient ("*to help reduce the effect on your life, we can refer you to our low visual aids team who can provide you with useful advice and practical support such as providing you with magnifying lenses and suggest changes you can make to your home. I can also register you today as severely sight impaired. This will make it easier for you to claim financial benefits, such as help with health costs*")
  - Promote healthy living ("*try to eat a balanced diet, exercise regularly, stop smoking*")
  - Driving ("*your current level of vision does not meet the legal requirements for driving and you must inform the DVLA*")
- Check that the patient is following your explanation and encourage patient feedback and questions ("*I appreciate that I have given you a lot of information. Would you like me to go over anything again or do you have any questions that you would like to ask me?*")
- Provide a summary of the main points of the discussion to provide the patient with any key take home messages (*"To summarise our discussion…..*")
- Provide the patient with a point of contact should he have any questions or concerns

6.3 Explaining Surgical Complications

6.3.1 Scenario

Re: Mr. Andrew Taylor, aged 72 years

You have just performed a cataract operation on Mr. Taylor that did not go according to plan. You ruptured the posterior capsule and dropped the lens into the vitreous during the operation. You have left the patient aphakic.

Your task is to explain the complication to Mr. Taylor, addressing his concerns

6.3.1.1 Approach

- Introduce yourself to the patient as the surgeon who performed the operation
- Explain that you had a problem during the surgery and apologise that it occurred ("*I had some trouble with the thin capsule that surrounds the lens. This thin capsule tore during the operation and the lens fell into the back of the eye and I was unable to put an artificial lens into your eye. You will need another operation to remove the lens that has dropped into the back of your eye and at the same time we will insert a new artificial lens into your eye. I am so sorry this has happened*")
- Inform the patient that you are working on the next steps and that you have a plan to take them safely forward ("*I will have to follow you more closely and I would like to see you again tomorrow in clinic to make sure that the pressure in the eye is ok. In the meantime, I will also arrange for you to see my retinal specialist colleague who will be performing your second operation*")
- Check that the patient is following your explanation and encourage patient feedback and questions ("*I appreciate that I have given you a lot of information. Would you like me to go over anything again or do you have any questions that you would like to ask me?*")
- Reassure the patient that his vision will be poor until after his second operation ("*Your vision will be poor when I see you in clinic tomorrow as you don't have an artificial lens in place. The vision will improve once the second operation has been performed. I know this is an inconvenience and difficult for you*")
- Reassure patient that you are going to be with them all the way and that you will stay in touch with them following their second operation
- Provide a summary of the main points of the discussion to provide the patient with any key take home messages (*"To summarise our discussion…..*")

- Provide the patient with a point of contact should he have any questions or concerns

6.4 Explaining Surgical Errors

6.4.1 Scenario

Re: Master Craig Burton, aged 3 years

You have just finished a routine squint operation on a 3-year old boy before you realised that you have operated on the wrong muscle in the wrong eye. His mother is in the waiting room and wants an update on how things went during the operation.

Your task is to explain the surgical error to the mother, addressing her concerns

6.4.1.1 Approach

- Introduce yourself to the mother as the surgeon who performed the operation
- Explain that you had an incident during the surgery and apologise that it occurred ("*after I finished the operation on your child, which was routine, I realised that I had operated on the wrong muscle in the wrong eye. I am so sorry this has happened*")
- Identify any concerns from the mother ("*I know that there must be some concerns on your part as a result of this incident, and I would like to find out what is worrying you the most*"). Listen and acknowledge any concerns from the mother. Allow her to say what she wants to, without interruption before addressing the concerns
- Inform the mother that you are keen to follow up on her son but would understand if she wanted you to refer her son to one of your colleagues for further care ("*Going forwards, I would like to follow up your son closely in clinic to see how his eyes are doing. However, given what has happened I would understand if you would prefer one of my colleagues to look after your son in the future*")
- Inform the mother that you are working on the next steps and that you have a plan to take them safely forward ("*your son will need to be seen more closely in clinic by our orthoptists to determine how his eyes are recovering from the operation. This will help us determine what the best course of action going forwards would be*")
- Give an assurance of further action in relation to the incident ("*the incident will be reported as a never event to the risk management team, who will investigate it further to determine why the event occurred and decide what actions might be taken to prevent this event from happening again*")
- Invite further questions from the patient's mother and provide further information if required
- Provide an opportunity for the mother to make a complaint ("*if you wish you can lodge a written complaint with our PALS department and it will be taken seriously*")
- Provide a summary of the main points of the discussion to provide the mother with any key take home messages ("*To summarise our discussion.....*")
- Provide the mother with a point of contact should she have any questions or concerns

6.5 Consent for Treatment

6.5.1 Scenario 1

Re: Mrs. Susan Spencer, aged 60 years

Mrs. Spencer has noticed a reduction in her vision and distortion in her left eye for 6 months. Clinical examination and OCT scan revealed an idiopathic stage 4 full thickness macular hole.

Your task is to explain the diagnosis and to counsel her for surgery

6.5.1.1 Approach

- Introduce yourself and confirm the patient's identity
- Take any relevant history from the patient that has not been provided
  - Driving status
  - Occupation
- Establish what the patient already knows ("*can you tell me what you understand about the problem with your eyes?*")
- Begin explaining the diagnosis ("*your eye examination and tests shows that you have a hole in the back of your left eye*")
- Explain the best way forward and explain any possible alternatives ("*the best way to close the hole and to try to improve your vision in the left eye would be to perform an operation called a vitrectomy. Without an operation the hole is very unlikely to close*")
- Explain the nature of the operation ("*a vitrectomy is where we surgically remove the jelly at the back of the eye. Following a vitrectomy, a thin layer of tissue surrounding the hole will be peeled. At the end of the operation, we will be injecting a temporary gas bubble into the back of your eye. You may need to spend several hours during the day face down after the operation for up to 5 days and will not be able to fly whilst the gas bubble is in the eye. The operation can be performed either with you awake where you will be given a local anaesthetic injection or with you asleep under a general anaesthetic*")
- Explain the risks and benefits of the operation ("*the operation is successful in closing the hole in 9 out of 10 people who have had the hole for less than 6 months, and 6 out of 10 people who have had the hole for a year or longer. Complications include the development of a cataract, failure of the hole to close and requiring a second operation, retinal detachment and much more rarely serious complications such as an infection and bleeding in the back of the eye*")
- Driving: if the patient drives then inform her that she will not be able to drive for 6 to 8 weeks after her operation while the gas bubble is present in her eye
- Work: if patient is still working then she will need some time off work—she will be provided with a sick note after the operation
- Check that the patient is following your explanation and encourage patient feedback and questions ("*I appreciate that I have given you a lot of information. Would you like me to go over anything again or do you have any questions that you would like to ask me?*")
- Seek permission to proceed ("*Would you like to proceed with the operation? Local or general anaesthetic?*")
- Provide the patient with a point of contact should she have any questions or concerns

6.5.2 Scenario 2

Re: Colin Kent, aged 40 years

Mr. Kent presents to clinic with a macular on rhegmatogenous retinal detachment in his right eye. He has previously lost all vision in his left eye from a previously unsuccessful retinal detachment repair. Mr. Kent works fulltime in a sales job and drives regularly. He suffers from anxiety and depression. He is due to go abroad on a holiday of a lifetime in a week's time.

Your task is to explain the diagnosis and counsel the patient for surgery

6.5.2.1 Approach

- Introduce yourself and confirm the patient's identity
- Establish what the patient already knows ("*can you tell me what you understand about the problem with your right eye?*")
- Begin explaining the diagnosis ("*examination of your right eye shows a retinal detachment from a retinal tear*")
- Explain the best way forward and explain any possible alternatives (*"similar to your left eye, you will need an operation in the right eye called a vitrectomy to fix the retinal detachment. Without an operation, you will eventually lose the vision in your right eye"*)
- Explain the nature of the operation ("*a vitrectomy is where we surgically remove the jelly at the back of the eye. Following a vitrectomy, any retinal tears will be closed with a freezing therapy. At the end of the operation, we will be either injecting a temporary gas bubble into the back of your eye or inserting silicone oil into the back of your eye*)
- Explain the risks and benefits of the operation ("*the operation is intended to repair the retinal detachment in your right eye. Complications include re-detachment with the need for further operations, cataract formation, high pressures in the eye and much more rarely serious complications such as infection or bleeding in the back of the eye*")
- Discuss patients upcoming holiday ("*if we insert gas into the eye then you will not be able to fly after the operation. If we insert silicone oil into the eye then you can still fly but you will require a second operation to remove the oil in the future*")
- Address patients driving ("*you will not be able to drive for 6 to 8 weeks after the operation while the gas bubble is present in the eye*"/"*you will not be able to drive after the operation until the oil has been removed from your eye and your vision has improved*")
- Work ("*you will need some time off work after the operation and you will be provided with a sick note after the operation*")
- Check that the patient is following your explanation and encourage patient feedback and questions ("*I appreciate that I have given you a lot of information. Would you like me to go over anything again or do you have any questions that you would like to ask me?*")
- Seek permission to proceed ("*Would you like to proceed with the operation? local or general anaesthetic? silicone oil or gas?*")
- Provide the patient with a point of contact should he have any questions or concerns

6.6 Encouraging Compliance with Treatment

6.6.1 Scenario

Re: Mr. Mark Davis, aged 70 years

Mr. Davis has primary open angle glaucoma in both eyes. His IOPs were previously stabilised on G Latanoprost once a night in both eyes and G Brinzolamide twice a day in both eyes. His intraocular pressures were 14 mmHg in both eyes 6 months ago, but today in clinic is IOPs were 32 mmHg in both eyes. His visual fields today show loss progression. He had mentioned to the visual field technician that he had not been taking his drops because he felt his eyes have been well.

Your task is to discuss ways to improve his intraocular pressure control

6.6.1.1 Approach

- Introduce yourself and confirm the patient's identity
- Explain to the patient that his intraocular pressures today are not well controlled and that his visual fields today show progression. Make it clear that achieving better control of his IOP's is the aim of the discussion ("*I am afraid to say that the pressures in your eyes today is very high and your field test shows that your glaucoma has progressed. We need to try to achieve lower pressures in your eyes*")
- Explore whether poor compliance could be a problem ("*how are you getting on with the current drops? do you take the drops regularly?*")
- Explore reasons for poor compliance ("*do you experience any problems with the drops*?")
- Counter misunderstandings ("*some drops can cause*
- Explain the importance of drop compliance and the risk of uncontrolled IOP ("*it is important to take your drops regularly as it keeps the pressure in your eyes under control. Without the drops, the pressures in your eyes will be very high which can lead to permanent loss of vision in your eyes*")
- Offer an alternative solution ("*if you find taking your drops difficult then we could perform a laser treatment as an alternative method to reduce the pressures in your eyes*")
- Check that the patient is following your explanation and encourage patient feedback and questions ("*I appreciate that I have given you a lot of information. Would you like me to go over anything again or do you have any questions that you would like to ask me?*")
- Agree a way forward, ensure follow-up arrangements are in place and reassure him that you will be happy to review him sooner if there are questions or concerns

6.7 Communicating with Angry Parents

6.7.1 Scenario

Re: Master Thomas Edwards, aged 1 year

You suspect NAI in a 1-year old boy, who was bought in by his mother. The child has multiple unexplained bruises. The paediatrician is not onsite until tomorrow and in the interest of the child, you had recommended admission for 'observation' despite the fact you are not doing anything active in terms of treatment of the eye. The mother is very angry at you for detaining the child for 'observation' and would like to take the child home.

Your tasks are to discuss with the mother, addressing any concerns

6.7.1.1 Approach

- Introduce yourself and confirm the patient's and mother's identity
- Explain you will need a chaperone (nurse or health care assistant) present
- Establish what the mother already knows ("*can you tell me what you understand about why your son has been bought into hospital today?*")
- Take any relevant history from the mother that has not been provided

  - History of events ("*when did you notice the bruises? how did the bruises occur? Any other witnesses around at the time?*")
  - *Who normally looks after the child at home?*
  - *Who is in the house? Do you have any other children? Where are your other children at present?*
- Be open and honest to the mother about your reasons for wanting admission. Be non-judgemental ("*I have some concerns that some of the bruises found on your son may have occurred in a non-accidental manner. I am not here to judge but when I find injuries like this then it is mandatory for me to ask a paediatrician to examine your child. This examination is performed nationwide in an effort to safeguard children and is a requested as part of a national guidance. Unfortunately, the paediatrician is not available until tomorrow and therefore the hospital protocol is to have your son admitted into hospital for observation*")
- Explore the mothers understanding and concerns ("*I appreciate that I have given you a lot of information. Would you like me to go over anything again or do you have any questions that you would like to ask me?*")
- Explain that admission is mandatory and not optional ("*I understand why you are feeling upset/angry by this and I know that this will be an inconvenience to you, but your son will have to admitted into hospital today as unfortunately the paediatrician is not available today to examine your son*")
- Explain possible consequences of refusal if the mother is insistent on leaving the hospital with her son despite your best efforts to convince her otherwise ("*My priority is to make sure your son is well and safe. If you decide to leave the hospital with your son then I won't restrain you. However, the police will be called immediately and they will then initiate a police protection order to admit your son to hospital*")
- Allow the mother time to think about what has been discussed and invite questions
- Agree a way forward

6.8 Breaching Confidentiality in the Public Interest

6.8.1 Scenario

Re Mrs. Emma Smith, aged 65 years

Mrs. Smith is a patient you have been seeing regularly in clinic for her advanced primary open angle glaucoma in both eyes. You performed an Estermann visual field test which she failed. Mrs. Smith is keen to continue to drive no matter what.

Your task is to explain to the patient that she should not be driving

6.8.1.1 Approach

- Introduce yourself and confirm the patient's identity
- Explain the test result ("*the visual field you performed today shows that you have lost a large proportion of your peripheral vision. Your visual fields do not meet the legal requirements for driving*"). Allow the patient time to digest this information
- Explore patient understanding and concerns ("*how do you feel about that?*")
- Explore the patient's reasons for not wanting to adhere to advice
- Explain the risks of continuing to drive and possible alternatives ("*With the amount of visual field you have lost, if you continue driving you will be at a high risk of threatening your own life as well as the lives of others. Would public transport work for you as an alternative method of getting around?*)"
- Explain possible consequences of refusal ("*I find myself with a dilemma of interests. Whilst my first concern is for you, I am concerned that should you continue driving, you would*

be at risk personally as well as a risk to other on the road. If you continue to drive despite my best efforts to dissuade you, then I may have to inform the DVLA's medical advisor")

- Offer a second opinion ("*I am happy to refer you to my colleague for a second opinion if that would help you. Please do not drive in the meantime*")
- Allow the patient time to think about what has been discussed and invite questions
- Agree a way forward together

Part II

Objective Structured Clinical Examination (OSCE)

7 OSCE Technique: Do's and Don'ts

Timothy H. M. Fung and Winfried M. K. Amoaku

Abstract

An objective structured clinical examination (OSCE) is a practical assessment that enables examiners to evaluate a candidate's clinical skills and knowledge in either a real or simulated clinical environment. To perform well in the OSCE, candidates must adopt a systematic approach to examining patients and communicate their findings clearly and concisely to the examiners. This chapter provides guidance on conducting patient examinations, presenting findings, and offers strategies for effectively answering questions from the examiners.

7.1 Formalities

- Ensure that you have adequate amounts of sleep and rest in the lead up to the exam
- Dress professionally on the day of the exam
- Arrive at the exam venue in good time
- Do not forget to alcohol gel your hands before examining each patient

7.2 Practice Examination Routines

- Develop your own system for examining
  - The anterior and posterior segment with the slitlamp
  - The posterior segment with the direct ophthalmoscope (practice viewing the optic disc in non-dilated pupils) and indirect ophthalmoscope
  - Eyelids
  - Orbits
  - Pupils
  - Confrontational visual fields
  - Ocular motility
- Practice the examinations at every opportunity again and again before the OSCE
- When you go into the OSCE you should appear as though you have performed your examination of each system of the eye hundreds of times (ideally because you have!)

7.3 Equipment

- Make sure that you bring the following equipment with you on the day of the OSCE
  - Pentorch (bring 2 in case one does not work during the exam!)
  - Visual field pins
  - Slit-lamp and indirect ophthalmoscopy lenses

T. H. M. Fung (✉)
University Hospitals of Derby & Burton NHS Foundation Trust, Royal Derby Hospital, Derby, UK
e-mail: timothy.fung@nhs.net

W. M. K. Amoaku
Eye, Ear, Nose and Throat Centre, Queens Medical Centre, Nottingham University Hospitals NHS Trust, Nottingham, UK

T. H. M. Fung, W. M. K. Amoaku (eds.), *Viva and OSCE Exams in Ophthalmology*,
https://doi.org/10.1007/978-3-031-97401-4_7

  - Clear ruler in mm (×2)
  - Occluder
  - Fixation stick
  - Direct ophthalmoscope (not mandatory)
  - Indirect ophthalmoscope (not mandatory)

7.4 What the Examiners Are Looking For

- The examiners need to be satisfied that you are a safe, competent doctor, suitable to be an independent consultant general ophthalmologist
- They are not looking for in depth sub-specialty knowledge (they are not looking for the next Professor of ophthalmology!)
- They do not want to see arrogance on the day of your exam. They respect a friendly and confident manner
- Examiners come with a wide range of personalities. Do not worry about what sort of examiners you get. They are not trying to catch you out but want to find out what you can do and know

7.5 Examining Patients

- Be nice and treat patients with respect at all times
- Always introduce yourself to the patient and ask the patient for permission to examine them
- Ensure patient is positioned correctly before you begin (e.g., ensure correct position of a patient on a slit-lamp before beginning to examine the anterior segment)
- Don't look for feedback from the examiners
- Whilst examining patients, look for signs, decide how best to interpret the signs and think about how you will present your findings to the examiner
- Tell patients what you will be doing, smile and show that you care
- Say thank you to the patient at the end of your examination

7.6 Examining and Presenting

- Listen carefully to the examiners instructions and just examine what they have asked you to examine. If in doubt, clarify with the examiner.
- Try to avoid the "running commentary" approach while examining a patient unless the examiner asks you to do it. The vast majority of examiners prefer you to present your findings at the end of the examination. A running commentary slows you down, and may disrupt the flow of your examination routine.
- Have a structured approach to presenting your findings to the examiner
  - Describe what you have seen. Make sure you are honest. Do not ever make up signs
  - Give the examiner either what you think is the diagnosis or 2 to 3 differential diagnosis (start with commonest things first before mentioning the rarities)
  - If the diagnosis is uncertain, describe what else you might have expected to find in support of your differential diagnosis. State what else you could do to help resolve the issue (history, further examination, investigations)
  - Remember that even if you don't know a diagnosis for a case, you can still give a good structured answer and pass
- Practice describing your findings: your technique, findings and interpretation are all under assessment!

7.7 Answering Examiners Questions

- Listen to the questions
- Answer the question that you have been asked
- Take a moment or two to gather your thoughts before answering the questions
- Maintain eye contact with the examiner when talking (and not at the floor!)
- Speak clearly and succinctly. Do not speak too quietly or too quickly
- Try to give a well-structured answer to the questions

- Be confident in your answer if you think you are right, but do not argue with the examiner!
- Avoid emotive words like "senile" in front of patients
- The examiner may ask "*are you sure*" in response to your answer. Have a think about your answer and do not feel afraid to stick to your answer or afraid to retract statements you feel were wrong
- If you do not know the answer to a question, be honest and say so
- Really important that you avoid saying anything that would pose a danger to patients

7.8 When You Think Things Are Going Wrong

- Remember that difficult cases are likely to be difficult to all candidates
- Remember that difficult questions often reflect a good performance
- Each case of an OSCE station is marked separately. Try to stay positive (easier said than done) if you feel you have performed badly in a case. A poor performance in a station does not necessarily mean that you will fail the exam overall. Try to maximise your marks in every case for every station.

Anterior Segment 8

Timothy H. M. Fung and Winfried M. K. Amoaku

Abstract

This chapter offers a comprehensive overview of a wide range of corneal and anterior segment pathologies that are commonly encountered in an OSCE exam for ophthalmologists.

8.1 Anterior Segment Examination Sequence

- Introduce yourself to patient
- Set patient up on slit lamp
- Examine lower eyelid—punctum first (ectropion, plug) then eyelashes and eyelid margin for anterior or posterior blepharitis, slide finger across lid to look for lumps
- Ask the patient to look up and pull lower eyelid down and look at conjunctiva for scars, symblepharon
- Ask patient to look down and lift upper eyelid—look for punctum first (ectropion, plug) then eyelashes and eyelid margin for anterior or posterior blepharitis, slide finger across lid to look for lumps

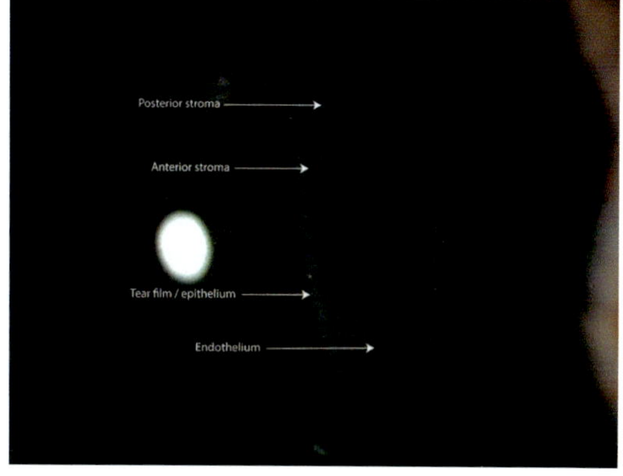

Fig. 8.1 Anterior segment image of a slit beam of the cornea

- Look at upper bulbar conjunctiva for blebs/tubes
- Ask the patient to look to the right to look at temporal conjunctiva and then to the left to look at nasal conjunctiva
- Ask the patient to look straight ahead and then examine cornea (epithelium, anterior stroma, posterior stroma, thickness of cornea, endothelium—see Fig. 8.1)
- Examine AC for cells
- Examine iris for PI, areas of atrophy (transillumination), PXF, PS, ectropion uveae, nodules, comment on any corectopia
- Examine lens and comment on position, aphakia, pseudophakia, PCO, previous Yag capsulotomy, cataract and its density, as may apply
- Examine anterior vitreous for cells, degenerations

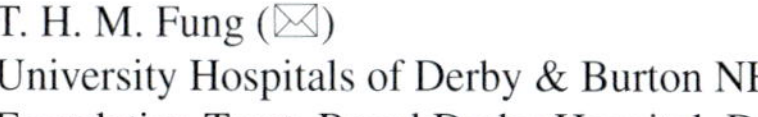
T. H. M. Fung (✉)
University Hospitals of Derby & Burton NHS Foundation Trust, Royal Derby Hospital, Derby, UK
e-mail: timothy.fung@nhs.net

W. M. K. Amoaku
Eye, Ear, Nose and Throat Centre, Queens Medical Centre, Nottingham University Hospitals NHS Trust, Nottingham, UK

T. H. M. Fung, W. M. K. Amoaku (eds.), *Viva and OSCE Exams in Ophthalmology*,
https://doi.org/10.1007/978-3-031-97401-4_8

8.2 Epithelial Basement Membrane Dystrophy (EBMD) (Table 8.1)

8.2.1 History

- Hx of RCES without previous trauma

8.2.2 Examination

- Findings should be present in both eyes
- Grayish-white maplike opacities in the superficial corneal epithelium ("maps") - characteristic and pathophysiologic feature and represent corneal epithelial basement membrane present within the epithelium itself—best seen on retroillumination (see Fig. 8.2)
- Parallel fingerprint-like lines in the corneal epithelium ("fingerprint")—represent parallel rows of thickened basement membrane within the epithelium—best seen on retroillumination (see Fig. 8.2)

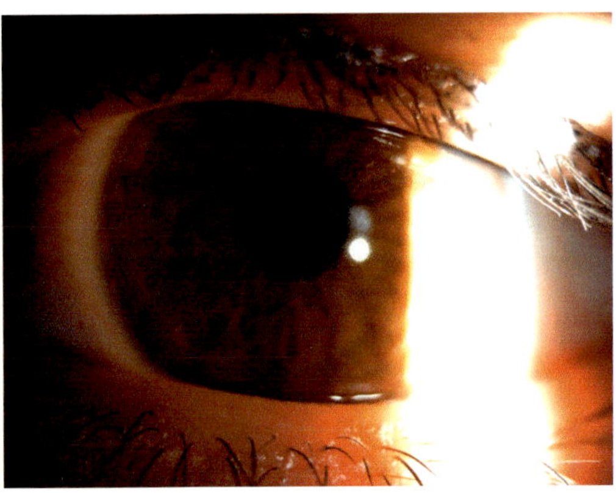

Fig. 8.2 Anterior segment image of a patient with the typical "dot" and "map" changes associated with EBMD

Table 8.1 Theoretical pathogenesis of EBMD

Epithelial cells produce abnormal multi-laminar basement membrane, both in normal location and intraepithelially, as the intraepithelial basement membrane thickens it blocks normal migration of epithelial cells toward the surface, trapped epithelial cells degenerate to form intraepithelial microcysts, abnormal intraepithelial basement membrane produces map and fingerprint changes

- Intraepithelial gray microcysts (most unusual finding—"dot")—represents individual small mounds of thickened basement membrane beneath the basal layer of epithelium—best viewed by retroillumination (see Fig. 8.2)

8.2.3 Treatment

- Management of RCES: lubricants, cycloplegia, patching, BCL insertion, mechanical debridement of the loosened epithelium, anterior stromal puncture for recalcitrant recurrent erosions below the visual axis (80% first time success rate), PTK for recurrent erosions in the visual axis—superficial ablation just into Bowman's layer ensuring that all abnormal epithelial basement membrane is removed, alcohol delamination

8.2.4 Other Diagnoses to Consider

- Meesman's dystrophy (see Sect. 8.3)
- Corneal dystrophies of Bowman's layer: Reis Bucklers/Thiel-Behnke dystrophy (see Sect. 8.4)

8.3 Meesman Dystrophy (Table 8.2)

Table 8.2 Key facts of Meesman dystrophy

A type of corneal epithelial dystrophy—defined as a corneal opacity or alteration which is most often bilateral and progressive, occurs after birth, and is not inflammatory
AD condition caused by mutations in the genes for cytokeratins CK3 and CK12
Microcysts contain "peculiar substance"—An electron dense accumulation of granular and filamentary material

8.3.1 History

- Positive FHx: AD condition
- Symptoms: reduction of vision, photophobia

8.3.2 Examination

- Multiple diffusely distributed tiny vesicles that extend all the way to the limbus
- Vesicles are more numerous in the interpalpebral area and are best visualised with retroillumination (see Fig. 8.3)
- The epithelium adjacent to the cysts is clear, but there can be whorled and wedge-shaped epithelial patterns
- Findings are bilateral and limited to the corneal epithelium

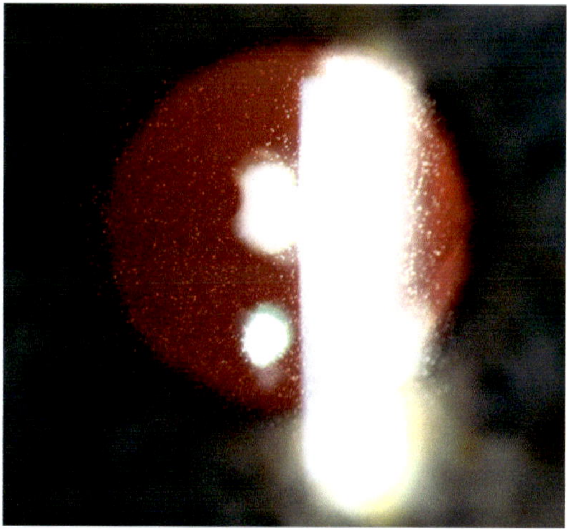

Fig. 8.3 Anterior segment image of a patient with Meesman corneal dystrophy showing the typical tiny vesicles distributed diffusely across the corneal epithelium

8.3.3 Treatment

- Rarely required as patients are usually asymptomatic or have minimal symptoms
- Indications for treatment: significant photophobia or visual impairment
- Treatment options
  - Superficial keratectomy
  - Excimer laser phototherapeutic keratectomy
  - Lamellar keratoplasty: DALK

8.3.4 Other Diagnoses to Consider

- "Dot" changes of epithelial basement membrane dystrophy (irregular round, oval, or comma-shaped, non-staining, gray-white intraepithelial opacities of various sizes in close proximity to the maplike patches): hx of recurrent corneal erosions (pain, lacrimation, photophobia), dots alone are never seen—look for maps (geographic circumscribed gray lesions best seen with broad oblique illumination) and fingerprint lines (branching refractile lines with club-shaped terminations—best seen in retroillumination)
- Lisch epithelial corneal dystrophy—x-linked dominant (FHx), densely crowded transparent epithelial microcysts in a feathery whorled pattern

8.4 Reis-Buckler Dystrophy (Table 8.3)

Table 8.3 Key facts of reis-buckler dystrophy

A corneal dystrophy of Bowman's layer
AD condition caused by mutations in the keratoepithelin gene (TGFB1)
Characterised by replacement of Bowman's layer with a fibrocellular scar tissue (stains blue with Masson trichrome)

8.4.1 History

- Hx of RCES since childhood

8.4.2 Examination

- Honeycomb shaped opacities in the Bowman's layer involving the center of the cornea with/without scarring (see Fig. 8.4)

8.4.3 Treatment

- RCES: lubricants, mechanical debridement, BCL with prophylactic topical antibiotics, anterior stromal puncture, PTK, alcohol delamination
- If vision reduced: PTK, lamellar or penetrating keratoplasty

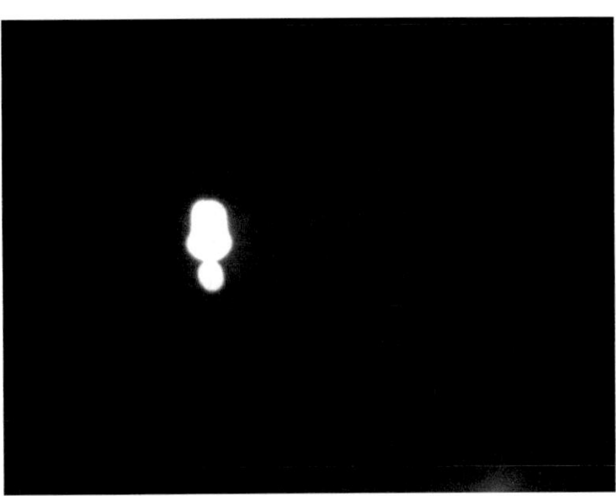

Fig. 8.4 Anterior segment image of a patient with Reis-Buckler dystrophy with typical honeycomb shaped opacities in the Bowman's layer

8.4.4 Other Diagnoses to Consider

- Thiel-Behnke corneal dystrophy: distinguished from Reis-Bucklers by electron microscopy looking a fibrocellular scar that is characterised by curly collagen fibers and a saw-tooth configuration.

8.5 Lattice Dystrophy (Table 8.4)

8.5.1 History

- Hx of RCES
- FHx of lattice dystrophy

8.5.2 Examination

- Refractile radially orientated branching lines that overlap one another creating a latticework pattern +/− a diffuse central anterior stromal haze (see Fig. 8.5)

Table 8.4 Key facts of lattice dystrophy

Bilateral AD inherited primary localised corneal amyloidosis with progressive deposition of amyloid in the corneal stroma
Type I: Mutation in the TGFβ1 gene on chromosome 5, isolated to the eye
Type II (Meretoja's syndrome): Mutation in the gelsolin gene, ocular and systemic features (cardiac conduction abnormalities, peripheral neuropathy)
Amyloid stains with Congo red and demonstrate apple green birefringence and dichroism at polarising microscopy

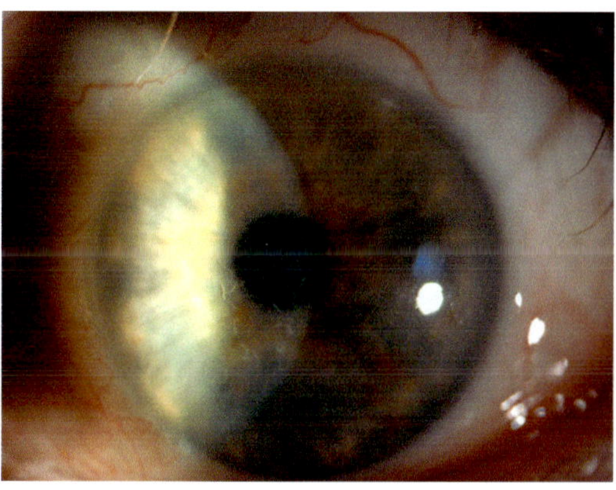

Fig. 8.5 Anterior segment image of a patient with lattice dystrophy with the typical refractile radially orientated branching lines that overlap one another

- Examine for facial paresis (lagophthalmos and exposure keratopathy), blepharochalasis, and laxity of the facial skin (Type II)

8.5.3 Treatment

- RCES: topical lubricants, BCL, patching, anterior stromal puncture, PTK, alcohol delamination
- VA impaired: lamellar or penetrating keratoplasty (highest rate of recurrence in lattice dystrophy compared to granular and macular dystrophy)
- Refer to medics If type II suspected for assessment of systemic involvement

8.5.4 Other Diagnoses to Consider

- Granular dystrophy (see Sect. 8.6)
- Macular dystrophy (see Sect. 8.7)
- Avellino dystrophy (see Sect. 8.8)
- Schnyder's crystalline dystrophy (see Sect. 8.9)

8.6 Granular Dystrophy (Table 8.5)

8.6.1 History

- Positive FHx
- Hx of RCES

8.6.2 Examination

- Small discrete sharply demarcated grayish white opacities in the anterior central stroma with intervening clear stroma and sparing of the periphery (see Fig. 8.6)
- Opacities vary in shape and can be grouped into 3 basic morphologic types: drop-shaped, crumb-shaped, and ring shaped.

Table 8.5 Key facts of granular dystrophy

AD condition involving the deposition of hyaline material in the corneal stroma (hyaline material in the stroma stains red with Masson trichrome)
Caused by a mutation in the keratoepithelin gene (TGFB1)

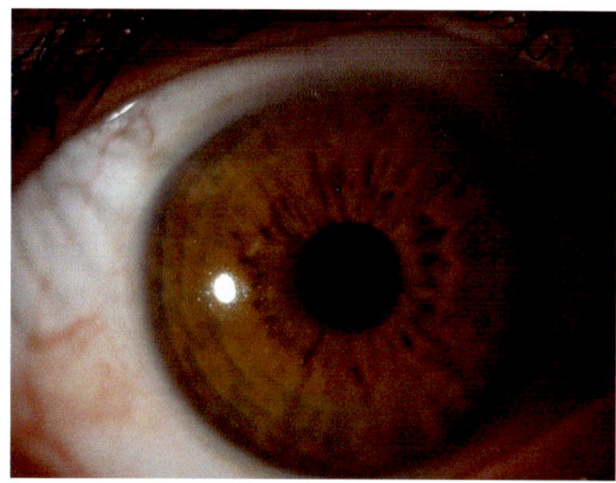

Fig. 8.6 Anterior segment image of a patient with granular dystrophy with typical multiple white anterior stromal opacities with clear intervening stromal spaces between each opacity

8.6.3 Treatment

- RCES: lubricants, BCL with prophylactic topical antibiotics, mechanical debridement, anterior stromal puncture, PTK, alcohol delamination
- If vision reduced: keratoplasty (PK or DALK) but high chance of recurrence

8.6.4 Other Diagnoses to Consider

- Macular dystrophy (see Sect. 8.7): recessive FHx, decreased CCT, involvement of peripheral stroma, early intervening stromal haze
- Avellino dystrophy (see Sect. 8.8): combination of lattice dystrophy and granular dystrophy
- Schnyder's crystalline dystrophy (see Sect. 8.9)

8.7 Macular Dystrophy (Table 8.6)

8.7.1 History

- Hx of RCES

8.7.2 Examination

- Multiple gray-white opacities in the anterior stroma on a background of diffuse clouding in the anterior stroma, extending from limbus to limbus (see Fig. 8.7). Guttae are commonly present.
- Associated with reduced CCT

8.7.3 Treatment

- RCES: lubricants, mechanical debridement, BCL with prophylactic topical antibiotics, anterior stromal puncture, PTK, alcohol delamination
- Photophobia: tinted glasses or tinted cosmetic CL
- Reduced vision: keratoplasty (DALK or PK)

Table 8.6 Key facts of macular dystrophy

AR disorder involving the deposition of a GAG (keratin sulphate) in the stroma (GAG stains with Alcian blue or colloidal iron)
Arises from mutations in the gene for carbohydrate sulfotransferase (CHST6)

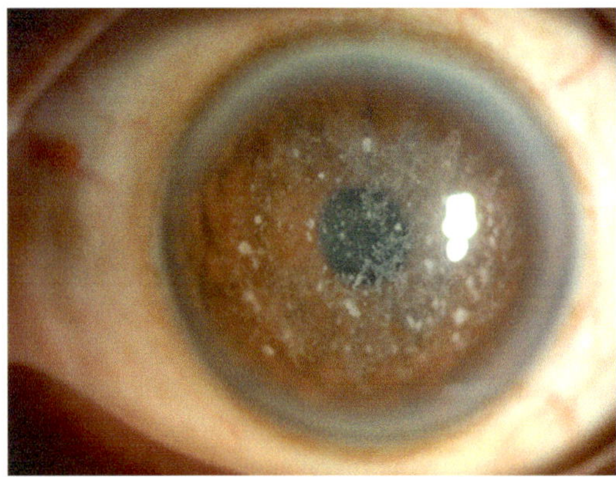

Fig. 8.7 Anterior segment image of a patient with macular dystrophy with multiple white opacities in the anterior stroma on a background of diffuse haze of the corneal stroma

8.7.4 Other Diagnoses to Consider

- Granular dystrophy (see Sect. 8.6)
- Avellino dystrophy (see Sect. 8.8)
- Schnyder's crystalline dystrophy (see Sect. 8.9)

8.8 Avellino Dystrophy

8.8.1 History

- Hx of RCES

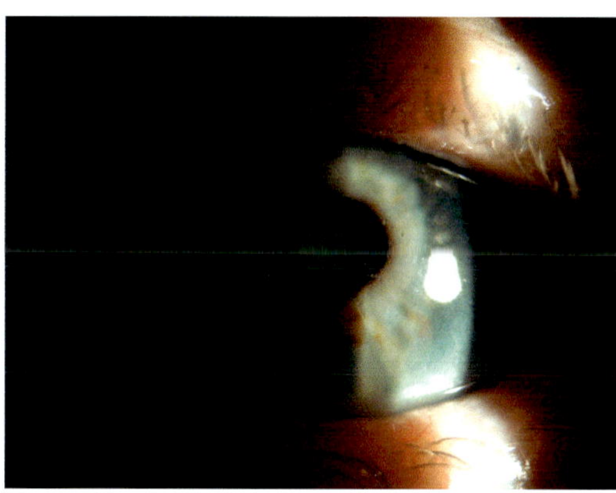

Fig. 8.8 Anterior segment image of a patient with Avellino dystrophy showing signs of both lattice dystrophy and granular dystrophy

8.8.2 Examination

- Anterior stromal, discrete gray-white granular deposits with anterior stromal haze (see Fig. 8.8)
- Mid to posterior stromal lattice lesions (see Fig. 8.8)

8.8.3 Treatment

- RCES: lubricants, mechanical debridement, BCL with prophylactic topical antibiotics, anterior stromal puncture, PTK, alcohol delamination
- Photophobia: tinted glasses or tinted cosmetic CL
- Reduced vision: PK

8.8.4 Other Diagnoses to Consider

- Lattice dystrophy/Granular dystrophy

8.9 Schnyder's Crystalline Dystrophy (SCD) (Table 8.7)

8.9.1 History

- Hx of hypercholesterolaemia
- Hx of paraproteinaemias

8.9.2 Examination

- Bilateral central refractile crystals/opacities in the central anterior stroma (see Fig. 8.9) with associated arcus lipoides
- Diffuse stromal haze, which may affect all levels of the stroma

8.9.3 Investigations

- Bloods: fasting cholesterol and triglyceride levels (SCD), leucocyte cysteine content (cystinosis), lymphocytosis (leukaemia)

Table 8.7 Key facts of SCD

AD stromal dystrophy caused by mutations in the UBIAD1 gene
Characterised by the deposition of cholesterol crystals and phospholipids in the corneal stroma (crystals stain red with Oil Red O)

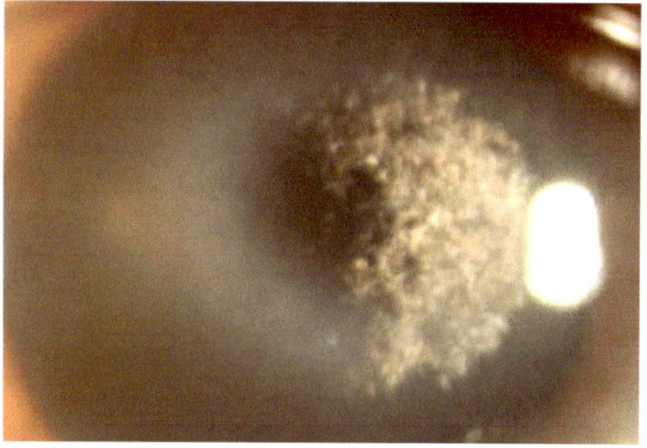

Fig. 8.9 Anterior segment image of a patient with Schnyder's crystalline dystrophy showing subepithelial crystalline deposition

8.9.4 Treatment

- If visual problems: keratoplasty (lamellar or penetrating) although recurrence of cholesterol crystals may occur

8.9.5 Other Diagnoses to Consider

- Cystinosis
- Dysproteinaemia's: multiple myeloma, Waldenstrom's macroglobulinaemia, Hodgkin's disease, leukaemia, benign monoclonal gammopathy, cryoglobulinaemia
- Medications: gold
- Bietti's peripheral crystalline dystrophy—peripheral location of crystals + retinal degeneration

8.10 Posterior Polymorphous Corneal Dystrophy (PPCD) (Table 8.8)

8.10.1 History

- Hx of Alport syndrome: 85% XR condition, anterior lenticonus, sensorineural deafness, dot & fleck retinopathy, glomerulonephritis

8.10.2 Examination

- Vesicular-like lesion (hallmark of PPCD): appears as sharply demarcated transparent round cysts surrounded by a grey halo at the level of DM and endothelium and commonly occur in lines or clusters
- Band lesions: typically horizontal, have parallel scalloped edges, and do not taper towards the ends (see Fig. 8.10)

Table 8.8 Key facts of PPCD

Bilateral, AD inherited corneal dystrophy
Normally non-progressive although has potential of decreasing vision due to corneal oedema and glaucoma

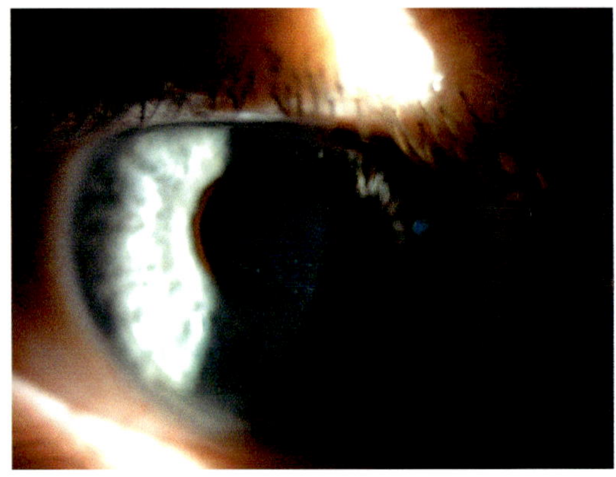

Fig. 8.10 Anterior segment image of a patient with PPCD with typical horizontal band lesions

- Diffuse deep stromal opacities: small, macular, gray-white lesions at the level of DM. There may be deep stromal haze adjacent to these lesions
- Endothelial guttae
- Corneal oedema occurs infrequently and ranges from minimal stromal thickening to bullous keratopathy
- PAS (characteristic feature of PPCD) seen with or without gonioscopy, corectopia, areas of iris atrophy
- Check IOP—open (compression of TM secondary to high iris insertion) and angle closure (endothelial cell migration across the TM onto the iris forming synechiae) glaucoma
- Look for trabeculectomy or glaucoma drainage implant
- Fundus examination: CDR (glaucoma), dot & fleck retinopathy (Alport syndrome)

8.10.3 Investigations

- Bloods: deranged renal function tests—glomerulonephritis—Alport syndrome
- Urinalysis: haematuria & proteinuria—glomerulonephritis—Alport syndrome
- Hearing test: sensorineural hearing loss—Alport syndrome

8.10.4 Treatment

- Observation: in the great majority of patients, PPCD is stable and asymptomatic
- Treat any glaucoma present: medical / surgical intervention
- PK: if significant reduced vision—presence of PAS visible without gonioscopy and increased IOP must be considered relative contraindications to corneal transplantation

8.10.5 Other Diagnoses to Consider

- ICE syndrome—unilateral, sporadic occurrence, female predilection, always has iridocorneal adhesions, displays iris atrophy, always has glaucoma, progressive and symptomatic
- Posterior corneal vesicle syndrome
- Early-onset CHED
- Congenital glaucoma
- Axenfeld-Rieger syndrome

8.11 Fuchs Endothelial Dystrophy (FED) (Table 8.9)

8.11.1 History

- Symptoms: reduced vision (most predominantly in the morning)

8.11.2 Examination

- Corneal guttae +/− melanin pigment pigmentation—appear as dark spots on the posterior corneal surface by direct illumination (beaten metal appearance—coalescence of central guttae) (see Fig. 8.11)
- Corneal stromal oedema with DM folds, microcystic epithelial oedema (seen as a stippled pattern that stands out in sclerotic scatter, using fluorescein stain the microcystic pattern is highlighted as a disruption in the tear film) that eventually coalesces to form bullae, which can lead to erosions and fingerprint lines
- In end stage disease, subepithelial fibrous scarring occurs between the epithelium and Bowman's membrane (best seen with tangential illumination) (see Fig. 8.12)

Table 8.9 Key facts of FED

Age of onset over age 50
Female: Male ratio of 3:1

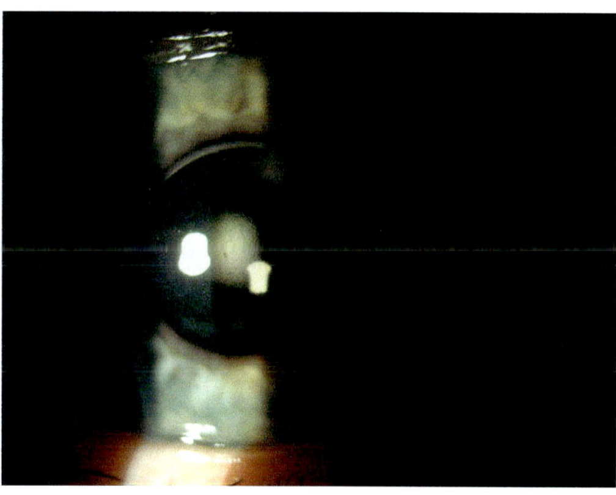

Fig. 8.11 Anterior segment image of a patient with FED showing multiple corneal guttae

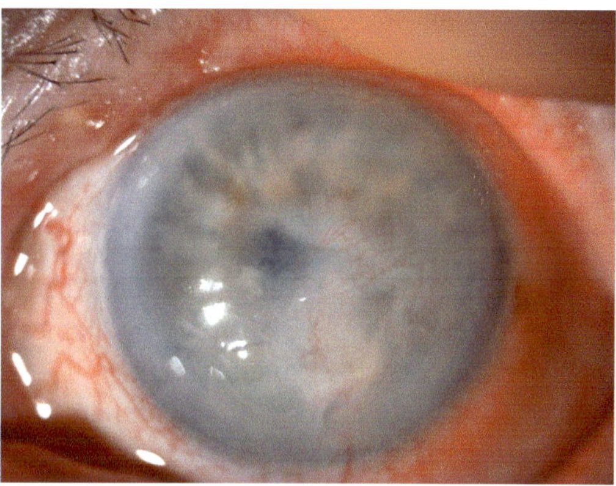

Fig. 8.12 Anterior segment image of a patient with end stage FED with diffuse corneal oedema and vascularised subepithelial fibrosis

- Measure IOP and examine the optic disc for glaucoma: increased incidence of primary open angle glaucoma (POAG) in FED

8.11.3 Investigations

- Specular microscopy—reduced endothelial cells counts, increased average cell volume, loss of hexagonality of the cells and increased variation of cell sizes
- Pachymetry—increased CCT

8.11.4 Treatment

- Medical
  - Indication(s): visually significant corneal oedema.
  - Options:
    - Topical hypertonic saline solutions
    - Dehydration of cornea by a blow dryer in the morning or throughout the day
    - Reduction of IOP (avoid topical carbonic anhydrase inhibitors)
    - BCL for treatment of recurrent erosions caused by epithelial bullae
- Surgical
  - Indication(s): blurring of vision in the morning, evidence of epithelial oedema on slitlamp examination
  - Options:
    - Lamellar keratoplasty (DSEK, DMEK)
    - Full thickness PK –preferred if significant corneal scarring present
- FED and cataract (see Table 8.10)
  - Staged cataract extraction followed by keratoplasty:
    - Advantages: IOL stability in the bag, easier to manage if complications occur, delay of graft procedure
    - Disadvantages: two operative procedures on separate occasions required for patient, longer visual rehabilitation procedure for patient
  - Triple procedure (keratoplasty with cataract extraction and IOL implant):
    - Indications(s): consider if CCT more than 650, endothelial cell count <1000, dense cataract present
    - Advantages: faster visual recovery and reduced number of operations
    - Disadvantages: may be unable to perform keratoplasty (with subsequent loss of valuable graft tissue) if complications arise from initial cataract surgery

Table 8.10 Management of a patient with FED and a cataract

If the patient has no cataract and mild corneal oedema—consider conservative medical management
If the patient has a dense cataract and severe corneal oedema—consider triple procedure
If the patient has no cataract but has severe corneal oedema—Consider keratoplasty first and cataract extraction if a visually significant cataract develops
If the patient has a dense cataract and no corneal oedema—Consider cataract extraction first and keratoplasty if corneal decompensation develops

8.11.5 Other Diagnoses to Consider

- Pseudophakic bullous keratopathy
- Chandler's syndrome—unilateral ICE syndrome with a hammered silver appearance of the corneal endothelium, corectopia, iridocorneal adhesions
- Posterior polymorphous dystrophy—corectopia, iridocorneal adhesions
- Central herpetic disciform keratitis—presence of underlying KP's
- Macular dystrophy
- Congenital hereditary endothelial dystrophy—present at birth (CHED 2—AR)
- Corneal pseudoguttae: post-trauma, post-intraocular inflammation—these apparent guttae are transient and disappear with resolution of underlying condition

8.12 Interstitial Keratitis (IK) (Table 8.11)

8.12.1 Causes of IK

- Infectious: bacterial (congenital—if bilateral or acquired—if unilateral syphilis, TB, leprosy, lyme disease, trachoma, brucellosis), viral (HSV, HZV, EBV, mumps, rubeola, HTLV-1), parasitic (acanthamoeba keratitis, microsporidiosis, leishmaniasis, onchocerciasis, trypanosomiasis)
- Non-infectious: cogan's syndrome, sarcoidosis, lymphoma

8.12.2 History

- Syphilis: hx of congenital syphilis or hx of parents being treated for STI, symptoms of meningism (headaches, photophobia, neck stiffness), hearing loss
- HSV: Hx of HSV keratitis, hx of herpetic "cold sores"
- HZV: Risk factors for immunosuppression: immunosuppressive drugs, organ transplant recipients, neoplastic diseases, HIV
- Acanthamoeba: Hx of CL wear (extended wear CL), poor CL hygiene (rinsing in tap water), swimming with CL in situ (ponds, hot tubs, swimming pools), corneal trauma (rural or agricultural setting)
- TB: fever, night sweats, weight loss, cough, hx of TB, recent travel to endemic areas, contacts of active TB
- Cogan's syndrome: acute tinnitus, vertigo (dizziness), bilateral hearing loss

Table 8.11 Key facts of IK

Defined as a nonsuppurative inflammation characterised by cellular infiltration and vascularisation of the corneal stroma with minimal primary involvement of the corneal epithelium or endothelium

8.12.3 Examination

- Vascularised corneal opacification is a sign of prior stromal inflammation. Look for ghost vessels (a tracery of intertwined phantom vessels forming a thread like network weaving through a stromal haze) from the limbus (see Fig. 8.13)
- Syphilis: bilateral in congenital and unilateral in acquired, cellular infiltration of stroma with stromal oedema, stromal neovascularisation (superficial capillaries bud from venules of the limbal arcades, deeper vessels arise as terminal branches of the anterior ciliary vessels), anterior and posterior uveitis, associated findings in congenital syphilis—salt & pepper retinopathy, Hutchinson's teeth (widely spaced teeth with notched incisors), frontal bossing, saddle shaped nose, sabre shins, associated findings in acquired syphilis—maculopapular rash (trunk, palms, soles), lymphadenopathy, painless chancre, painless ulcer of mouth or conjunctiva, light-near dissociation (Argyll Robertson pupil—neurosyphilis)
- HSV: stromal oedema (suggested by increased width of slit beam and DM folds), stromal neovascularisation, stromal cellular infiltration (3 hallmarks of IK) +/− scleritis or uve-

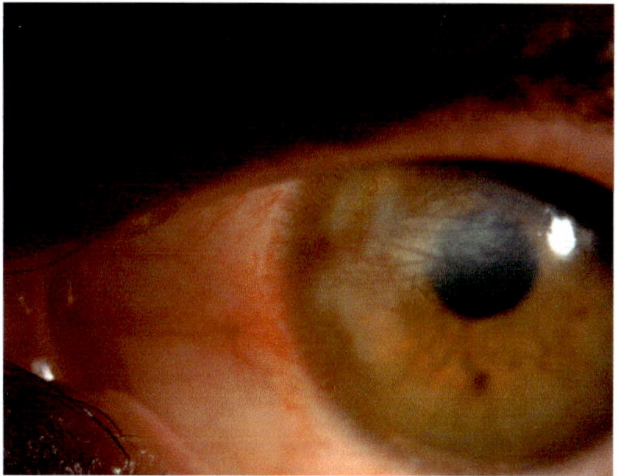

Fig. 8.13 An anterior segment image of a patient with interstitial keratitis. Note the ghost vessels in the corneal stroma arising from the limbus

itis, pattern of stromal infiltration may be central or peripheral, focal or multifocal, superficial or full-thickness, wessely-type immune rings (if present supports the diagnosis—best seen on sclerotic scatter), look for anterior stromal scars (footprints or ghost dendrites) from previous HSV disease, raised IOP, sectoral iris atrophy, check for reduced corneal sensation

- HZV: stromal infiltration with stromal oedema, pseudodendrites (lack central ulceration, have blunt ends, raised epithelial cells), vesicular eruption of periocular skin and eyelids (look for scabbed lesions), uveitis
- Acanthamoeba: stromal oedema with infiltration, ring infiltrate, perineural infiltrates, pseudodendrites
- TB: unilateral, cellular infiltration of stroma is often peripheral or quadrantic and is followed by localised oedema, and later stromal vascularisation +/− scarring or thinning. May have additional uveitis, particularly choroiditis.
- Cogan's syndrome: patchy cellular infiltration of the mid-stroma with stromal oedema, stromal neovascularisation from the limbus, stromal scarring and ghost vessels (late-finding)

8.12.4 Investigations

- Syphilis: non-treponemal tests (VDRL, RPR—better for screening), treponemal tests (FTA-ABS, hemagglutination, enzyme immunoassay—ELISA), HIV test (check for co-infection, HIV antibody detection via ELISA. +ve ELISA results are confirmed with western blot), LP (if active intraocular disease or neuro-syphilis—leukocytosis, raised protein levels). Treponemal tests remains reactive for life in pt's with congenital or acquired syphilis. Over time, the non-treponemal test titres decrease, ultimately becoming undetectable.
- Acanthamoeba: corneal scrape and stain with calcofluor white (stain cysts visualised under UV light) and culture on non-nutrient agar with E.coli overlay +/− PCR, in-vivo confocal microscopy with direct visualisation of cysts
- TB: CXR, tuberculin skin test, Interferon gamma release assay (IGRA—T-spot or QuantiFERON), sputum culture for AFB, early morning urine sample for AFB, corneal scraping for culture and histopathological evaluation
- Cogan's syndrome: bloods for FBC (leukocytosis, eosinophilia), ESR (raised), p-ANCA (PAN), c-ANCA (GPA), hearing test (sensorineural hearing loss), VDRL/RPR (to rule out syphilis)

8.12.5 Treatment

- Syphilis: topical steroids, GU referral with contact tracing, benzylpenicillin, PK for corneal scarring
- HSV: topical steroids with topical antivirals (prevent breakout of epithelial keratitis)—no benefit of adding oral aciclovir (HEDS I), oral acyclovir 400 mg BD reduced the probability of stromal keratitis recurrence by 50% from 28% to 14% at the 1 year time point (HEDS II), cycloplegia (for uveitis), PK for corneal scarring
- HZV: topical steroids, oral aciclovir 800 mg 5x/day (IV aciclovir if pt. is immunocompromised to avoid complication of disseminated infection), cycloplegia (for uveitis), PK (high risk of failure) or Boston keratoprosthesis for corneal scarring. PK only generally performed for tectonic reasons.
- Acanthamoeba: admit, topical biguanide (PHMB 0.02% or chlorhexidine 0.02%) + diamidine (propamidine 0.1% or hexamidine 0.1%), PK for corneal scarring
- TB: topical steroids, systemic anti-TB medication (rifampicin, isoniazid, pyrazinamide, ethambutol), cycloplegia (for uveitis), PK for corneal scarring
- Cogan's syndrome: low dose topical steroids for IK, high dose systemic corticosteroids for inner ear disease

8.12.6 Other Diagnoses to Consider

- Microbial keratitis—bacterial (pseudomonas, syphilis, chlamydia), viral (HSV. HZV), fundal (candida, aspergillus, fusarium), parasitic (onchocerca)

- Traumatic corneal scarring from chemical burns
- LESC failure
- OCP
- SJS
- Terrien's marginal degeneration
- Ocular rosacea
- Atopic keratoconjunctivitis

8.13 Lipid Keratopathy

8.13.1 Causes

Secondary lipid keratopathy is more common than primary lipid keratopathy and occur in corneal neovascularisation.

- Primary: no hx of trauma, corneal vascularisation, or known disorders of lipid metabolism
- Secondary: interstitial keratitis, trauma: surgical—corneal intacs implantation, corneal ulceration, corneal hydrops, mustard gas injuries, disorders of lipid metabolism (fish eye disease, tangier disease, familial LCAT deficiency, apolipoprotein A1 deficiency)

8.13.2 Examination

- Primary lipid keratopathy: lipid deposition centrally or peripherally
- Secondary lipid keratopathy: gray to yellow-white infiltrates (often at edge of scars/lesions) associated with the presence of an adjacent corneal blood vessel (see Figs. 8.14 and 8.15)

8.13.3 Treatment

- Indications: vision, cosmesis
- Options
  - Argon laser to limbal feeder vessel or needle point cautery to induce absorption of the lipids through destruction of the feeder vessels

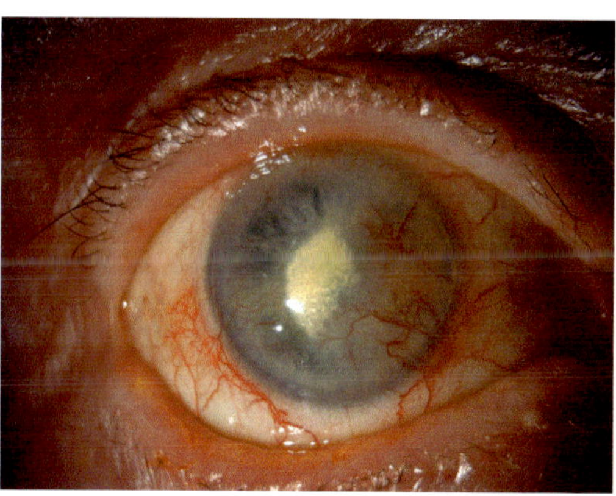

Fig. 8.14 Anterior segment image of a patient with lipid keratopathy in a region of corneal scarring and stromal neovascularisation resulting from previous herpes simplex keratitis

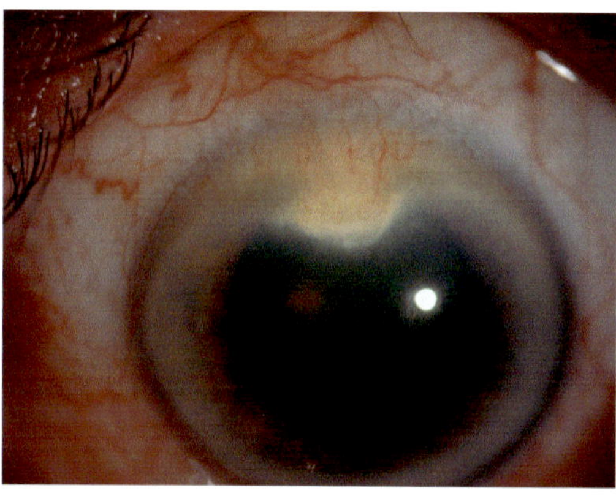

Fig. 8.15 Anterior segment image of a patient with lipid deposition at the leading edge of the superior pannus associated with Terrien marginal degeneration

  - Intrastromal anti-VEGF agents with off license avastin
  - Keratoplasty: PK or DALK

8.14 Radial Keratotomy (RK) (Tables 8.12 and 8.13)

8.14.1 Examination

- Radial incision lines (from center to peripherally) (see Fig. 8.16)
- Star shaped iron deposit forming centrally (tear star—no effect on vision)

Table 8.12 Cataract surgery considerations in patients who have undergone a previous radial keratotomy refractive procedure

IOL power calculation may be problematic and may result in undercorrection and hyperopia
Calculation of implant power for cataract surgery after RK should be done using a third-generation formula (Haigis, Hoffer Q, Holladay 2, or SRK/T) rather than a regression formula (SRK I or II)
Keratometric power is determined in 1 of 3 ways: Direct measurement using corneal topography; application of pre-RK keratometry minus the refractive change; or adjustment of the base curve of a Plano contact lens by the overrefraction.
Scleral tunnel incisions preferred (clear corneal incisions increase the risk of the blade transecting the RK incision, which can induce irregular astigmatism)
Place incision in the steep meridian of the cornea or use of toric IOLs to reduce preoperative astigmatism
Prevent overhydrating the cataract incision in order to avoid rupture of the RK incision

Table 8.13 Measuring intraocular pressures in patients who have undergone a previous radial keratotomy refractive procedure

Changes in the corneal shape without corneal thinning can lead to falsely low IOP values with central applanation tonometry
In eyes that have undergone RK, non-Goldmann measurement of IOP and continued examination of the optic nerve and possibly VF is recommended.

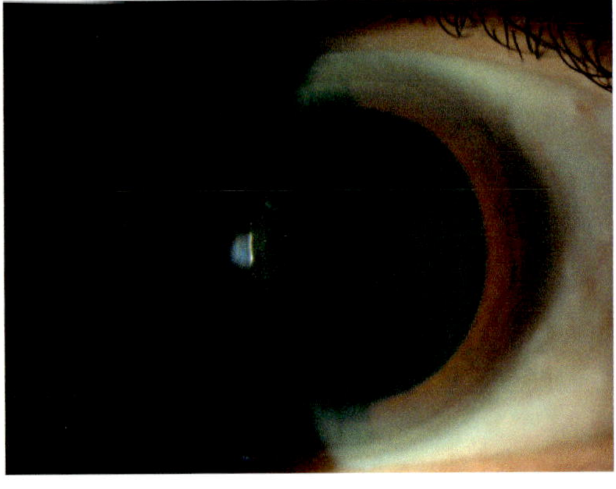

Fig. 8.16 Anterior segment image of a patient who previously underwent a radial keratotomy refractive procedure to correct an underlying myopic refractive error

8.14.2 Indications of RK

- Refractive surgery procedure to correct myopia (−1.00 to −4.00 D)

8.14.3 Complications of RK

- Intraoperative: penetration into AC causing iris/lens damage
- Postoperative: irregular astigmatism (visual glare + distortion) due to wound gape and epithelial plugs, epithelial downgrowth, endophthalmitis, traumatic cataract, starburst effects (starburst patterns around lights at night—light scattering off radial incisions), perforation of the cornea, progressive hyperopic shift (can be corrected with LASIK or PRK)

8.15 Vortex Keratopathy

8.15.1 History

- Use of medications (dose and duration): amiodarone, hydroxychloroquine, chloroquine, phenothiazines (chlorpromazine), tamoxifen, indomethacin
- Hx of Fabry's disease: x-linked recessive disorder, deficiency of alpha-galactosidase A enzyme, renal failure, cardiovascular disease, neurologic changes, cutaneous angiokeratomas

8.15.2 Examination

- Pattern of non-elevated white to brown whorl-shaped opacities within the basal corneal epithelium, consisting of fine lines emanating from a central nodal point (most commonly located in the inferior paracentral region—typically bilateral and symmetric) (see Fig. 8.17)
- Look for aneurysmal dilatations and tortuosity of the conjunctival and retinal vessels and a spoke-like posterior subcapsular cataract: Fabry's disease
- Look for bulls eye maculopathy (ring of depigmentation surrounded by an area of hyperpigmentation seen centered on the fovea): hydroxychloroquine toxicity, chloroquine toxicity

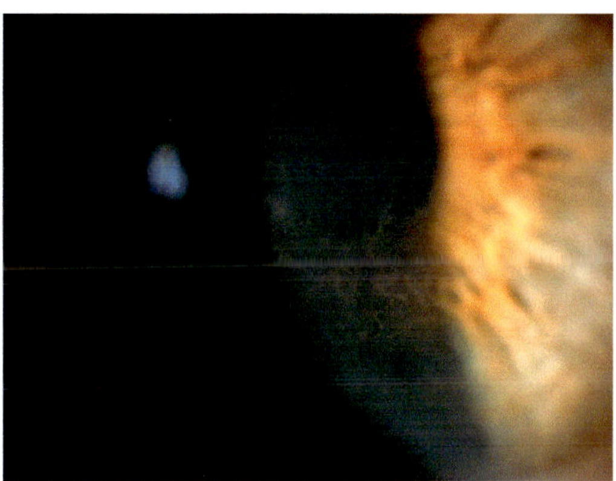

Fig. 8.17 Anterior segment image of a patient with vortex keratopathy who was on long term amiodarone treatment

- Look for optic neuropathy (VA, RAPD, colour vision, VF), retinopathy, and anterior subcapsular lens opacities: amiodarone

8.15.3 Investigations

- Screening for greatly deficient or absent alpha-galactosidase A activity in plasma or peripheral leukocytes or gene sequencing: Fabry's disease

8.15.4 Treatment

- Cornea verticillata is visually insignificant and is not an indication for stopping any associated medications.
- Discontinuation or reduction of the dose of amiodarone should be considered if optic neuropathy is observed.

8.15.5 Other Diagnoses to Consider

- Corneal iron lines (faint yellow to dark brown discolouration in the corneal epithelium): tear star after RK, Hudson-Stahli line (horizontal line located in the lower third of the cornea), Ferry line (appears on cornea anterior to filtering bleb), Stocker's line (advancing edge of pterygium), Fleischer ring (base of the cone of KC)
- Corneal stromal deposits: gold (chrysiasis—gold to violet like fine deposits scattered from the corneal epithelium to the deep stroma +/− bulbar conjunctiva), silver (argyrosis—lids and conjunctiva have a light to dark slate-grey appearance, deposits of blue-gray material in the peripheral deep stroma of the cornea), antacid, retinoid deposition

8.16 Calcific Band Keratopathy (BK) (Table 8.14)

8.16.1 Causes of BK

- Ocular: chronic anterior uveitis, JIA, herpetic keratouveitis, long standing interstitial keratitis, phthisis bulbi, prolonged corneal oedema, silicone oil in AC
- Systemic: hypercalcaemic states (CKD, hyperparathyroidism, sarcoidosis), hyperphosphataemia (CKD), hyperuricaemia (CKD), x-linked ichthyosis

8.16.2 History

- Hx of uveitis
- Hx of RD repair requiring the use of silicone oil
- Hx of chronic kidney disease (CKD)
- Hx of gout
- Symptoms suggestive of hypercalcaemia: abdominal pain, depression, renal stones
- Use of vitamin D and calcium supplements

8.16.3 Examination

- White and chalky band of opacity beginning peripherally at the 3 and 9 o'clock positions, with a sharply demarcated peripheral edge separated from the limbus by a lucent zone (see Fig. 8.18)

Table 8.14 Key facts about BK

Calcific BK is a deposition of calcium hydroxyapatite across the cornea at the level of Bowman's layer

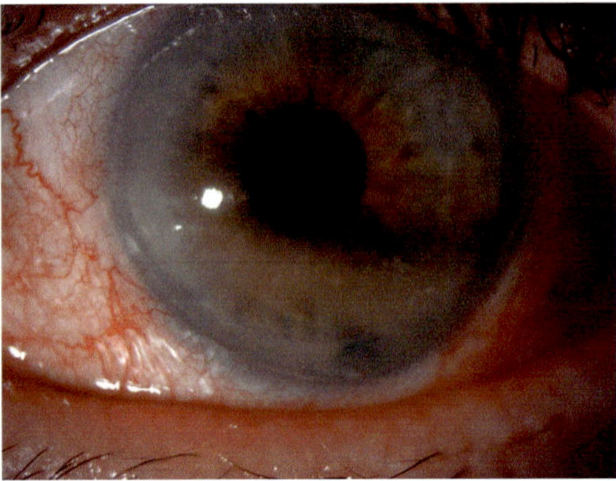

Fig. 8.18 Anterior segment image of a patient with calcific band keratopathy

- Lucent holes are scattered throughout the opacity and represent penetrating corneal nerves through Bowman's layer
- Exclude the presence of uveitis and the presence of silicone oil in AC.
- Exclude phthisis bulbi: hypotony, small eye

8.16.4 Investigations

- Bloods: U&E's, calcium, phosphorus, uric acid, ACE (if sarcoidosis suspected), PTH levels (if hyperparathyroidism suspected)
- CXR: sarcoidosis

8.16.5 Treatment

- Indication: patient becomes symptomatic with reduced VA, FB sensation, tearing or photophobia
- Options:
  - Lubricants and BCL for comfort (temporary measure)
  - Removal of epithelium followed by application of ethylenediaminetetraacetic acid (ETDA) to calcific areas. No.15 blade used to remove any residual calcium
  - Excimer laser phototherapeutic keratectomy (PTK)

8.16.6 Other Diagnoses to Consider

- Spheroidal degeneration (climatic droplet keratopathy): bilateral golden-yellow globular deposits within the interpalpebral area, deposits located within Bowman's layer and the anterior stroma
- Urate keratopathy: brown scintillating crystal deposits in the superficial cornea

8.17 Infectious Crystalline Keratopathy (ICK) (Table 8.15)

8.17.1 History

- ICK: hx of keratoplasty, hx of chronic use of topical steroids
- Multiple myeloma: backache
- Waldenstrom's macroglobulinaemia: epistaxis, bleeding gums
- Cryoglobulinamia: raynaud's phenomenon, urticaria, ulceration of the skin
- Drug Hx: gold

8.17.2 Examination

- ICK: crystalline fine needle like branching opacities in the anterior or mid-stroma (resembling a snowflake) occurring beneath an intact epithelium in the absence of clinically evident stromal inflammation (see Fig. 8.19)
- Cystinosis: myriad of fine needle shaped, highly refractile opacities present in the conjunctiva and corneal epithelium, stroma, and endothelium (see Fig. 8.20)
- Multiple myeloma: prominent corneal nerves, presence of numerous scintillating polychromatic crystals scattered throughout the corneal stroma and conjunctiva, BRVO/CRVO
- Waldenstrom's macroglobulinaemia: needle-like crystals scattered throughout the corneal stromal and conjunctiva, BRVO/CRVO
- Cryoglobulinaemia: superficial scattered crystalline corneal deposits
- Benign monoclonal gammopathy: diffuse deposition of gray-white, yellow, gray-brown,

Table 8.15 Key facts about ICK

A non-inflammatory intrastromal microbial colonization of a graft: Bacterial (S. *viridans*, S. *pneumoniae*, coagulase negative *streptococcus*. P. *aeruginosa*), fungal (*Candida*)
Diagnosis of ICK can be made clinically based upon a hx of keratoplasty, a hx of topical steroid use, and the clinical appearance of the lesion

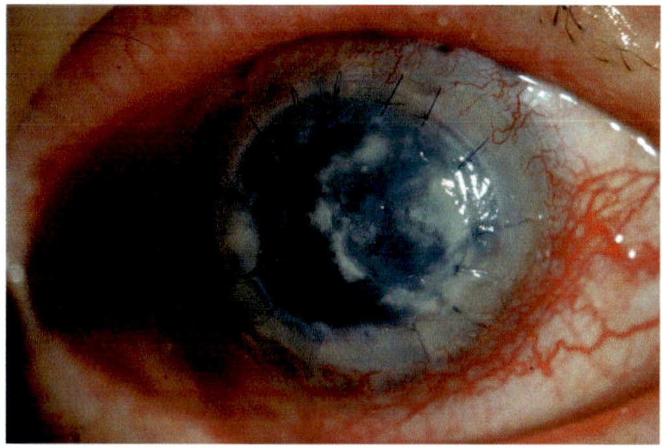

Fig. 8.19 Anterior segment image of a patient with infectious crystalline keratopathy secondary to Candida

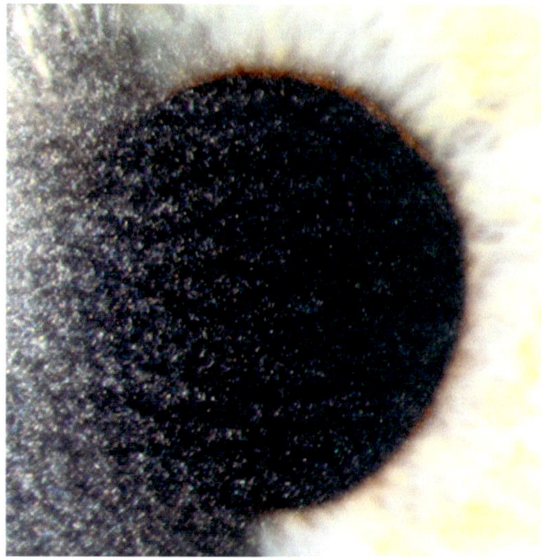

Fig. 8.20 Anterior segment image of a patient with cystinosis showing the diffuse presence of needle-shaped crystals throughout the corneal surface

or polychromatic iridescent dot-like opacities with a diffuse, fine stippled appearance

8.17.3 Investigations

- ICK: corneal scrapings for cultures and smears (help select appropriate antibiotics)
- Corneal biopsy: histopathologic analysis of the crystalline deposition
- Cystinosis: measure the leucocyte cysteine content, U&E's, conjunctival biopsy to measure the extracted free cysteine, electron microscopy to detect the characteristic crystals
- Multiple myeloma: bloods—hypercalcaemia & pancytopenia, XR spine—vertebral fractures and lytic punched out lesions, serum and urine electrophoresis, bone marrow biopsy

8.17.4 Treatment

- ICK: fortified intensive topical antibiotic drops—coverage for S.viridans includes topical vancomycin, stop topical corticosteroids, repeat PK in order to eradicate the infection or to treat scar formation that may have caused decreased VA
- Cystinosis: oral and topical cysteamine

8.17.5 Other Diagnoses to Consider

- Lipid keratopathies: Schnyder's crystalline dystrophy, Tangier disease, familial lipoprotein disorders, lecithin-cholesterol acyltransferase (LCAT) deficiency
- Errors of protein metabolism: cystinosis, tyrosinaemia, hyperuricaemia
- Acquired immunoprotein keratopathies: multiple myeloma, benign monoclonal gammopathy, cryoglobulinaemia, Waldenstrom's macroglobulinaemia
- Drug deposition: chrysiasis

8.18 Bullous Keratopathy (Table 8.16)

8.18.1 Causes (Table 8.17)

- FED
- Trauma from cataract surgery
- Angle-closure glaucoma (ACG)
- PXF keratopathy
- HSV endotheliitis
- Chandler's syndrome
- PPCD

8.18.2 Examination

- Diffuse epithelial microcysts with the presence of adjacent epithelial bullae (see Fig. 8.21)
- Examine for aphakia or pseudophakia: ABK/PBK
- Examine for guttae: FED
- Examine for a fixed and dilated pupil, iris atrophy (transillumination defect), presence of patent PI's (transillumination), shallow AC (using gonioscopy or Van Herrick's method—narrow slit beam at angle of 60 degrees onto cornea just anterior to the limbus—narrow if distance between iris and posterior cornea is < ¼ of the corneal thickness), glaukomflecken, increased CDR, defects on HVF testing: ACG
- Examine for whitish dandruff-like material on pupillary margin and anterior lens capsule centrally and peripherally with clear intermediate zone (if phakic), peripupillary transillumination defects, iridodonesis/phaco- or pseudo-phacodonesis: PXF
- Examine for KP's overlying stromal and epithelial oedema (pattern of KP's and distribution of oedema—diffuse, disciform, linear) and anterior uveitis: HSV endotheliitis (stromal infiltrate and neovascularisation, which are signs of stromal inflammation, are absent in endotheliitis)

Table 8.16 Characteristics of bullous keratopathy

Bullous keratopathy is characterised by corneal oedema with formation of epithelial bullae. It is secondary to loss or dysfunction of the corneal endothelial cells

Table 8.17 Causes of pseudophakic bullous keratopathy

Pre-operative factors: Pre-existing endothelial disease—FED, PXF, trauma, ACG, HSK
Intraoperative factors: Phacoemulsification in the AC, IOL-to-cornea touch, vitreous loss +/− nuclear loss, instrumentation, ultrasound damage
Postoperative factors: Retained lens fragment in the AC, IOL dislocation—Touch, vitreous-to-endothelial touch, flat AC (immediate with wound leakage or delayed with pupil block) with IOL touch to cornea, chronic post-op uveitis, ACIOL (chronic uveitis, IOL-to-cornea—Touch)

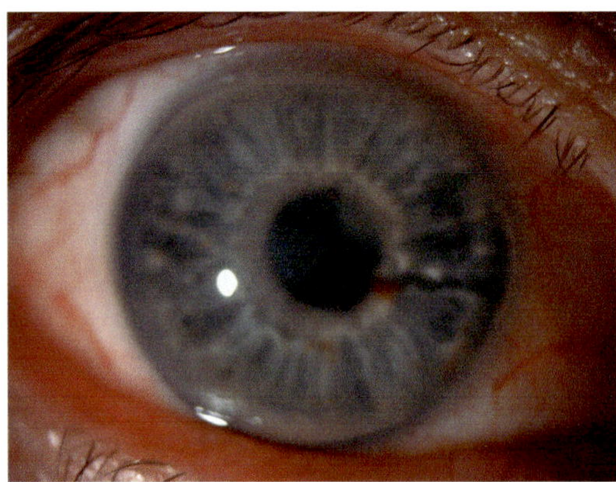

Fig. 8.21 Anterior segment image of a patient with pseudophakic bullous keratopathy with diffuse epithelial microcysts with several larger epithelial bullae

8.18.3 Treatment

- Medical management: topical corticosteroids for inflammation, reduction of IOP if raised, hypertonic agents (5% NaCL), BCL, anterior stromal puncture (form adhesions between epithelium and stroma, decreasing formation of bullae)—reserved for eyes that have poor visual potential or are poor surgical candidates
- Surgical management: repositioning or exchange of IOL if IOL subluxed or dislocated, removal of retained lens fragment if

present, endothelial keratoplasty when visual loss and discomfort becomes medically untreatable, conjunctival flap—reserved for eyes with poor visual potential or patients who are not candidates for corneal transplantation

8.19 Salzmann Nodular Degeneration (Table 8.18)

8.19.1 Causes

- Vernal keratoconjunctivitis
- Phlyctenular keratitis
- IK
- Post-corneal surgery
- MGD/Ocular Rosacea
- Trachoma

8.19.2 History

- Hx of allergic eye disease, dry eye, rosacea, or trachoma
- Hx of previous corneal surgeries

8.19.3 Examination

- Single or multiple white or blue elevated nodular lesions adjacent to areas of corneal scarring or a corneal pannus (see Fig. 8.22)
- An iron line may be seen at the edge of the nodules (indicate chronicity)
- Examine for rosacea
- Examine for ghost vessels
- Examine everted upper eyelid for papillary changes, Horner-trantas dots (VKC)
- Examine everted upper eyelid for Herbert pits or Arlt line

Table 8.18 Key facts about Salzmann nodular degeneration

Dense collagen plaques with hyalinisation are located between the epithelium and Bowman's layer
Female predilection

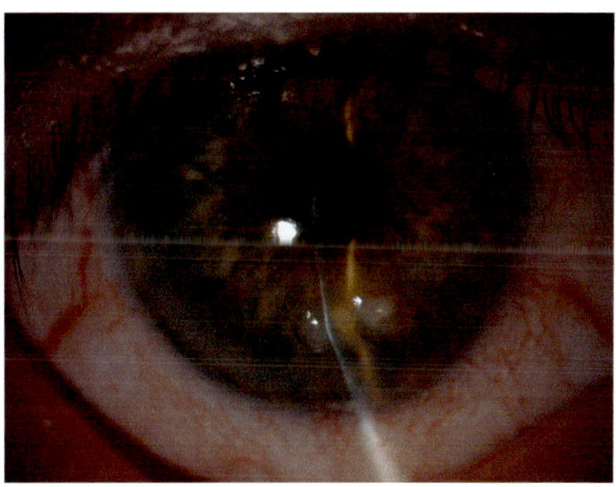

Fig. 8.22 Anterior segment image of a patient with Salzmann nodular degeneration with multiple elevated nodules inferiorly

8.19.4 Treatment

- Indications: comfort and vision
- Options:
  - Lubricants and BCL for comfort
  - Superficial keratectomy by manual dissection or PTK for nodules involving visual axis and causing decreased vision

8.19.5 Other Diagnoses to Consider

- Corneal keloids: more frequently in men, younger age group, occur post-trauma or in association with chronic ocular surface inflammation
- Spheroidal degeneration

8.20 Laser In-Situ Keratomileusis (LASIK)

8.20.1 LASIK Surgical Technique

- Two stage procedure:
  - Creation of a thin flap (consists of epithelium, Bowman's layer, and superficial stroma) (see Fig. 8.23) on the surface of the cornea using a microkeratome blade or using a FemtoSecond laser

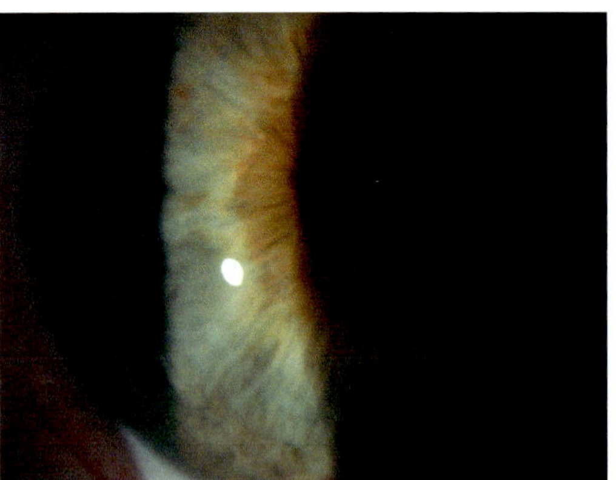

Fig. 8.23 Anterior segment image of a patient who previously had a LASIK refractive procedure to correct myopia. The LASIK flap can be seen as a fine white line in the anterior corneal stroma

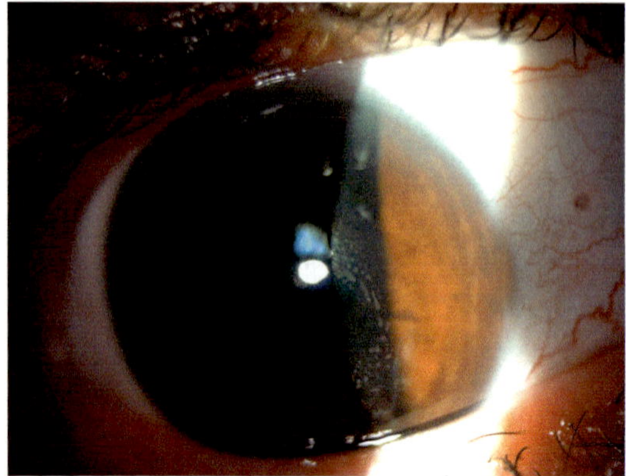

Fig. 8.24 Anterior segment image of a patient who previously had a LASIK refractive procedure which has been complicated with epithelial downgrowth

  - Flap is lifted and the stromal bed is then reshaped with the excimer laser

8.20.2 Complications of LASIK

- Intraoperative:
  - Creation of the flap with the microkeratome related problems:
    - Incomplete or irregular cut flap
    - Button hole
    - Corneal perforation
  - Photoablation-related problems:
    - Treatment decentration
    - Interface debris
    - Wrinkles
- Postoperative
  - Early:
    - Dislodged flaps:
      - First 24 hours
      - Emergency repositioning +/− sutures + BCL to prevent fixed folds and epithelial ingrowth
    - Diffuse lamellar keratitis (shifting sands of Sahara):
      - First 24 hours
      - Diffuse inflammation at flap interface without microbial cause
      - White sand-like deposits in lamellar cut plane in absence of both epithelial defect and AC activity
      - Aggressive topical steroid leads to rapid resolution
    - Infectious keratitis:
      - ≤10d—gram +ve organisms, >10/7d- mycobacteria
      - Flap lift, scrape, frequent topical antibiotics
    - Epithelial downgrowth (see Fig. 8.24):
      - Flap lift and scrape
  - Late
    - Iatrogenic keratectasia
    - Dry eye

8.21 Keratoconus (KC) (Table 8.19)

8.21.1 Associations of KC

- Ocular: retinitis pigmentosa (RP), vernal keratoconjunctivitis (VKC), leber's congenital amarousis (LCA), floppy eyelid syndrome

Table 8.19 Key facts about KC

Clinical term used to describe a bilateral condition in which the cornea assumes a conical shape because of thinning and protrusion
Process is non-inflammatory with no cellular infiltration and vascularisation
Onset occurs at about the age of puberty, where the cornea begins to thin and protrude, resulting in irregular astigmatism

- Systemic: *atopic disease* (asthma, eczema, hayfever), *Down's syndrome* (habitual ocular massage), *craniosynostosis* (Crouzon's syndrome, Apert syndrome), *connective tissue disorders* (Marfan's syndrome, Ehlers-Danlos syndrome, Osteogenesis Imperfecta)

8.21.2 History

- Atopic disease—asthma, eczema, hayfever
- Hx of connective tissue disorders—Marfan syndrome, Ehlers-Danlos syndrome, Osteogenesis Imperfecta
- Hx of Down's syndrome
- Hx of craniosynostosis
- Previous laser refractive surgery

8.21.3 Examination

- Corneal thinning from one-half to one-fifth of normal thickness is observed at the cone apex, the point of maximal protrusion (see Fig. 8.25)
- Prominent corneal nerves
- Munson's sign: angulation of the lower lid in downgaze
- Vogt's striae (ruptures in Bowman's layer): fine vertical posterior stromal folds, which disappear when external pressure is applied to the globe
- Fleischer ring (provides a landmark for the peripheral edge of the cone): partial or complete annular iron line commonly seen at the base of the cone—cobalt blue illumination in the widest possible slit beam can enhance the appearance of a subtle iron ring
- Rizutti's sign: conical reflection on nasal cornea when pentorch is shone temporally

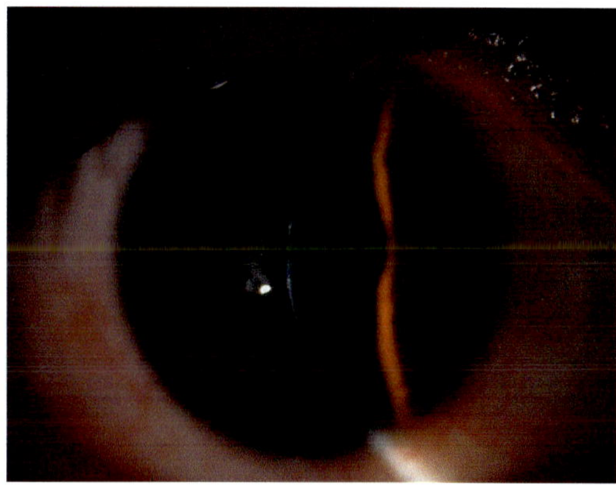

Fig. 8.25 Anterior segment image of a patient with KC showing thinning and scarring of the corneal stroma

- Charleaux oil droplet sign: dark reflex in area of cone on observation of the cornea with the pupil dilated using a direct ophthalmoscope set on plano
- Corneal hydrops (ruptures in DM): stromal imbibition of aqueous and result in marked corneal oedema
- Deep stromal scarring of cornea: suggestive of previous hydrops
- Examine lids for upslanting of palpebral aperture (Down's syndrome) and floppy eyelid syndrome (easily everted upper eyelid tarsal plates + upper palpebral conjunctival papillary reaction)
- Examine for conjunctival papillae, Horner-Trantas dots (raised white accumulations of eosinophils at the limbus), shield ulcer: VKC
- Examine for blue sclera (results from visualisation of the underlying choroid through a thin sclera): Osteogenesis Imperfecta, Ehlers-Danlos syndrome
- Examine for ectopia lentis: Marfan's syndrome (superotemporal lens subluxation), Ehlers-Danlos syndrome
- Dilated fundus examination for mid-peripheral bone spicule retinal pigmentation, waxy pallor of the optic disc, arteriolar attenuation (RP), retinal detachment (Marfan's syndrome, Ehlers-Danlos syndrome)
- Examine for nystagmus: LCA

8.21.4 Investigations

- Refraction: scissoring on retinoscopy (see Table 8.20), irregular astigmatism, high myopia (Marfan Syndrome)
- Keratometer: inability to superimpose the central keratometric rings suggest irregular astigmatism, look for inferior corneal steepening (early sign of KC) by performing central keratometry followed by keratometry in upward gaze
- Placido disc: a focal area of increased corneal curvature appears as an isolated area of smaller ring spacing and distortion—look for decreased ring spacing inferiorly in early KC. As the condition progresses, the ring spacing decreases overall and becomes increasingly irregular
- Corneal topography (see Sect. 2.9.4)

8.21.5 Treatment

- Spectacle correction
- Rigid gas permeable (RGP)/scleral/mini-scleral CL fitting
- Intacs (see Fig. 8.26): improves VA by flattening the central cornea, reducing astigmatism and centering the cornea, indicated for mild to moderate KC without corneal scarring—goal of procedure is to improve CL fit and comfort +/− improve BCVA, ideal candidates have low spherical equivalent and average K readings of <53D, ring segments do not prevent progression of the underlying disease, CCT needs to be ≥450 μm
- CXL: slows or halts progression of the underlying disease + improves CL fit, improves VA by decreasing both corneal curvature and astigmatism, CCT needs to be >400 μm thick. Failure of CL is not an indication for CXL (Table 8.21)

Table 8.20 Causes of a scissoring reflex on retinoscopy

Causes
Corneal ectasias: KC, pellucid marginal degeneration
Corneal scars
Tilted lens
Irregular retina (e.g. from a RD)

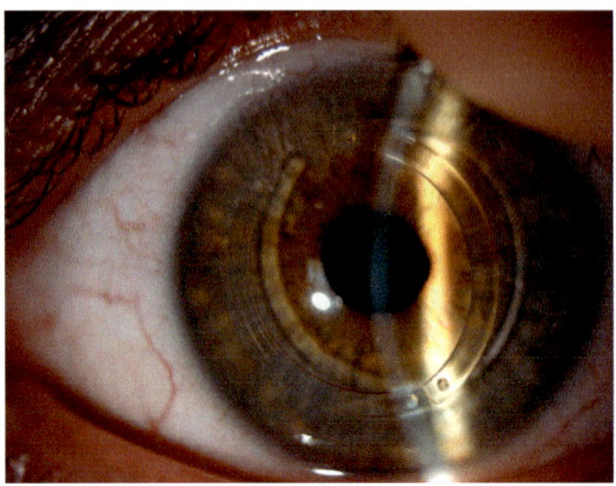

Fig. 8.26 Anterior segment image of a patient with KC who had corneal intacs implanted into the mid-peripheral corneal stroma to improve vision

Table 8.21 Dresden protocol for CXL

Dresden protocol
Gold standard protocol for CXL
Technique:
Topical anaesthesia
Central 9 mm of corneal epithelium removed
0.1% riboflavin every 1–5 minutes for 30 minutes
Exposure to UVA light (3 mW/cm^2, 365 nm wavelength) for 30 minutes (total energy 5.4 J/cm^2)
Topical antibiotic
BCL insertion
Contraindications:
CCT <400
Age >35 years old

- Keratoplasty (PK or DALK—if normal DM): Indications—intolerance to CL wear or severe irregular astigmatism with poor vision despite gls or CL or significant stromal scarring involving the visual axis
- Corneal hydrops: hypertonic NaCL drops &/or ointment, BCL, topical steroids, cycloplegia, intracameral gas—20% SF6 (acts as a mechanical barrier, reducing aqueous flow into the stroma through the rupture in DM)

8.21.6 Other Diagnoses to Consider

- Pellucid marginal degeneration: bilateral inferior corneal thinning (typically from 4 to 8 o'clock position) with maximal protrusion occurs just superior to the area of thinning (see Fig. 8.27), shift in axis of astigmatism

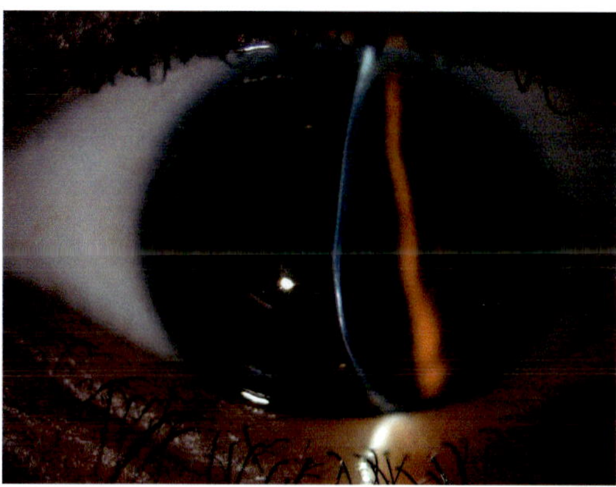

Fig. 8.27 Anterior segment image of a patient with pellucid marginal degeneration with inferior corneal thinning and corneal protrusion above the area of inferior thinning

from against-the-rule superiorly to with-the-rule near the point of maximal protrusion, crab-claw appearance on power map of corneal topography (see Fig. 2.82)
- Keratoglobus: bilateral globular protrusion of the cornea results from generalised thinning most marked in the periphery, prone to corneal rupture after minimal trauma, corneal topography reveals diffuse steepening on the power map and diffuse thinning on the pachymetric map
- Post-traumatic ectasia e.g. post-LASIK ectasia
- Protrusion of cornea subsequent to corneal thinning from ulceration

8.22 Ocular Cicatricial Pemphigoid (OCP)

8.22.1 Causes of Symblepharon Formation

- Steven-Johnson syndrome (SJS)/Toxic epidermal necrolysis (TEN)
- Chemical burns
- Trachoma
- Avitaminosis A
- Severe chronic keratoconjunctivitis caused by bacteria or viruses
- Medications (causing cicatricial conjunctivitis): systemic—penicillamine, topical—pilocarpine, timolol, gentamicin 1.5%)

8.22.2 History

- Exclude SJS/TEN: drug Hx (sulfonamides, anti-convulsants, allopurinol) and previous or current infections (mycobacteria, HSV)
- Exclude avitaminosis A: nyctalopia, hx of cystic fibrosis or hx of jejunoileal bypass (fat malabsorption)
- Ask about previous chemical injury to eye
- Ask about Hx of trachoma

8.22.3 Examination

- OCP
  - Subepithelial conjunctival fibrosis (stage I)
  - Fornix foreshortening (stage II)
  - Symblepharon formation (stage III) (see Fig. 8.28)
  - Ankyloblepharon and surface keratinisation of ocular surface (stage IV)
  - Progressive sicca syndrome with unstable tear film (obstruction of lacrimal ductules and meibomian gland ducts), trichiasis and entropion occur from subepithelial fibrosis with eventual corneal neovascularisation, corneal ulceration and scarring

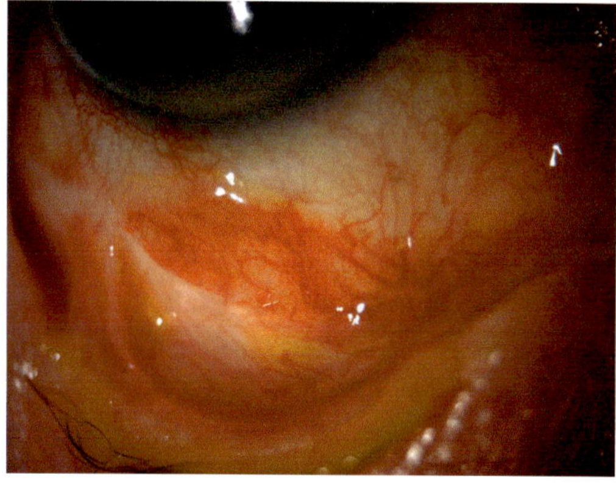

Fig. 8.28 Anterior segment image of a patient with OCP with symblepharon formation

- SJS/TEN
  - Acute eye findings (bilateral): pseudomembranous conjunctivitis +/− secondary purulent bacterial conjunctivitis, corneal ulceration, anterior uveitis
  - Chronic eye findings (bilateral): lid margin keratinisation, scarring (subconjunctival fibrosis), symblepharon formation, & cicatrization of the conjunctiva—leads to entropion formation, trichiasis, & instability of tear film (goblet cell dysfunction), keratoconjunctivitis sicca (KCS), persistent ED, corneal scarring & stromal neovascularisation, LESC failure
  - Non-ocular findings:
    - *SJS*: erythematous macules that develop central necrosis to form vesicles, bullae, and areas of denudation on the face, trunk, and extremities, 2 or more mucosal surfaces are involved (conjunctiva, oral cavity, upper airway or oesophagus, GI tract, anogenital mucosa), less than 20% of body surface area involved,
    - *TEN*: involvement of more than 30% of the body surface area, positive Nikolsky's sign (friction applied to healthy areas of skin, causing epidermis is wrinkle and separate), mucous membranes are usually involved with severe erosions of the lips, oral surface, conjunctiva, and genital areas.
- Trachoma (*C. trachomatis* Serovars A-C): follicular conjunctivitis, Herbert's pits (breakdown of follicles around limbus with subsequent tissue necrosis), Artl's line (linear scarring on the upper tarsus), cicatricial lid changes with tarsal plate contraction with accompanying trichiasis—lead to superior pannus, scarring or opacification of cornea (see Table 8.22).
- Avitaminosis A: conjunctival xerosis (metaplastic keratinised surface) and Bitot spots (foamy), corneal xerosis (localised or generalised oedema with a typical dry, lackluster appearance, later the cornea may develop a "peau d'orange" appearance from keratinization), corneal ulceration/keratomalacia (frank necrosis or sloughing of the corneal stroma)

Table 8.22 WHO grading system for Trachoma

TF grade: 5 or more 0.5 mm or more in diameter follicles in upper tarsal conjunctiva
TI grade: Inflammatory thickening of tarsal conjunctiva that obscures more than half of normal deep tarsal vessels
TS grade: Scarring in tarsal conjunctiva
TT grade: Trichiasis
CO grade: Corneal opacity over pupil

8.22.4 Investigations

- OCP: conjunctival biopsy to look for linear immune deposits (must be demonstrated before treatment initiated) along the epithelial basement membrane zone (immunofluorescence microscopy—Michel's transport medium)
- SJS/TEN: bloods for raised inflammatory markers, conjunctival biopsy to look for absence of goblet cells in SJS, referral to dermatologists/plastic surgery for skin biopsy in TEN
- Avitaminosis A: vitamin A levels
- Trachoma: swabs for immunofluorescent staining, cell culture, PCR, ELISA

8.22.5 Treatment

- OCP
  - Treat sicca syndrome (artificial tears, ointments, punctal occlusion if Schirmer values less than 5 mm/5 min)
  - Treat chronic blepharitis and meibomitis (warm compresses, lid hygiene, oral doxycycline 100 mg OD 3/12 then 50 mg OD)
  - Immunomodulatory therapy if cases that are active and rapidly progressive (mild: dapsone + oral prednisolone, moderate: MTX, AZT or MMF + oral prednisolone, severe: IV/PO cyclophosphamide + oral prednisolone)
  - Keratoprosthesis for stage IV disease
- SJS/TEN
  - Systemic disease: refer to intensive burn care unit for monitoring of fluid balance, respiratory function, nutritional requirements, and wound care

– Ophthalmic disease—acute stage: frequent conjunctival irrigation + prophylactic topical antibiotics to prevent secondary infection, frequent PF topical lubricants (lubricate conjunctival and corneal epithelium), cycloplegics (anterior uveitis), topical steroids but monitor for secondary bacterial keratitis (anterior uveitis), lamellar keratoplasty or PK if perforation impending or occurs, conjunctival flap (Gunderson flap) for an impending perforation, daily lysis of the symblepharon or placement of a symblepharon ring
– Ophthalmic disease—chronic stage: repair cicatricial entropion and treat trichiasis (epilation, electrolysis, cryotherapy), frequent PF topical lubricants to treat KCS, fornix reconstruction through mucous membrane grafts, BCLs, AMG or tarsorrhaphy for persistent ED, limbal stem cell transplant for LECS failure, keratoprosthesis for end stage corneal scarring and neovascularisation

- Avitaminosis A
  - Vitamin A supplementation
- Trachoma
  - TF grade—azithromycin 1 g PO, TT grade—bilamellar tarsal rotation, TI grade—azithromycin 1 g PO, TS grade—lubricants (infection no longer present at TS stage and so antimicrobial therapy is not useful), CO grade—PK

8.23 Penetrating Keratoplasty (PK)

8.23.1 Definition

- Transplant procedure in which full-thickness host corneal tissue is replaced with donor tissue

8.23.2 Examination

- Examine for a full thickness graft with no graft-host interface present to identity patients who have had a PK surgical procedure

8.23.3 Indications

- Visual (restoration of corneal clarity): keratoconus, pseudophakic/aphakic corneal oedema, FED, deep stromal corneal dystrophies, corneal scarring secondary to herpes simplex keratopathy, infections, trauma
- Tectonic (restoration of structural integrity): corneal thinning, actual or threatened perforation
- Therapeutic: infective keratitis

8.23.4 Contraindications

- Relative
  - Epithelial dysfunction secondary to limbal stem cell deficiency (aniridia, chemical injuries), severe neurotrophic, and dry eye states
  - Stromal vascularisation, especially when involving more than 2 quadrants
  - Multiple (2 or more) graft failures

8.23.5 Advantages of PK

- Familiarity

8.23.6 Disadvantages of PK

- Higher risk of graft rejection
- Risk of suture-related complication
- Risk of traumatic wound dehiscence and globe rupture

8.23.7 Complications

- Intraoperative
  - Scleral perforation from bridal suture placement or scleral ring placement
  - Damage to donor cornea
  - Trephine reversal: causes unwanted hyperopia and difficulty in closing wound
  - Retained Descemet's membrane: suggested by presence of double AC on post-op day 1 (patient will need re-grafting)

  - Iris-lens damage during trephination
  - AC haemorrhage from iris damage
  - Suprachoroidal expulsive haemorrhage
- Early postoperative
  - Wound leaks (shallow AC, seidel +ve): if leak controlled with BCL resuturing is not necessary
  - Epithelial defect: treat with lubricants, topical antibiotics +/− BCL +/− tarsorrhaphy, decrease application of topical steroids
  - Filamentary keratitis: treat with lubricants and removal
  - Suture-related complications:
    - Infection
    - Immune infiltrates: multiple on recipient side of cornea and treated with intensive topical steroids and removal of suture
    - Endophthalmitis
    - Kaye dots: small epithelial dots a short distance from sutures on the donor side—not pathologic and usually disappear after suture removal
  - Glaucoma
  - Anterior synechiae: increases graft oedema and risk of rejection—postop dilatation increases AC depth
  - Pupillary block: shallow AC, raised IOP, intact wound—aqueous misdirection, choroidal detachment
  - Urrets-Zavalia pupil: irregular pupil a few days post PK for KC—iris stromal atrophy, ectropion uvea, multiple posterior synechiae, discrete subcapsular opacities
- Late postoperative
  - Graft failure (see Fig. 8.29): causes include immunologic rejection, poor donor quality, intraoperative trauma to donor endothelium, prolonged flat AC in the immediate postoperative period, HSV reactivation
  - Immunologic rejection (risk of an immunologic rejection episode is constant over the first 3 years after transplantation):
    - Epithelial rejection: elevated epithelial rejection line those stains with fluorescein—responds to topical steroids
    - Subepithelial infiltrates: immune reaction seen only in the donor tissue without associated conjunctivitis—responds to topical steroids
    - Endothelial rejection line (khodadoust line): does not extend beyond graft-host junction with KP's at the leading edge with an overlying hazy and oedematous stroma +/− DM folds—if left untreated this line will proceed across the donor endothelium from the point of origin at the graft wound leaving damaged endothelium behind it—treat with intensive topical steroids or IV methylprednisolone
    - Diffuse endothelial rejection: isolated or diffuse KP's are scattered across the endothelium and are limited to the donor endothelium and often associated with an AC reaction—treat with intensive topical steroids or IV methylprednisolone)
    - Post-operative astigmatism

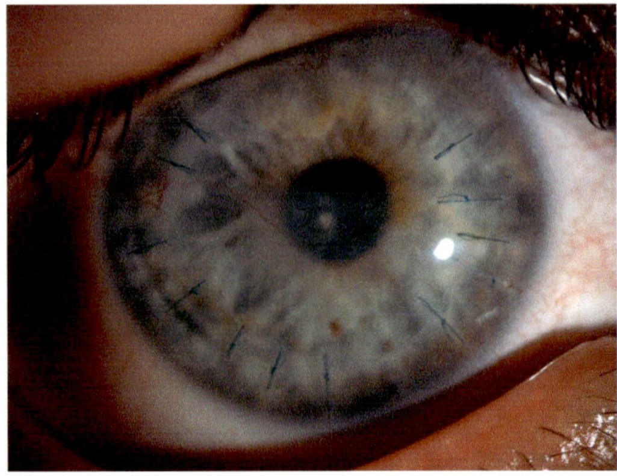

Fig. 8.29 Anterior segment image of a patient with a failed penetrating keratoplasty showing diffuse corneal haze with stromal neovascularisation

8.23.8 Risk Factors for Immunologic Rejection (Poor Prognostic Factors)

- Corneal stromal vascularisation
- Reduced corneal sensation
- Ocular surface disease (Dry eye, OCP, SJS)
- Previous graft failure
- Large graft size (8–8.5 mm) and eccentric grafts

- Uncontrolled glaucoma
- Active or recurrent herpetic inflammation

8.23.9 Penetrating Keratoplasty in Children

- Preoperative complications
  - Need for frequent topical drop applications
  - Requirement of frequent postoperative visits
  - Commitment to amblyopia therapy
- Intraoperative complications
  - Higher posterior pressure: forward displacement of lens and iris with increased risk of iris prolapse, lens extrusion, suprachoroidal haemorrhage
  - Smaller donor grafts and more pliable tissue with more difficulty with suturing
- Postoperative complications
  - Stronger inflammatory response to surgery than adults: increased risk of graft rejection and failure, contraction of tissue at the 360-degree interface between host and donor tissue can lead to loosening of the sutures which is a risk factor for suture abscesses and neovascularisation of the corneal tissue
  - Frequent application of topical steroids to reduce high risk of rejection
  - High risk of infection: loose sutures, wound dehiscence, high dose of topical steroids—longer use of prophylactic topical antibiotics
  - Amblyopia: high rate of vision loss despite clear graft
- Prognosis
  - Only about 33% of the grafts performed for Peter's anomaly, Sclerocornea, or intrauterine infection were clear at 1 year
  - In infants less than 1 year old, only 25% of grafts were clear at 1 year
  - In children between 1–4 years old, about 50% were clear at 1 year
  - In children older than 4 years, about 65% were clear at 1 year

8.24 Deep Anterior Lamellar Keratoplasty (DALK)

8.24.1 Definition

- Surgical technique whereby the majority of the corneal stroma down to the Descemet's membrane is replaced by donor tissue, leaving the host endothelium intact (see Fig. 8.30)

8.24.2 Examination

- Examine for a graft-host interface to identify patients who have had a DALK surgical procedure

8.24.3 Indications

- Visual: corneal ectasias, stromal dystrophies sparing Descemet's membrane and endothelium, corneal stromal scars from previous infections or chemical injuries
- Tectonic: descemetocoele, pellucid marginal degeneration, advanced Terrien's marginal degeneration, peripheral corneal melts from autoimmune disorders (e.g. rheumatoid arthritis)

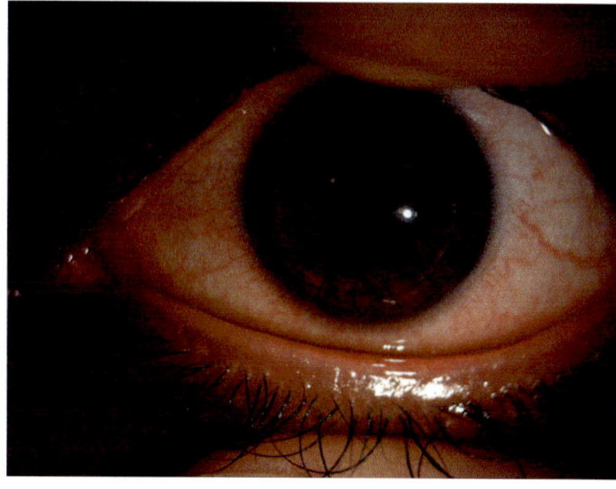

Fig. 8.30 Anterior segment image of a patient who had a DALK procedure

8.24.4 Contraindications

- Absolute: endothelial dysfunction
- Relative: epithelial dysfunction

8.24.5 Advantages of DALK

- Preserve host endothelium
- Lower incidence of graft rejection

8.24.6 Disadvantages of DALK

- Working near or at Descemet's membrane with potential risk for perforation

8.24.7 Complications

- Intraoperative
  - Perforations and ruptures of Descemet's membrane during trephination, stromal dissection or with a suture needle
- Postoperative
  - Urrets-Zavalia syndrome (fixed dilated pupil from irreversible damage to the iris sphincter): associated with air/gas injection into the AC at the end of surgery
  - Suture-related complications:
    - Loosening of sutures
    - Suture abscesses
  - Stromal rejection

8.25 Descemet Stripping Automated Endothelial Keratoplasty (DSAEK)

8.25.1 Definition

- Partial thickness cornea transplant procedure that involves selective removal of recipient Descemet's membrane and endothelium, followed by transplantation of donor corneal endothelium, Descemet's membrane and posterior stroma

8.25.2 Examination

- DSAEK grafts can be visualised as a subtle ring (see Fig. 8.31) in the diffuse illumination and can be seen protruding posteriorly from the cornea in the inferior aspect of the slit beam

8.25.3 Indications

- Endothelial dystrophy: FED, posterior polymorphous corneal dystrophy
- Bullous keratopathy: aphakia, pseudophakia
- Endothelial failure: trauma, previous surgery, angle closure, tubes
- ICE syndrome
- Failed PK—if acceptable refractive result was achieved

8.25.4 Contraindications

- Stromal opacity or scarring that limits visual potential
- Keratoconus, ectasia
- Hypotony/pre-phthisical eye

8.25.5 Advantages of DSAEK

- No suture-related complications
- Reduced incidence of graft rejection
- Rapid visual rehabilitation

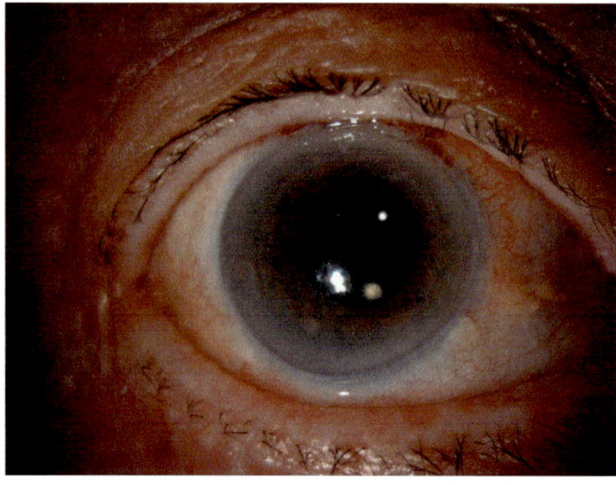

Fig. 8.31 Anterior segment image of a patient who had a DSAEK procedure

8.25.6 Disadvantages of DSAEK

- Possible interface haze and deposits
- Potential significant loss of donor endothelium during surgical procedure
- Risk of graft dislocation

8.25.7 Complications

- Intraoperative
  - Complications with donor tissue preparation: damaged donor tissue, eccentric trephination, thin donor tissue (increase chance of graft striae)
  - Retained Descemet's membrane: prevents proper attachment of the DSAEK graft
  - Air management: donor tissue attachment appears to be dependent on the maintenance of air in the AC (challenge in aphakic eyes or pseudophakic eyes with an open posterior capsule and in patients with previous trabeculectomy or glaucoma drainage implants)
- Postoperative
  - Donor dislocation (methods to avoid: cornea surface massage with a flap roller, vents are made in the midperipheral recipient cornea down to the graft interface)
  - Primary graft failure (graft failing to clear within the first 2 weeks after the op):
    - Primary failure: unhealthy donor endothelial, inadequate preservation of the corn, or traumatic pre- or intraoperative technique
    - Secondary failure: graft rejection, detached donor from residual fluid or viscoelastic in interface, retained Descemet's membrane
  - Graft rejection: presence of AC cells +/– KP's and concomitant corneal oedema
  - Pupillary block glaucoma: due to placement of excessively large gas bubble in the AC or migration of the air bubble behind the iris—tx by partial evacuation of the air bubble and concurrent replacement with BSS to maintain the AC
  - Endothelial cell loss
  - Refractive change: hyperopic refractive shift post DSAEK
  - Interface deposits and epithelial ingrowth: epithelial cells may be dragged onto stromal surface during insertion of the donor tissue—if epithelial ingrowth does not progress to the visual axis and if the donor is well attached to the recipient surface, the patient can be followed closely without surgical intervention

8.26 Descemet Membrane Endothelial Keratoplasty (DMEK)

8.26.1 Definition

- Partial thickness cornea transplant procedure that involves selective removal of recipient Descemet's membrane and endothelium, followed by transplantation of donor corneal endothelium and Descemet's membrane

8.26.2 Examination

- DMEK grafts can be visualised as a subtle ring in the diffuse illumination

8.26.3 Indications

- Endothelial dystrophy: FED, PPMD, CHED
- Bullous keratopathy: pseudophakic
- Endothelial failure: failed endothelial keratoplasty
- ICE syndrome

8.26.4 Contraindications

- Stromal scarring
- Keratoconus, ectasia
- Hypotony
- Inability to lie flat
- Aniridia, Aphakia, ACIOL
- Previous glaucoma surgery (trabeculectomy/GDI)

8.26.5 Advantages of DMEK

- Superior visual outcomes and faster visual rehabilitation compared to DSAEK
- Lower immunologic graft rejection rate compared to DSAEK

8.26.6 Disadvantages of DMEK

- Higher rate of primary graft failure compared to DSAEK

8.26.7 Complications

- Intraoperative:
- Damage to donor tissue during preparation
- Upside down graft
- Postoperative:
- Graft detachment
- Graft rejection and failure
- Raised IOP and secondary glaucoma

8.27 Anterior Scleritis (Table 8.23)

8.27.1 Associations of Scleritis

- Non-infectious: systemic diseases (RA, GPA, relapsing polychondritis, PAN, IBD, SLE, Churg-Strauss syndrome), surgically induced (strabismus surgery, trabeculectomy, cataract extraction, RD repairs, pterygium excisions)

Table 8.23 Causes of a blue sclera

Scleritis
Osteogenesis Imperfecta: hx of fractures (brittle bones), hyperextensibility of the joints, sensorineural hearing loss, hyperopia
Connective tissue disorders: Ehlers-Danlos syndrome (ectopia lentis, RD, hyperelasticity and fragility of the skin), Marfan's syndrome (ectopia lentis, RD, myopia, arachnodactyly, high arched palate), pseudoxanthoma elasticum—PXE (angioid streaks +/− CNV, optic disc drusen, yellowish lumps on the skin of the neck, axillae, and antecubital fossa)
Keratoconus/Keratoglobus

- Infectious: traumatic +/− FB, post-surgical, extension from other structures (keratitis, choroiditis, endophthalmitis, conjunctivitis, orbital cellulitis, sinusitis, dacryocystitis)

8.27.2 History

- Scleritis: severe pain enough to awaken patient at night
- Episcleritis: mild discomfort or FB sensation
- POHx of previous ocular surgeries
- PMHx of any systemic diseases (GPA—sinusitis, bloody nasal discharge, saddle nose, relapsing polychondritis—degenerative pinna cartilage)

8.27.3 Examination

- Anterior scleritis (no blanching with topical phenylephrine): diffuse (distortion and tortuosity of both episcleral and scleral vascular networks, post resolution the sclera appears translucent or bluish-gray suggesting thinning of the sclera), nodular (firm, immobile, and tender yellow to deep red nodule to palpation), necrotising with inflammation (white avascular areas of sclera and conjunctiva, with surrounding scleral oedema and congestion, blue-black uveal tissue may appear as the overlying sclera becomes thin and translucent—see Fig. 8.32), necrotising without inflammation (scleromalacia perforans—complete lack of symptoms with thinned and avascular areas of episclera and sclera with no surrounding inflammation)
- Posterior scleritis: choroidal folds, choroidal effusions, exudative RD, CMO, optic disc oedema
- Examine hands for RA: swollen MCP, PIP, wrist, or MTP joints, Z-deformity of thumb, swan-neck and Boutonniere deformity of fingers
- Examine for skin rashes: SLE (discoid rash, malar rash), PAN (livedo reticularis)

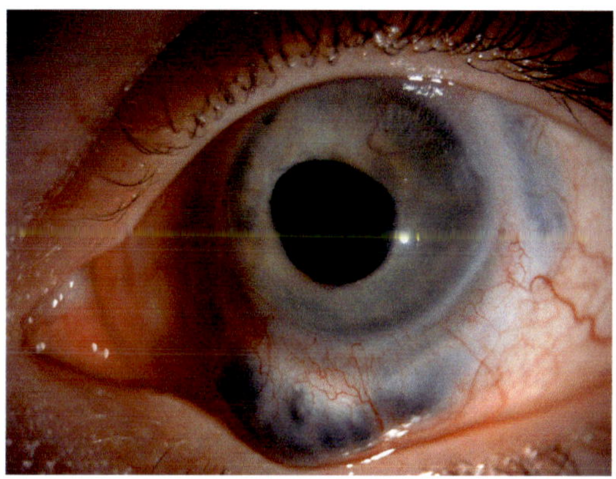

Fig. 8.32 Anterior segment image of a patient with multiple previous episodes of scleritis showing severe scleromalacia with diffuse purple hue from increased uveal visibility. There is a large area of uveal protrusion with only a thin layer of conjunctiva overlying the uvea

8.27.4 Investigations

- B-scan: T-sign—posterior scleritis
- Bloods: c-ANCA (GPA, PAN), p-ANCA (Churg-Strauss syndrome), ANA (SLE), rheumatoid factor (RA), anti-CCP (RA), HLA-B27 (IBD)
- CXR: GPA (pulmonary haemorrhage), Churg-Strauss syndrome
- Urinalysis: proteinuria & haematuria (GPA)

8.27.5 Treatment

- Oral NSAIDS: reduce pain and inflammation in non-necrotising scleritis
- Systemic corticosteroids: indicated in severe non-necrotising scleritis unresponsive to oral NSAIDs and in necrotising scleritis—oral prednisolone at a starting dose of 1 mg/kg/day followed by a slow taper according to response
- Systemic immunosuppresants: indicated in cases of necrotising scleritis and scleritis of any type in the setting of GPA (cyclophosphamide) or PAN, or when maintenance dose of oral prednisolone ≤7.5 mg OD is not possible without recurrence of disease

8.27.6 Other Diagnoses to Consider

- Episcleritis: simple: sectoral or diffuse redness which blanches with topical phenylephrine, globe non-tender, no Ix required unless hx suggestive of systemic disease, tx with topical lubricants, oral NSAIDS, topical corticosteroids, nodular: red nodule arising from episclera that can be moved separately from the sclera and conjunctiva, globe non-tender, blanches with topical phenylephrine, no Ix required unless Hx suggestive of systemic disease, tx as for simple episcleritis
- Peripheral ulcerative keratitis (PUK): unilateral crescent-shaped peripheral corneal ulceration with overlying epithelial defect and stromal thinning, sectoral or diffuse scleritis, tx involves ensuring adequate tear film (lubricants, punctal plugs, punctal cautery), prophylactic topical antibiotics, oral doxycycline and oral vitamin C (inhibit proteases and free radicals, respectively), systemic immunosuppression (liaise with rheumatologist, corticosteroids—IV methylprednisolone or oral prednisolone, MTX, AZT, MMF, ciclosporin, cyclophosphamide), BCL + cyanoacrylate glue for pending/actual perforation, conjunctival recession, tectonic freehand lamellar keratoplasty, conjunctival flaps
- Mooren's ulcer: diagnosis of exclusion (rule out Hepatitis C), unilateral peripheral ulceration with stromal melt with leading edge undermining epithelium, ulcer advances centrally and circumferentially, no associated scleritis (but conjunctiva and episcleral inflammation), tx similar to PUK—nay require interferon if coexistent hepatitis C (as directed by hepatologist)

8.28 Limbal Epithelial Stem Cell (LESC) Deficiency

8.28.1 Causes

- LESC deficiency occurs when there is sufficient disturbance or destruction of the limbal stem cells of the corneal epithelium, resulting in disruption of the normal physiologic regenerative process and repopulation of corneal epithelium
- Typical causes include
  - Aniridia
  - Chemical (alkali injury) or thermal injury
  - Chronic contact lens wear
  - Preservative drop toxicity
  - OCP
  - SJS/TEN
  - Ocular surgery: multiple previous pterygium excisions

8.28.2 History

- History of ocular chemical injuries
- History of contact lens wear
- History of ocular surgeries e.g. pterygium surgery
- History of aniridia

8.28.3 Examination

- Examine for loss of palisades of Vogt, late staining of the corneal epithelium with fluorescein, persistent epithelial defects, corneal neovascularisation, corneal scarring, and the development of a peripheral pannus
- A "whorled" appearance of the corneal epithelium (results from conjunctivalisation of the corneal epithelium—invasion of conjunctival epithelium onto the corneal surface—occurs when <25–33% of LESC remain)

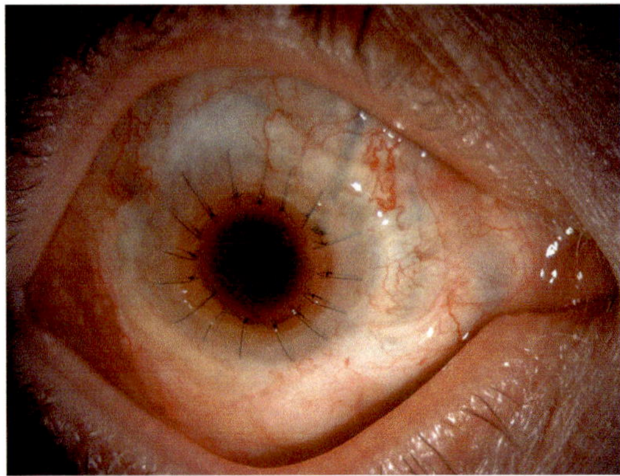

Fig. 8.33 Anterior segment image of a patient with congenital aniridia who had a limbal stem cell transplantation

- Examine for a limbal stem cell transplant graft (see Fig. 8.33)

8.28.4 Investigations

- Impression cytology (nitrocellulose paper is pressed onto cornea and examined under the microscope): presence of mucin-containing goblet cells on the corneal epithelium and the absence of normal differentiation markers of corneal epithelium (CK 3 and 12)

8.28.5 Treatment

- Any chronic inflammation of the conjunctiva, conjunctival scarring, symblepharon formation, trichiasis, and MGD must be identified and treated prior to limbal stem cell grafting
- Partial: conjunctivalised metaplastic epithelium on cornea—if visual axis affected: sequential sector conjunctival epitheliectomy + AMG, if visual axis is not affected: sequential sector conjunctival epitheliectomy, with fibrovascular pannus—sector limbal transplant + AMG

- Total: unilateral—conjunctival limbal autograft (CLAU) from contralateral better eye, bilateral—living-related keratolimbal allograft (CLAL), cadaveric CLAL

8.29 Gundersen Flap

8.29.1 Definition

- A Gundersen flap (see Fig. 8.34) is a surgical technique that uses a thin, bipedicle, total conjunctival bridge flap to achieve a number of purposes including
  - To restore the integrity of a compromised ocular surface
  - To provide a metabolic and mechanical support for corneal healing
  - To relieve pain
  - To provide an alternative to invasive surgery or enucleation

8.29.2 Indications

- Persistent corneal epithelial defect
- Unresponsive ulcerative microbial keratitis
- Corneal thinning and perforation

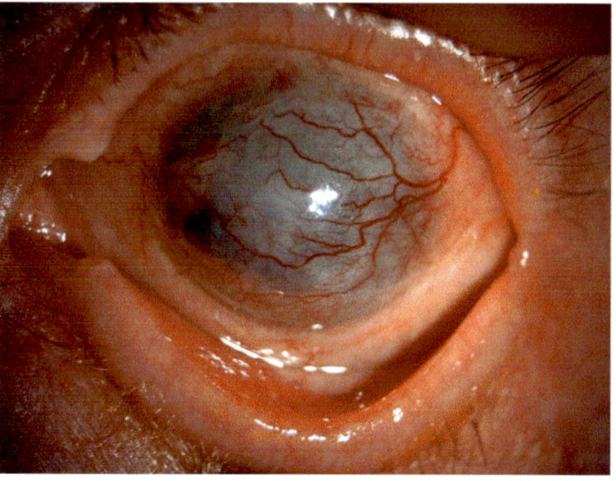

Fig. 8.34 Anterior segment image of a patient with a Gundersen flap

8.29.3 Advantages

- Can improve quality of life in patients with an eye with poor visual potential and a chronically irritated anterior segment
- Can eliminate the need for chronic medication and bandage lenses

8.29.4 Disadvantages

- Vision significantly decreased by the conjunctival flap that covers the visual axis
- Prevents monitoring of disease progression by obstructing any view of the cornea and anterior chamber
- Poor cosmetic appearance

8.29.5 Complications

- Intraoperative
  - Buttonhole formation
  - Dissection of an inadequate flap
  - Excessive haemorrhage
- Postoperative
  - Ptosis
  - Retraction of the flap
  - Vascularisation and opacification of the underlying cornea

9 Glaucoma & Lid

Timothy H. M. Fung, Mong-Loon Kuet, and Winfried M. K. Amoaku

Abstract

This chapter offers a comprehensive overview of a wide range of glaucoma and eyelid pathologies that are commonly encountered in an OSCE exam for ophthalmologists.

9.1 Pseudoexfoliation (PXF) Syndrome (Table 9.1)

9.1.1 Risk Factors

- Female sex
- Increasing age
- Polymorphisms in LOXL1 (lysyl oxidase-like 1) gene

Table 9.1 Useful information about PXF syndrome

A systemic condition in which white dandruff like material is deposited over the anterior segment of the eye and other organs such as the heart, skin, lungs, kidneys

9.1.2 Examination

- Whitish dandruff-like material on pupillary border and anterior lens capsule (centrally and peripherally with clear intermediate zone) (see Fig. 9.1)
- Peripupillary transillumination defects
- Poor mydriasis

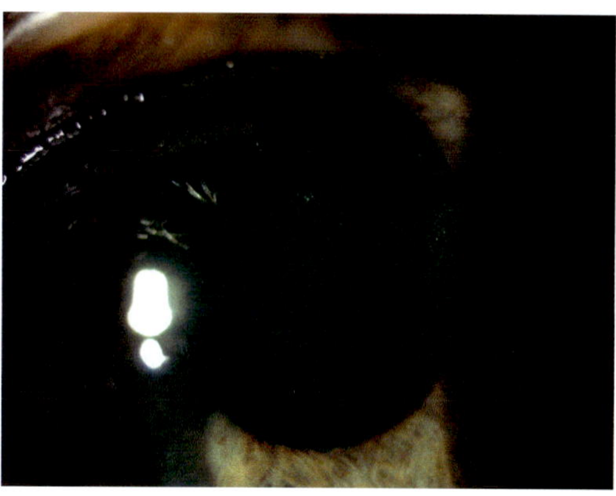

Fig. 9.1 Anterior segment image of a patient with PXF syndrome showing the whitish dandruff-like material on the lens capsule

T. H. M. Fung (✉)
University Hospitals of Derby & Burton NHS Foundation Trust, Royal Derby Hospital, Derby, UK
e-mail: timothy.fung@nhs.net

M.-L. Kuet
Moorfields Eye Hospital, London, UK

W. M. K. Amoaku
Eye, Ear, Nose and Throat Centre, Queens Medical Centre, Nottingham University Hospitals NHS Trust, Nottingham, UK

T. H. M. Fung, W. M. K. Amoaku (eds.), *Viva and OSCE Exams in Ophthalmology*,
https://doi.org/10.1007/978-3-031-97401-4_9

Table 9.2 Locating Schwalbe's line on gonioscopy

Finding Schwalbe's line on gonioscopy: dark room, short narrow slit beam at oblique angle, identified by the corneal wedge that is created at the junction between the inner light beam along the corneal endothelium and the outer light beam along the corneoscleral junction

- Iridodonesis/phacodonesis
- Cataract: nuclear, PSC
- Check IOP
- Perform gonioscopy (Table 9.2)
  - Open angle
  - Closed angle from weak zonules with anterior movement of lens-iris diaphragm
  - Increased but irregular TM pigmentation
  - Flecks of PXF material
  - Sampaolesi's line—pigmented line anterior to Schwalbe's line
- Examine the optic nerves to look for signs of glaucoma:
  - Generalised signs: CDR 0.7 or more, asymmetry of CDR of 0.2 or more, progressive enlargement of cup
  - Focal signs: rim thinning/notching (ISNT rule), regional pallor, NFL haemorrhage, NFL loss

9.1.3 Investigations

- HVF
  - Early: paracentral defect, nasal step—IT or ST rim thinning, temporal wedge—nasal disc thinning
  - Late: arcuate defect, double arcuate defect, central vision only
  - Ensure VF defects correlate with optic nerve head findings

9.1.4 Treatment

- If raised IOP: medical, SLT, trabeculectomy (higher complication rate but similar overall success to trabeculectomy in POAG)
- Cataract extraction if IOP controlled: weak zonules (CTR), small pupil (intracameral phenylephrine, iris hooks/malyugin ring/I-Ring pupil expander)

9.1.5 Prognosis

- Compared to POAG, the disease course is more severe, with poorer response to medical therapy and more frequent need for surgery
- Glaucoma risk: 1% at 1 year, 5% at 5 years, 15% at 15 years

9.2 Pigment Dispersion Syndrome (PDS) (Table 9.3)

9.2.1 Risk Factors for PDS

- Myopia
- Age 20–40
- Male sex
- Caucasian ethnicity

9.2.2 Risk Factors for Conversion of PDS to Pigmentary Glaucoma

- Male gender
- Black race
- Higher degrees of myopia
- Krukenberg spindle (see Fig. 9.2)

9.2.3 Examination

- Krukenberg spindle: pigment on the endothelium in a vertical line
- Mid-peripheral spoke like iris transillumination defects
- Scheie strip: pigment deposit along the insertion of the zonular fibers to the anterior lens capsule

Table 9.3 Useful information about PDS

A condition characterised by the release of pigment from the mid-peripheral posterior surface of the iris, from where it is distributed around the anterior segment
Pigment release is thought to occur as a result of posterior bowing of the mid peripheral iris rubbing against the zonules
Reverse pupillary block: AC pressure greater than PC pressure (pushing peripheral iris backwards against the lens zonules)

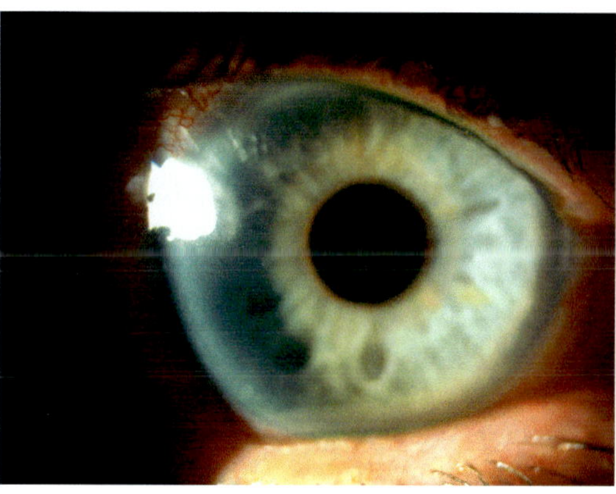

Fig. 9.2 Anterior segment image of a patient with PDS showing a Krukenberg spindle

- Check IOP
- Perform gonioscopy
  - Open angle
  - 360 degrees of homogenous pigmentation of TM (see Fig. 9.3)
  - Sampaolesi's line
  - Posterior bowing of the iris
  - Dilated fundus exam:
    - Look at optic disc for signs of glaucoma:
      - Generalised signs: CDR 0.7 or more, asymmetry of CDR of 0.2 or more, progressive enlargement of cup
      - Focal signs: rim thinning/notching—ISNT rule, regional pallor, NFL haemorrhage, NFL loss
    - Look at the peripheral retinal for lattice degeneration

9.2.4 Investigations

- HVF
  - Early: paracentral defect, nasal step (IT or ST rim thinning), temporal wedge (nasal disc thinning)
  - Late: arcuate defect, double arcuate defect, central vision only

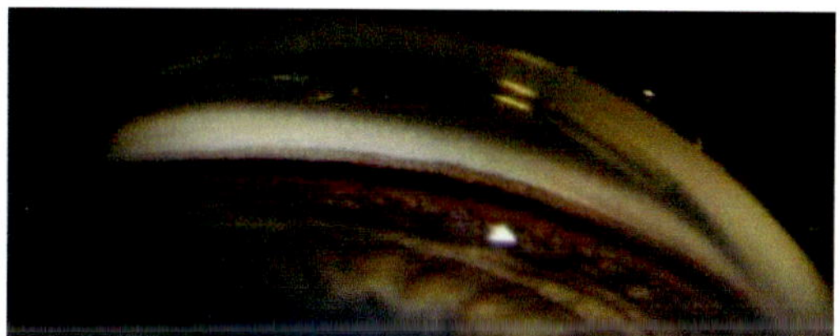

Fig. 9.3 Gonioscopic view of a patient with PDS syndrome showing homogenous pigmentation of the TM

9.2.5 Treatment

- If IOP raised
  - Medical
  - SLT: relatively contraindicated as the TM is heavily pigmented, increasing the risk of significant post-SLT elevations in IOP (NICE Guidance—NG81) [3]
  - Trabeculectomy: increased risk of post-op hypotonus maculopathy
- With increasing age, there is an apparent improvement or at least an arrest in the disease process—postulated to result from an increasing AL of the lens over time, which lifts the peripheral iris off the lens zonules, preventing the rubbing between iris and zonules and the subsequent release of pigment granules

9.2.6 Role of PI in PDS/Pigmentary Glaucoma

- Insufficient evidence of high quality on the effectiveness of PI for pigmentary glaucoma or PDS

9.2.7 Other Diagnoses to Consider

- Trauma: surgical (pigment dispersion with PCIOL—rubbing of lens haptic and optic against posterior iris—transillumination defects corresponding to position of lens haptic and edges of optic) and non-surgical (angle-recession)

- Uveitis: photophobia, KP's, cells / flare, PS, gonioscopy (PAS, increased TM pigmentation but is seen as irregular clumps of pigment randomly dispersed, usually in the inferior quadrants / widened ciliary body band in angle recession)
- POAG with increased pigmentation: TM pigmentation tends to be more segmental, pt's typically older

9.3 Neovascular Glaucoma (NVG)

9.3.1 Causes of NVG

- Retinal ischaemic diseases: Ischaemic CRVO (50% risk of conversion to NVG), DR, OIS, chronic RD, BRVO, CRAO, SCR
- Inflammatory diseases: Uveitis
- Tumours: iris (melanoma), retinal or choroidal

9.3.2 Examination

- Iris rubeosis: small, fine tortuous vessels at the pupillary margin, mid and peripheral anterior surface of the iris (see Fig. 9.4)
- Ectropion uvea
- Check the IOP
- Perform gonioscopy
  - Look for NVA (see Fig. 9.5)—vessels on the TM and ciliary body band
  - Open angle or closed angle with PAS (typically ends at Schwalbe's line)
- Examine the optic nerve for signs of glaucoma:
  - Generalised signs: CDR 0.7 or more, asymmetry of CDR of 0.2 or more, progressive enlargement of cup
  - Focal signs: rim thinning/notching (ISNT rule), regional pallor, NFL haemorrhage, NFL loss)
- Dilated fundus examination to look for any underlying retinal ischaemic diseases

9.3.3 Investigations

- Carotid doppler US: if no retinal pathology or asymmetric DR (rule out OIS)
- B-scan US: if poor/no fundal view from dense cataract (tumours, RD)
- HVF: early: paracentral defect, nasal step—IT or ST rim thinning, temporal wedge—nasal disc thinning / late: arcuate defect, double arcuate defect, central vision only

9.3.4 Treatment

- Treat underlying cause: RD repair for RD, carotid endarterectomy for OIS

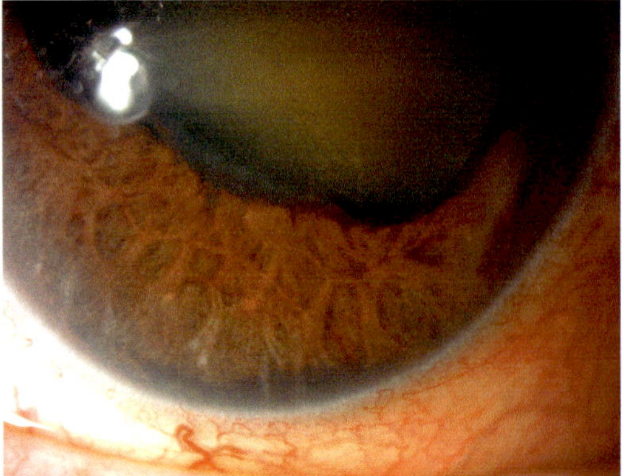

Fig. 9.4 Anterior segment image of a patient with neovascular glaucoma with NVI

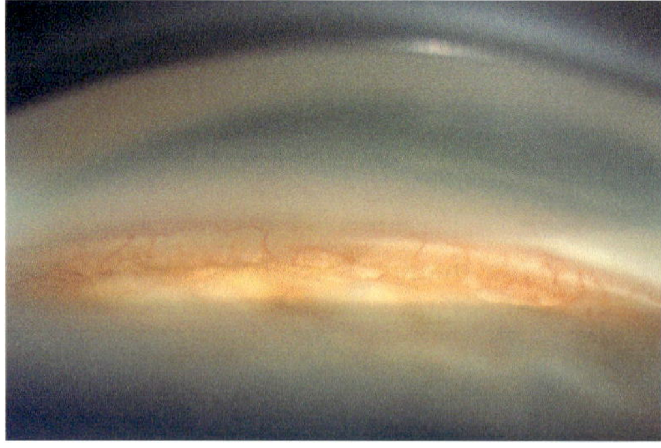

Fig. 9.5 Gonioscopic view of a patient with neovascular glaucoma with NVA

- Neovascularisation: PRP +/− anti-VEGF injection
- IOP control: reduction of raised IOP with medical treatment and surgical treatment if medical treatment fails (GDI, trabeculectomy, cyclodiode—visual potential of eye will determine best surgical option for patient)
- Pain control: reduction of IOP if raised, cycloplegia, topical steroids, if vision poor and eye phthisical—retrobulbar alcohol, evisceration/enucleation

9.4 Primary Congenital Glaucoma (PCG) (Table 9.4)

9.4.1 Examination

- Enlargement of globe/cornea if onset less than age 4 years: Buphthalmos
- Dense corneal stromal opacification
- Curvilinear lines in Descemet's membrane (from stretching of the cornea): Haab striae
- Measure the corneal diameter (more than 13 mm)
- Check IOP
- Perform gonioscopy: high iris insertion, indistinct angle landmarks, fine iris processes
- Examine the optic disc for signs of glaucoma
  - Generalised signs: CDR 0.7 or more, asymmetry of CDR of 0.2 or more, progressive enlargement of cup
  - Focal signs: rim thinning/notching (ISNT rule), regional pallor, NFL haemorrhage, NFL loss

Table 9.4 Useful information about PCG

Angle dysgenesis causes reduced aqueous outflow
Typically diagnosed within 1st year of life but not usually at birth
2% chance of affected parent having affected child if no FHx of PCG
Bilateral in 70% and more common in males
PCG (CYP1B1 gene): 1st 3 years of age
Primary juvenile glaucoma (MYOC gene): 4–16 years of age

9.4.2 Investigations

- HVF: early: paracentral defect, nasal step (IT or ST rim thinning), temporal wedge (nasal disc thinning) / late: arcuate defect, double arcuate defect, central vision only

9.4.3 Treatment

- If IOP raised/glaucoma
  - Medical treatment to lower IOP acutely
  - Surgical treatment options:
    - Goniotomy
    - Trabeculotomy
    - Trabeculectomy
    - GDI (see Fig. 9.6)
    - Cyclodiode
- Corneal opacification
  - PK

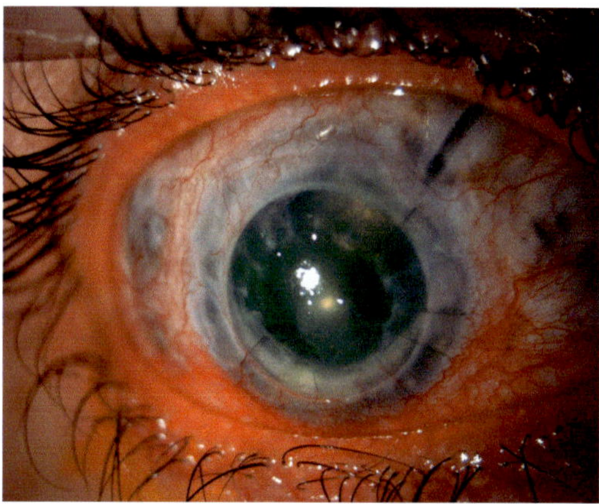

Fig. 9.6 Anterior segment image of a patient with congenital glaucoma with a tube and a failed PK graft

9.5 Aphakic Glaucoma

9.5.1 Causes of Aphakia

- Removal of congenital cataracts without subsequent IOL implantation
- Complicated cataract surgery without IOL implantation
- Dislocated lens: trauma or connective tissue disorders
- Previous ICCE with spectacle rehabilitation
- Primary congenital aphakia

9.5.2 Mechanism of IOP Elevation in Aphakia

- Distortion of AC angle
- PAS: flat AC post-op, inflammation
- Pigment dispersion post cataract surgery
- Pupil block (post ICCE): adherence between the iris and anterior vitreous face after a transient flat AC secondary to a wound leak

9.5.3 Complications of Aphakia

- Glaucoma
- Retinal detachment (RD): vitreous traction on retina (complicated surgery)

9.5.4 Examination

- Aphakic (see Fig. 9.7)
- Check IOP
- Perform gonioscopy: open angle, PAS
- Examine the optic disc for signs of glaucoma
  - Generalised signs: CDR 0.7 or more, asymmetry of CDR of 0.2 or more, progressive enlargement of cup
  - Focal signs: rim thinning/notching (ISNT rule), regional pallor, NFL haemorrhage, NFL loss
- Perform a dilated fundus examination to look for a RD

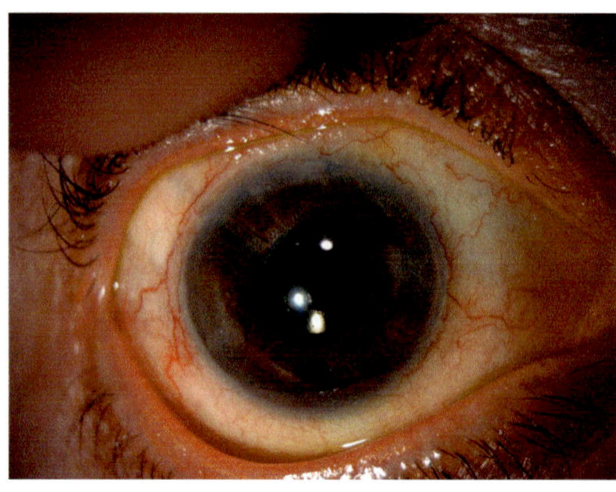

Fig. 9.7 Anterior segment image showing a GDI implant in an aphakic eye

9.5.5 Investigations

- HVF: early: paracentral defect, nasal step (IT or ST rim thinning), temporal wedge (nasal disc thinning) / late: arcuate defect, double arcuate defect, central vision only

9.5.6 Treatment

- Medical
- Surgical options
  - GDI's (initial surgical intervention) (see Fig. 9.7)
  - Trabeculectomy

9.6 Sturge-Weber Syndrome (Encephalotrigeminala angiomatosis) (Table 9.5)

9.6.1 Examination

- Naevus flammeus of the face (port-wine stain) along distribution of CN V (see Fig. 9.8)
- Dilated and tortuous episcleral and conjunctival vessels
- Check IOP

Table 9.5 Key facts about Sturge-Weber syndrome

Type of phakomatosis (group of disorders characterised by hamartomas: congenital tumours arising from tissue that is normally found in the involved area) that occurs sporadically (no inheritance pattern)
No race or sex predilection
Tumours are present at birth
Mechanism of glaucoma: developmental anomaly AC angle before the first decade of life, elevated episcleral venous pressure after the first decade of life

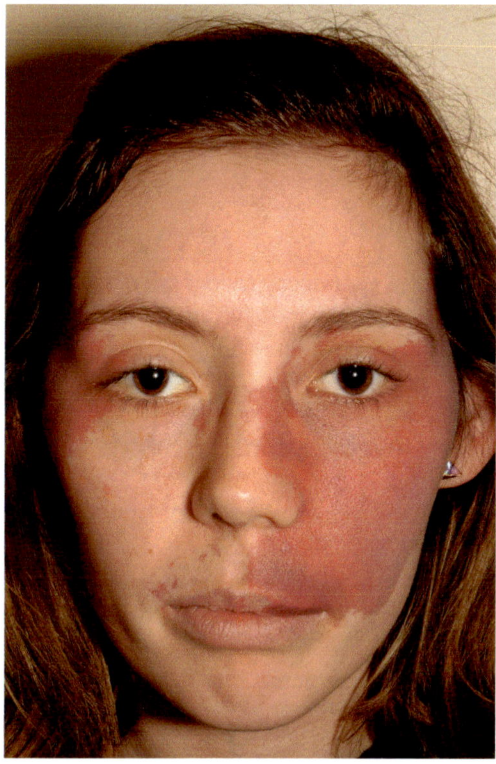

Fig. 9.8 Facial photograph of a patient with Sturge-Weber syndrome with a naevus flammeus (port-wine stain) of the face

- Perform gonioscopy: open angle or lack of anatomical landmarks
- Examine the optic disc for signs of glaucoma
  – Generalised signs: CDR 0.7 or more, asymmetry of CDR of 0.2 or more, progressive enlargement of cup
  – Focal signs: rim thinning/notching (ISNT rule), regional pallor, NFL haemorrhage, NFL loss

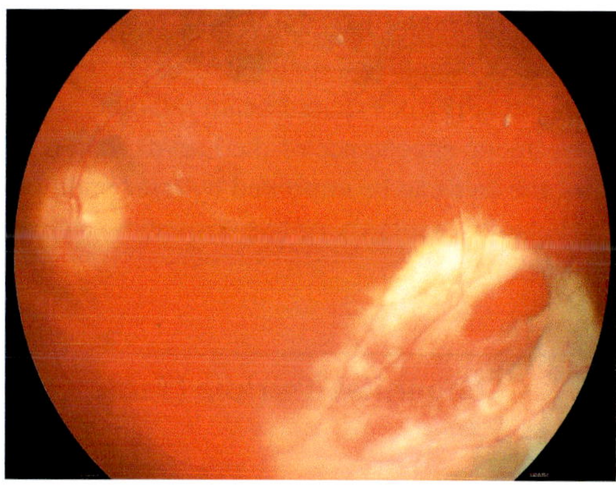

Fig. 9.9 Colour fundus image of the patient in Fig. 9.8 showing an area of chorioretinal scarring from previous external beam radiotherapy treatment for a circumscribed choroidal haemangioma

- Perform a dilated fundus examination to look for a diffuse (tomato ketchup red appearing fundus) or circumscribed choroidal haemangioma (see Fig. 9.9)

9.6.2 Investigations

- HVF: early: paracentral defect, nasal step (IT or ST rim thinning), temporal wedge (nasal disc thinning) / late: arcuate defect, double arcuate defect, central vision only
- MRI head: look for CNS haemangiomas

9.6.3 Treatment

- If IOP high
  – Medical treatment: topical medications
  – Surgical treatment if medical treatment fails:
    - Trabeculotomy
    - Goniotomy
    - Trabeculectomy (associated with intra-operative choroidal effusion +/– expulsive haemorrhage) with prior prophylactic posterior sclerostomies
    - GDI
    - Cyclodiode

- Treat choroidal haemangiomas if associated with a secondary exudative RD: options include PDT or external beam radiotherapy
- Cosmetic appearance of the naevus flammeus of the face can be improved by laser photocoagulation in infancy or late cosmetics to cover the defect

9.7 Congenital Aniridia (Table 9.6)

9.7.1 History

- Positive FHx of aniridia (AD inheritance)
- Always ask about FHx as if case is sporadic there is a risk of WAGR syndrome (Wilms tumour—nephroblastoma, aniridia, GU abnormalities, reduced IQ)

9.7.2 Examination

- Nystagmus
- Corneal opacification with subepithelial fibrosis and peripheral pannus—LESC deficiency
- Iris hypoplasia (rudimentary iris stump) (see Fig. 9.10)
- Cataracts
- Check IOP
- Examine optic nerve
  - Look for optic nerve hypoplasia
  - Look for signs of glaucoma:
    - Generalised signs: CDR 0.7 or more, asymmetry of CDR of 0.2 or more, progressive enlargement of cup
    - Focal signs: rim thinning/notching (ISNT rule), regional pallor, NFL haemorrhage, NFL loss

Table 9.6 Useful information about congenital aniridia

Congenital aniridia is a bilateral disease with complete or partial absence of iris as well as other ocular abnormalities
AD with variable expressivity in two-thirds and sporadic in one-third
Caused by mutations in PAX6 gene

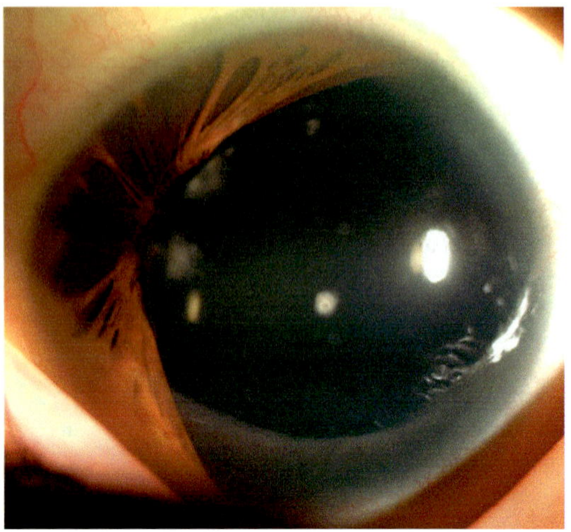

Fig. 9.10 Anterior segment image of a patient with congenital aniridia

- Perform gonioscopy to look for chronic angle closure caused by blockage of TM by rudimentary iris stump rotating forward

9.7.3 Investigations

- OCT: foveal hypoplasia (see Fig. 9.11)
- Renal US: nephroblastoma
- HVF: early: paracentral defect, nasal step—IT or ST rim thinning, temporal wedge—nasal disc thinning / late: arcuate defect, double arcuate defect, central vision only

9.7.4 Treatment

- If IOP raised / glaucoma: topical medication, goniotomy (if clear cornea)—useless of advanced cases, trabeculotomy (if cornea cloudy), trabeculectomy—usually first surgical procedure in cases of aniridic glaucoma refractory to medical tx, GDI's, Cyclodiode in cases refractory to trabeculectomy or GDI
- Keratopathy: Scleral CL, keratolimbal allograft (KLAL), Boston keratoprosthesis (KPro) for severe aniridia associated keratopathy
- Dry eye: lubricants, ointments, punctal occlusion

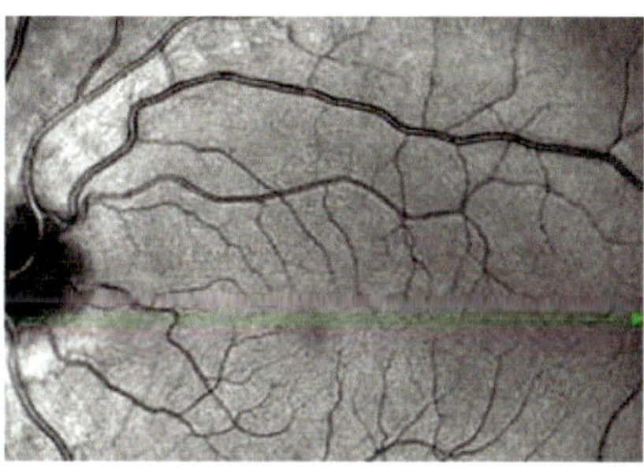
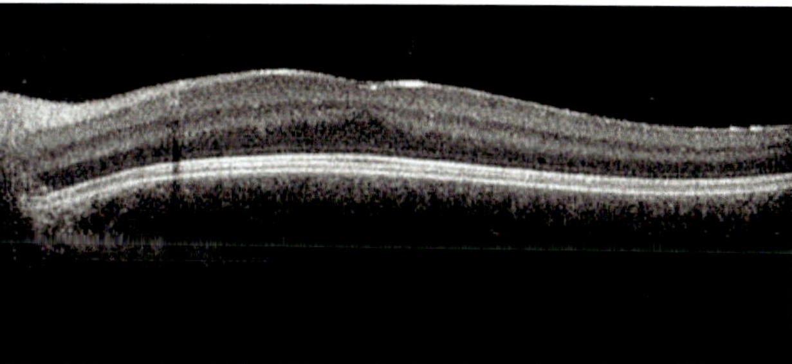

Fig. 9.11 OCT image of a patient with Rieger syndrome showing foveal hypoplasia

- Cataract extraction for visually significant cataracts—beware of fragile anterior capsule
- If patient has significant glare or photophobia (from iris atrophy, polycoria, corectopia): painted or tinted CL

9.7.5 Other Diagnoses to Consider

- Trauma: post-surgical or non-surgical
- Rieger syndrome (see Sect. 9.8)
- ICE syndrome (findings are unilateral)
  - Essential iris atrophy: corectopia, iris atrophy with polycoria (iris hole formation), guttata (fine hammered silver appearance) +/− corneal oedema, ectropion uveae, gonioscopy shows broad based PAS extending to and beyond Schwalbe line
  - Cogan-Reese syndrome: unilateral multiple diffuse brown nodules on anterior surface of iris, guttata (fine hammered silver appearance) +/− corneal oedema, ectropion uveae, iridocorneal adhesions, pupil distortion +/− corectopia, gonioscopy shows broad based PAS extending to and beyond Schwalbe line
- Gillespie syndrome: AR, ataxia

9.8 Rieger Syndrome

- Anterior segment dysgenesis (failure of the normal development of the anterior segment of the eye)

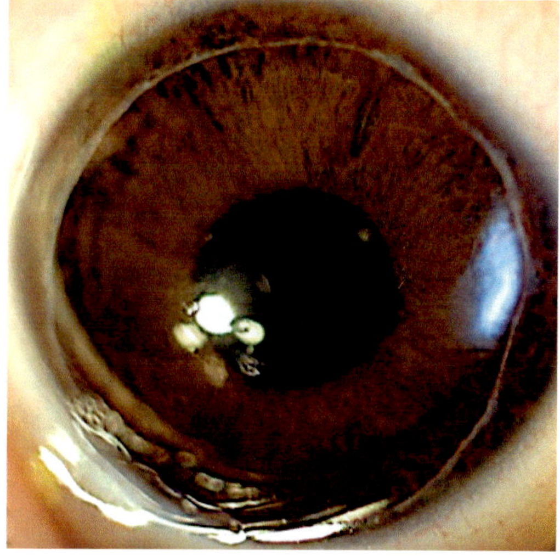

Fig. 9.12 Anterior segment image of a patient with Rieger syndrome showing a posterior embryotoxin and iris atrophy

9.8.1 History

- Positive FHx (AD)

9.8.2 Examination

- Findings tend to be bilateral
- Posterior embryotoxin (see Fig. 9.12)
- Iris atrophy / iris hypoplasia
- Corectopia
- Polycoria (multiple holes in the iris)
- Visible pupil sphincter against the hypoplastic iris stroma
- Check IOP

- Perform gonioscopy: prominent Schwalbe line, iris strands bridging the AC angle from the peripheral iris to the prominent ridge
- Examine the optic disc for signs of glaucoma
- Systemic examination to look for redundant periumbilical skin, microdontia, oligodontia

9.8.3 Investigations

- HVF: early: paracentral defect, nasal step—IT or ST rim thinning, temporal wedge—nasal disc thinning / late: arcuate defect, double arcuate defect, central vision only

9.8.4 Treatment

- If IOP raised / glaucoma: medical, surgical—goniotomy, trabeculotomy, trabeculectomy, GDI, Cyclodiode
- If pt. has significant glare or photophobia (from iris atrophy, polycoria, corectopia): painted or tinted CL

9.8.5 Other Diagnoses to Consider

- ICE syndrome: unilateral, guttata, lack of systemic abnormalities, manifestation in middle age, female predominance
- Peters anomaly: central corneal opacity with absence of DM and endothelium, iridocorneal adhesions

9.9 Trabeculectomy (Table 9.7)

9.9.1 Indications

- Failure to control IOP with MTMT
- Pt intolerant of topical medications
- Pt wishes to be drop free
- First line treatment if patient has advanced disease and needs lower IOP's or if patient is at high risk of progression

Table 9.7 Useful information about trabeculectomies

A filtering surgical procedure that creates an opening, or fistula, at the limbus, which allows a direct communication between the AC and subconjunctival space, with the subsequent formation of a filtering bleb (elevation of conjunctiva at the surgical site) (see Fig. 9.13)
Fistula bypasses the TM, Schlemm canal, and collecting channels

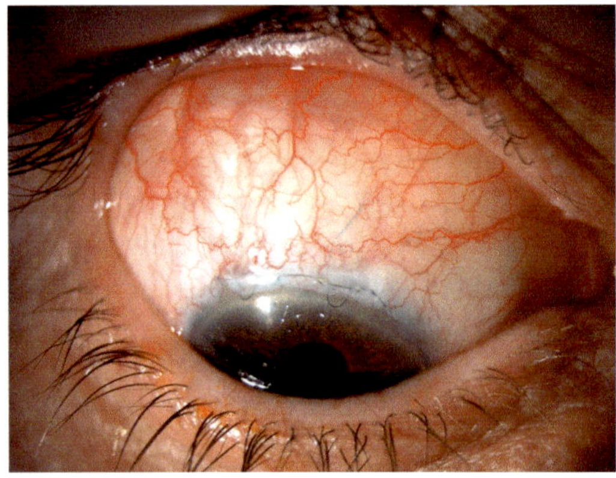

Fig. 9.13 Anterior segment image of a patient with a trabeculectomy with visible releasable sutures

9.9.2 Description of Bleb Morphology

- Area
  - Diffuse: thin-walled blebs with large surface area and low elevation
  - Flat: blebs showing no important signs of bleb development such as elevation or microcysts
- Vascularity
  - Avascular
  - Similar to adjacent conjunctiva
  - Increased
  - Massive
- Corkscrew vessels
  - None
  - In one third
  - In two thirds
  - Entire bleb
- Microcysts
  - None
  - Over the scleral flap

- Lateral or medial aspect of the scleral flap
- Entire bleb

- Encapsulation (thick-walled blebs with cystic appearance, high elevation and a well demarcated area—see Fig. 9.14)
  - None
  - In one-third
  - In two-thirds
  - Entire bleb

9.9.3 Complications

- Intraoperative: tearing or buttonholing of the conjunctival flap, haemorrhage (episcleral, choroidal), choroidal effusion, vitreous loss, lens injury, tearing of scleral flap from its limbal hinge
- Early postoperative
  (a) Hypotony with or without Bowmans folds (IOP < 6 mmHg) (see Fig. 9.15) and flat/shallow AC:
    (1) Conjunctival defect / leak (flat bleb)—pressure patching (check leak again in 1–2 hours post patching), temporarily tapering topical steroids, BCL, cyanoacrylate tissue adhesive or autologous fibrin glue, injection of autologous blood inside or around a bleb, surgical re-suturing
    (2) Excessive filtration (extensive bleb)—decreasing the frequency of postoperative topical steroids, reform AC with viscoelastic, resuturing of scleral flap if choroidal detachments present with maculopathy
    (3) Ciliary body shutdown (flat bleb)—reform AC with viscoelastic, treat excessive inflammation with topical steroids

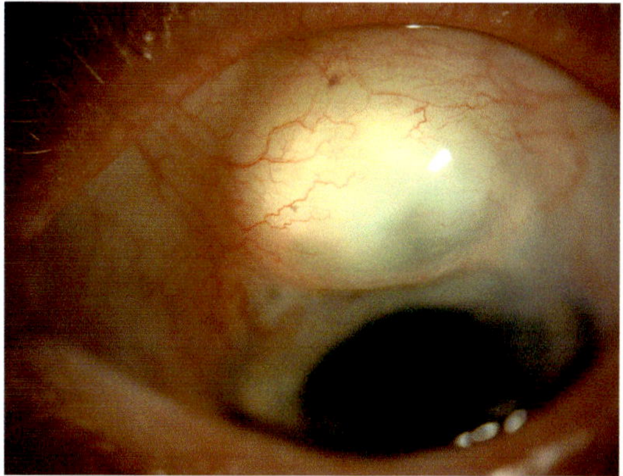

Fig. 9.14 Anterior segment image of a patient with an encapsulated bleb

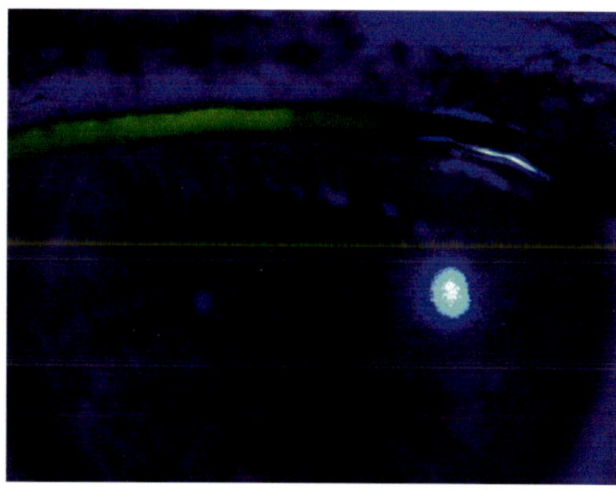

Fig. 9.15 Anterior segment image of a patient with hypotony post trabeculectomy. Fluorescein staining shows Bowman's folds, an early sign of ocular hypotony

  (b) Elevated IOP and flat/shallow AC
    (1) Suprachoroidal haemorrhage—surgical drainage (anterior sclerostomies 7 to 10 days post haemorrhage to enable clot to liquefy) indicated if RD and 360-degree suprachoroidal haemorrhage, kissing choroidal detachments, vitreous incarceration, vitreoretinal adhesions
    (2) Malignant glaucoma (shallow central & peripheral AC)—atropine, disruption of anterior hyaloid face with Yag Laser or vitrectomy
    (3) Incomplete iridectomy with pupil block—perform new Yag PI followed by topical steroids and atropine
  (c) Elevated IOP and deep AC:
    (1) Inadequate filtration (tight scleral flap or obstruction of fistula by iris, ciliary processes, lens, blood, or vitreous): laser suture lysis or release of suture, Yag laser to remove obstructing iris or ciliary processes from ostium, revision of filter

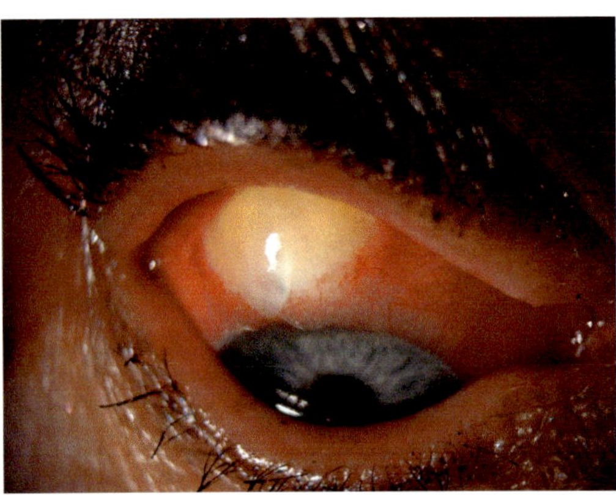

Fig. 9.16 Anterior segment image of a patient with a blebitis

(d) Loss of vision ("wipe out")—risk factors include older age, preoperative macular splitting in the VF, hypotony
(e) Bleb-related infections—blebitis (milky bleb—see Fig. 9.16): intensive topical antibiotics and systemic antibiotics (ciprofloxacin 750 mg BD) / bleb-related endophthalmitis (BRE): intravitreal tap + injection of antibiotics, systemic antibiotics (ciprofloxacin 750 mg BD)

- Late postoperative
  (a) Late filtration failure—bleb encapsulation (highly elevated, smooth dome-shaped bleb with large vessels but intervening avascular spaces and no microcysts): resume topical medications, digital pressure, bleb needling +5-FU
  (b) Leaking bleb (risk factors: blebs with large avascular area)—aqueous suppressants, BCL, cyanoacrylate glue or autologous fibrin glue, autologous blood, bleb revision surgery
  (c) Bleb-related infections
  (d) Loss of vision—cataract
  (e) Eyelid changes—upper eyelid retraction (adrenergic effect of aqueous humour on Muller muscle), ptosis (trauma to levator)

9.10 Glaucoma Drainage Implants (GDI's) (Table 9.8)

9.10.1 Types of GDI

- Valved: Ahmed implant
- Non-valved: Baerveldt implant, Molteno implant, Paul implant

Table 9.8 Useful information about GDIs

Basic design: silicone tube that extends from the AC (see Figs. 9.17 and 9.18) to a plate, disc, or encircling element beneath the conjunctiva and Tenon capsule
Successful outcome of a GDI is most dependent on size of the plate

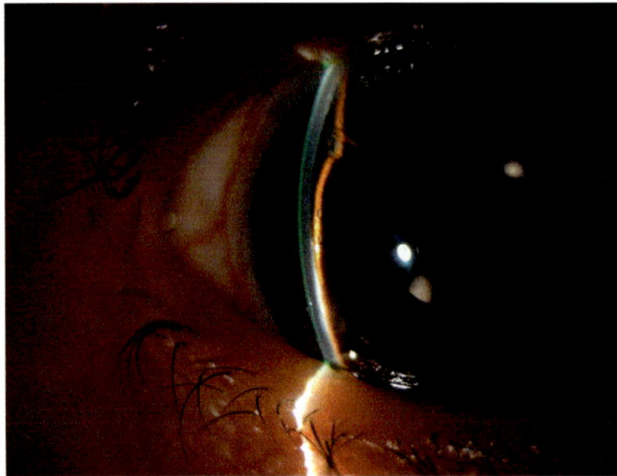

Fig. 9.17 Anterior segment image of a patient with a GDI with the tube visible in the AC. Note also the presence of a shallow AC

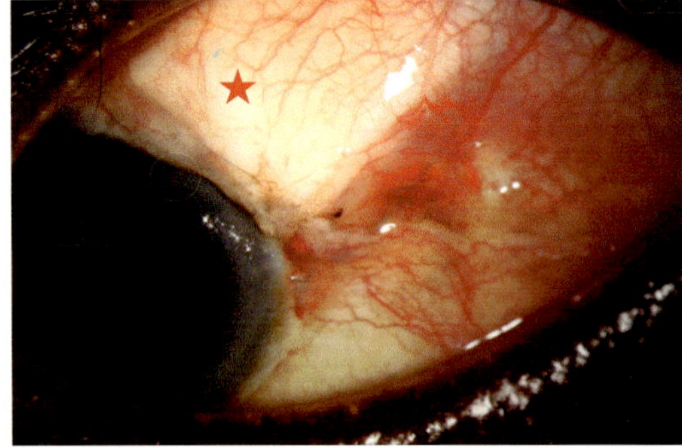

Fig. 9.18 Anterior segment image of a patient with a GDI showing the presence of a tube in the AC (white circle) and a patch graft (red star) over the tube plate to reduce the risk of tubal erosion through the overlying conjunctiva

9.10.2 Mechanism of Action

- Fibrous capsule forms (after 6 to 8 weeks) a filtering bleb around the external portion of the draining device

9.10.3 Indications

- Classically performed for conditions where a filtering surgery would have a high likelihood of failure
  - Conjunctival scarring (from previous VR surgeries or glaucoma from chemical burns)
  - Uveitic glaucoma
  - Neovascular glaucoma
  - Aphakic glaucoma
  - Angle recession glaucoma
  - Childhood glaucomas (e.g. Sturge Weber syndrome)
  - Previous failed trabeculectomy

9.10.4 Complications

- Intraoperative
  - (a) Avulsion of rectus muscles.
  - (b) Globe perforation while suturing the plate to the sclera
- Post-operative
  - (a) Hypotony with flat AC: injection of dense viscoelastic into AC, removal of tube from AC with subsequent repositioning of tube, permanent ligation of tube
  - (b) Elevated IOP: medical tx initially, if encapsulated drainage implant from thick fibrous capsule—needling beneath conjunctiva
  - (c) Tube migration, implant extrusion, and erosion of silicone tube through the overlying conjunctiva
  - (d) Endophthalmitis: removal of GDI, intravitreal tap and injection of antibiotics
  - (e) Visual loss
  - (f) Corneal decompensation: tube-cornea touch
  - (g) Diplopia: acquired Brown syndrome, SO palsy

9.11 Minimally Invasive Glaucoma Surgery (MIGS)

9.11.1 Types of MIGS and Their Mechanisms of Action

- Creating a subconjunctival drainage pathway e.g. XEN implant (see Fig. 9.19), InnFocus Microshunt
- Increasing trabecular outflow by bypassing the TM by stent placement e.g. iStent (see Fig. 9.20), Hydrus micro-stent
- Increasing trabecular outflow by bypassing the TM by tissue excision e.g. Gonioscopy Assisted Transluminal Trabeculotomy (GATT), OMNI (see Fig. 9.21)
- Increasing aqueous outflow through Schlemm's canal e.g. OMNI, Ab Interno Canaloplasty (ABiC)
- Increasing uveoscleral outflow via suprachoroidal pathways e.g. CyPass micro-stent

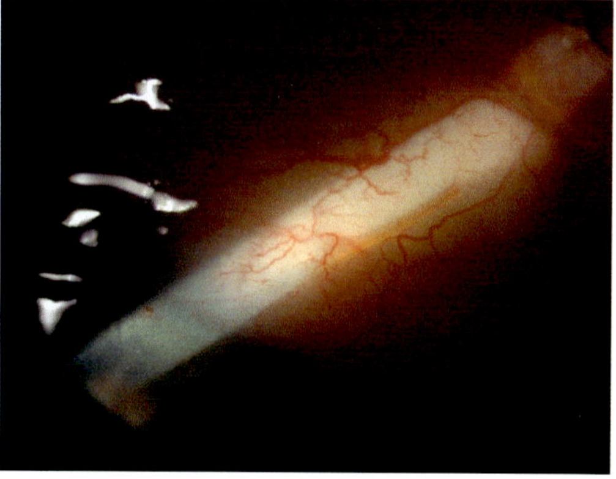

Fig. 9.19 Anterior segment image of a patient with a XEN implant in the superonasal subconjunctival space

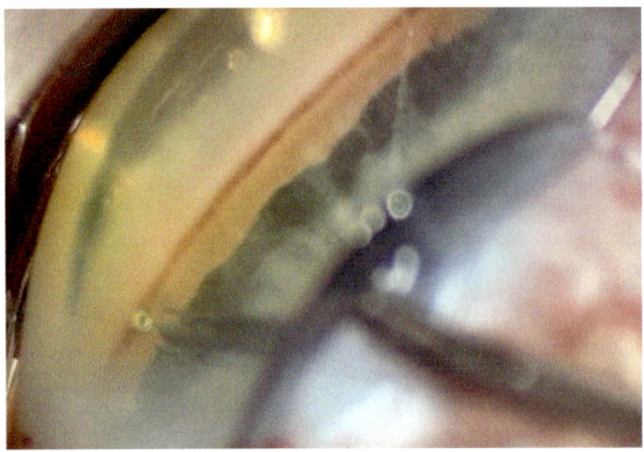

Fig. 9.20 Gonioscopic view showing the placement of an iStent into the TM

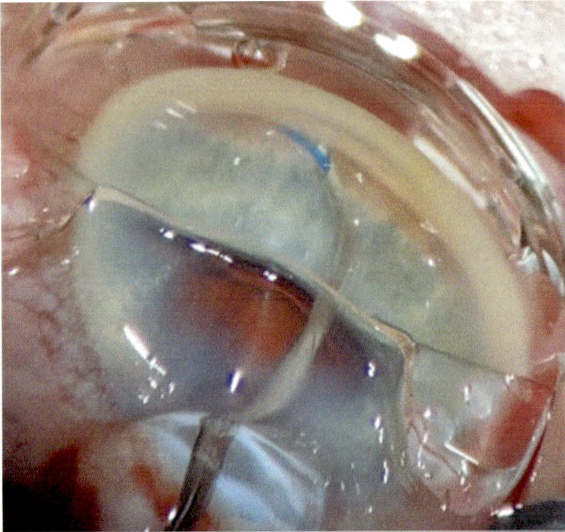

Fig. 9.21 Gonioscopic view showing the placement of a microcatheter into the Schlemm's canal using the OMNI surgical system

9.11.2 Indications

- There is currently little robust high-quality RCT evidence comparing the efficacy and safety of one MIGS technique over another for OAG
- At present there is no guidelines on the use of MIGS in clinical practice
- Possible indications
  - Patients with OAG (POAG, PXF glaucoma, pigmentary glaucoma) that is manageable with drops but who have poor drop compliance
  - Patients with OAG and a clinically significant cataract, as surgery may be performed simultaneously (Phaco-Plus)

9.12 PreserFlo Ab-Externo MicroShunt

9.12.1 Mechanism of Action

- The PreserFlo MicroShunt is an implantable device measuring 8.5 mm in length and 0.35 mm in width, with a lumen diameter of 70 μm and a pair of 0.375 mm fins for intrascleral fixation
- The tube length and lumen diameter were selected to provide sufficient resistance to limit IOP reduction and minimise the risk of hypotony
- The MicroShunt is implanted subconjunctivally via an ab-externo approach and provides filtration from the AC to the subconjunctival space without the need for scleral flap formation, sclerostomy, or iridectomy (see Figs. 9.22, 9.23, 9.24, and 9.25)

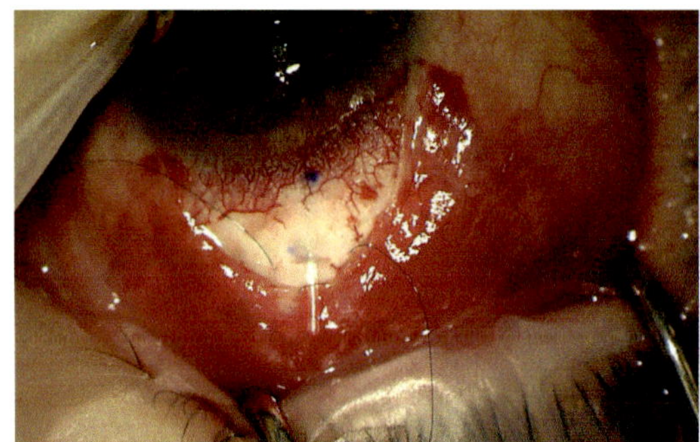

Fig. 9.22 Intraoperative view showing the insertion of a PreserFlo MicroShunt through a scleral tunnel. The distal end of the shunt is visible

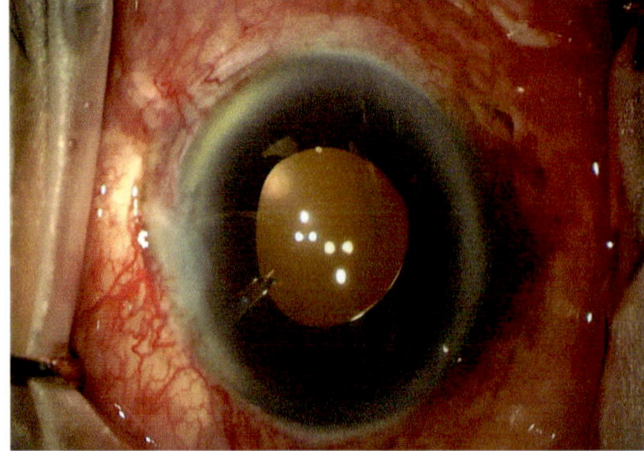

Fig. 9.23 Intraoperative view of the same eye as shown in Fig. 9.22 with the proximal end of the PreserFlo MicroShunt visible in the AC

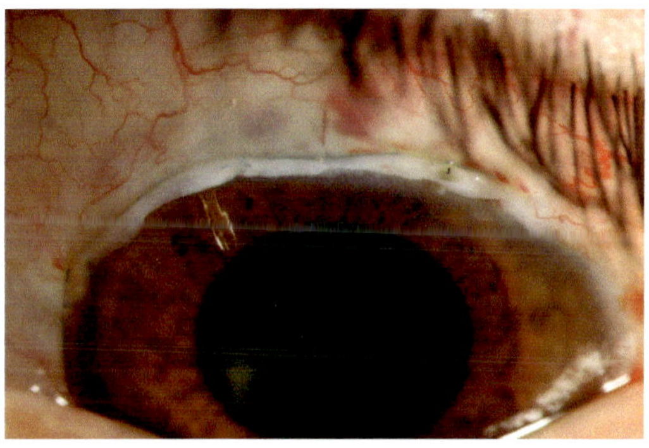

Fig. 9.24 Slit-lamp image showing the presence of the proximal tip of the PreserFlo MicroShunt in the AC. There is a visible releasable suture placed inside the distal end of the shunt, which helps control the initial drainage flow and minimise the risk of postoperative hypotony

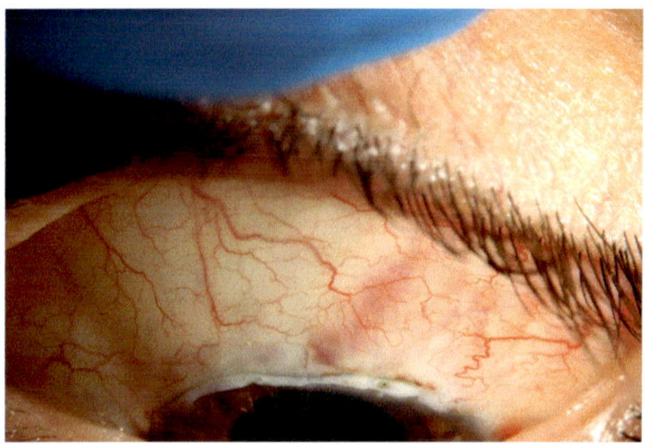

Fig. 9.25 Slit-lamp image of the same patient as shown in Fig. 9.24 showing the absence of a scleral flap. The Preserflo MicroShunt is well covered by the Tenon capsule and conjunctiva

9.12.2 Indications

- There is a large prospective, randomised, multicenter study that compared the effectiveness and safety of the MicroShunt versus trabeculectomy in patients with POAG [1, 2]
- Eligible patients were aged 40–85 years with mild-to-severe POAG inadequately controlled on MTMT, with IOP ≥15 and ≤ 40 mmHg and a visual field mean deviation of −3.00 decibels or worse [1, 2]
- The study demonstrated greater surgical success and a lower mean IOP at 1 year with trabeculectomy compared with MicroShunt implantation [1]. At 2 years, both the MicroShunt and trabeculectomy provided significant reductions in IOP and medication use, with trabeculectomy continuing to result in greater surgical success [2].
- There was a significantly lower incidence of transient and persistent hypotony in the MicroShunt implantation group compared to the trabeculectomy group [1, 2]

9.13 Lid Examination Sequence

- Introduce oneself
- Sit in front of patient with patient's eyes at your eye level
- Quick inspection for any obvious ptosis, brow ptosis, frontalis overaction, eyelid scars from previous surgeries, eyelid malpositions (e.g. ectropion's or entropions), CN VII palsy
- Ask patient to look straight ahead at a distance target and measure the palpebral aperture (PA): distance from the upper lid margin to the lower lid margin (normal range 9–11 mm)
- Shine a penlight at the patient's eye and measure the marginal reflex distance 1 (MRD1): distance from central corneal light reflex to the upper lid margin (normal range 4–5 mm)
- Ask patient to look down and measure the upper eyelid skin crease height: distance from lid margin to skin crease (normal range 6–8 mm for men and 8–10 mm for women)
- Measure levator function (LF): block action of patient's brow with your thumb and measure excursion of the upper lid from extreme downgaze to extreme upgaze (normal range 13–16 mm)
- Check for the presence of any lagophthalmos by asking patient to close their eyes
- Check orbicularis function by asking patient to squeeze their eyes shut without letting you open their eyes
- Hold a pen above the patient's eye level and check for fatiguability by asking a patient to look up at your pen for at least 30–60 seconds (ask examiner if they want you to do this in the

exam): if fatiguability is present the eyelid will slowly drop as the patient stares at your pen

- Check for lid lag by asking a patient to follow your pen from upgaze to downgaze
- Hold a pen below the patient's eye level and check for a Cogan's lid twitch by asking the patient to look down at your pen for 20 seconds before asking them to look straight ahead: a positive Cogan's twitch is present if the upper eyelid overshoots following the sudden return of the eye to the primary position
- Ask patient to open and close the mouth and move the jaw around to check for a Marcus-Gunn jaw winking ptosis (see Sect. 9.26)
- Check ocular motility and pupils

9.14 Ectropion (Table 9.9)

Table 9.9 Useful information about ectropions

Ectropion occurs when the lid margin everts or turns away from the eyeball
Any type of ectropion may cause tearing as a result of reflex tearing, punctal eversion, or inadequate lacrimal pump

9.14.1 Classification

- Lower eyelid
  - Involutional (see Fig. 9.26): horizontal lid laxity
  - Paralytic: loss of orbicularis muscle support of the lower eyelid, associated with lower facial paralysis and brow ptosis (CN VII palsy)
  - Cicatricial (see Fig. 9.27): shortening of the anterior lamella from trauma or skin changes
- Upper eyelid
  - Cicatricial
  - There is no upper eyelid equivalent for paralytic or involutional ectropion

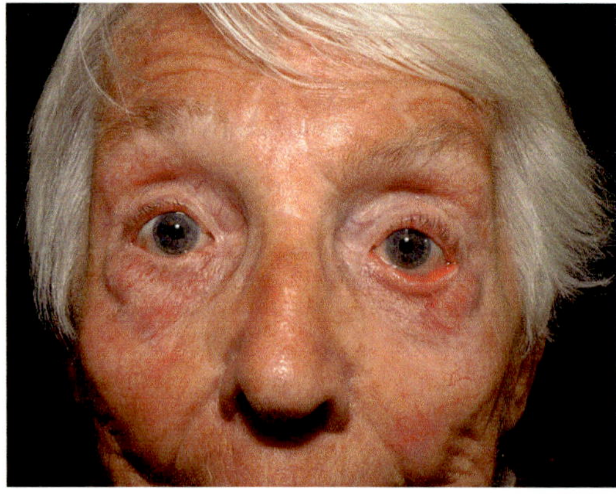

Fig. 9.26 Facial photo of a patient with an involutional ectropion

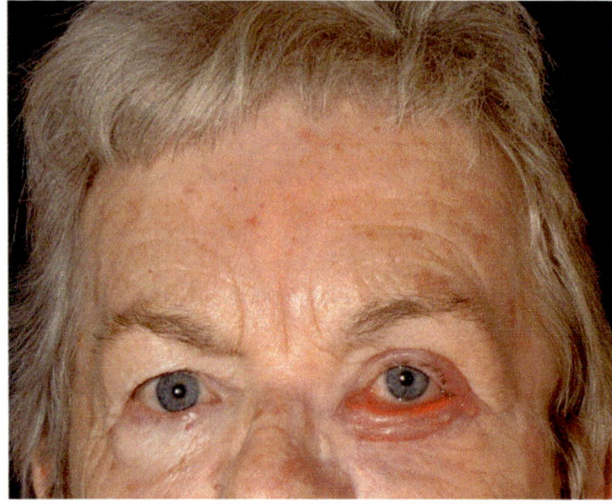

Fig. 9.27 Facial photo of a patient with a left cicatricial ectropion with visible scar tissue in the lower eyelid from a previous full thickness skin graft procedure

9.14.2 History

- Hx of trauma or cicatrising skin disease—ichthyosis (anterior lamellar shortening)
- Hx of previous excision of skin cancer or repair of laceration in the periocular area (anterior lamellar shortening)
- Hx of CN VII palsy

9.14.3 Examination

- Location—medial lid, lateral lid, entire lid, punctal eversion only
- Examine for scarring of the periocular area: indicate previous accidental or surgical trauma as a cause for cicatricial ectropion

- Examine for generalised tightness of the skin: indicates skin shrinkage as a cause for cicatricial ectropion
- Examine for CN VII palsy suggesting paralytic ectropion: facial asymmetry, flattening of nasolabial folds, co-existing brow ptosis, corneal exposure
- Examine for horizontal eyelid laxity (see Fig. 9.28): eyelid distraction test (manually pull lower eyelid away from eyeball, the lower lid should not move more than 6 mm off the eyeball), eyelid snap test (pulling lower eyelid inferiorly toward the inferior orbital rim, an eyelid without lower eyelid laxity will spring back into position without a blink)
- Examine for medial canthal tendon laxity: if lateral traction of lower eyelid displaces the punctum to or beyond the limbus, then medial canthal tendon laxity exists

9.14.4 Treatment

- Horizontal lid shortening procedures
  (a) Lateral tarsal strip (LTS): prepare the patient (inject LA), perform a lateral canthotomy, perform a lateral cantholysis, form the strip (splitting the anterior and posterior lamella, cut along inferior margin of tarsus, remove skin and conjunctiva from the strip), shorten the strip, reattach the strip, trim redundant anterior lamella, close the canthotomy

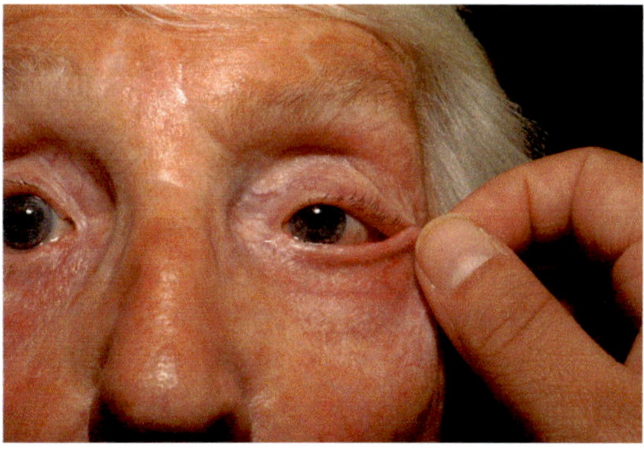

Fig. 9.28 Facial photo of the same patient in Fig. 9.26 showing the presence of horizontal lid laxity

  (b) Pentagonal wedge resection: choice of procedure for upper eyelid with floppy eyelid syndrome
  (c) Kuhnt-Szymanowski: wedge resection and lower lid blepharoplasty
- Vertical lid shortening procedures
  (a) Medial spindle procedure (excision of a diamond of conjunctiva inferior to the lower puntum and closure with a suture): procedure for punctal ectropion alone or combined with LTS if lid laxity present (perform medial spindle procedure before eyelid is tightened with a LTS).
- Combined lid shortening procedures
  (a) Lazy T: diamond excision (medial spindle procedure) and wedge resection
- Involutional ectropion: lid shortening procedures
- Paralytic ectropion: correction of corneal exposure with lubricants and ointments, lid shortening procedures
- Cicatricial ectropion: lengthening of anterior lamella with full-thickness skin graft (pre-auricular, post-auricular, supraclavicular area, inner upper arm, inguinal area)

9.15 Entropion (Table 9.10)

9.15.1 Classification

- Lower eyelid
  - Involutional: disinsertion or laxity of the lower eyelid retractors (primary cause of involutional entropion as it allows the inferior edge of the tarsus to rotate away from the eye), horizontal lid laxity, overriding preseptal orbicularis muscle
  - Cicatricial (see Fig. 9.29): shortening of the posterior lamella (pulls eyelid margin inwards) from scarring of the conjunctiva (e.g. alkali burns, surgical or accidental trauma, OCP, SJS, trachoma)

Table 9.10 Useful information about entropions

Lid margin inverts or turns against the eyeball
Keratinised skin of the eyelid margin and eyelashes rub against the cornea and conjunctiva, causing irritation

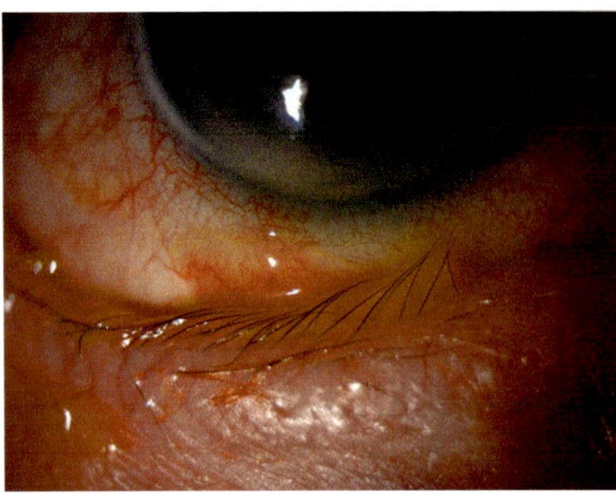

Fig. 9.29 Anterior segment image of a patient with a cicatricial entropion from OCP

  - Spastic: squeezing of the lids in association with ocular pain or inflammation, entropion resolves once discomfort disappears, occurs in patients who have predisposing factors to involutional entropion such as horizontal lid laxity and lax lower lid retractors
  - Congenital
- Upper eyelid
  - Cicatricial

9.15.2 History

- Intermittent symptoms of irritation: suggest an involutional cause
- Constant symptoms of irritation: suggests a cicatricial cause
- Hx of previous surgical or accidental trauma
- Hx of chemical injuries, OCP, SJS, trachoma

9.15.3 Examination

- For subtle entropions, look for a slightly rolled appearance of the posterior angle of the lid margin (should be a flat platform with well-defined right-angled anterior and posterior edges). For intermittent entropions not seen on examination initially, ask patient to squeeze eyes to elicit entropion
- Examine to determine if entropion is cicatricial: with your finger, return the inverted lid to its normal position. If cicatricial changes are present, there is resistance to placing the lid in the normal position and after you release the lid it will immediately return to its inverted position, examine the conjunctiva for signs of fornix shortening or scarring
- Examine the degree of conjunctival scarring: identify the position of the meibomian gland orifices in the least inverted part and follow to most inverted part, in severe scarring the meibomian gland openings may be on the posterior surface of tarsus
- If not cicatricial, the entropion must be involutional: lid returns to normal position with your finger and it will remain there for a blink or two. If entropion does not recur with a few blinks, ask the patient to squeeze the lids closed for a moment, lower eyelid may ride above the lower limbus suggesting some laxity of the lower eyelid retractors
- Examine for horizontal lid laxity if involutional entropion present: eyelid distraction test (manually pull lower eyelid away from eyeball, the lower lid should not move more than 6 mm off the eyeball), eyelid snap test (pulling lower eyelid inferiorly toward the inferior orbital rim, an eyelid without lower eyelid laxity will spring back into position without a blink)

9.15.4 Treatment

- Involutional (aim is to restore the normal tension of the lower lid retractors and to correct any co-existing horizontal lid laxity)
  - Retractor reinsertion procedure: Jones procedure—lower lid subciliary incision, identify lower lid retractors (landmark is the preaponeurotic fat), dissect retractors from anterior fat and posterior conjunctiva, advance lower lid retractors onto the tarsus, skin closure
  - Horizontal lid shortening procedure: LTS, wedge excision, Kuhnt-Szymanowski

- Cicatricial (aim is to restore normal length of the posterior lamella using either incisions alone or incisions with mucous membrane grafts)
  - Tarsal fracture (tarsotomy—requires a contact lens post op for a few weeks to avoid irritation of cut tarsus) if mild-moderate cicatricial changes,
  - Terminal tarsal rotation operation for upper eyelid entropion
  - Mucous membrane grafts if severe cicatricial changes
- Spastic
  - Treat cause of underlying irritation causing spasm
  - If not possible to eliminate the cause of irritation:
    - Quickert sutures: topical & local anaesthetic, load a double armed suture, pass the arms of the suture thought the lid from deep in the fornix passing anteriorly and superiorly to emerge from the skin just below the eyelashes, repeat so that there are medial, central, and lateral sutures in position, tie the sutures so that there is a slight overcorrection

9.16 Facial Nerve (CN VII) Palsy

9.16.1 Causes of CN VII Palsy

- Bell's palsy (diagnosis of exclusion)
- Acoustic neuroma (cerebellopontine angle tumour)
- Facial tumour (parotid gland mass)
- Trauma
- Ramsay-Hunt syndrome (VZV): otalgia, vesicular rash on ear canal, tympanic membrane
- Sarcoidosis (CN VII palsy tends to be bilateral)
- Lyme disease (CN VII palsy tends to be bilateral)

9.16.2 History

- Hx of otalgia, hearing loss, or vestibular complaints (if present pt. needs scanning)
- Find out likelihood of recovery from ENT colleagues—perhaps tumour resection required cutting the facial nerve, meaning there is no chance of recovery

9.16.3 Examination

- Look for incomplete blink
- Look for brow ptosis (see Fig. 9.30)
- Look for lower eyelid ectropion (see Fig. 9.30)

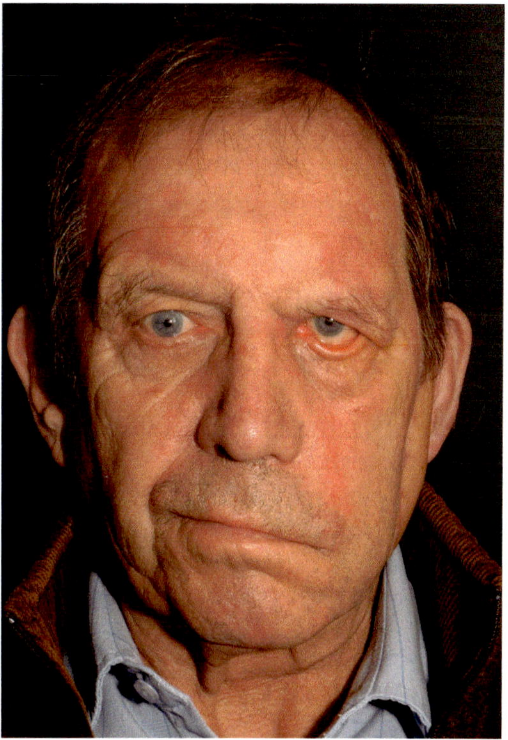

Fig. 9.30 Facial photo of a patient with a left-sided lower motor neurone facial nerve palsy with a brow ptosis and a paralytic ectropion

- Look for lagophthalmos with corneal exposure
- Examine for Bell's phenomenon: if good, patients may have little or no corneal exposure despite incomplete closure
- Examine for aberrant regeneration: narrowing of palpebral fissure on pursing of lips/showing of teeth
- Examine corneal sensation: may be reduced if CN VII palsy is due to acoustic neuroma resection (resection may compromise CN V as CN V, VII, VIII leave the brainstem in close proximity)—reduced corneal sensation makes corneal exposure more difficult to manage

9.16.4 Investigations

- ENT referral to establish cause for all new-onset CN VII palsy
- MRI for UMN facial palsy, recurrent CN VII palsy or pts. with otalgia, vestibular symptoms, or hearing loss to exclude inflammatory or neoplastic (cerebellopontine angle) causes

9.16.5 Treatment

- Treatment depends on how permanent the palsy is likely to be, the degree of anatomic dysfunction (Bells phenomenon), and the patient's needs
- Corneal exposure
  - (a) Medical treatment:
    - Hourly artificial tears or ointments
    - Eyeglasses outdoors to protect the eye from the wind
    - Avoidance of moving air from fans or heating vents indoors
    - Taping lid closed at night
  - (b) Surgical treatment (if corneal exposure cannot be managed medically or the facial paralysis is likely to be long term e.g. no improvement in 18 months):
    - Static procedures (narrow the palpebral aperture a fixed amount):
      - Tarsorrhaphy: temporary (see Table 9.11) or permanent
      - Elevation of lower eyelid (retractor disinsertion +/− graft)
    - Dynamic procedures (improve lid closure):
      - Botox:
        - Technique: 25G needle passed through central aspect of upper lid immediately inferior to the superior orbital rim, needle passed against orbital roof for 1-2 cm, 5 to 10 units are injected, after 48 hours the upper lid rests closed
        - Side-effects: ocular surface dryness (temporary paralysis of orbicularis and decreased blinking), upper eyelid ptosis and diplopia (botox induced paresis of the levator muscle or extraocular muscles)—may last for 6 weeks
      - Upper eyelid gold weight implantation
- Ectropion—LTS +/− medial spindle procedure
- Brow ptosis—browplasty
- Aberrant regeneration: treat if narrowing of palpebral fissure affects vision. Options include Botox and levator aponeurosis advancement

Table 9.11 Surgical technique for a temporary suture tarsorrhaphy

Can be placed anywhere along the lid margins. The nylon suture can be left in place for 2 weeks
Topical anaesthetic and inject local anaesthetic into the eyelids
Cut two 5 mm pieces of a narrow red rubber catheter to use as bolster material
Pass 1 arm of a double ended 5/0 nylon suture through the bolster material, then into the lower lid skin 5 mm below the lid margin, emerging out the lid margin through the meibomian glands, into the opposite lid margin, out the skin 5 mm above the upper eyelid margin, and through the second bolster
Repeat this procedure with the other arm of the suture
Tie a slip knot over the bolster on the upper eyelid

- For Bell's palsy—oral prednisolone (25 mg BD) for 10 days starting within 72 hours after the onset of symptoms has increased complete recovery rates from 64% to 83% at 3 months and from 82% to 94% at 9 months

9.17 Simple Congenital Ptosis

9.17.1 History

- Present at birth with no associated ocular or systemic problems
- For a child: Is the lid above the pupil? How many times is lid above the pupil?
- Hx of previous ptosis surgery +/− secondary lagophthalmos
- Hx of CN VII palsy
- Hx of dry eye/use of topical lubricants

9.17.2 Examination

- Reduced/poor levator function
- Absent or weak upper eyelid crease (see Fig. 9.31)
- Lid lag on downgaze +/− lagophthalmos
- Examine for amblyopia (astigmatism or deprivation) in a child
- Examine for risk factors that would increase the chance of post-operative corneal exposure: poor Bell's phenomenon, lagophthalmos
- Examine anterior segment for dry eye: assess tear lake height, fluorescein staining of cornea, Schirmer's I test, TBUT
- Normal ocular motility (or SR weakness alone in 5%) and pupil examination

9.17.3 Treatment

- If levator function <4 mm, a frontalis sling procedure is appropriate
- If levator function ≥4 mm, a levator aponeurosis advancement is appropriate

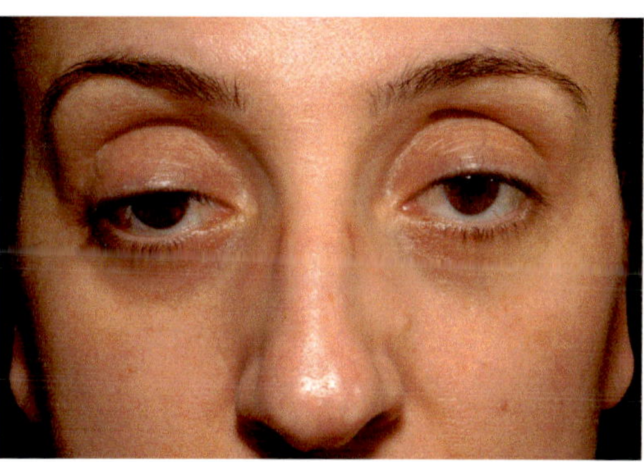

Fig. 9.31 Facial photo of a patient with a simple congenital ptosis

9.18 Involutional Ptosis

9.18.1 History

- Indefinite onset
- Gradual progression
- No associated ocular or systemic problems
- Ptosis usually about the same severity throughout the day
- Hx of previous ptosis surgery +/− secondary lagophthalmos
- Hx of CN VII palsy
- Hx of dry eye/use of topical lubricants

9.18.2 Examination

- Normal (13–16 mm) or near normal (12 mm) levator function
- High skin crease (8–10 mm in women, 6–8 mm in men)
- Lid drop on downgaze (lid margin remains low throughout downgaze)
- Frontalis overaction (see Fig. 9.32)
- Examine for dermatochalasis or brow ptosis: combined surgery with levator aponeurosis advancement may be required
- Examine for risk factors that would increase the chance of post-operative corneal exposure: poor Bell's phenomenon, lagophthalmos

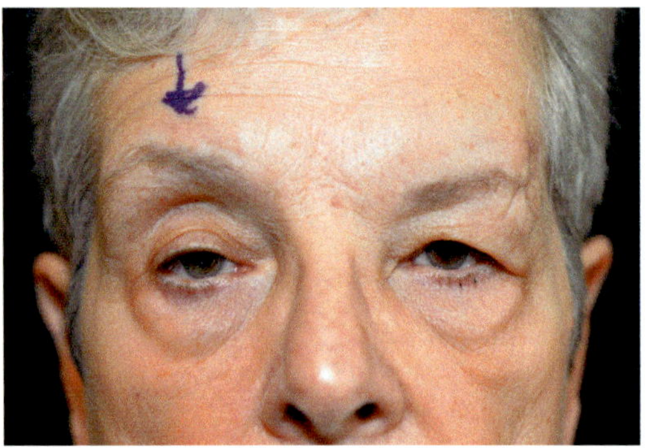

Fig. 9.32 Facial photo of a patient with a right involutional ptosis with frontalis overaction

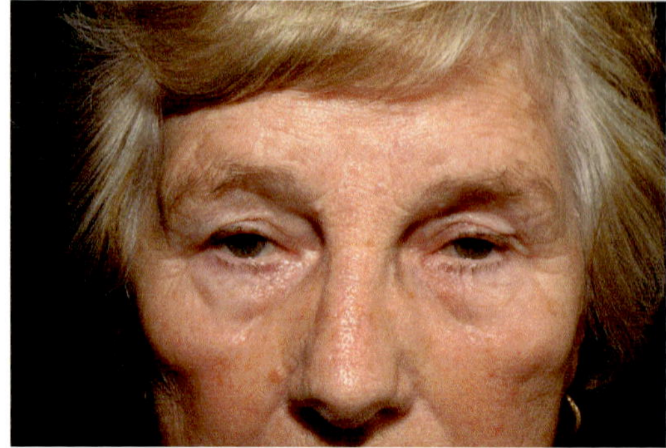

Fig. 9.33 Facial photo of a patient with CPEO showing bilateral symmetrical ptosis

- Examine anterior segment for dry eye: assess tear lake height, fluorescein staining of cornea, Schirmer's I test, TBUT
- Normal ocular motility and pupil examination

9.18.3 Treatment

- Levator aponeurosis advancement procedure +/− brow plasty +/− blepharoplasty

9.19 Chronic Progressive External Ophthalmoplegia (CPEO)

9.19.1 History

- Ask about FHx to rule out myotonic dystrophy and oculopharyngeal dystrophy

9.19.2 Examination

- Bilateral progressive symmetrical ptosis (see Fig. 9.33) with poor levator function (CPEO), good levator function initially with oculopharyngeal dystrophy
- CN VII weakness especially orbicularis weakness (CPEO)
- Test fatigability (MG): ask patient to look up for 30–60 seconds and upper eyelid will fatigue and slowly drop
- Look for Cogan's eyelid twitch (MG): ask patient to look down for 20 seconds and then at object in the primary position—positive if lid overshoots
- Progressive symmetrical advanced loss of ocular motility (eyes virtually immobile with secondary fibrotic changes in advanced stages)—reduced pursuits and always reduced (hypometric) saccadic velocities (CPEO), check for improvement in ocular motility with Dolls head testing (Supranuclear gaze palsy), normal saccadic velocities in MG, down and out eye in complete CN III palsy
- Normal pupil reactions and accomodation (CPEO), mydriasis with poor reactions (CN III palsy)
- Examine for x-mas tree cataract, frontal balding, slow-release grip (myotonic dystrophy)
- Fundus exam: pigmentary retinopathy (Kearns-Sayre syndrome / myotonic dystrophy)
- Ask patient to drink glass of water quickly (oculopharyngeal dystrophy)

9.19.3 Investigations

- ECG (Kearns-Sayre syndrome / myotonic dystrophy): heart conduction defects
- Fields of uniocular fixation (CPEO)
- Tensilon test (MG): ensure IV atropine, resuscitation equipment, and trained staff is on hand, cardiac monitoring (ECG) essential. Give 2 mg edrophonium IV and if no ill effects at 30 s, give further 8 mg edrophonium IV. Compare pre- and post-test ptosis or motility disorder

- Ice pack test (MG): measure ptosis, ice cubes in rubber glove with pt. holding it over their eyelid for 2 mins, re-measure ptosis: positive if ≥2 mm improvement
- Serum antibodies (MG): anti-Ach receptor antibodies (50% ocular myasthenia, 95% generalised myasthenia)
- Single fiber EMG (MG); reduction in action potential amplitude
- Hess chart (CN III palsy)
- Skeletal muscle biopsy: ragged red fibers with peripheral concentration of mitochondria (CPEO)
- Bloods: Mitochondrial DNA mutations (CPEO), expanded CTG repeat in the dystrophica myotonica protein kinase (DMPK) gene (myotonic dystrophy), expanded GCG repeat (oculopharyngeal dystrophy)

9.19.4 Treatment

- Prisms if diplopia present (CPEO)
- Strabismus surgery if eyes in grossly eccentric position (CPEO)
- Ptosis props (CPEO)
- Ptosis surgery: risk of causing serious exposure keratitis due to the associated poor orbicularis function and absent Bell's phenomenon (CPEO)

9.19.5 Other Diagnoses to Consider

- Myasthenia gravis
- Myotonic dystrophy
- Oculopharyngeal dystrophy
- CN III palsy
- Supranuclear gaze palsy

9.20 Floppy Eyelid Syndrome

9.20.1 History

- Unilateral/bilateral ocular injection and irritation (nocturnal eversion of the extremely lax upper eyelid rubbing on the pillow)
- Hx of obstructive sleep apnoea (OSA) +/− wearing a CPAP mask at night
- If no hx of OSA ask about snoring, sleepless nights, daytime fatigue

9.20.2 Examination

- Papillary conjunctivitis
- Upper eyelid laxity, eyelid can be folded on itself and easily turned inside out (see Fig. 9.34)

9.20.3 Investigations

- If pt. symptomatic from OSA, refer to sleep specialist

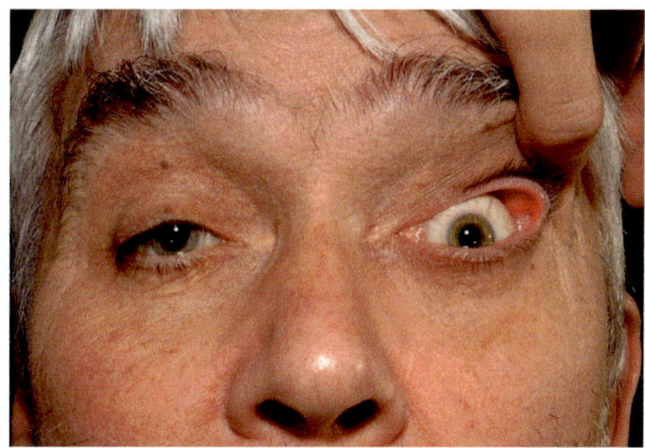

Fig. 9.34 Facial photo of a patient with floppy eyelid syndrome

9.20.4 Treatment

- Protecting eye with an eye shield at night (trial for a few weeks is a good test to see if lid tightening will improve the irritation)
- Horizontal lid tightening of the upper eyelid (usually pentagonal wedge resection)

9.21 Dermatochalasis (Table 9.12)

9.21.1 History

- Hx of dry eye (sensitivity to moving air, from ceiling fans, air vents, or windshield defrosters) and use of artificial tears: relative contraindication for blepharoplasty procedures—less skin and muscle removal required
- Hx of CN VII palsy
- Hx of previous blepharoplasty: any remaining ptosis is likely from brow ptosis

9.21.2 Examination

- Examine height and contour of brow (normal male brow is at the rim and relatively flat; the normal female brow is above the rim and arched temporally). Judge height by palpating brow between your index finger and thumb relative to the orbital rim. (Look for ptotic brow hanging over the superior orbital rim); is there a generalised ptosis of the brow or is there more of a mild temporal droop? Brow furrows indicate that the pt. is trying to see by using the brows to elevate the lids
- Examine for extra-tissues in the upper skin fold (see Fig. 9.35): estimate the amount of redundant skin and muscle in the skin fold by lifting the brow into the normal position at or above the rim, if you lift the brow higher you can see any fullness of sulcus if there is prolapsed orbital fat present (central or nasal fat)
- Examine the upper eyelid height: determine MRD1 (normal MRD1 as redundant upper eyelid skin does not change the eyelid position) by elevating the upper skin fold slightly to check the position of the upper eyelid margin, record levator function (not necessary if ptosis repair is not being considered)
- Examine the lower eyelid: look for prolapsed orbital fat (medially/laterally), look for redundant skin and muscle (any lower eyelid malar bags or festoons), estimate lower lid laxity (lid distraction test—normally the eyelid should not pull more than 6 mm away from eyeball, snap test with lower eyelid pulled down and released—normally lid returns to position without a blink or with one blink)
- Examine anterior segment: Look at size of tear lake and the presence of any corneal staining

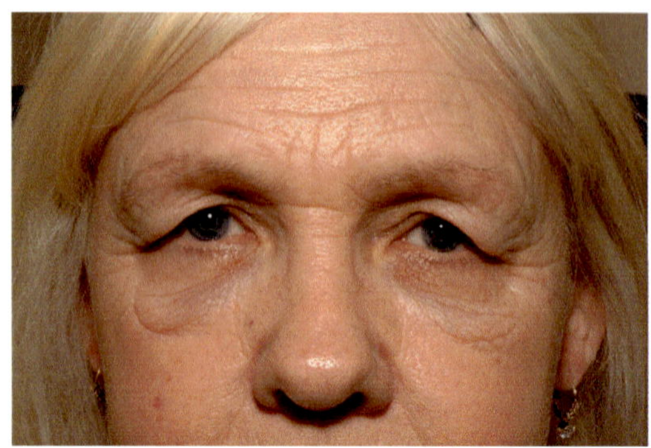

Fig. 9.35 Facial photo of a patient with dermatochalasis

Table 9.12 Causes of a pseudo-ptosis

Excessive skin: brow ptosis, dermatochalasis
Inadequate globe size: microphthalmos, phthisis bulbi, prosthesis
Incorrect globe position: enophthalmos, hypotropia
Contralateral lid retraction
Contralateral large globe
Contralateral proptosis

9.21.3 Investigations

- 24-2 HVF: performed with eyelids in relaxed ptotic position and with the eyelids taped open. An improvement in the superior visual field defect of at least 12 degrees is required

9.21.4 Treatment

- Browplasty: entire brow, temporal brow
- Upper lid blepharoplasty (removes redundant skin and muscle from the upper skin fold with variable amounts of fat excised depending on the amount of fat prolapse)
  - Indications:
    - Functional (vision blocked by redundant skin fold)
    - Cosmetic
  - Surgical technique: skin marking (skin crease, upper limit of skin excision—should leave between 10 and 15 mm of skin between the eyebrow hairs and the skin crease), anaesthesia, skin incision, skin and muscle excision, fat excision, closure
  - Complications:
    - Postoperative: asymmetry, reoperation, scarring, corneal exposure, lagophthalmos, blindness (retrobulbar haemorrhage—requires opening of surgical wound)
- Lower lid blepharoplasty

9.22 Marcus-Gunn Jaw Winking Syndrome

9.22.1 Definition

- A congenital miswiring of the CN V (pterygoid muscles) gets misdirected to CN III (levator muscle)

9.22.2 History

- Ptosis onset from birth
- Hx of amblyopia

9.22.3 Examination

- Partial ptosis (mild to severe) in primary position
- Poor levator function in majority of patients. A few patients will have good levator function
- Elevation of ptotic lid with movements of the mouth (see Fig. 9.36)

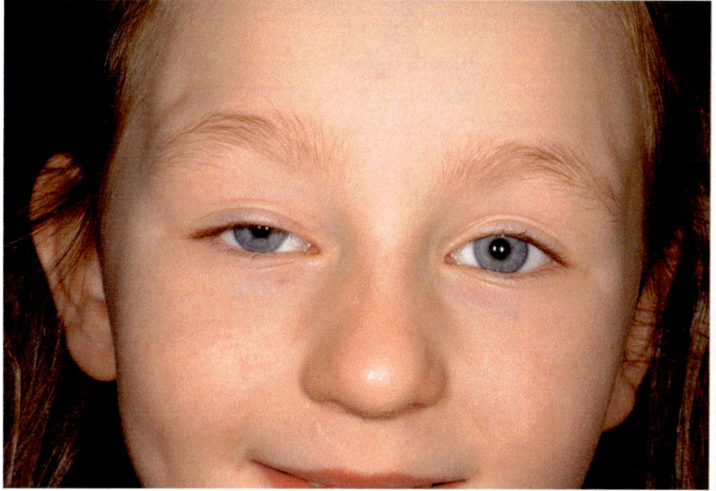
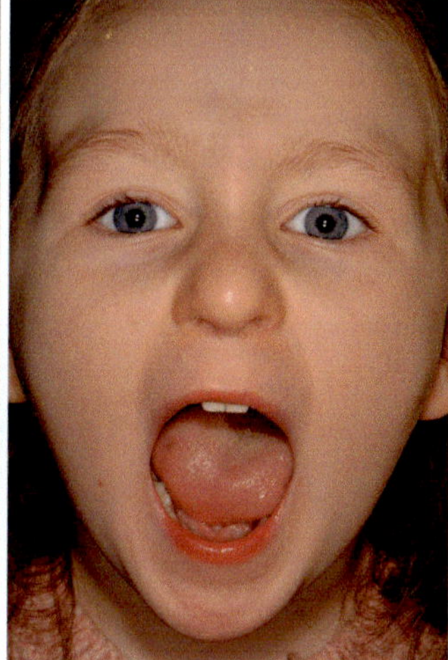

Fig. 9.36 Facial photos of a patient with Marcus-Gunn jaw winking phenomenon

9.22.4 Treatment

- If poor levator function and significant synkinesis: extirpation of the levator to eliminate the abnormal movements and a frontalis sling operation to elevate the upper lid
- If good levator function and minimal synkinesis: levator aponeurosis advancement

9.23 Myasthenia Gravis

9.23.1 History

- Variable ptosis and diplopia (worse towards the evening / with exercise)
- Any breathlessness, swallowing problems or choking episodes

9.23.2 Examination

- Unilateral ptosis +/− contralateral pseudo-lid retraction (consequence of Hering's law) or bilateral ptosis
- Fatigability: ask patient to look up for 30–60 seconds and upper eyelid will fatigue and slowly drop (see Fig. 9.37)
- Cogan's eyelid twitch: pt. to look down for 20 seconds and then at object in the primary position—positive if lid overshoots
- Normal pupil exam
- Ocular motility disturbance (any pattern) with always normal saccadic velocities (see Fig. 9.38)

9.23.3 Investigations

- Tensilon test
  - Pretreatment requirements—ensure IV atropine, resuscitation equipment, and trained staff is on hand, cardiac monitoring (ECG) essential
  - Technique—give 2 mg edrophonium IV and if no ill effects at 30 seconds, give further 8 mg edrophonium IV. Compare pre- and post-test ptosis or motility disorder (Hess)
  - Possible side-effects—increased salivation, sweating, bronchospasm, hypotension, bradycardia, arrhythmia
- Ice pack test—measure ptosis, ice cubes in rubber glove with patient holding it over their eyelid for 2 minutes, re-measure ptosis: positive if ≥2 mm improvement
- Serum antibodies—anti-Ach receptor antibodies (50% ocular myasthenia, 95% generalised myasthenia)—negative test does not rule out MG
- Single fiber EMG—reduction in action potential amplitude
- Bloods—TFT (MG associated with Graves disease in 4–10%)
- CT chest—thymoma

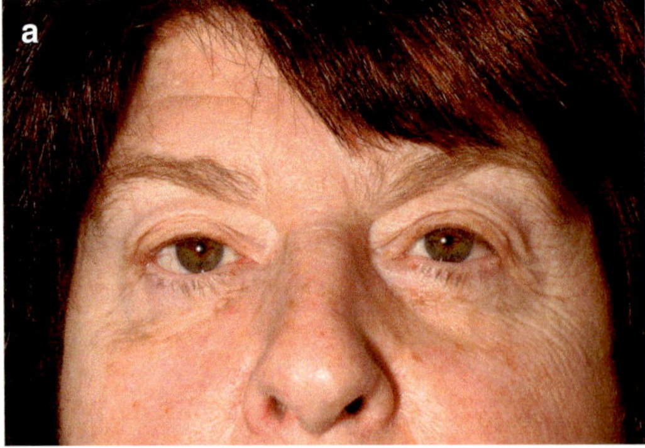

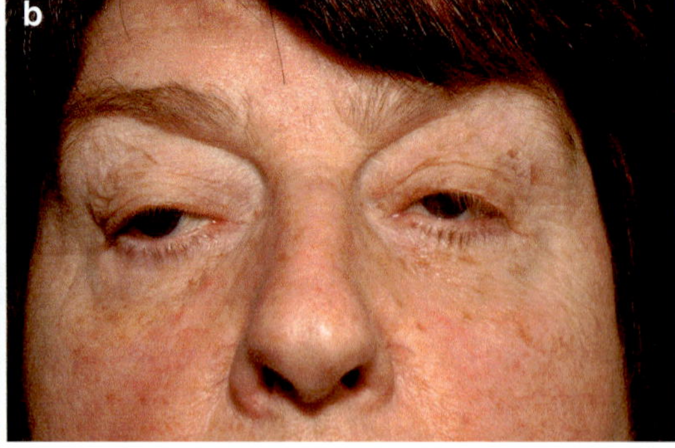

Fig. 9.37 Facial photos of a patient with myasthenia gravis showing minimal ptosis initially (**a**) and fatiguability of the upper eyelids after prolonged upgaze (**b**)

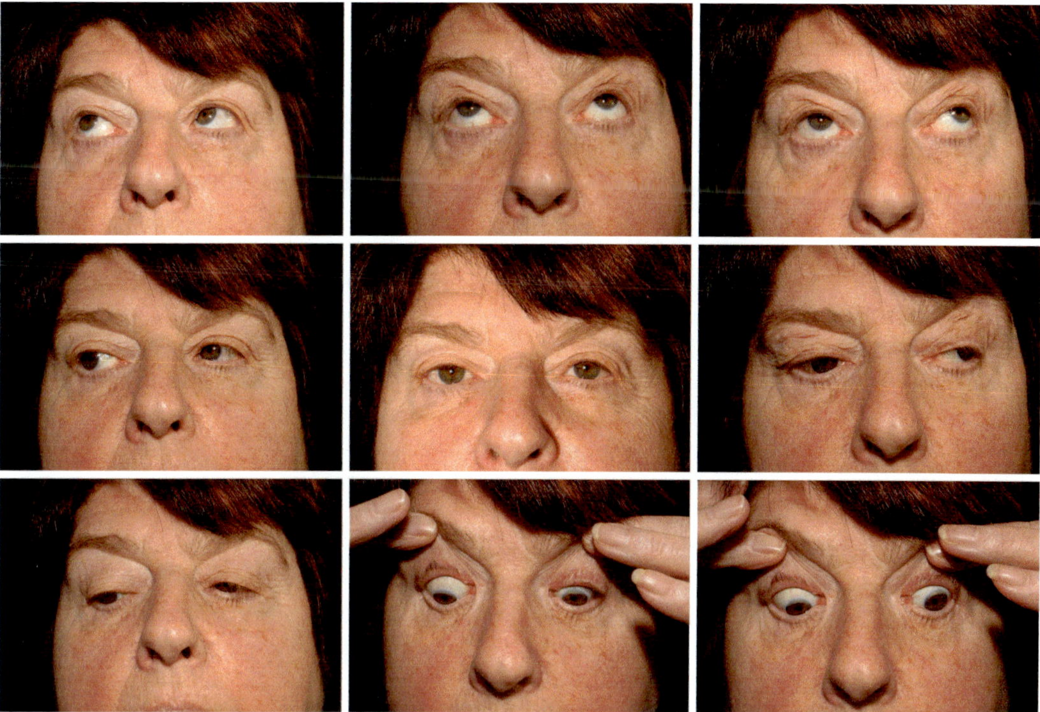

Fig. 9.38 Nine positions of gaze for the same patient as shown in Fig. 9.37 showing a limitation of adduction in the right eye

9.23.4 Treatment

- Co-manage with a neurologist
- Ocular manifestations: Lid crutches for ptosis, surgical ptosis correction if medical treatment unsuccessful although variability remains, prisms for diplopia
- Systemic manifestations:
  - Medical tx—pyridostigmine (anti-acetylcholinesterase), immunosuppression (oral prednisolone to reduce dose of pyridostigmine, azathioprine, AZT, plasmapheresis and IV immunoglobulin for myasthenic crisis)
  - Surgical tx—thymectomy

9.24 Basal Cell Carcinoma (BCC)

9.24.1 Classification of BCC

- Nodular (see Fig. 9.39)
- Morpheaform: sclerotic plaques or papules, border not defined
- Superficial: scaly patches or papules (mimics eczema or psoriasis)

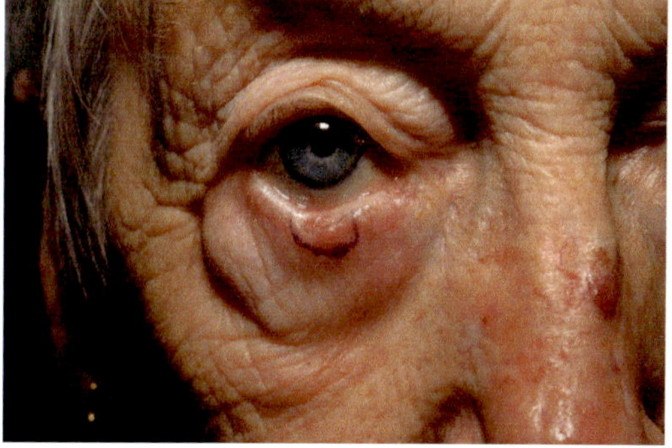

Fig. 9.39 Facial photo of a patient with a lower eyelid nodular BCC

- Pigmented: areas of brown and black pigment seen in lesion along with signs similar to nodular

9.24.2 History

- Hx of sun exposure
- Positive FHx of BCC: Gorlin's syndrome (basal cell naevus syndrome)—AD, predisposes patients to multiple BCCs, associated

with jaw cysts, palmar pits, skeletal abnormalities (syndactyly of the digits, sprengel deformity—scapula displacement and limitation of shoulder movement)
- Hx of xeroderma pigmentosum

9.24.3 Examination (Tables 9.13)

- Firm nodule with pearly borders with telangiectasia +/− central ulceration (lesions are not tender and not painful to touch)
- Destruction of normal lid margin architecture when the lesion involves the lid margin—lashes are often lost
- Examine for signs of actinic skin damage: skin appears thin with deep wrinkles and furrows, changes in pigmentation include diffuse mottling or brownish patches known as solar lentigo, vessels of the dermis are visible due to loss of surrounding collagen in elastic tissue, tight skin with no wrinkles despite advancing age
- BCCs most commonly present in the lower lid, then the medial canthus, then the upper lid and then the lateral canthus

Table 9.13 Characteristics suggestive of eyelid skin malignancy

Ulceration: often associated with bleeding, malignant lesions do not tend to be painful, nor are they tender to touch
Induration: all malignancies tend to be firm or indurated
Irregularity: irregular margins and asymmetric shapes
Pearlypof BCC, heaped up edges often surround an area of central ulceration
Loss of eyelid margin architecture: malignancy may destroy the normal architecture of the lid margin, suspect malignancy when an area of lash loss or lid margin destruction is present

9.24.4 Investigations

- Incisional biopsy (only portion of lesion is removed): used to sample a lesion for diagnosis—best place to sample the tumour is at the periphery of the lesion and include areas of normal tissue, centre of lesion should not be sampled, especially if there is central ulceration—histopathological interpretation may yield only necrotic tissue
- Genetic testing: mutations in PTCH1 and SUFU genes (Gorlin's syndrome)

9.24.5 Treatment

- Topical imiquimod 5% cream for small superficial BCCs
- Wide local excision using Moh's micrographic tumour excision technique followed by eyelid reconstruction (see Table 9.14): after removal of a debulking layer, narrow margins of surrounding tissue including the sides and the base of the tumour bed are removed for frozen section analysis, the frozen section are interpreted by the excising surgeon, if any tumour remains the surgeon goes back to the exact site and removes more tissue, the process is repeated with small areas of excision until all tumour tissue has been excised

9.24.6 Referrals of BCCs into Secondary Care (NICE Guidance [NG12] [4])

- Consider routine referral for people if they have a skin lesion that raises the suspicion of a BCC
- Only consider a suspected cancer pathway referral (for an appointment within 2 weeks) for people with a skin lesion that raises the suspicion of a BCC if there is particular concern that a delay may have a significant impact, because of factors such as lesion site or size

Table 9.14 Eyelid reconstruction

Repair of full-thickness eyelid defects up to 25%:
Primary/direct eyelid margin repair:
The primary eyelid margin repair begins with identifying the appropriate anatomic landmarks of the eyelid, especially the landmarks of the lid margin.
The strength of the closure is in sutures placed in the tarsal plate
Eyelid wound margin eversion is necessary to prevent lid notching
Steps of eyelid margin repair are:
Inject local anaesthetic
Align the lid margin (7/0 vicryl vertical mattress suture passed through the meibomian gland orifices to align and evert the lid margin)
Suture the tarsal plate (use 2 to 3 interrupted 5/0 vicryl sutures passed in a lamellar fashion to align the tarsal plate)
Suture the lid margin (place a 7/0 vicryl vertical mattress suture anterior to the gray line—this suture should align the eyelashes and provide eversion of the lid margin)
Close the skin (5/0 vicryl interrupted sutures)
If the closure is under too much tension or the lower lid retracts inferiorly under the globe do a lateral canthotomy and cantholysis—If there is still too much tension
Perform a Tenzel flap procedure, advancing tissue from the temple to form a new lid margin
If the defect involves most of the lower eyelid, you should start with a Hughes flap procedure
If the defect involves most of the upper eyelid, you should start with a cutler beard procedure
Repair of full-thickness eyelid defects of 25% to 50%:
Canthotomy, cantholysis, and eyelid margin closure:
The canthotomy (angle canthotomy incision slightly superiorly for lower eyelid and angle canthotomy incision slightly inferiorly for upper eyelid) and cantholysis are used to release the lateral aspect of the lid to allow the lid margin to be closed under less tension
Perform a primary lid margin repair and close the canthotomy
Repair of lid defects of 50% to 75%:
The Tenzel semi-circular flap:
Steps of the Tenzel procedure are:
Inject local anaesthetic: draw an arched line extending superiorly (lower lid) or inferiorly (upper lid) from the lateral canthus in a curve
Perform lateral canthotomy and cantholysis: angle canthotomy superiorly as the canthotomy incision will continue as the Tenzel flap.
Form and mobilise the Tenzel flap: dissect a myocutaneous flap posterior to the orbicularis muscle in the preseptal plane
Perform a primary lid margin repair and close the flap
Repai of lower lid defects of 75% or greater:
(A) The Hughes procedure:
Used to reconstruct the posterior lamella of a full thickness lower eyelid defect that is too wide for the use of a Tenzel flap (no lashes on lower eyelid)
Procedure provides a flap of tarsus and conjunctiva from the upper eyelid, which is sewn into the lower eyelid. This tarsoconjunctival flap carries its own blood supply because it remains attached to the upper eyelid for 4 weeks
An anterior lamella is provided using a myocutaneous advancement flap or FTSG
Steps of the Hughes procedure:
Inject local anaesthetic
Measure the lower eyelid defect
Form the tarsoconjunctival flap: leave 3 mm of intact superior lid margin to prevent upper lid entropion, make a horizontal cut parallel to the lid margin full thickness through the tarsus, dissect tarsus off the underlying orbicularis muscle and levator aponeurosis superiorly to the top edge of the tarsus, dissect a tissue plane between Muller's muscle and the conjunctiva up to the superior fornix, make vertical cuts in the conjunctiva to bring down the tarsal flap,
Suture the flap into the lower eyelid defect
Complete the anterior lamellar repair
4 weeks later, open the eyelids by excising the flap. Cut slightly above the lower lid margin
(B) Free tarsal graft:
Harvested from the contralateral upper lid to be used as a posterior lamellar replacement for lower eyelid defects
Advantage is that it is a one staged procedure
Disadvantage is that it does not have a blood supply, so it must be covered with a myocutaneous advancement flap

(continued)

Table 9.14 (continued)

Repair of upper lid defects of 50% or greater:
(A) The Cutler Beard procedure:
Used to repair large full thickness defects of the upper lid.
Two-stage lid sharing procedure
A width of full thickness lower eyelid below the tarsal plate is used to reconstruct the upper eyelid defect
The eyelids are sewn closed for several weeks before the second stage procedure (6–8 weeks later) to open the eyelids is performed
(B) Free tarsal graft and bipedicle flap:
Use a free tarsal graft from contralateral upper lid to fill the posterior lamellar defect
Make a horizontal incision in the upper lid anterior lamella and advance a bipedicle flap of skin and muscle inferiorly to vascularise the free tarsal graft
Place a free skin graft over the defect where you borrowed the tissue for the bipedicle flap.

Table 9.15 Useful information about actinic keratosis

Premalignant skin lesion, the precursor to squamous cell carcinoma
Lesions appear in the context of sun damaged skin on the face, hands, bald scalp, and ears

9.25 Actinic Keratosis (Table 9.15)

9.25.1 Examination

- Multiple flesh coloured, yellowish, or brownish macules or papules +/− cutaneous horn (see Fig. 9.40), depending on the degree of hyperkeratosis, which are rough to touch
- Upper lid is rarely a site of actinic keratosis because of shading of the skin by the prominence of the superior brow

9.25.2 Investigations

- Perform an incision biopsy if there is any doubt of the underlying diagnosis
- If a keratin horn is present, perform a deep excision biopsy including the base of the horn to determine the diagnosis

9.25.3 Treatment

- Monitor for formation of squamous cell carcinoma (see Fig. 9.41)
- Treatment options: excision, topical application of imiquimod or 5-FU, cryotherapy

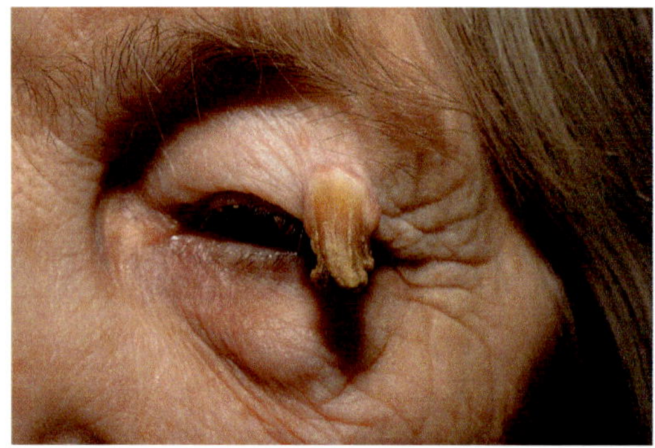

Fig. 9.40 Facial photo of a patient with an upper eyelid keratin horn

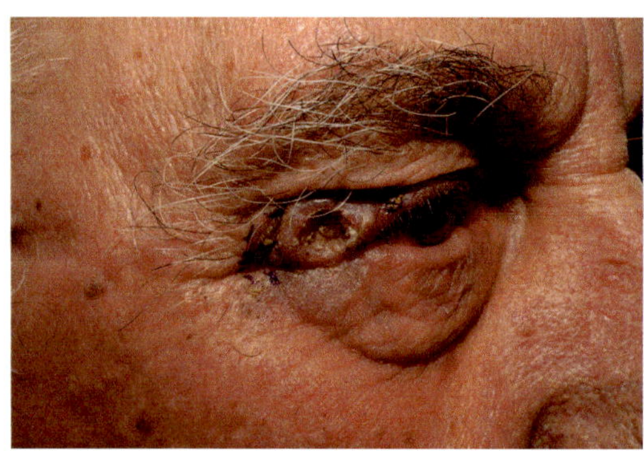

Fig. 9.41 Facial photo of a patient with a right upper lateral lid squamous cell carcinoma

9.26 Melanocytic Naevus (Table 9.16, 9.17 and 9.18)

9.26.1 History

- Presentation age: at birth—congenital naevus, teenaged child—junctional or compound naevus, older adult—intradermal naevus

Table 9.16 Life cycle of a melanocytic naevus

Junctional naevus: flat small oval or round light to dark brown macules—at border of epidermis and dermis
Compound naevus: raised and dome shaped—extending from epidermis into dermis
Intradermal naevus: raised with loss of colour returning to light brown or flesh colour—within dermis

Table 9.17 Characteristics of benign pigment cell tumours (e.g. naevus)

Uniform in colour (small variations from light brown to brown are normal)
Regular smooth borders (smooth edges)
Symmetric shape (lesion can be folded on itself)

Table 9.18 Characteristics of malignant pigment cell tumours (e.g. melanoma)

Recent onset of pigmented lesion
Change in existing pigmented lesion (shape, size, colour)
Irregular margins
Asymmetric shape (lesion cannot be folded on itself)
Large size greater than 6 mm in diameter
Colour change or presence of multiple colours

9.26.2 Examination

- Junctional naevus: brown flat lesion (see Fig. 9.42)
- Compound naevus: darker dome-shaped lesion
- Intradermal naevus: elevated non-pigmented lesion

9.26.3 Investigations

- Punch biopsy (incisional biopsy technique where a disposable skin dermatome, like a corneal trephine, is used to "core" out a sample of the lesion) should be performed if a naevus shows a dramatic change in colour or shape

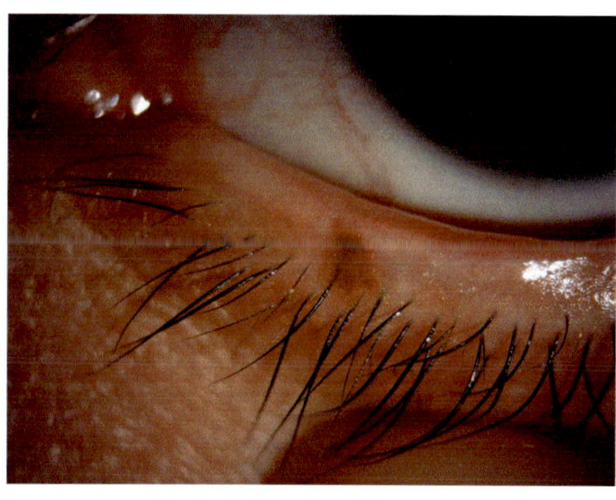

Fig. 9.42 Anterior segment photo of a patient with an eyelid melanocytic naevus

9.26.4 Treatment

- No treatment required for majority of naevi
- For intradermal naevus (elevated nonpigmented naevus) causing irritation or disfigurement: shave biopsy (incisional biopsy technique with lesion shaved off flush with the lid margin)

References

1. Baker ND, Barnebey HS, Moster MR, Stiles MC, Vold SD, Khatana AK, Flowers BE, Grover DS, Strouthidis NG, Panarelli JF. Ab-Externo MicroShunt versus trabeculectomy in primary open-angle glaucoma. One-year results from a 2-year randomized, multicenter study. Ophthalmology. 2021;128:1710–21.
2. Panarelli JF, Moster MR, Garcia-Feijoo J, Flowers BE, Baker ND, Barnebey HS, Grover DS, Khatana AK, Lee B, Nguyen T, Stiles MC, Sadruddin O, Khaw PT. Ab-Externo MicroShunt versus trabeculectomy in primary open-angle glaucoma. Two-year results from a randomized, multicenter study. Ophthalmology. 2024;131:226–76.
3. National Institute for Health and Care Excellence. Glaucoma: diagnosis and management [NG81]. [Online]. London: NICE; 2017. Available at https://www.nice.org.uk/guidance/ng81. Accessed 10 Dec 2024.
4. National Institute for Health and Care Excellence. Suspected cancer: recognition and referral [NG12]. [Online]. London: NICE; 2015. Available at https://www.nice.org.uk/guidance/ng12. Accessed 15 Dec 2019.

Posterior Segment 10

Timothy H. M. Fung and Winfried M. K. Amoaku

Abstract

This chapter offers a comprehensive overview of a wide range of posterior segment pathologies that are commonly encountered in an OSCE exam for ophthalmologists

10.1 Posterior Segment Examination Sequence

10.1.1 Indirect Slit-Lamp Biomicroscopy

- Introduce yourself to the patient
- Set patient up on the slit-lamp
- Focus and center a slit beam (use the brightest light intensity that the patient can easily tolerate) in the center of the corneal surface and hold a condensing lens (e.g. +90 D) stationary between your thumb and index finger approximately 5–10 mm from the patient's cornea
- Keeping the slit beam centered on both the patient's cornea and the condensing lens, pull the slit-lamp joystick with your freehand away from the patient until the patient's red reflex becomes a focused fundus image
- Ask the patient to look at your ear or shoulder to begin examining the optic disc. Proceed temporally circumferentially around the posterior pole and ending at the fovea. Examine different aspects of the peripheral retina by asking the patient to look in different directions of gaze

10.1.2 Indirect Ophthalmoscopy

- For the exam the patients will likely be lying flat on a bed with the pupils dilated
- Introduce yourself to the patient
- Ask for room lights to be dimmed (if not already dimmed)
- Begin by asking the patient to stare at a distance target on the ceiling just above and beyond your shoulder (your right shoulder when examining the patient's right eye and your left shoulder when examining the patient's left eye)
- Examine each eye in turn. Direct the indirect ophthalmoscopes light source into the center of the patient's pupil. Hold the condensing lens, and position it just in front of the patient's eye and center the pupil in it. Pull the lens slowly away from the patient's eye by flexing your wrists and by bending your fingers holding the lens until you see a focused image of the fundus
- Shift the field of view to different areas of the eye by walking around the patient and by asking the patient to look in different directions of gaze

T. H. M. Fung (✉)
University Hospitals of Derby & Burton NHS Foundation Trust, Royal Derby Hospital, Derby, UK
e-mail: timothy.fung@nhs.net

W. M. K. Amoaku
Eye, Ear, Nose and Throat Centre, Queens Medical Centre, Nottingham University Hospitals NHS Trust, Nottingham, UK

T. H. M. Fung, W. M. K. Amoaku (eds.), *Viva and OSCE Exams in Ophthalmology*,
https://doi.org/10.1007/978-3-031-97401-4_10

- Remember that the image of the patient's fundus is reversed and inverted

10.2 Stargardt Disease (Table 10.1)

10.2.1 Examination

- Bilateral symmetrical changes often confined to the posterior pole
- Yellowish white flecks (see Fig. 10.1) (differ from drusen in that they are more elongated than round and they often contact each other at angles that create a branching or net-like appearance) at the level of the RPE—pisciform flecks (2 adjacent flecks form an obtuse angle)
- Relative sparing of the peripapillary retina and RPE
- Circular area of RPE atrophy centered at the fovea with a metallic sheen (crystalline deposits overlying this atrophy) +/− clumps of dark pigment within the atrophic lesion
- Vermillion or light-brown colour to the fundus with complete obscuration of the underlying choroidal vessels

Table 10.1 Key facts about Stargardt disease

AR macular dystrophy (onset in childhood)
Mildest of the ABCA4 phenotypes

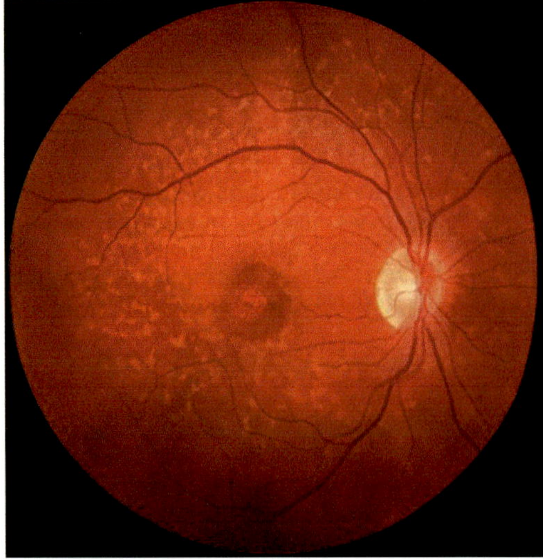

Fig. 10.1 Colour fundus image of a patient with Stargardt disease showing the typical yellowish-white flecks in the posterior pole

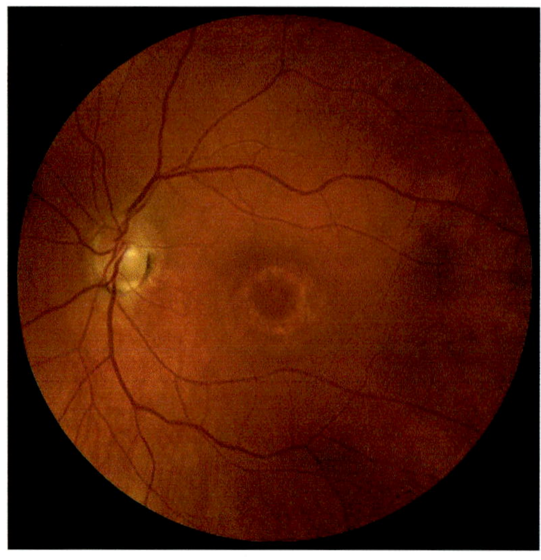

Fig. 10.2 Colour fundus image of a patient with Stargardt disease with a typical bull's eye maculopathy

Table 10.2 Causes of Bulls eye maculopathy

Stargardt disease
Hydroxychloroquine toxicity
Cone dystrophy / Cone-rod dystrophy
Batten disease (neuronal ceroid lipofuscinosis—ERG severely reduced or extinguished before age of 10 years)

- Bull's eye maculopathy (see Fig. 10.2 and Table 10.2): ring of atrophic RPE surrounding the fovea

10.2.2 Investigations

- FAF: loss of autofluorescence in areas of atrophy (including the atrophic fovea and bull's eye maculopathy)
- FFA: dark choroid (see Fig. 10.3)—masking of the choroidal circulation with dye filled retinal vessels lying upon a completely hypofluorescent background +/− hyperfluorescence of flecks and areas of atrophy
- OCT: RPE atrophy and outer retinal loss (loss of ellipsoid zone)
- Molecular testing: ABCA4 gene
- EDTs: full field ERG- typically normal in Stargardt disease, pattern ERG (PERG)—group 1 (severe PERG abnormality with normal full field ERG), group 2 (additional loss

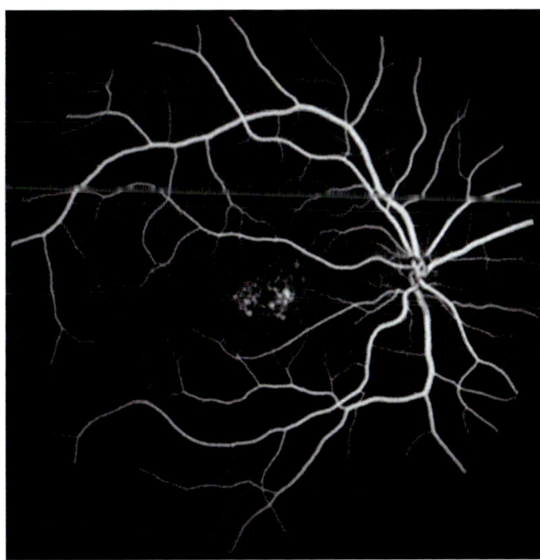

Fig. 10.3 Fundus fluorescein angiogram of a patient with Stargardt disease showing a typical dark choroid with hyperfluorescence of flecks

of photopic function), group 3 (additional loss of both photopic and scotopic function)

10.2.3 Treatment

- There is currently no proven treatment for ABCA4 disease

10.2.4 Other Diagnosis to Consider

- Fundus flavimaculatus: AR, adult onset, pisciform flecks, peripapillary sparing, relative preservation of vision (no macular atrophy)
- Stargardt like autosomal dominant macular dystrophy (SLDMD): +ve FHx, pisciform flecks, peripapillary sparing, macular atrophy, normal ERG
- Pattern dystrophy (group of inherited conditions characterised by changes at the level of the RPE)—reticular pattern: AD (+ve FHx), gene testing for PRPH2 mutations, low risk of CVN development
- Cone dystrophy / Cone-rod dystrophy
- Central areolar choroidal dystrophy: AD (+ve FHx), earliest change is a fine mottled depigmentation in the macula of both eyes and gradually evolves into symmetric, sharply outlined oval or round areas of GA of the RPE, normal full field ERG

10.3 Best Macular Dystrophy (BMD) (Table 10.3)

10.3.1 History

- Positive FHx (autosomal dominant)

10.3.2 Examination

- Solitary round oval yellow slightly elevated lesion centered on the fovea (egg-yolk like lesion) (see Fig. 10.4) +/− pseudohypopyon (yellow material gravitates inferiorly in the subretinal space) +/− subretinal fibrosis +/− RPE atrophy +/− RPE hyperpigmentation
- Subretinal haemorrhage in the macula—suggestive of a CNV membrane (20%)

Table 10.3 Key facts about BMD

AD macular dystrophy caused by mutations in BEST1 gene
Onset usually in childhood
BMD refers to the "classic" form of a single symmetric egg-yolk like lesion centered on the fovea of each eye

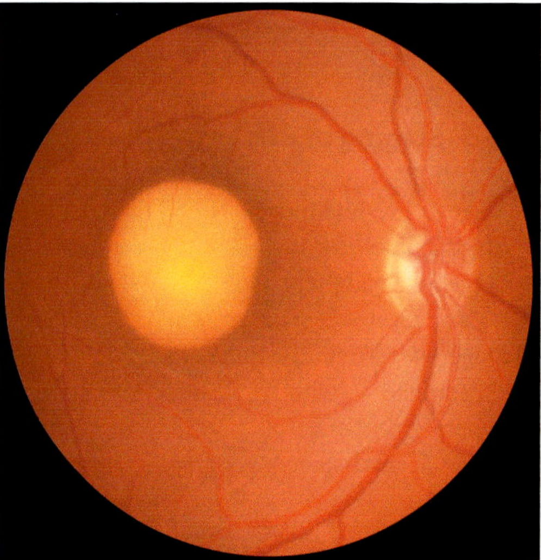

Fig. 10.4 Colour fundus image of a patient with BMD showing the typical egg-yolk like lesion

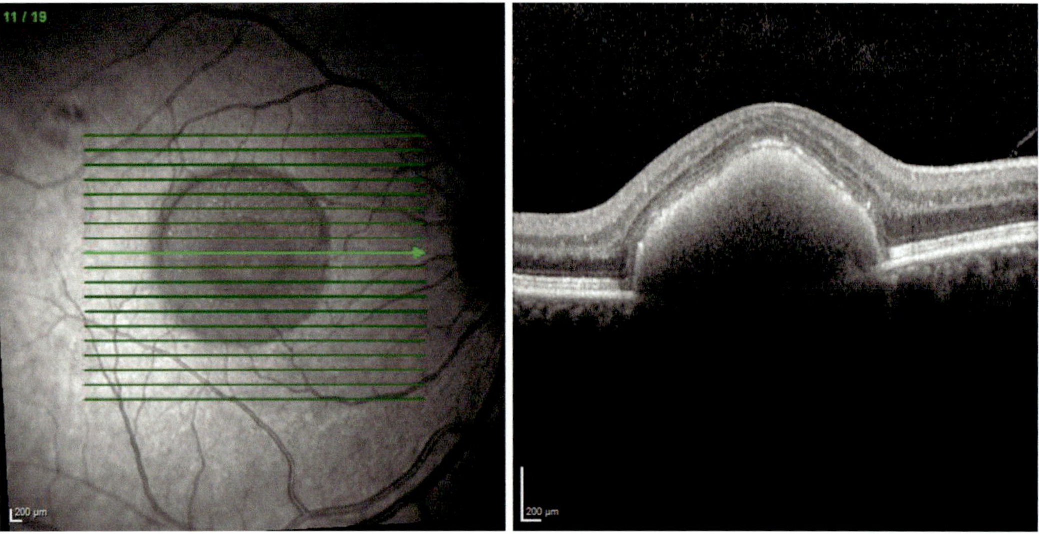

Fig. 10.5 OCT image of a patient with BMD showing the typical sub-RPE hyper-reflective lesion

10.3.3 Investigations

- OCT: sub-RPE hyper-reflective lesion (see Fig. 10.5)
- FFA: look for leakage suggestive of a CNV membrane
- EDT: EOG—reduced Arden ratio (less than 1.5), ERG—normal full field ERG

10.3.4 Treatment

- Treatment of CNV with anti-VEGF therapy

10.3.5 Staging of BMD

- Stage 1: Pre-vitelliform—EOG findings only
- Stage 2: Vitelliform—yolk-like macular lesion
- Stage 3: Pseudohypopyon—partial absorption leaving level
- Stage 4: Vitellidisruptive—scrambled egg appearance with RPE atrophy + hyperpigmentation
- Stage 5: End-stage—geographic atrophy of the RPE

10.3.6 Other Diagnoses to Consider

- Adult-onset foveomacular vitelliform pattern dystrophy—smaller (less than 1/3 DD) vitelliform lesions than BMD, normal EOG

10.4 Sorsby Macular Dystrophy (Table 10.4)

10.4.1 History

- Positive FHx

10.4.2 Examination

- In the early stages, yellow-to-grey material (similar in appearance to drusen) is present at the level of Bruch's membrane
- Bilateral subfoveal CNV membranes with extensive disciform scarring (see Figs. 10.6 and 10.7), which can extend peripherally (unlike AMD which rarely extends beyond the temporal vascular arcades) in the late stages

Table 10.4 Key facts about Sorsby macular dystrophy

AD condition caused by a mutation in the TIMP3 gene
Progressive atrophy of the peripheral choroid and RPE is common
Most commonly presents in the 4th or 5th decade of life

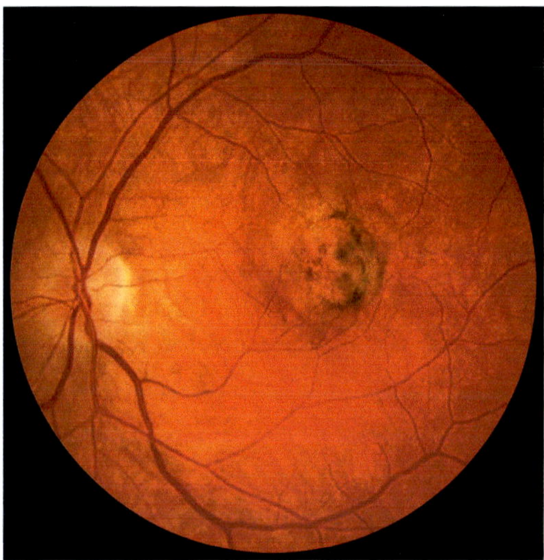

Fig. 10.6 Colour fundus image of a patient with Sorsby macular dystrophy showing subfoveal disciform scarring

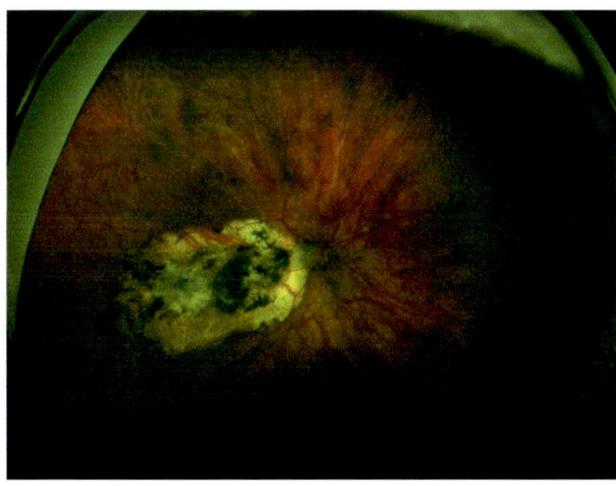

Fig. 10.7 Ultra-widefield pseudocolour fundus image of another patient with Sorsby macular dystrophy showing extensive subfoveal disciform scarring

10.4.3 Investigations

- Genetic testing for mutation in TIMP3 gene
- OCT-A—detect CNV membrane

10.4.4 Treatment

- CNV: anti-VEGF therapy

10.4.5 Other Diagnoses to Consider

- AMD

10.5 Retinitis Pigmentosa (RP) (Table 10.5)

10.5.1 Classification

- Based on inheritance (50% have no FHx): AD (later onset and less severe), AR, XL recessive (both AR and XL recessive RP have an earlier onset and more severe)

10.5.2 History

- Positive FHx
- Symptoms: nyctalopia, loss of peripheral visual field, loss of central vision, photopsias

10.5.3 Examination

- In typical RP, there is a high degree of symmetry of fundus abnormalities between the 2 eyes
- Bone spicule intraretinal pigmentation (see Figs. 10.8 and 10.9)—represent RPE migration into the retina

Table 10.5 Key facts about RP

Term used for a group of disorders that are characterised by inherited, progressive dysfunction, cell loss, and eventual atrophy of retinal tissue
Initial involvement of photoreceptors leads to subsequent damage to inner retinal cells. Eventually there is widespread atrophy of several, if not most, layers of the retina
RP may be seen in isolation (typical RP) or in association with systemic disease in <25% of cases (syndromic RP)

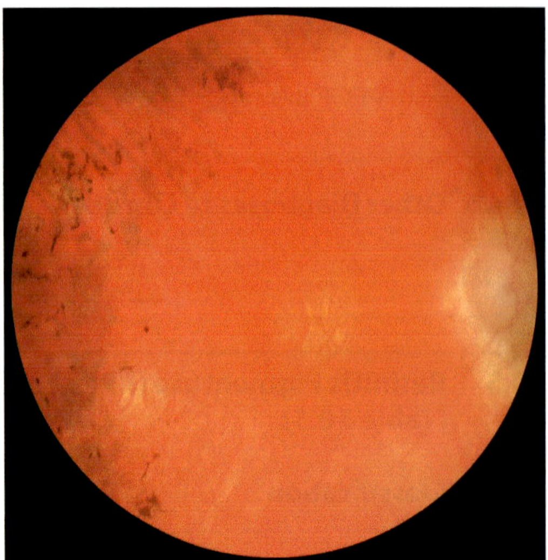

Fig. 10.8 Colour fundus image of a patient with RP showing a disc pallor, attenuated retinal vessels, bone spicules and foveal and peripheral atrophy of the RPE and choriocapillaris

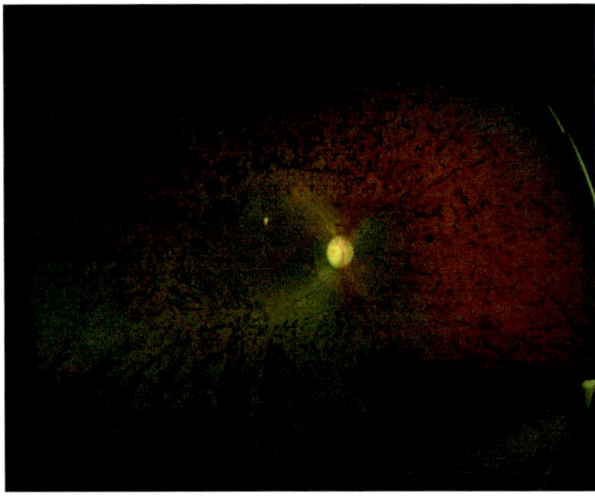

Fig. 10.9 Ultra-widefield pseudocolour fundus image of another patient with RP showing disc pallor, attenuated retinal vessels and extensive bone spicules

- Optic nerve head pallor (from atrophy +/− gliosis) +/− optic disc drusen
- Attenuated retinal vessels
- Mottling and granularity of the RPE
- Atrophy of RPE and choriocapillaris with fundus pallor and visible large choroidal vessels in advanced disease (see Fig. 10.8)
- Check IOP: RP patients at risk of open angle glaucoma
- Perform an anterior segment examination: look for cataracts (posterior subcapsular cataract) and keratoconus

10.5.4 Investigations

- Refraction: high myopia and astigmatism
- Kinetic VF: scotomas in the mid-periphery which coalesce to form a ring of VF loss (ring scotoma)
- EDT: scotopic ERG is more affected than photopic ERG, ERG extinguished in advanced RP, abnormal EOG
- OCT: CMO, ERM, decreased thickness of the ONL, loss of the ELM and IS/OS junction
- Genetic testing especially for RPE65 gene mutations

10.5.5 Treatment

- Refractive error correction
- Cataract extraction when indicated
- Treatment of CMO when present: topical / oral CAI's
- Visual impairment registration and referral for low vision aids
- Voretigene neparvovec if RPE65 gene mutations are present (NICE Guidance [HST11])

10.5.6 Syndromic RP

- Usher syndrome: AR sensorineural deafness (most commonly congenital), pigmentary retinopathy indistinguishable from typical RP, ERG is profoundly abnormal to undetectable—cochlear implantation
- Kearns-Sayre syndrome: mitochondrial DNA deletion syndrome, pigmentary retinopathy, CPEO, ptosis, cardiac conduction block, cerebellar ataxia—muscle biopsy shows red ragged fibers by light microscopy
- Refsum disease (infantile or adult-onset): AR, pigmentary retinopathy, peripheral neuropathy, ichthyosis, cardiac conduction defects,

ERG responses are severely abnormal or unrecordable at all ages, high phytanic acid levels in blood and urine—restriction of dietary phytanic acid (dairy products)
- Bardet-Biedl syndrome: AR, pigmentary retinopathy, polydactyly, congenital obesity, mental retardation, hypogonadism

10.6 Sector Retinitis Pigmentosa (Sector RP) (Table 10.6)

10.6.1 History

- Positive FHx

10.6.2 Examination

- Bone-spicule like pigmentary changes limited to one or two quadrants (see Fig. 10.10) with minimal or no extension of the retinal area involved with time +/− chorioretinal atrophy
- Retinal arteriolar attenuation in the affected quadrants only
- Cataract: posterior subcapsular lens opacity
- Sector RP can be differentiated from acquired pigmentation by its symmetry between the 2 eyes

Table 10.6 Key facts about sector RP

Specific subtype of RP: usually AD but can be AR
Usually bilateral and symmetrical

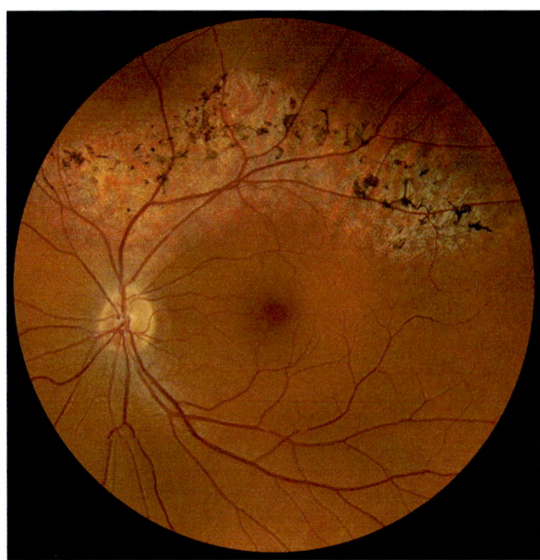

Fig. 10.10 Colour fundus image of a patient with superior sector RP

10.6.3 Investigations

- Refraction
- VF: defects usually only in the regions of retinal pigmentation
- ERG: relatively good responses—relative preservation of amplitudes, with mild to moderate sub-abnormalities of both rod- and cone-mediated responses with normal implicit times
- Genetic testing
- OCT: look for CMO

10.6.4 Treatment

- Refractive error correction
- Cataract extraction when indicated
- Treatment of CMO when present: topical / oral CAI's
- Visual impairment registration and referral for low vision aids

10.6.5 Other Diagnoses to Consider

- Prior trauma (e.g. surgical such as a prior RD repair)
- Inflammation or infection: syphilis (congenital or acquired), congenital rubella (normal ERG, cataracts, hearing loss, no arteriolar attenuation), toxoplasmosis, DUSN
- Retinal toxicity: thioridazine, chlorpromazine, chloroquine, hydroxychloroquine, quinine
- Neoplasm (retinal or choroidal) and CAR (autoimmune paraneoplastic retinopathy)

10.7 Age-Related Macular Degeneration (AMD)

10.7.1 Classification of AMD

NICE Guidance [NG82] [43]

- Early AMD
  (a) Low risk of progression
    - Medium drusen (63–124 μm)
    - Pigmentary abnormalities
  (b) Medium risk of progression
    - Large drusen (≥ 125 μm)
    - Reticular drusen
    - Medium drusen with pigmentary abnormalities
  (c) High risk of progression
    - Large drusen with pigmentary abnormalities
    - Reticular drusen with pigmentary abnormalities
    - Vitelliform lesion without significant visual loss (BCVA better than 6/18)
    - Atrophy smaller than 175 μm and not involving the fovea
- Late AMD (indeterminate)
  (a) RPE degeneration and dysfunction (presence of degenerative AMD changes with SRF or IRF in the absence of neovascularisation)
  (b) Serous PED without neovascularisation
- Late AMD (dry)
  (a) Geographic atrophy (in the absence of neovascular AMD)
  (b) Significant visual loss (6/18 or worse) associated with:
    - Dense or confluent drusen
    - Advanced pigmentary changes and/or atrophy
    - Vitelliform lesion
- Late AMD (wet active)
  (a) Classic CNV
  (b) Occult (fibrovascular PED and serous PED with neovascularisation)
  (c) Mixed (predominantly or minimally classic CNV with occult CNV)
  (d) RAP
  (e) PCV
- Late AMD (wet inactive)
  (a) Fibrous scar
  (b) Subfoveal atrophy or fibrosis secondary to an RPE tear
  (c) Atrophy (absence or thinning of RPE and/or retina)
  (d) Cystic degeneration (persistent IRF or tabulations unresponsive to treatment)

The Age-Related Eye Disease Study (AREDS) Severity Scale [62]

- Group 1 (No AMD): none or a few small drusen (<63 μm)
- Group 2 (Early AMD): any or all of the following—multiple small drusen; few intermediate drusen (63–124 μm); RPE abnormalities (increased pigmentation or depigmentation but not geographic atrophy)
- Group 3 (Intermediate AMD): any or all of the following—extensive intermediate drusen; at least 1 large drusen (≥ 125 μm, equivalent to the width of a major retinal vein at the optic disc edge), geographic atrophy that does not extend under the center of the macula
- Group 4 (Advanced AMD): presence of geographic atrophy extending under the center of the macula and/or presence of neovascular AMD

Rotterdam Classification System [74]

- Grade 0 (no AMD): no signs of AMD at all **OR** hard drusen (<63 μm) only
- Grade 1 (preliminary early AMD): soft distinct drusen (≥ 63 μm) only **OR** pigmentary abnormalities only
- Grade 2 (early AMD): soft indistinct drusen (yellow lesions with indistinct borders and ≥ 125 μm in size) / reticular pseudodrusen only **OR** soft distinct drusen (≥ 63 μm) **AND** pigmentary abnormalities
- Grade 3 (early AMD): soft indistinct drusen (yellow lesions with indistinct borders and ≥ 125 μm in size) / reticular pseudodrusen **AND** pigmentary abnormalities
- Grade 4 (late AMD): atrophic, neovascular, or mixed AMD

10.7.2 History

- Ask about risk factors for AMD (NICE Guidance [NG82]) [43]:
  - Older age
  - Smoking
  - Positive FHx of AMD
  - HTN
  - Presence of AMD in other eye
  - BMI of 30 kg/m^2 or higher
  - Diet high in fat
  - Lack of exercise

10.7.3 Examination

- Non-neovascular (see Fig. 10.11): confluent pale yellow poorly defined soft drusen (intermediate 63–124 µm, large ≥125 µm [width of a retinal vein at the disc edge]) +/− RPE focal hyperpigmentation (intraretinal pigment clumping from RPE migration associated with drusen) +/− RPE hypopigmentation (associated with drusen) +/− RPE atrophy (sharply delineated round or oval area of hypopigmentation or depigmentation with visible choroidal vessels)
- Neovascular (see Fig. 10.12): subretinal (red) or sub-RPE (grey) haemorrhage, subretinal or sub-RPE exudates, retinal or RPE detachment, subretinal fibrosis (disciform scar)

10.7.4 Investigations

- OCT (see Sect. 2.1.4.5)
- OCT-A: enables qualitative and quantitative analysis of CNV membranes and to follow-up structural changes after intravitreal injections
- FFA (see Sect. 2.3): perform if late AMD (wet active) suspected to confirm presence of CNV membrane
- ICG: branching vascular network (BVN) in PCV, “hot hyperfluorescent spot” in RAP

10.7.5 Treatment

- Non-neovascular
  (a) Visual impairment registration and referral to low vision aid service
  (b) Referral to support groups
  (c) Refraction with increased near add

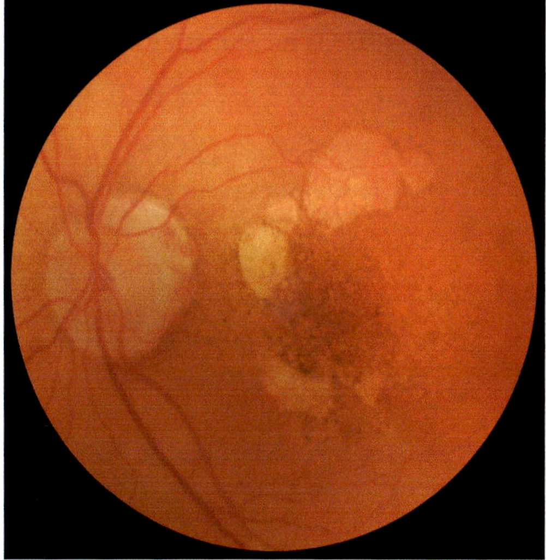

Fig. 10.11 Colour fundus image of a patient with late AMD (dry) showing the presence of geographic atrophy and advanced pigmentary changes

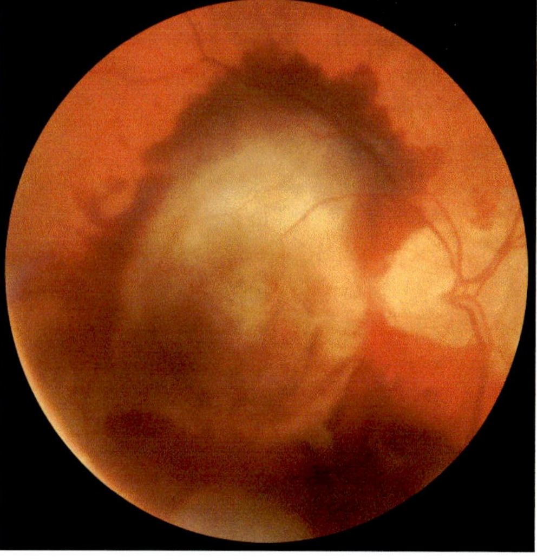

Fig. 10.12 Colour fundus image of a patient with late AMD (wet active) showing the presence of a subretinal haemorrhage with a disciform scar

(d) Amsler grid: advise patients about new or progressive metamorphopsia
(e) Lifestyle changes: smoking cessation, increased intake of food rich in macular carotenoids (spinach, broccoli, cabbage) and omega-3 fatty acids (oily fish such as salmon, mackerel, sardines), exercise
(f) Vitamin supplementation (indications—advanced AMD in 1 eye, ≥1 large druse or extensive intermediate drusen in 1 or both eyes): AREDS 1 (vitamin C & E, β-carotene, zinc, copper)—25% reduced risk of progression to advanced AMD at 5 years [2], AREDS 2 (vitamin C & E, zinc, copper, lutein, zeaxanthin)—18% reduced risk of progression to advanced AMD at 5 years [63]
(g) Discharge from outpatient department

- Neovascular
  (a) Visual impairment registration and referral to low vision aid service
  (b) Referral to support groups
  (c) Refraction with increased near add
  (d) Amsler grid: advise patients about new or progressive metamorphopsia
  (e) Lifestyle changes: smoking cessation, increased intake of food rich in macular carotenoids (spinach, broccoli, cabbage) and omega-3 fatty acids (oily fish such as salmon, mackerel, sardines), exercise
  (f) Laser photocoagulation: extrafoveal or peripapillary CNV
  (g) Anti-VEGF therapy:
    - Eligibility criteria (NICE Guidance [NG82]) [43] in the UK:
      - The BCVA is between 6/12 and 6/96
      - There is no permanent structural damage to the central fovea
      - Greatest linear dimension of lesion size ≤12DD
      - Evidence of recent presumed disease progression (recent VA changes or blood vessel growth on FFA)
      - In eyes with BCVA worse than 6/96 consider anti-VEGF treatment for late AMD (wet active) only if a benefit in the person's overall visual function is expected (e.g. if the affected eye is the persons better seeing eye)
    - Ranibizumab:
      - NICE approved [TA155] [31]
      - Clinical trials:
        - **MARINA** [57]**:** monthly Lucentis compared with sham injection for minimally classic or occult (see Sect. 5.4.2)
        - **ANCHOR** [10]: monthly Lucentis compared with vPDT for predominantly classic CNV (see Sect. 5.4.1)
        - **PrONTO** [20, 28]**:** PRN dosing (see Sect. 5.4.3)
        - **PIER** [1, 56]**:** quarterly dosing (see Sect. 5.4.4)
    - Aflibercept:
      - NICE approved [TA294] [37]
      - Clinical trials:
        - **VIEW 1** & **VIEW 2** [23]: see Sect. 5.4.6
    - Brolucizumab:
      - NICE approved [TA672] [45]
      - Clinical trials:
        - **HAWK** and **HARRIER** [17]: see Sect. 5.4.8
    - Faricimab:
      - NICE approved [TA800]
      - Clinical trials:
        - **TENAYA** and **LUCERNE** [24]: see Sect. 5.4.9
    - Bevacizumab Gamma:
      - NICE approved [TA1022] [50]
      - Clinical trial:
        - **NORSE TWO** [50] see Sect. 5.4.10
    - Bevacizumab:
      - Clinical trials:
        - **CATT** [66]: see Sect. 5.4.5
        - **IVAN** [14]: see Sect. 5.4.7

10.7.6 Defining Risk for the Development of Advanced AMD

- The AREDS investigators devised a clinical scoring system defining risk categories for development of advanced AMD (The [3])
- The scoring system tabulates a person score by assigning 1 risk factor to each eye of an individual for the presence of at least 1 large druse (within 2-disc diameters of the foveal center) and 1 risk factor for the presence of any pigment abnormality (increased pigmentation thought to be attributed to AMD, RPE depigmentation, or areas of noncentral geographic atrophy)
- Risk factors are summed across both eyes on which the 5-year risk of developing advanced AMD in at least one eye can be approximated
- Risk of developing advanced AMD is as follows: total score 0, 0.5% risk; 1 factor, 3%; 2 factors, 12%; 3 factors, 25%, and 4 factors, 50%
- Modifications of the scale award persons without any large drusen 1 risk factor if medium sized drusen are present in both eyes and individuals with advanced AMD in their first eye receive a score of 2 for that eye when tabulating the person score to estimate the risk for their fellow eye

10.7.7 Geographic Atrophy Secondary to AMD

- Avacincaptad pegol (Izervay; Astellas Pharma Inc) is a pegylated RNA aptamer, which functions as an inhibitor of complement C5 cleavage. The GATHER2 trial demonstrated monthly Avacincaptad pegol 2 mg significantly slowed non-centrepoint-involving geographic atrophy growth over 12 months than sham treatment [27]. This treatment was FDA approved in 2023 but has not yet received NICE approval

10.7.8 Other Diagnoses to Consider

- Polypoidal choroidal vasculopathy (PCV—see Fig. 10.13):
  - More prevalent among black and asian populations
  - Appearance of reddish-orange polypoidal lesions
  - Presents as serosanguineous exudative maculopathy characterised by RPE detachment, serous exudation, and haemorrhage in multiple layers
  - The presence of a branching vascular network (BVN) appear as a shallow elevation of the RPE, while the polypoidal lesions appear as sharper protuberances.
  - OCT features of PCV:
    (a) Subretinal fluid (see Fig. 10.14)
    (b) Notched PED—a high PED connected with PEDs of lower height—“M-shaped” PEDs (see Fig. 10.15)
    (c) Polyps can be seen as round or oval structures connected to the outer surface of PEDs (see Fig. 10.16)

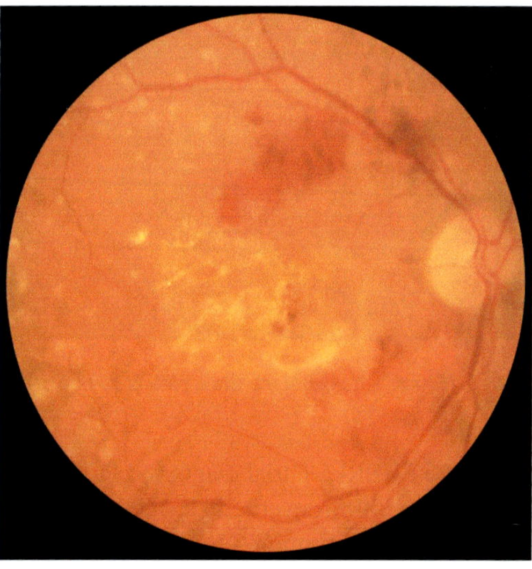

Fig. 10.13 Colour fundus image of a patient with PCV showing a peripapillary and macula subretinal haemorrhage

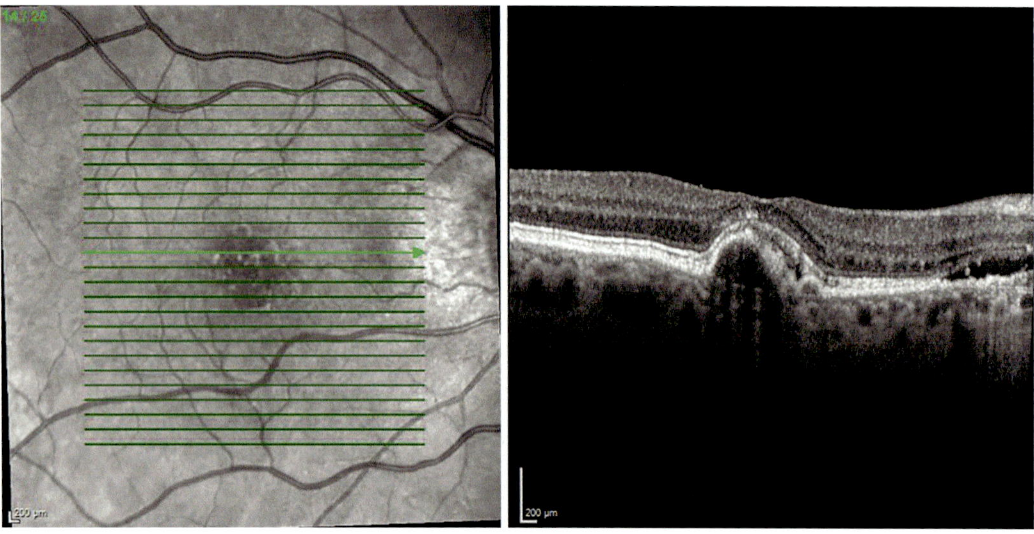

Fig. 10.14 OCT image of a patient with PCV showing peripapillary and macula subretinal fluid

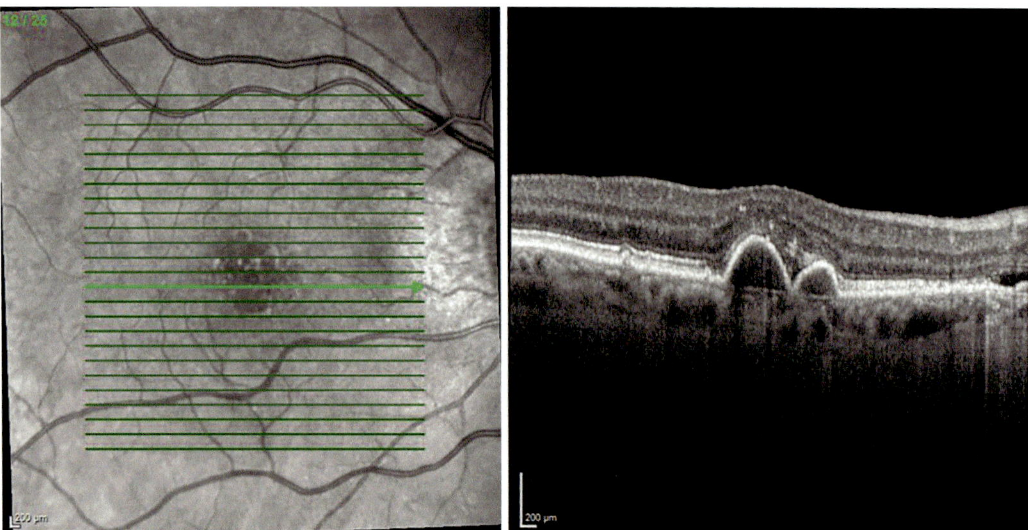

Fig. 10.15 OCT image of the same patient as Fig. 10.14 showing a notched "M-shaped" PED

- The EVEREST trial diagnosed PCV based on the following criteria [60]:
  - (a) Early subretinal ICGA hyperfluorescence appearing within the first 5 minutes of ICG dye injection (see Fig. 10.17) and at least one of the following diagnostic criteria:
    - (1) Nodular appearance of the polyp on stereoscopic viewing
    - (2) Hypofluorescent halo around the nodule
    - (3) Abnormal vascular channel(s) supplying the polyps
    - (4) Pulsatile filling of polyps
    - (5) Orange subretinal nodules corresponding to the hyperfluorescent area on ICGA
    - (6) Massive submacular haemorrhage
- The LAPTOP study [55] was a RCT that showed 3 monthly injections followed by as-needed injections of ranibizumab can achieve better 24-month visual outcomes than PDT

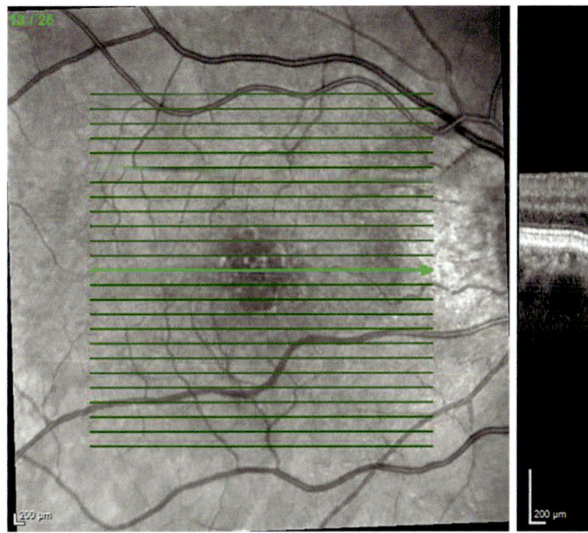

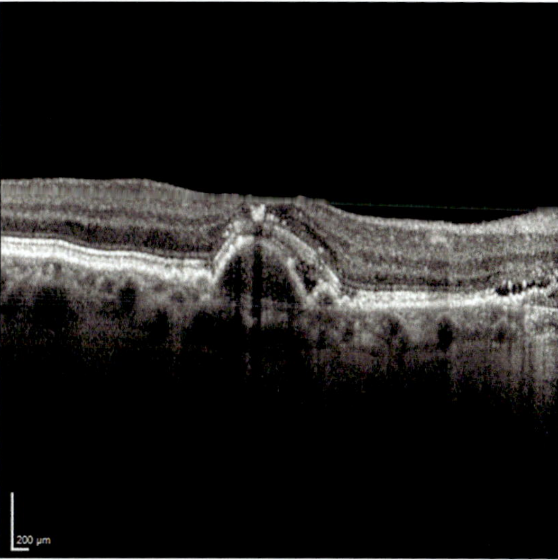

Fig. 10.16 OCT image of the same patient as Figs. 10.14 and 10.15 showing the presence of polyps connected to the outer surface of the PEDs

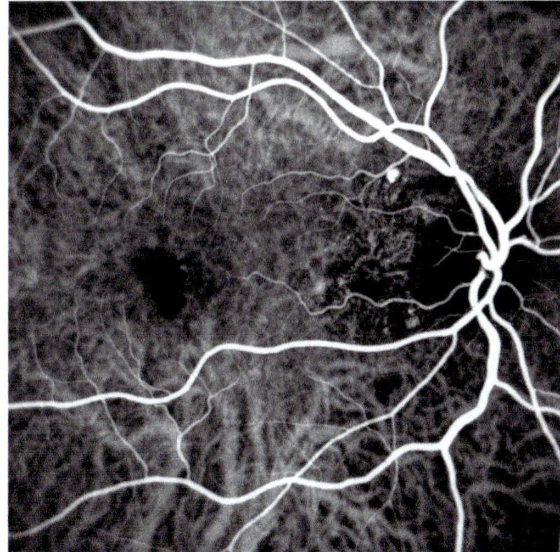

Fig. 10.17 ICGA image of the same patient as shown in Figs. 10.14, 10.15, and 10.16 with PCV showing nodular areas of hyperfluorescence appearing within 30 seconds after dye injection. A branching vascular network is seen adjacent to the optic disc

- The PLANET study [29] was a large scale RCT that showed at 12 months improvement in visual acuity and/or functional outcomes in more than 85% of participants with PCV who had monotherapy with intravitreal aflibercept

10.8 Peripapillary Choroidal Neovascular (CNV) Membrane (Table 10.7)

10.8.1 Causes of Peripapillary CNV Membrane

- Degenerative
  - AMD
  - Angioid streaks
  - Degenerative myopia
  - Laser photocoagulation scars
  - Traumatic choroidal ruptures
- Vascular
  - PCV
- Inflammatory
  - Birdshot chorioretinopathy
  - POHS
  - Sarcoidosis
  - Serpiginous choroiditis
- Optic nerve malformations
  - Optic disc drusen
  - Optic disc pits
  - Retinochoroidal colobomas
- Neoplastic
  - Choroidal naevi
  - Choroidal osteoma
- Idiopathic (up to 39% of cases)

Table 10.7 Key facts about peripapillary CNV membrane

Key facts
Peripapillary CNV membranes are defined as a collection of new choroidal blood vessels, any portion of which lies within 1DD of the nerve head
Account for 10% of all CNV membranes
Clinical manifestations only occur if the membrane extends over the macula, if the vessels haemorrhage into the subretinal space, or fluid exudation occurs within the macula
2 types of peripapillary CNV membranes: type 1—CNV membrane is sub- RPE (e.g. AMD), type 2—CNV membrane in the subretinal space (e.g. POHS)

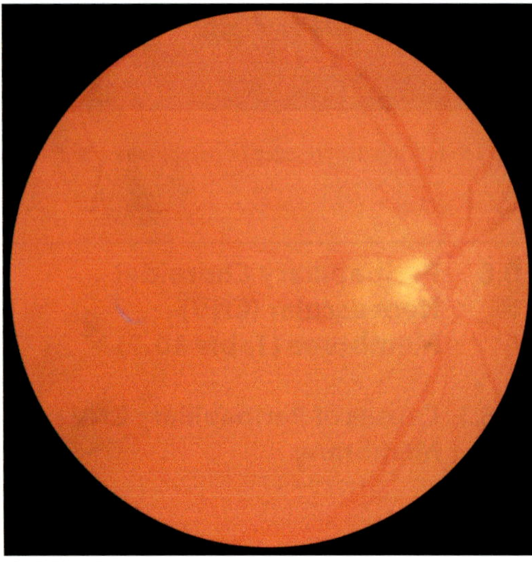

Fig. 10.18 Colour fundus image of a patient with a temporal peripapillary CNV membrane

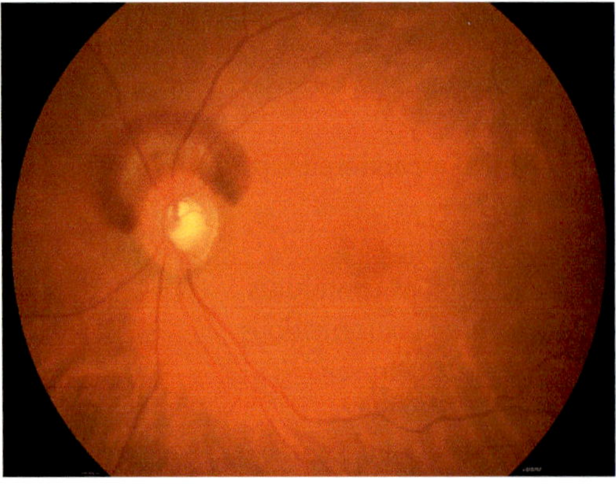

Fig. 10.19 Colour fundus image of a patient with a superior peripapillary CNV membrane

10.8.2 Examination

- Peripapillary (within 1DD) SRF +/− subretinal haemorrhages (see Figs. 10.18 and 10.19)
- Peripapillary fibrotic scar

10.8.3 Investigations

- OCT (see Fig. 10.20): look for presence of SRF
- OCT-A: detect CNV membrane
- FFA: look for leakage confirming presence of a CNV membrane
- ICG: look for PCV (see Fig. 10.17)

10.8.4 Treatment

- Indication: treat when fluid threatening or involving the fovea with reduction of vision
- Options:
  - Anti-VEGF agents: maintains the integrity of the papillomacular bundle
  - Laser photocoagulation: induce scar formation, thermal injury, vitreous haemorrhage, BRAO, damage to the papillomacular bundle

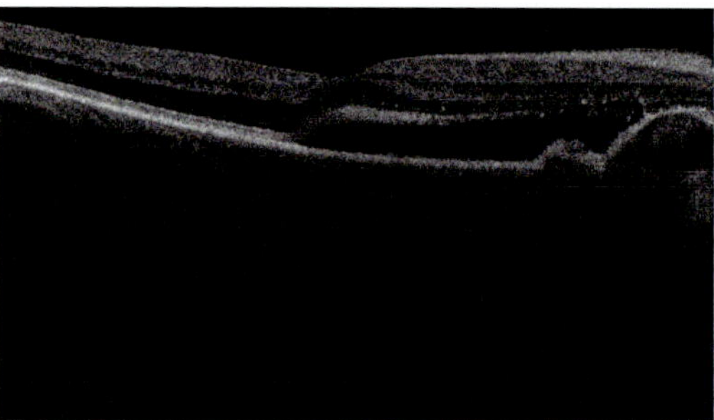

Fig. 10.20 OCT image of a patient with a peripapillary CNV membrane showing SRF tracking to the fovea

10.9 Myopic Macular Degeneration (Tables 10.8 and 10.9)

10.9.1 Examination

- Tilted optic discs
- Peripapillary atrophy (predominantly temporal to optic disc)
- Patchy or diffuse chorioretinal atrophy: visibility of choroidal vessels
- Lacquer cracks (ruptures of Bruch's membrane): yellowish linear lesions
- Posterior staphyloma: outward protrusion of all layers of the posterior eye globe
- Macular CNV (macular haemorrhage) +/− elevated pigmented forster fuchs spot (see Fig. 10.21)

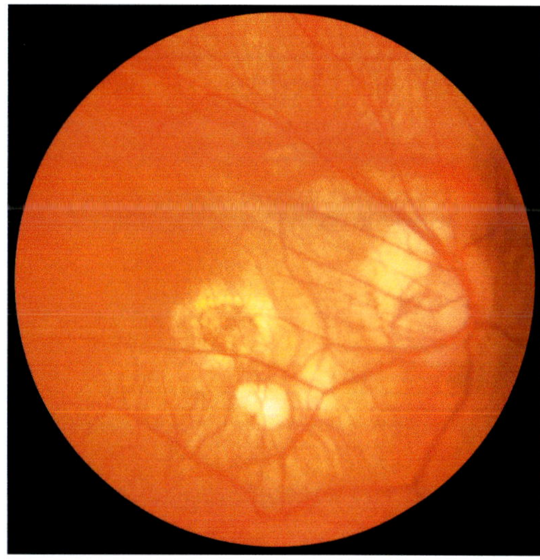

Fig. 10.21 Colour fundus image of a patient with myopic macular degeneration showing diffuse chorioretinal atrophy, tilted optic disc, peripapillary atrophy and a forster fuchs spot

10.9.2 Investigations

- Refraction
- B-scan US: posterior staphyloma
- OCT: posterior staphyloma, myopic foveoschisis (split layers have bridge columns between them, ILM detachment, well preserved IS/OS junction—see Fig. 10.22), macular hole
- OCT-A: detect CNV membrane
- FFA: classic CNV membrane

Table 10.8 Myopia definitions

High myopia is defined as myopia −6.00 D or more or an axial length ≥ 26.5 mm
Pathologic myopia is defined as myopia over −8.00D or an axial length > 32.5 mm

Table 10.9 Associations of myopia

Connective tissue disorders:
Sticklers syndrome
Marfan syndrome
Ehlers-Danlos syndrome
Infectious:
Congenital rubella
Chorioretinal dystrophies:
Gyrate atrophy
Others:
Albinism
Downs syndrome

10.9.3 Treatment

- CNV
  (a) Laser photocoagulation for extrafoveal CNV
  (b) Anti-VEGF therapy for subfoveal CNV:
  - Ranibizumab:
    - NICE Guidance [TA298] [36]: ranibizumab is recommended as an option for treating visual impairment due to choroidal neovascularisation secondary to pathological myopia
    - *RADIANCE* study [76]: comparison of vPDT and Lucentis—after 3/12 of treatment Lucentis showed significantly greater gain in no. of ETDRS letters
  - Aflibercept:
    - NICE Guidance [TA486] [42]: aflibercept is an option treating visual impairment because of myopic choroidal neovascularisation in adults

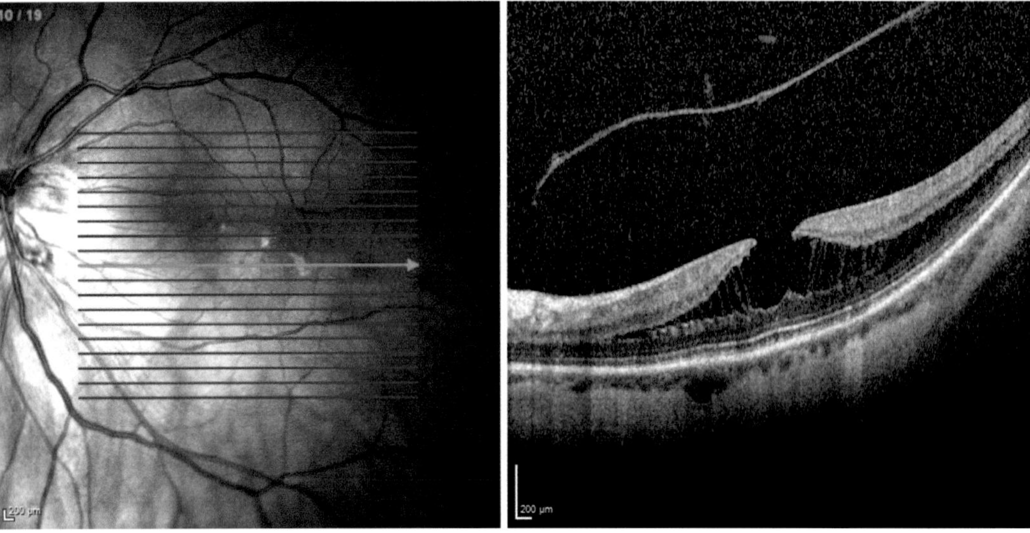

Fig. 10.22 OCT image of a patient with myopic foveoschisis

- MYRROR study [26]: comparison of Eylea and sham injection—at week 24 a gain of 12.1 letters and loss of 2 letters was seen in the Eylea and sham group, respectively.

- Myopic foveoschisis
  (a) If foveal detachment is found on OCT images, macular hole formation is likely to start in the near future and surgery must be planned soon (1–2 months)
  (b) If retinoschisis present with no foveal retinal detachment—not an indication for surgery

10.10 Branch Retinal Vein Occlusion (BRVO) (Table 10.10)

10.10.1 Risk Factors

- Arteriosclerosis: HTN, DM, smoking, hyperlipidaemia (including secondary to hypothyroidism)
- Glaucoma

Table 10.10 Key facts about BRVO

Mostly occurs at arteriovenous crossings
Retinal artery and vein share a common adventitial sheath—lumen of vein compressed by arteriosclerotic artery at the crossing site
Venous obstruction leads to elevation of venous pressure that may overload the collateral drainage capacity and lead to macular oedema and ischaemia

- Ocular inflammatory disease: Behcet's disease, PAN, sarcoidosis, SLE
- Haematological: Protein C, protein S or anti-thrombin deficiency, activated protein C resistance, factor V Leiden, myeloma, Waldenstrom's macroglobulinaemia, antiphospholipid syndrome

10.10.2 Examination

- Acute: wedge shaped segmental distribution of intraretinal haemorrhage in a quadrant of the fundus (see Fig. 10.23), narrowed branch retinal vein passing under a retinal artery, dilated and tortuous retinal vein, cotton wool spots

- Chronic: telangiectatic vessels (dilation of capillaries) forming collaterals that cross the horizontal raphe, microaneurysms, exudates, sclerosed retinal vein +/− NVE > NVD > NVI (see Fig. 10.24)
- Check for RAPD
- Check the IOP
- Look for NVI on anterior segment examination
- Perform gonioscopy for NVA

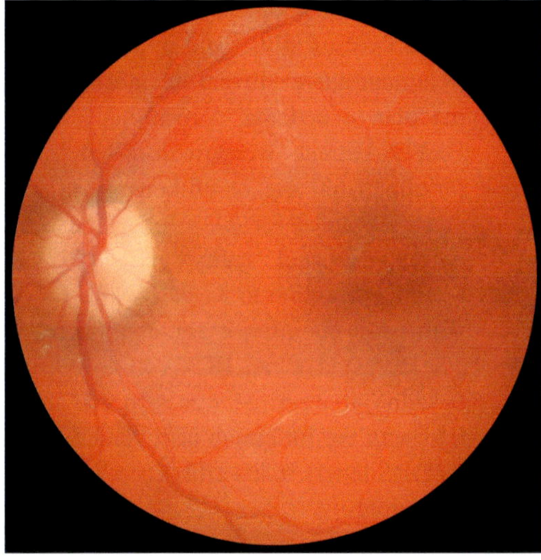

Fig. 10.23 Colour fundus image of a patient with a superior macular BRVO

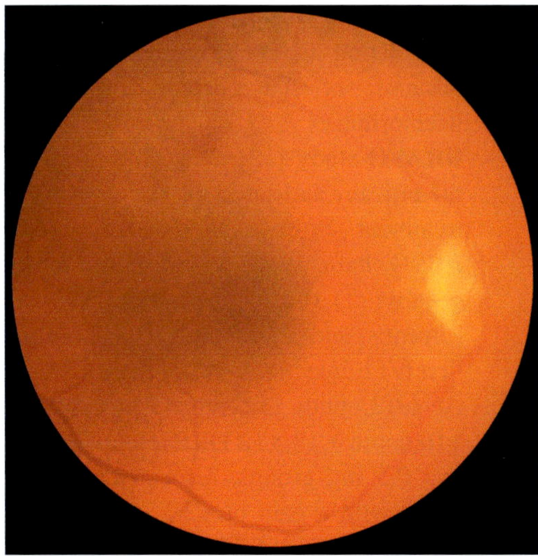

Fig. 10.24 Colour fundus image of a patient with a superotemporal BRVO with NVE

10.10.3 Investigations

RCOphth Retinal Vein Occlusion (RVO) Guidelines 2022: [70]

- BP
- Bloods: FBC (leukaemia/lymphoproliferative disorders), ESR (paraprotein), glucose
- OCT: CMO
- FFA (if uncertain diagnosis): delayed filling of the occluded retinal vein, capillary non-perfusion—>5 DD is defined as an ischaemic BRVO [64, 65], macular ischaemia, telangiectatic vessels forming collaterals that cross the horizontal raphe
- OCT-A is recommended to assess retinal non-perfusion

10.10.4 Treatment

- Control of cardiovascular risk factors: HTN, hyperlipidaemia, smoking, DM
- Neovascularisation: sectoral PRP—branch vein occlusion study—BVOS [64, 65] recommended that laser photocoagulation be applied only after NV is observed, which reduces the likelihood of vitreous haemorrhage from about 60% to 30%
- Macular oedema
  (a) Laser photocoagulation
    - **BVOS** [64, 65]:
      - An RCT that aimed to answer 3 questions: (1) can laser photocoagulation improve VA compared to observation in eyes with macular oedema from BRVO that reduces the vision to 6/12 or worse; (2) Can sectoral PRP prevent the development of NV; (3) Can sectoral PRP prevent vitreous haemorrhage
      - Wait for at least 3/12 if VA 6/12 or worse before considering laser therapy to allow clearing of intraretinal haemorrhages to permit FFA and evaluation of macular oedema and macular ischaemia

- If perfused macular oedema accounts for the visual loss, and vision continues to be 6/12 or worse without spontaneous improvement, consider grid macular photocoagulation (0.1 s duration, 100 μm spot size, power titrated to produce a "medium" white burn) to the leaking area demonstrated by FFA
- After 3 years of follow-up, 65% of treated eyes gained 2 or more lines of vision compared to 37% of untreated eyes

– RCOphth RVO Guidelines 2022: [70]
- If laser photocoagulation is contemplated, it should be performed in those eyes with macular oedema secondary to BRVO of at least 3 months duration with VA of 6/12 or worse and without significant macular haemorrhage and with a FFA showing capillary perfusion in the absence of blood involving the fovea.
- Those with severe visual loss (less than 6/60 vision) and those in whom symptoms have been present for more than 1 year are unlikely to benefit from the treatment

(b) Dexamethasone intravitreal steroid implant (Ozurdex)
– NICE Guidance [TA 229] [32]: recommend as an option for treatment of macular oedema due to a BRVO when treatment with laser photocoagulation has not been beneficial or treatment with laser photocoagulation is not considered suitable because of the extent of retinal haemorrhages
– **GENEVA** study [22]: A RCT that evaluated the effects of a single dexamethasone implant compared to sham injection for the treatment of macular oedema secondary to BRVO and CRVO. Increase in BCVA of ≥15 ETDRS letters was achieved in 30% of the Ozurdex 0.7 mg group, 26% of the Ozurdex 0.35 mg group, and 13% of the sham group 60 days after injection (peak response) and was maintained through day 90 in BRVO patients. There was no difference between either Ozurdex groups and the sham group at day 180.

(c) Faricimab
– NICE Guidance [TA1004] [49]: recommended as an option for treatment of visual impairment caused by macular oedema following BRVO
– **BALATON** study [59]: A RCT to evaluate the 24-week efficacy and safety of faricimab versus aflibercept in patients with treatment-naïve foveal center-involved macular oedema resulting from BRVO. Patients were randomised 1:1 to faricimab 6.0 mg or aflibercept 2.0 mg every 4 weeks for 24 weeks. The best-corrected visual acuity gains (BCVA) from the baseline to week 24 with faricimab were noninferior versus aflibercept. The adjusted mean BCVA change from baseline at week 24 was +16.9 ETDRS letters in the faricimab arm versus +17.5 ETDRS letters in the aflibercept arm.

(d) Ranibizumab
– NICE Guidance [TA283] [34]: recommend as an option for treatment of macular oedema due to a BRVO when treatment with laser photocoagulation has not been beneficial or treatment with laser photocoagulation is not considered suitable because of the extent of retinal haemorrhages
– **BRAVO** study [12]: A RCT to evaluate the efficacy and safety of Lucentis in the treatment of macular oedema from BRVO. Patients were randomised into 3 groups: (1) sham injection; (2) 0.3 mg Lucentis; and (3) 0.5 mg Lucentis. In the first 6/12, injections were given monthly. At 6/12, both Lucentis groups gained +16.6 and + 18.3 ETDRS letters (0.3 mg and 0.5 mg groups, respectively) compared with a gain of +7.3 letters in the control group. At 6/12, 55.2% and 61.1% of patients receiving Lucentis 0.3 mg and 0.5 mg gained ≥3 ETDRS lines com-

pared to 28.8% in the sham injection group

(e) Aflibercept (Eylea)
   - NICE Guidance [TA305] [38]: recommend as an option for treatment of visual impairment caused by macular oedema following BRVO
   - **VIBRANT** study [13]: A RCT that evaluated the efficacy and safety of Eylea compared to macular grid laser in the treatment of macular oedema from BRVO or HRVO. After 6/12 of treatment, 26.7% of the laser group gained ≥3 ETDRS lines compared to 52.7% in the Eylea group. Mean change in letters from baseline was +6.9 letters in the laser group compared to +17.0 letters in the Eylea group.

10.10.5 Prognosis

- BVOS [64, 65]
  - Only eyes with ischaemic BRVO (> 5 DD of retinal capillary non-perfusion) are at risk of developing NV—40% of these eyes develop NV, and of these 40%, 60% will experience periodic vitreous haemorrhage
  - Retinal or disc NV, or both, may develop at any time within the first 3 years after an occlusion but are most likely to appear within the first 6–12 months after the occlusion
  - Up to 10% of patients with BRVO in one eye will develop any type of RVO in the fellow eye

10.10.6 Other Diagnoses to Consider

- Macular telangiectasia
- Susac syndrome: BRAO, sensorineural hearing loss, subacute encephalopathy, hyperintense lesions in the corpus callosum on T2 MRI
- Diabetic retinopathy
- Radiation retinopathy
- Retinal inflammation: Sarcoidosis, Behcet

10.11 Central Retinal Vein Occlusion (CRVO)

10.11.1 Risk Factors

- Arteriosclerosis: HTN, DM, smoking, hyperlipidaemia (including secondary to hypothyroidism)
- Glaucoma
- Ocular inflammatory disease: Behcet's disease, PAN, sarcoidosis, SLE
- Haematological: Protein C, protein S or antithrombin deficiency, activated protein C resistance, factor V Leiden, myeloma, Waldenstrom's macroglobulinaemia, antiphospholipid syndrome
- Pharmacological: oral contraceptive pill

10.11.2 Examination

- Acute: retinal haemorrhages (flame shaped and deep blot type) in all 4 quadrants of the fundus with a dilated tortuous retinal venous system, cotton wool spots, optic disc swelling, CMO
- Chronic: optociliary shunt vessels (collateral vessels connecting the choroidal and the retinal vasculature—do not leak on FFA-see Table 10.11) (see Figs. 10.25 and 10.26), telangiectatic capillary bed, persistent dilatation and tortuosity (see Fig. 10.27), perivenous sheathing, NVI > NVD > NVE, CMO, glaucomatous optic neuropathy
- Check for a RAPD (see Table 10.12)
- Check the IOP
- Look for NVI on anterior segment examination
- Perform gonioscopy for NVA

Table 10.11 Causes of optociliary shunt vessels

CRVO
Chronic glaucoma
Chronic papilloedema
Optic nerve sheath meningioma

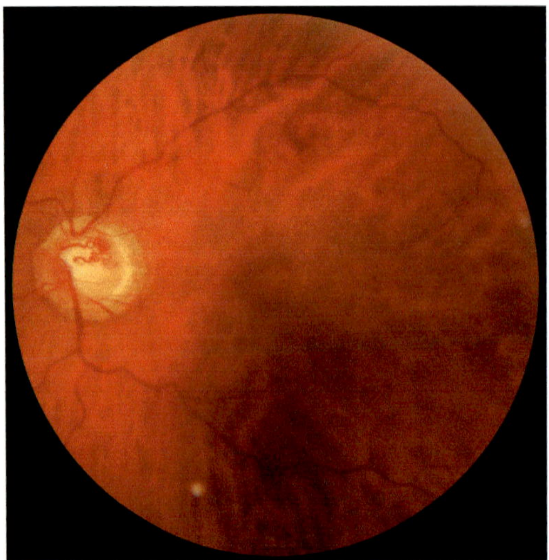

Fig. 10.25 Colour fundus image of a patient with a chronic CRVO showing the presence of telangiectatic vessels and optociliary shunt vessels

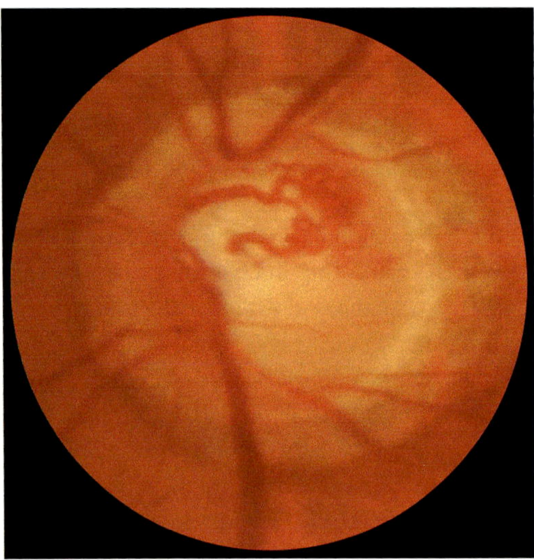

Fig. 10.26 Colour fundus image of a patient with optociliary shunt vessels from a chronic CRVO

10.11.3 Investigations

RCOphth RVO Guidelines 2022 [71]:

- BP
- Bloods—FBC (leukaemia/lymphoproliferative disorder), ESR (paraprotein), glucose
- OCT—CMO

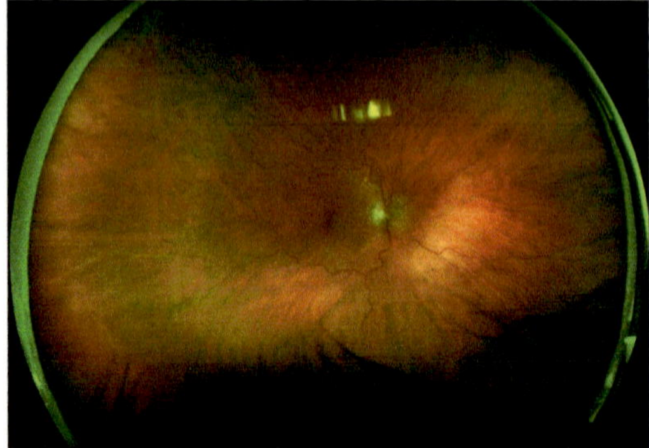

Fig. 10.27 Pseudocolour ultra-widefield image of a patient with a chronic CRVO showing the presence of tortuous retinal vessels and peripheral retinal ghost vessels

Table 10.12 Features suggestive of an ischaemic CRVO

Poor VA (CVOS—44% of eyes with vision of <6/60 develop rubeosis)
RAPD
Presence of multiple dark deep intraretinal haemorrhages
Presence of multiple cotton wool spots
Degree of venous dilation and tortuosity
FFA showing greater than 10-disc areas of capillary non-perfusion on 7 field FFA (CVOS)
ERG: reduced b wave amplitude, reduced b:a ratio (negative ERG) and prolonged b-wave implicit time

- FFA (uncertain diagnosis)—delayed filling of the occluded retinal vein, capillary non-perfusion, macular ischaemia, telangiectatic vessels forming collaterals that cross the horizontal raphe
- Widefield OCT-A where available is recommended to assess macular ischaemia or posterior pole non-perfusion to aid the identification of eyes with ischaemic CRVO

10.11.4 Treatment

- Control of cardiovascular risk factors: HTN, hyperlipidaemia, smoking cessation, DM
- RCOphth RVO guideline 2022 [71] recommends that oestrogen containing HRT and OCP should not be commenced in women with history of RVO. However, the continued use in a patient who develops RVO does not

appear to be associated with a higher rate of recurrence

- Neovascularisation:
  (a) Full scatter PRP—central vein occlusion study **CVOS** [67] recommended that laser photocoagulation be applied only after NV is observed, with greater resolution of NVI/NVA by 1 month after PRP in 56% of no early treatment eyes (no NVI or NVA present) compared with 22% of early treatment eyes (NVI or NVA present)
- Macular oedema:
  - Delay in initiating treatment up to 6 months results in fewer visual gains compared to immediate initiation of treatment. Therefore, treatment should be initiated as soon as the diagnosis is established [71]
  - Anecdotal clinical experience indicates that eyes with Snellen VA less than 6/96 can do well with treatment providing there is no gross afferent pupillary defect. Careful consideration should be given to further therapy in such eyes that do not improve in terms of Snellen VA or OCT central subfield thickness after 3 loading injections at monthly intervals and treatment is not recommended if no response occurs after 6 injections [71]
  - No robust data on outcomes of switching steroid to an anti-VEGF agent or switching between anti-VEGF agents or combining steroids with anti-VEGF agents for macular oedema due to CRVO
  - Intravitreal therapies:
    (a) <u>Ozurdex</u>
      - NICE Guidance [TA229] [32]: recommend as an option for the treatment of macular oedema following CRVO
      - **GENEVA** study [22]: A RCT that evaluated the effects of a single dexamethasone implant compared to sham injection for the treatment of macular oedema secondary to BRVO and CRVO. Increase in BCVA of ≥15 ETDRS letters was achieved in 29% of the Ozurdex 0.7 mg group and 9% of the sham group 60 days after injection but not at 90 or 180 days.

    (b) <u>Faricimab (Vabysmo)</u>
      - NICE Guidance [TA1004] [49]: recommended as an option for treatment of visual impairment caused by macular oedema following CRVO
      - **COMINO** study [59]: A RCT to evaluate the 24-week efficacy and safety of faricimab versus aflibercept in patients with treatment-naïve foveal center-involved macular oedema resulting from CRVO or HRVO. Patients were randomised 1:1 to faricimab 6.0 mg or aflibercept 2.0 mg every 4 weeks for 24 weeks. The best-corrected visual acuity gains (BCVA) from the baseline to week 24 with faricimab were noninferior versus aflibercept. The adjusted mean BCVA change from baseline at week 24 was +16.9 ETDRS letters in the faricimab arm versus +17.3 ETDRS letters in the aflibercept arm.

    (c) <u>Ranibizumab</u>
      - NICE Guidance [TA283] [34]: recommend as an option for treatment of visual impairment caused by macular oedema following CRVO
      - **CRUISE** study [5]: A RCT to evaluate the efficacy and safety of Lucentis in the treatment of macular oedema from CRVO. Patients were randomised into 3 groups: (1) sham injection; (2) 0.3 mg Lucentis; and (3) 0.5 mg Lucentis. In the first 6/12, injections were given monthly. At 6/12, both Lucentis groups gained +12.7 and + 14.9 ETDRS letters (0.3 mg and 0.5 mg groups, respectively) compared with a gain of +0.8 letters in the control group. At 6/12, 46.2% and 47.7% of patients receiving Lucentis 0.3 mg and 0.5 mg gained ≥3 ETDRS lines

compared to 16.9% in the sham injection group

(d) Aflibercept (Eylea)
- NICE Guidance [TA305] [38]: recommend as an option for treatment of visual impairment caused by macular oedema following CRVO
- **CORPERNICUS** study [9]: comparison of Eylea and sham injection—the proportion of patients who gained ≥15 letters from baseline in the Eylea and sham groups was 56.1% and 12.3% at week 24, respectively
- **GALILEO** study [25]: comparison of Eylea and sham injection—the proportion of patients who gained ≥15 letters from baseline in the Eylea and sham groups was 60.2% and 22.1% at week 24, respectively

10.11.5 Follow Up

- Non-ischaemic CRVO (may resolve completely without any complications): follow up every 3 months is recommended in the first 6 months in eyes not requiring treatment. Discharge from HES can be considered after a minimum of 18 months if no intervention is required or 18 months from the last intravitreal injection [71].
- Ischaemic CRVO: monthly monitoring recommended for 6 months and subsequently every 3 months for a year if anti-VEGF therapy is not commenced. Follow-up can be extended in the second and third year. In eyes that received anti-VEGF therapy, 1–2 monthly reviews are recommended in the first year. Follow up is recommended for 3 years from the last intervention, if any [71]
- RCOphth RVO guidelines 2022 [71] recommends that oestrogen containing HRT and OCP should not be commenced in women with history of RVO. However, the continued use in a patient who develops RVO does not appear to be associated with a higher rate of recurrence.

10.11.6 Prognosis

- At 3 years, there was a 45% chance of developing neovascular glaucoma after onset of ischaemic CRVO—highest risk if VA <6/60 or > 10 DD of non-perfusion on FFA (The Central Retinal Vein Occlusion Study Group 1997) [67]
- Overall, 34% of initially perfused eyes converted to non-perfused status after 3 years (The Central Retinal Vein Occlusion Study Group 1997) [67]
- Risk of CRVO in contralateral eye is 5% by 1 year [71]

10.12 Central Retinal Artery Occlusion (CRAO)

10.12.1 Risk Factors

- Arteriosclerosis: HTN (60%), DM (25%), smoking, hyperlipidaemia
- Embolic sources: carotid artery disease, aortic disease (dissection), cardiac valve vegetations (infective endocarditis), cardiac tumours (atrial myxoma), arrhythmias, cardiac septal defects
- Inflammatory disease: GCA, PAN, GPA, SLE
- Haematological: antiphospholipid syndrome, leukaemia, lymphoma,

10.12.2 Examination

- Acute (see Fig. 10.28)—retinal whitening in the posterior pole (ischaemic damage to the inner half of the retina), cherry red spot (normal appearing retina and is observed in high contrast against the surrounding opacified retina), box carring of retinal arteries, retinal emboli (Hollenhorst plaque—yellow refractile cholesterol embolus frequently found at bifurcation sites, calcific emboli—white, non-refractile, proximal to optic disc, platelet-fibrin clot—elongated), optic disc oedema
- Chronic (fundus may appear featureless) (see Fig. 10.29)—optic atrophy, retinal arterial

attenuation, cilioretinal collaterals, macular RPE changes, cotton wool spots, NVD (2%), NVE, NVI (18%)

- Check for a RAPD
- Check the IOP
- Look for NVI on anterior segment examination

10.12.3 Investigations

- BP
- Glucose
- FBC, CRP, ESR +/− temporal artery biopsy (TAB): rule out GCA if pt. age > 50 years
- OCT: inner retinal oedema in acute CRAO(see Fig. 10.30), inner retinal atrophy with outer retinal preservation in chronic CRAO (see Fig. 10.31)
- FFA: delayed filling of the retinal arteries (see Fig. 10.32)
- HVF: altitudinal defect
- ERG: negative ERG with the scotopic white stimulus

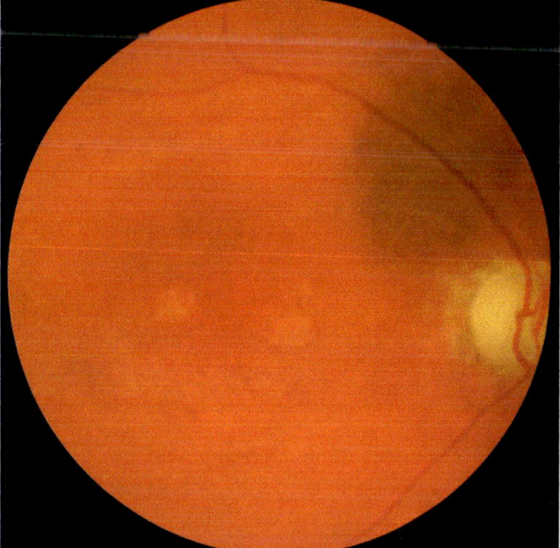

Fig. 10.29 Colour fundus image of a patient with a chronic CRAO

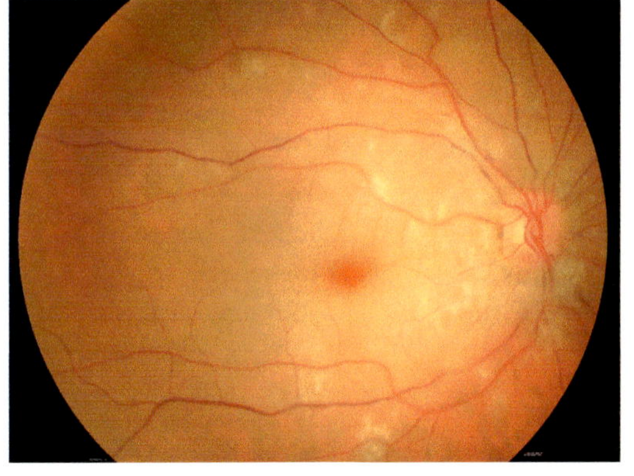

Fig. 10.28 Colour fundus image of a patient with an acute CRAO with a visible cherry red spot

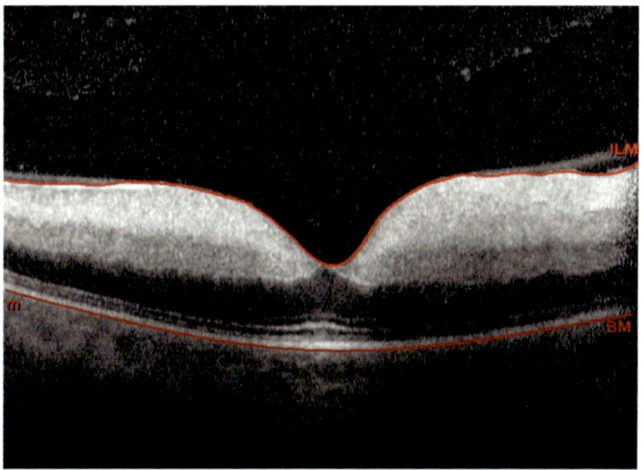

Fig. 10.30 OCT image of a patient with an acute CRAO with inner retinal oedema

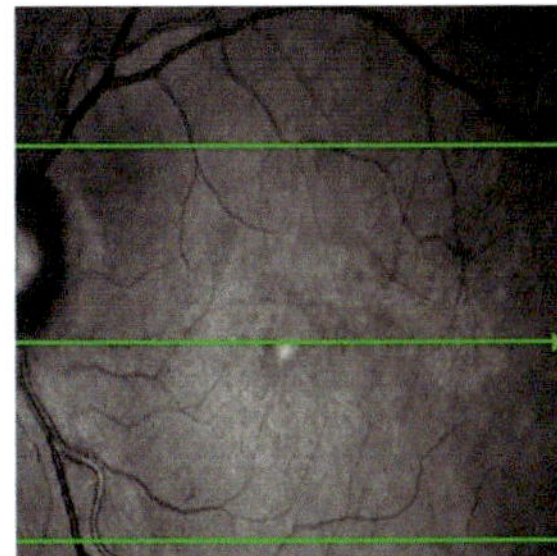

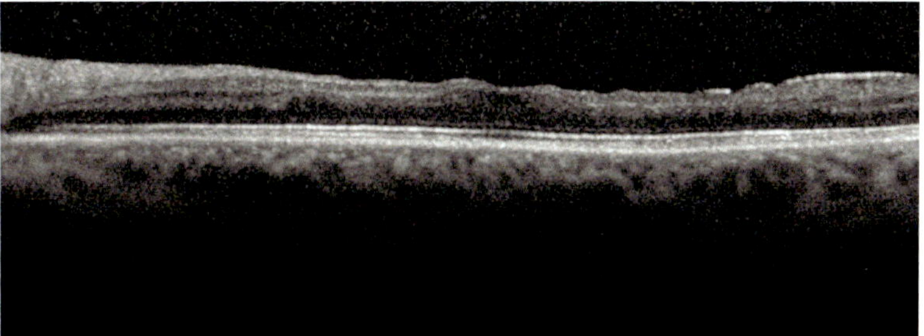

Fig. 10.31 OCT image of a patient with a chronic CRAO with inner retinal atrophy

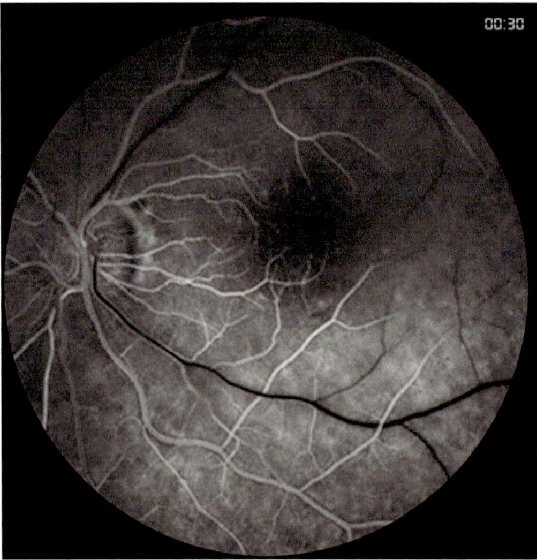

Fig. 10.32 Fundus fluorescein angiogram of a patient with CRAO showing delayed filling of the retinal arteries

10.12.4 Treatment

- If within 4 hours of onset: reduce IOP with 500 mg IV diamox, ocular massage (dislodge emboli), AC paracentesis (not proven benefit)
- If GCA suspected: start steroids and arrange TAB
- If embolic, refer to stroke (TIA) clinic for carotid doppler +/– echocardiography
- Treat NV: PRP

10.13 Diabetic Retinopathy (DR)

10.13.1 Proposed International Clinical Diabetic Retinopathy and Diabetic Macular Edema Severity Scales 2003 [75]

- Mild Non-proliferative DR (NPDR)
  - Microaneurysms (Mas) only
- Moderate NPDR
  - More than just Mas but less than severe NPDR
- Severe NPDR (4-2-1 rule)
  (a) One or more of the following:
    - More than 20 intraretinal haemorrhages in each of 4 quadrants
    - Definite venous beading in in 2 or more quadrants
    - Prominent intraretinal microvascular abnormalities (IRMA) in 1 or more quadrants
- Very severe NPDR
  - 2 or more features of severe NPDR present
- Proliferative DR (PDR)
  (a) 1 or more of the following:
    - Extraretinal neovascularisation (see Fig. 10.33)
    - Vitreous or preretinal haemorrhage
- Mild DMO
  - Some retinal thickening or hard exudates in the posterior pole, distant from the center of the macula
- Moderate DMO:
  - Retinal thickening or hard exudates near the center of the macula but not involving the center
- Severe DMO:
  - Retinal thickening or hard exudates involving the center of the macula

10.13.2 High-Risk PDR

- Defined by the Diabetic Retinopathy Study [68] with patients at higher risk of visual loss and requires prompt PRP treatment

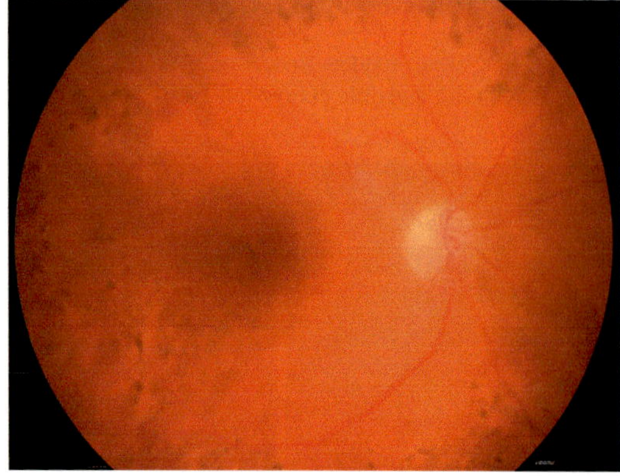

Fig. 10.33 Colour fundus image of a patient with active PDR; PRP commenced but incomplete

- Neovascularisation of the disc (NVD—new vessels on or within 1-disc diameter of the optic disc): NVD ≥ ¼ disc area or any size NVD with vitreous &/or preretinal haemorrhage
- Neovascularisation elsewhere in the retina (NVE): NVE ≥ ½ disc area with vitreous &/or preretinal haemorrhage

10.13.3 Clinically Significant Macular Oedema (CSMO)

- Defined by the Early Treatment of Diabetic Retinopathy Study (Early Treatment Diabetic Retinopathy Study Research Group. ETDRS Report number 9. 1991) [18]:
  - Retinal thickening at or within 500 μm of the centre of the macula &/or
  - Hard exudates at or within 500 μm of the centre of the macula, if associated with thickening of the adjacent retina &/or
  - Zone or zones of retinal thickening 1-disc area or larger, any part of which is within 1 disc diameter of the center of the macula

10.13.4 Examination

- NPDR
  (a) Mas (small red dots)
  (b) Intraretinal haemorrhages: dot and blot haemorrhages, flame haemorrhages (located in NFL)
  (c) Hard exudates: sharply demarcated yellow-white deposits within the retina
  (d) Cotton wool spots (CWS—patches of relative ischaemia affecting the NFL of the retina): small white patches with wispy borders situated in the inner retina
  (e) Venous beading: localised areas of change in vessel calibre with alternating regions of relative dilation and constriction
  (f) Venous loops
  (g) IRMA (see Fig. 10.34): segments of dilated and tortuous retinal vasculature without crossing both arterioles or veins in the underlying retina

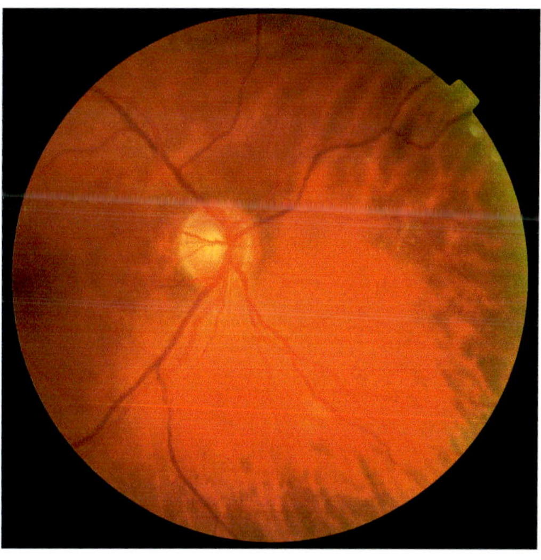

Fig. 10.34 Colour fundus image of a patient with severe NPDR showing the presence of IRMA

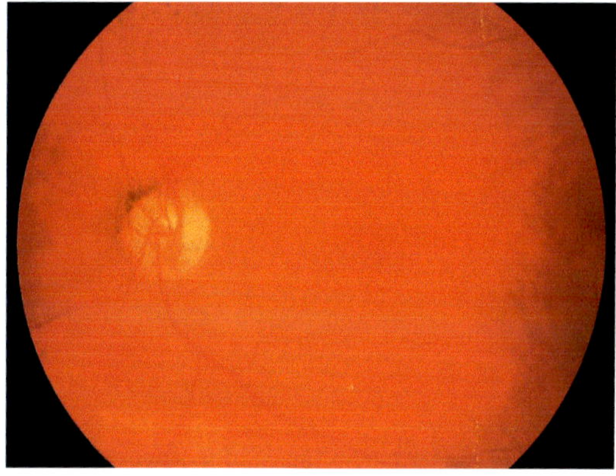

Fig. 10.35 Colour fundus image of a patient with PDR with active NVD, and incomplete PRP

  (h) Subretinal fibrosis
- PDR
  (a) NVD (see Fig. 10.35): wheel like network of vessels on or within 1DD of the disc
  (b) NVE (see Fig. 10.36): superficial location lying over retinal veins, formation of wheel-like networks, cross both arterioles and veins in the underlying retina, regressing new vessels appear to become sheathed
  (c) NVI/NVA
  (d) Concave tractional RD (see Fig. 10.37) +/− distortion or displacement (dragging) of the macula

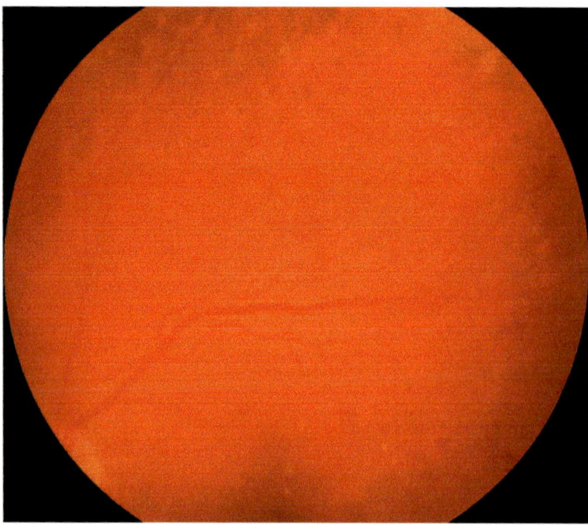

Fig. 10.36 Colour fundus image of a patient with PDR with active NVE (PRP commenced)

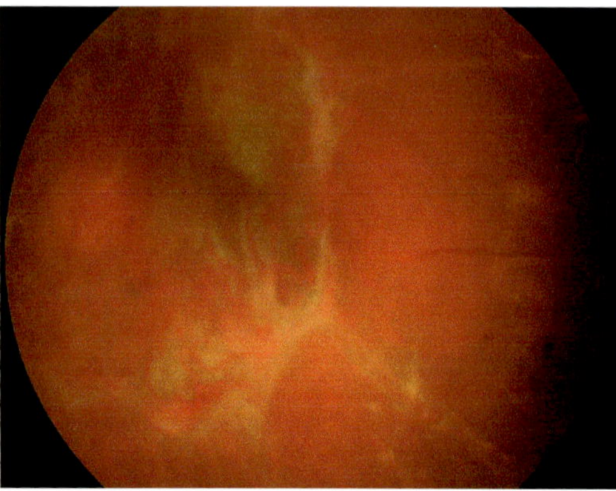

Fig. 10.37 Colour fundus image of a patient with PDR with a tractional RD involving the fovea

10.13.5 Investigations

- Venous fasting glucose ≥7.0 mmol/L +/− oral glucose tolerance test (75 g anhydrous glucose) with a 2-hour value ≥11.1 mmol/L +/− random venous glucose ≥11.1 mmol/L
- OCT
  (a) Hard exudates appear as hyperreflective foci within the retina
  (b) Macular oedema
  (c) Traction from ERM or VMT causing underlying macular oedema in the absence of retinal vascular leakage demonstrable by FFA
- OCT-A
  (a) Identify neovascular complexes, quantify foveal avascular zone and non-perfused areas
- FFA
  (a) Mas appear as hyperfluorescent dots visible during the arteriovenous transit phase
  (b) Intraretinal haemorrhages appear hypofluorescent blocking normal fluorescence from the underlying choroid
  (c) Hard exudates appear hypofluorescent
  (d) CWS appear hypofluorescent
  (e) IRMA appear hyperfluorescent during the arteriovenous transit phase and are often situated at the borders of areas of capillary non-perfusion
  (f) Macular oedema: petaloid pattern of leakage
  (g) NVD/NVE: leakage

10.13.6 Treatment

- NPDR
  (a) Modification of life-style:
    - Smoking cessation
    - Weight loss
    - Exercise
  (b) Modification of systemic risk factors:
    - Hyperglycaemia control:
      (a) **DCCT** ([16]): type 1 DM—tight control of HbA1C at mean of 7.2% was associated with 76% reduction in onset of retinopathy and slowed progression of DR by 54%, 60% reduction in onset of neuropathy, and 54% reduction in onset of nephropathy at 6.5 years
      (b) **UKPDS** [73]: type 2 DM—tight control of HbA1C at mean of 7% was associated with a 25% reduction in the onset of microvascular disease
      (c) **ACCORD** [61]: type 2 DM—intensive control of HbA1C reduced progression of DR by 42% and reduced development of PDR from 10.2% to 6.5%: avoid Pioglitazone in the presence of macular oedema, personalized HbA1c target should be set,

usually between 48–58 mmol/mol (6.5–7.5%)

(d) **NICE Guidance [NG242]** [51]: if a diabetic treatment is likely to result in a rapid, substantial drop in a person's HbA1C, an ophthalmologist should assess a person's eyes before treatment begins and check for changes afterwards

(e) **NICE Guidance [NG28]** [52]: for adults whose type 2 DM is managed either with lifestyle and diet, or lifestyle and diet combined with a single drug not associated with hypoglycaemia, aim for a HbA1C level of 48 mmol/mol (6.5%). For adults on a drug associated with hypoglycaemia, aim for a HbA1C level of 53 mmol// mol (7.0%)

– BP control:

(a) **UKPDS** [73]: type 2 DM—tight control of BP at mean of 144/82 was associated with a 37% reduction in the onset of microvascular disease and 32% reduction in diabetes related deaths

(b) **NICE Guidance [NG136]** [53]: For adults with hypertension aged under 80 with type 1 or type 2 DM, reduce clinic BP to below 140/90 mmHg and ensure it is maintained below that level. For adults with hypertension aged 80 and over with type 1 or type 2 DM, reduce clinic BP to below 150/90 mmHg and ensure it is maintained below that level

– Lipid control:

(a) **ACCORD** [61]: type 2 DM—40% reduction in the odds of having progression of DR over 4 years in patients allocated to fenofibrate in combination with a statin, compared to simvastatin alone): consider adding fenofibrate to a statin for NPDR in type 2 DM, avoid statins in pregnancy

(b) **NICE Guidance [NG242]** [51]: Ophthalmologists should consider fenofibrate for people with NPDR and type 2 DM to reduce the progression of DR

- CSMO

(a) Offer treatment to people with CSMO (centre involving and non-centre involving) and discuss the benefits and potential side-effects of macular laser treatment, intravitreal anti-VEGF treatment, intravitreal steroid treatment, vitrectomy and observation (NICE Guidance [NG242]) [51]

(b) Focal/grid laser:

– Indications: offer macular laser treatment to people with non-centre involving CSMO (NICE Guidance [NG242]) [51]. Consider macular laser treatment for people with centre-involving CSMO and good vision (79 ETDRS letters or better) (NICE Guidance [NG242]) [51]. For people with centre-involving CSMO, visual impairment (78 ETDRS letters or worse / snellen acuity of 6/9 or worse) and CMT < 400 μm, consider macular laser treatment (NICE Guidance [NG242]) [51]

– Clinical trial:

- **ETDRS** (Early Treatment Diabetic Retinopathy Study Research Group. ETDRS Report number 9. 1991) [18]: focal/grid laser reduced the risk of moderate vision loss (loss of ≥15 letters from baseline) by 50% at 3 years in eyes with mild or moderate NPDR with CSMO

(c) Anti-VEGF therapy:

– Indications (NICE Guidance [NG242]) [51]: offer anti-VEGF treatment for people with centre-involving CSMO, visual impairment (78 ETDRS letters or worse / snellen acuity of 6/9 or worse) and CMT ≥ 400 μm. Consider anti-VEGF treatment for people with centre-involving CSMO, visual impairment and CMT < 400 μm

– Anti-VEGF treatment options:

1. Faricimab (Vabysmo)

  - NICE Guidance [TA799] [46]: option for treatment of DMO if CMT ≥ 400 μm at the start of treatment
  - Regimen: a single injection every 4 weeks for 4 months, followed by 1 injection every 4–16 weeks
  - Clinical trials:
    - **YOSEMITE** study [77]
    - **RHINE** study [77]
2. Brolucizumab (Beovu)
  - NICE Guidance [TA820] [48]: option for treatment of DMO if CMT ≥ 400 μm at the start of treatment
  - Regimen: a single injection every 6 weeks for the first 5 doses, followed by 1 injection every 8–12 weeks
  - Clinical trials:
    - **KITE** study [6]
    - **KESTREL** study [6]
3. Aflibercept (Eylea)
  - NICE Guidance [TA346] [39]: option for treatment of DMO if CMT ≥ 400 μm at the start of treatment
  - Regimen: a single injection every month for 5 consecutive months, followed by 1 injection every 2 months with no requirement for monitoring between visits for the first 12 months
  - Clinical trials:
    - **VIVID** study [8]
    - **VISTA** study [8]
4. Ranibizumab
  - NICE Guidance [TA274] [33]: option for treatment of DMO if CMT ≥ 400 μm at the start of treatment
  - Regimen: given monthly and continued until maximum VA is reached—VA stable for 3 consecutive months:
  - Clinical trials:
    - **RISE** study [7, 54]
    - **RIDE** study [7, 54]
    - **RESTORE** study [30]

– Assessing response (NICE Guidance [NG242]) [51]: after the loading phase of anti-VEGF treatment, assess response and consider using macular laser as adjuvant treatment if the response is suboptimal. Treatment response is suboptimal if there is reduced vision or increased macular oedema or no change or increase in retinal thickness. Twelve months after starting anti-VEGF treatment, assess response to treatment and consider switching to an intravitreal steroid implant if the response is suboptimal. At any time after the start of treatment, if a person does not want to continue with regular anti-VEGF treatment, consider switching treatment to an intravitreal steroid implant

(a) Steroid therapy:

– Indications (NICE Guidance [NG242]) [51]: consider an intravitreal steroid implant when people with centre-involving CSMO have visual impairment and cannot have non-corticosteroid therapy

– Intravitreal steroid implants:

1. Dexamethasone intravitreal steroid implant (Ozurdex)
  - NICE Guidance [TA349] [40]: option for treatment of DMO if eye is pseudophakic and CSMO does not respond to non-corticosteroid treatment or such treatment is unsuitable
  - Regimen: A single implant is injected into the vitreous and remains in the vitreous for up to 270 days before fully dissolving

- Clinical trials:
  - **PLACID** study [11]
  - **BEVORDEX** study [21]
  - **MEAD** study [4]

2. Fluocinolone intravitreal steroid implant (Iluvien)
   - NICE Guidance [TA301] [35]: option for the treatment of chronic CSMO that is insufficiently responsive to available therapies if an eye is pseudophakic
   - Regimen: A single 190 μm of Fluocinolone Acetonide implant is injected with daily release of 0.2 μg/day for 36 months
   - Clinical trials:
     - **FAME** study [15]

(b) Vitrectomy:

- Indications (NICE Guidance [NG242]) [51]: for people with CSMO that do not respond to anti-VEGF treatment and also have either VMT or ERM. Check for warning signs of permanent damage (photoreceptor cell loss, macular atrophy or lamellar macular holes) and consider vitrectomy before any permanent damage occurs

(c) Observation:

- Consider observation for people with good vision (79 ETDRS letters or better) and centre-involving macular oedema (NICE Guidance [NG242]) [51]

- PDR
  (a) Modification of life-style:
  - Smoking cessation
  - Weight loss
  - Exercise

  (b) Modification of systemic risk factors (same as for NPDR)

  (c) Pan-retinal photocoagulation (PRP):
  - Indications [70]: presence of NVD/NVE/NVI/NVA—PRP performed on same day or within 2 weeks of diagnosis, consider PRP for severe/very severe NPDR in older patients with type 2 DM, where retinal view is difficult, prior to cataract surgery, in only eye where first eye lost to PDR, where regular clinic attendance is likely to be poor, difficult to examine patient for other reasons
  - NICE Guidance [NG242] [51]: Offer PRP to people when they are first diagnosed with PDR. If possible, start treatment within 4 weeks of offering. If it cannot be started within 4 weeks, start it within 6 weeks of offering. Complete PRP within 4 weeks of starting treatment. For people with high-risk characteristics or who have difficulty attending appointments, offer to start PRP on the same day.
  - Prognosis [68]: PRP reduces severe vision loss (<5/200 at 2 consecutive visits) from high-risk PDR by 50% at 2 years

  (d) Anti-VEGF therapy
  - In August 2024, the only anti-VEGF treatment licensed for PDR was ranibizumab and use of any other anti-VEGF treatment would be off-label (NICE Guidance [NG242]) [51]
  - Indications (NICE Guidance [NG242]) [51]: offer anti-VEGF treatment for people whose PDR remains active after complete PRP. Consider anti-VEGF treatment as a temporary treatment for people with PDR who have vitreous haemorrhage that is preventing PRP and/or need cataract surgery and the severity of the cataract is preventing PRP.

  (e) Vitrectomy:
  - Indications [70]: non-clearing (within 3 months for type 2 diabetic and 1 month for a type 1 diabetic) severe vitreous haemorrhage (confirmation of attached retina not possible with ophthalmoscopic examination), significant recurrent vitreous haemorrhage despite maximal PRP, tractional RD involving or threatening the fovea, combined tractional rhegmatogenous RD which

involves or threatens to involve the fovea, diffuse CSMO associated with posterior hyaloidal traction
  - NICE Guidance [NG242] [51]: consider vitrectomy for people with PDR and vitreous haemorrhage that has not cleared within 3 months. Perform vitrectomy within 3 months of offering it. Offer vitrectomy to people with PDR and macula involving or macula-threatening RD. Consider vitrectomy for people with non-macula-involving or non-macula-threatening RD who, despite complete PRP, have PDR that is active or recurring vitreous haemorrhages related to active PDR or VMT
  - Prognosis [69]: early vitrectomy (for those with severe vitreous haemorrhage with VA 5/200 or worse) increased chance of 20/40 vision from 12% to 36% in type 1 diabetics

10.13.7 Diabetic Retinopathy in the Context of Cataract Surgery

- Coexisting PDR should be treated with laser PRP preoperatively where possible if visualisation is allowed, otherwise indirect laser treatment may be performed at the conclusion of the cataract surgery

10.13.8 Diabetic Maculopathy in the Context of Cataract Surgery

- Maculopathy should ideally be fully treated (macular laser treatment and/or anti-VEGF treatment) with resolution of oedema prior to cataract surgery
- For cases in which macular oedema persists despite treatment at the time of cataract surgery, it is reasonable to consider adjunctive treatment with intravitreal triamcinolone injected at the completion of cataract surgery

10.14 Von Hippel Lindau (VHL) Syndrome (Table 10.13)

10.14.1 History

- Positive FHx (AD)

10.14.2 Examination

- Peripheral capillary haemangioblastoma (red nodular lesion) with the majority located in the ST midperipheral retina (Fig. 10.38) +/− optic nerve capillary haemangioblastoma (see Fig. 10.39)
- Normal to dilated and tortuous afferent and efferent vessels (paired retinal arteriole and venule) that may extend all the way posterior to the disc
- Intraretinal and subretinal exudation: formation of circinate retinopathy and exudative RD—exudates may accumulate preferentially in the macula (centripetal flow of subretinal fluid)

10.14.3 Investigations

- Standard colour fundus photography: assist with follow up to confirm growth, stability or regression following treatment
- FFA: rapid sequential filling of artery, haemangioma, and vein with diffuse leakage of fluorescein in the mid and late frames

Table 10.13 Key facts about VHL syndrome

Retinal capillary haemangioblastomas are benign hamartomas of the retinal (or optic disc) vasculature, consisting of capillary-like vessels—may be isolated or may be multiple and bilateral as part of a systemic disease (VHL syndrome)
VHL is an AD, multisystem, familial cancer syndrome caused by germline mutations in the VHL tumour suppressor gene
VHL is characterised by ocular retinal capillary haemangioblastomas as well as systemic tumours such as cerebellar or spinal cord haemangioblastomas, renal cell carcinoma, phaechromocytomas, and islet cell carcinoma
Diagnosis of VHL can be made in an individual with multiple tumours or isolated tumours with a positive FHx

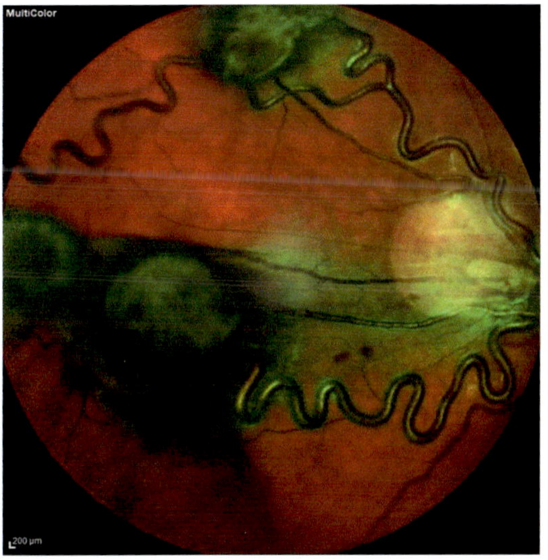

Fig. 10.38 MultiColour fundus image of a patient with VHL syndrome with multiple retinal haemangioblastomas

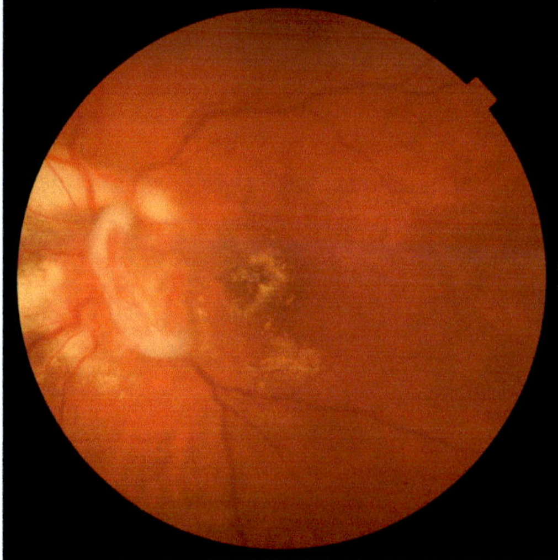

Fig. 10.39 Colour fundus image of a patient with VHL syndrome with an optic nerve capillary haemangioblastoma with subsequent intraretinal and subretinal exudation

- BP: HTN from phaechromocytomas
- 24-hour urine collection: vanillylmandelic acid (VMA) and metanephrines
- Abdominal US scan: renal cell carcinoma, islet cell carcinoma
- MRI brain/spinal cord: cerebellar or spinal cord haemangioblastomas

10.14.4 Treatment

- Refer to geneticist, physician or oncologist for systemic evaluation
- Laser photocoagulation (most suited for small tumours <1DD): burns of large size (>500 μm), low intensity, and long duration (0.2–0.5 s) are applied directly to surface of the angioma +/− feeder vessels
- Trans-scleral cryotherapy (for larger lesions, when media clarity poor, tumours located to anterior equator): 2 to 3 freeze-thaw cycles
- Radiotherapy

10.14.5 Other Diagnoses to Consider

- Retinal vascular disorders: acquired vasoproliferative retinal tumours, Coats disease, retinal artery macroaneurysm, racemose haemangioma, retinal cavernous haemangioma
- Tumours: retinal astrocytoma, retinoblastoma, malignant melanoma
- Inflammatory disorders: toxoplasmosis, toxocariasis

10.15 Angioid Streaks (Table 10.14)

10.15.1 Causes of Angioid Streaks

- Pseudoxanthoma elasticum (PXE or Gronbald-Strandberg syndrome—AR connective tissue disorder, optic disc drusen)
- Ehlers-Danlos syndrome
- Paget's disease
- Sickle cell retinopathy / β-thalassaemia
- Idiopathic
- Acromegaly

Table 10.14 Key facts about angioid streaks

Angioid streaks are breaks in an abnormally thickened and calcified Bruch's membrane

10.15.2 Examination

- Irregular reddish brown subretinal lines of varying widths that radiate out from the optic nerve to the retinal periphery (see Figs. 10.40 and 10.41)
- CNV membrane +/− subfoveal haemorrhage +/− choroidal rupture (after minor trauma)
- Optic disc drusen
- Perform a systemic examination to look for papular skin lesions and skin laxity of the neck (see Fig. 10.42), axilla, and antecubital fossa

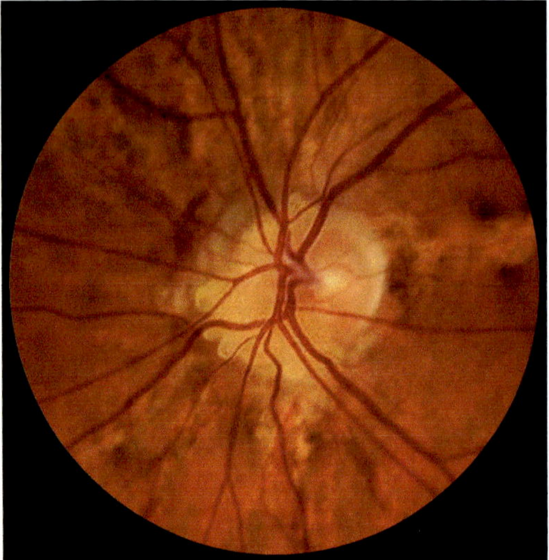

Fig. 10.40 Colour fundus image of a patient with angioid streaks radiating from the optic disc as well as optic disc drusen

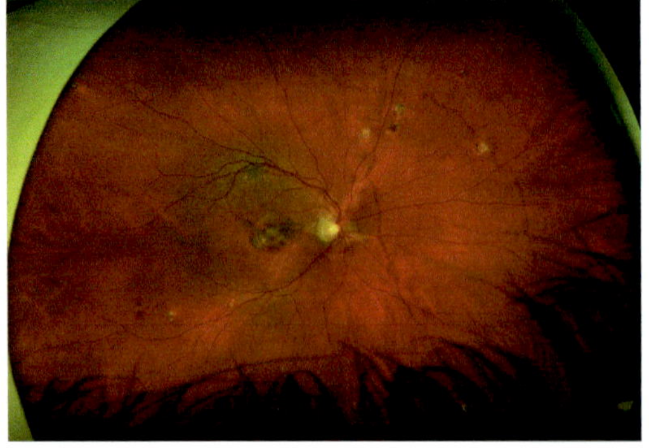

Fig. 10.41 Ultra-widefield pseudocolour fundus image of a patient with angioid streaks as well as macular scarring from a CNV membrane

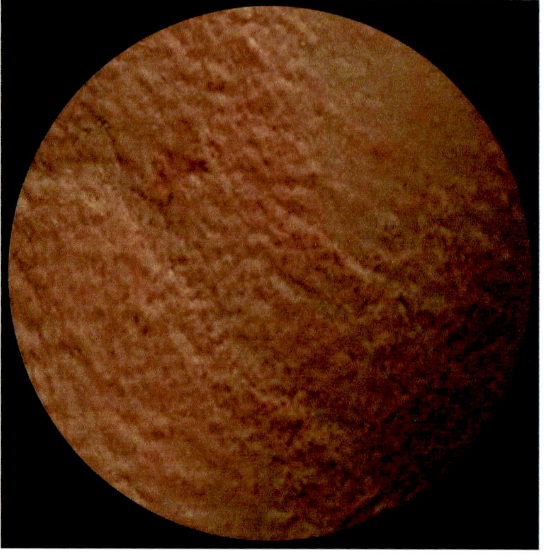

Fig. 10.42 Colour photo of the neck of a patient with PXE showing the typical papular skin lesions

10.15.3 Investigations

- OCT-A: detect CNV membrane
- FFA: look for leakage for CNV membrane, hyperfluorescence of angioid streaks in the early phase with late staining

10.15.4 Treatment

- Avoid contact sports
- CNV: subfoveal—anti-VEGF therapy, extra-foveal—laser photocoagulation

10.16 Optic Disc Pit (Table 10.15)

10.16.1 Examination

- Small hypopigmented yellow or whitish oval or round excavated defect (see Fig. 10.43), most often within the inferior temporal portion of the optic cup

Table 10.15 Key facts about optic disc pits

40–60% of patients with optic disc pits develop non-rhegmatogenous serous macular detachments

10.16.2 Investigations

- OCT: defect in the lamina cribrosa with herniation of nerve tissue into the pit (see Fig. 10.44), serous macular detachment

10.16.3 Treatment

- Serous macular detachment:
  - (a) Conservative: observation—25% of optic disc pit maculopathies resolve spontaneously
  - (b) Laser photocoagulation along temporal disc margin
  - (c) Surgical: PPV +/− ILM peeling +/− Endolaser + long-acting gas tamponade

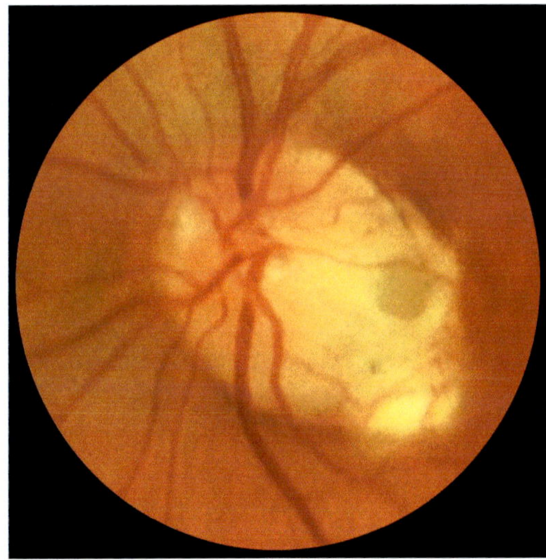

Fig. 10.43 Colour fundus image of a patient with an optic disc pit

10.17 Choroidal Folds

10.17.1 Causes of Choroidal Folds

- Ocular
  - Hypotony
  - Posterior scleritis
  - Uveitis
  - Choroidal lesions—tumours, disciform scars
- Orbit
  - TED
  - Retrobulbar mass
  - Idiopathic orbital inflammatory disease
- Intracranial:
  - Raised ICP
- Idiopathic:
  - Hypermetropia—bilateral in asymptomatic individuals

10.17.2 Examination

- Parallel alternating yellow and dark bands on the posterior pole (see Fig. 10.45)

Fig. 10.44 OCT image of a patient with an optic disc pit showing a defect in the lamina cribrosa with herniation of nerve tissue into the pit

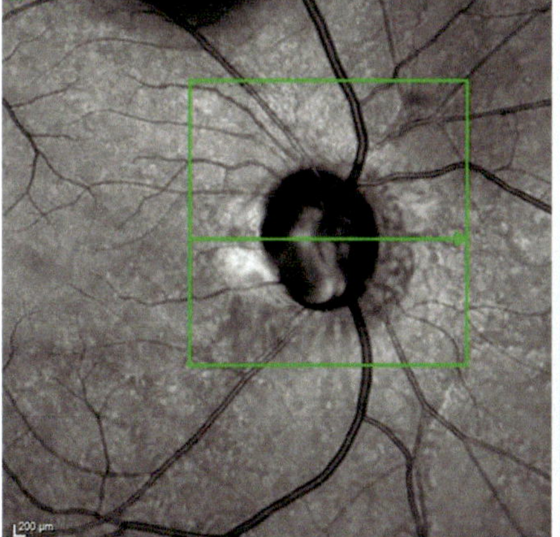

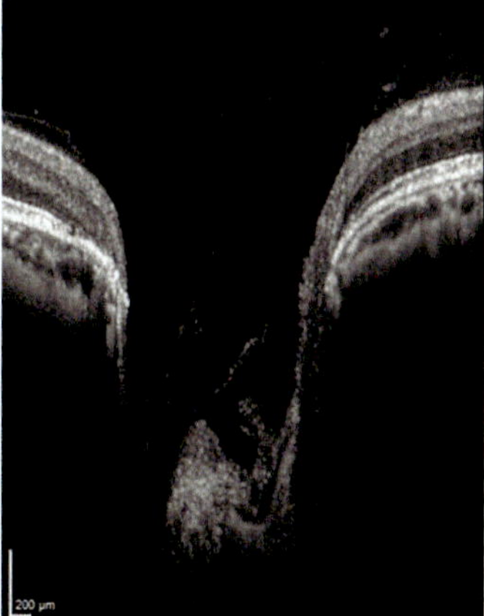

10.17.3 Investigations

- OCT (see Fig. 10.46)—undulations of the RPE

10.17.4 Treatment

- Treat underlying cause

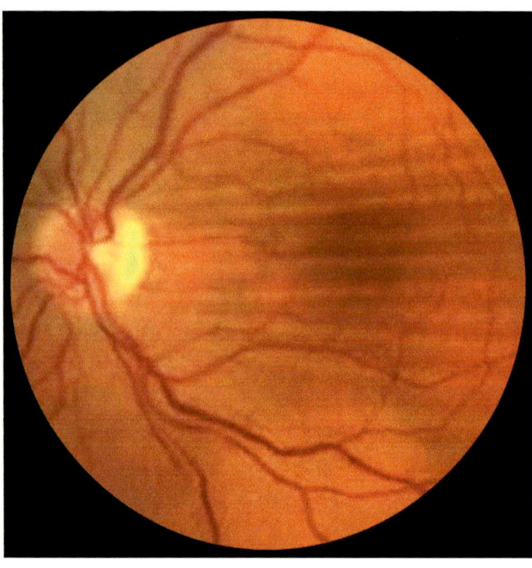

Fig. 10.45 Colour fundus image of a patient with choroidal folds

10.18 Choroideraemia (Table 10.16)

10.18.1 Examination

- RPE and choroidal atrophy with exposure of bare sclera: may get preservation of the choroid and RPE in the macula (see Fig. 10.47)
- Relative sparing of retinal vessels and optic disc

10.18.2 Investigations

- VF—constricted
- Genetic testing
- ERG—reduced or absent scotopic (affected first) and photopic responses

10.18.3 Treatment

- There is currently no licensed treatment available for choroideraemia

Table 10.16 Key facts about Choroideraemia

X-linked recessive condition characterised by generalised degeneration of the retina and choroid

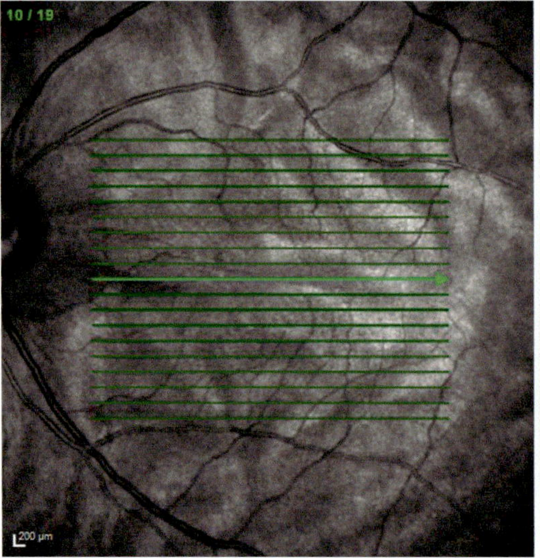

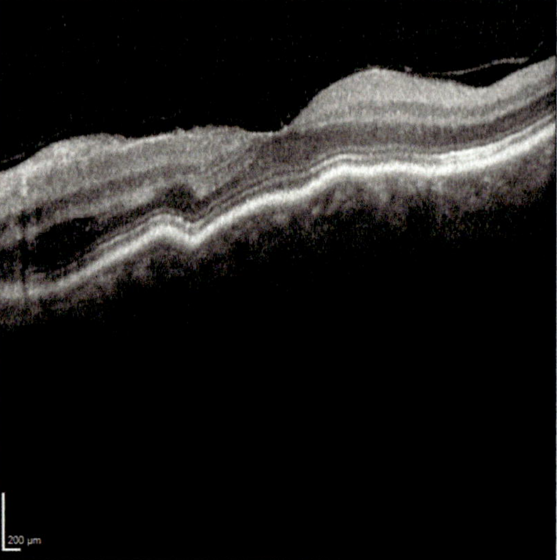

Fig. 10.46 OCT image of a patient with choroidal folds showing the characteristic undulations of the RPE

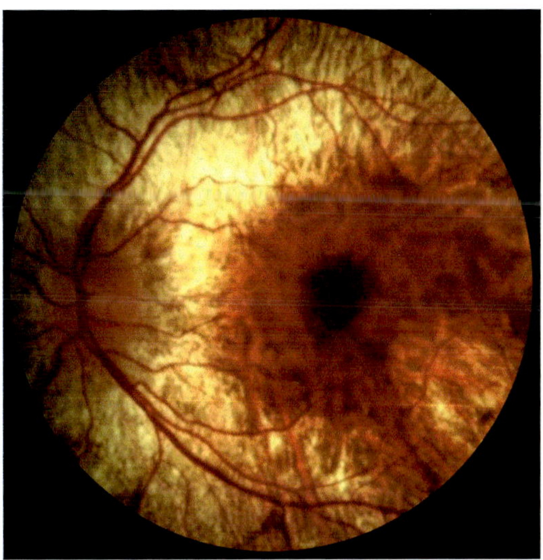

Fig. 10.47 Colour fundus image of a patient with choroideremia showing diffuse chorioretinal atrophy of the peripheral retina with preservation at the

10.19 X-Linked Retinoschisis (Table 10.17)

10.19.1 History

- Positive FHx—X-linked recessive inheritance

10.19.2 Examination

- Foveal schisis: spokewheel pattern of folds radiating out from the fovea (see Fig. 10.48)
- Peripheral retinoschisis: often in the inferotemporal region

10.19.3 Investigations

- OCT—splitting of the foveal neurosensory retina in the NFL
- EDT—negative ERG—reduced b-wave amplitude with preservation of a-wave amplitude
- FFA—absence of leakage—differentiates foveal schisis from CMO

Table 10.17 Key facts about X-linked retinoschisis

Inherited retinal degenerative disease
Most common form of juvenile onset retinal degeneration in males

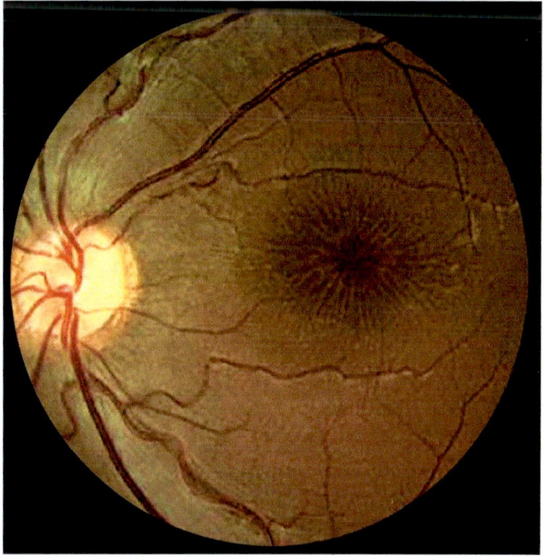

Fig. 10.48 Colour fundus image of a patient with X-linked retinoschisis showing the typical spokewheel pattern of folds radiating out from the fovea

10.19.4 Treatment

- Genetic counselling
  - Carrier women have 50% chance of transmitting the mutation in each pregnancy
  - Males with the mutation will be affected and females with the mutation will be carriers
  - Affected males pass the disease-causing mutation to all of their daughters and none of their sons
- Medical—carbonic anhydrase inhibitors
- Surgical—if tractional or rhegmatogenous RD or vitreous haemorrhage present

10.19.5 Other Diagnosis to Consider

- CMO—late hyperfluorescence in a petaloid pattern

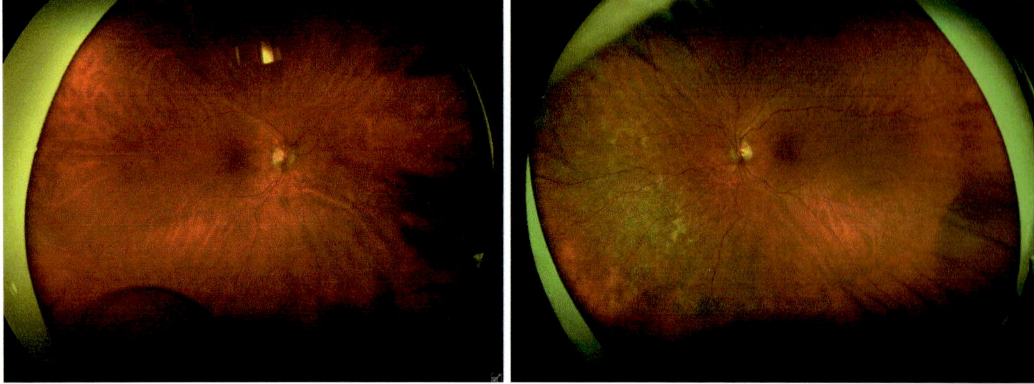

Fig. 10.49 Ultra-widefield pseudocolour fundus images of a patient with bilateral inferotemporal retinoschisis

- Degenerative retinoschisis (see Fig. 10.49)—bilateral, hypermetropes, smooth convex elevation, inferotemporal region, laser take up, absolute scotoma in schitic areas, split retina within OPL
- Goldmann Favre vitreoretinal degeneration—AD inheritance, foveal schisis, marked VF loss, pigmentary clumping, absence of vitreous veils, markedly reduced a-waves and b-waves

10.20 Macular Telangiectasia (MacTel) Type 2 (Table 10.18)

Table 10.18 Key facts about MacTel type 2

Disease characterised by telangiectatic vessels in the Juxtafoveal region, which tends to be bilateral but asymmetrical
Middle aged and older persons
All lesions begin temporal to the fovea but may subsequently involve the entire parafoveolar area
Other diagnoses to consider: MacTel type 1—developmental or congenital, usually unilateral vascular anomaly (may be part of the larger spectrum of Coats disease) Diabetic retinopathy Vascular occlusion Eales disease Radiation retinopathy ROP Sickle cell retinopathy

10.20.1 Examination

- Subtle loss of retinal transparency in the perifoveal region, beginning temporally
- Dilation of the parafoveal capillaries in the temporal parafoveal area, which may extend to surround the fovea (see Fig. 10.50)
- Crystalline deposits at the vitreoretinal interface
- Right angled venules +/− RPE hyperplasia and intraretinal pigment migration
- CNV or associated sequelae—subretinal or intraretinal haemorrhage, intraretinal oedema, retinal hard exudates, fibrovascular disciform scar

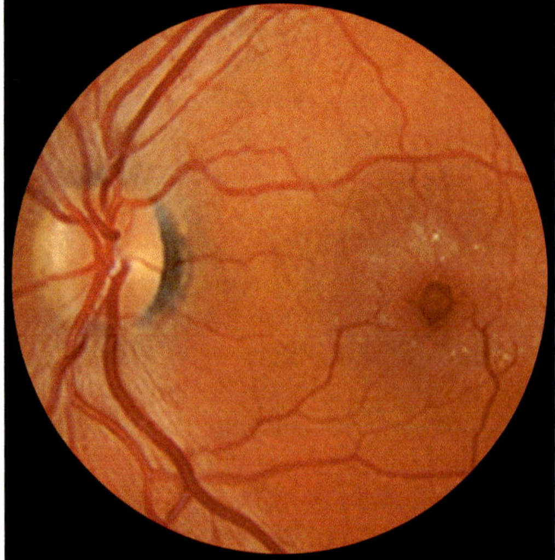

Fig. 10.50 Colour fundus image of a patient with MacTel type 2 showing dilation of capillaries in the temporal parafoveal region

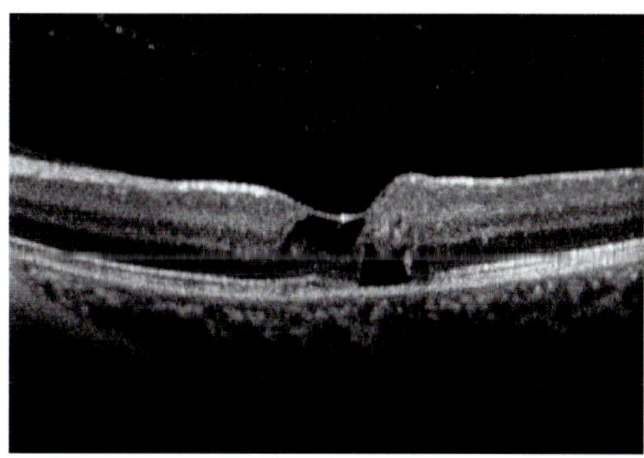

Fig. 10.51 OCT image of a patient with MacTel type 2 showing subfoveal cystoid cavities

10.20.2 Investigations

- OCT—subfoveal cystoid cavities (retinal cavity formations) (see Fig. 10.51) +/− photoreceptor disruption (ellipsoid zone) +/− outer retinal atrophy
- OCT-A—identification of the dilated, irregular telangiectatic vessels +/− choroidal communication
- FAF—loss of normal hypofluorescence at the fovea with abnormally increased autofluorescence at the fovea
- FFA—telangiectatic vessels starting predominantly temporal to the fovea with eventual involvement of entire parafoveal area with early hyperfluorescence and late leakage

10.20.3 Treatment

- CNV—anti-VEGF therapy

10.20.4 Other Diagnoses to Consider

- BRVO—segmental capillary changes, involves an area distal to an arteriolar-venular crossing, and does not cross the horizontal raphe unless there is already collateral formation
- Radiation retinopathy—involves larger area of retina, cotton wool spots, preretinal NV, hx of radiation to the eye, orbit or head
- Neovascular AMD—drusen, RPE changes, uncommon to have retinal capillary disease

10.21 Birdshot Chorioretinopathy (Table 10.19)

10.21.1 Examination

- Multiple small (1/4—½ DD) oval or round cream-coloured lesions scattered around the optic disc that radiate out to the equator (see Fig. 10.52)—lesions become atrophic but not pigmented
- Optic disc oedema leading to atrophy
- Vitritis (≤2+ vitreous haze)
- Retinal vasculitis (phlebitis)
- CMO
- ERM
- CNV (5% of eyes)

10.21.2 Investigations

- OCT—CMO, ERM
- OCT-A—detect CNV

Table 10.19 Key facts about birdshot chorioretinopathy

Key facts
Bilateral condition
Middle aged Caucasian adults with a slight female preponderance
Chronic inflammation with natural course of 6–10 years

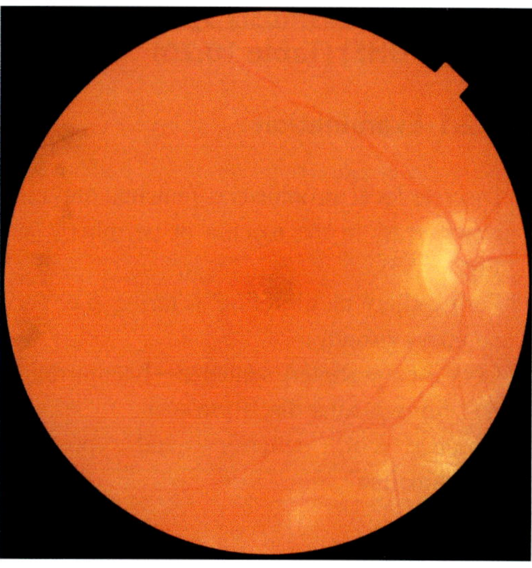

Fig. 10.52 Colour fundus image of a patient with birdshot chorioretinopathy with multiple scattered cream-coloured oval lesions and an ERM

- FFA—look for CNV and retinal vasculitis
- ICG—hypofluorescent (choroidal ischaemia or blockage from inflammatory infiltrates) birdshot lesions during active disease with diffuse late hyperfluorescence
- HLA-testing—positive HLA-A29
- VF—peripheral constriction, enlarged blind spot, central or paracentral scotomas
- ERG—negative ERG (reduced B wave amplitude and latency), delay in implicit time of 30 Hz flicker (to assess progression)

10.21.3 Treatment

- CMO—corticosteroids + long term immunosuppresants
- CNV—anti-VEGF therapy

10.21.4 Other Diagnoses to Consider

- Sarcoidosis
- Syphilitic chorioretinitis
- Multifocal choroiditis and panuveitis
- Sympathetic ophthalmia / VKH
- Intraocular B-cell lymphoma

10.22 Presumed Ocular Histoplasmosis Syndrome (POHS) (Table 10.20)

10.22.1 Examination

- Discrete focal atrophic (i.e. punched out) choroidal scars in the macula or periphery (see Fig. 10.53)
- Peripapillary chorioretinal scarring (i.e. peripapillary atrophy)
- CNV or associated sequelae—haemorrhagic RD, fibrovascular disciform scar
- Absence of anterior and posterior inflammation

Table 10.20 Key facts about POHS

An inflammatory disorder that has been postulated to result from systemic infection with the dimorphic fungi *Histoplasma capsulatum*
Only presumed, not proven
Histoplasma occurs mainly in Mississippi Valley; not identified in UK
A clinical diagnosis is based on the presence of at least 2 of the following fundus lesions in 1 or both eyes in the absence of ocular inflammation

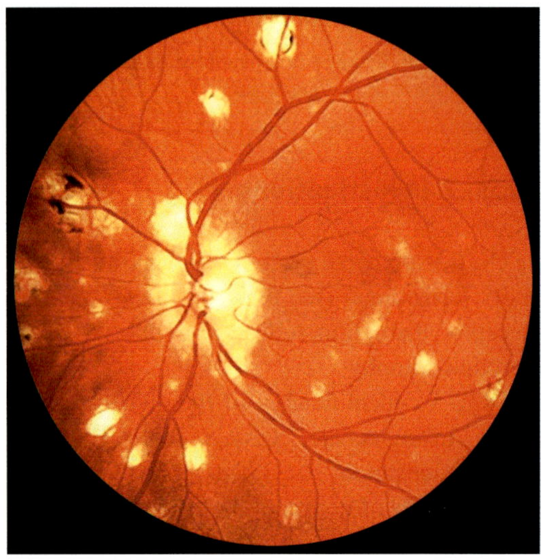

Fig. 10.53 Colour fundus image of a patient with POHS with multiple punched out atrophic chorioretinal spots and peripapillary atrophy

10.22.2 Investigations

- OCT-A—detect CNV membrane
- FFA—look for leakage to confirm presence of a CNV

10.22.3 Treatment

- Steroid therapy if inflammation active, and vision threatening
- CNV—anti-VEGF therapy

10.22.4 Other Diagnoses to Consider

- Multifocal choroiditis with panuveitis: multiple chorioretinal scars, significant anterior and posterior inflammation present in the active phase +/− CNV, bridging scars, subretinal fibrosis, clustering of lesions (e.g. macula, equator), narrow or sheathed vessels, progressive growth of lesions
- Sarcoidosis—usually accompanied by anterior and posterior inflammation, no peripapillary atrophy or CNV, elevated ACE, hilar adenopathy on CXR or CT chest
- Punctate inner choroidopathy (PIC)—predominantly seen in women, no anterior/posterior inflammation, no peripapillary atrophy, atrophic scars, CNV
- Myopic degeneration—peripapillary atrophy, CNV, small white focal areas of chorioretinal atrophy along with linear atrophic areas (e.g. lacquer cracks) in the posterior pole

10.23 Toxoplasmosis (Table 10.21)

10.23.1 Examination

- Acute lesions—intensely white focal lesions with overlying vitreous inflammatory haze adjacent ("headlight in the fog") to old hyperpigmented scars (satellite lesions), periphlebitis
- Chronic lesions—hyperpigmented scars with an atrophic center devoid of all retinal and choroidal elements (see Fig. 10.54)—the underlying sclera gives the lesion its white center
- Check the IOP
- Perform an anterior segment examination to look for any visually significant cataract

Table 10.21 Key facts about toxoplasmosis

Caused by T. gondii
Acquired from ingestion of oocyte from contaminated soil or the cyst form in undercooked infected meat—high risk of contamination from contact with cat faeces, litter boxes, or potentially contaminated outdoor sand and soil

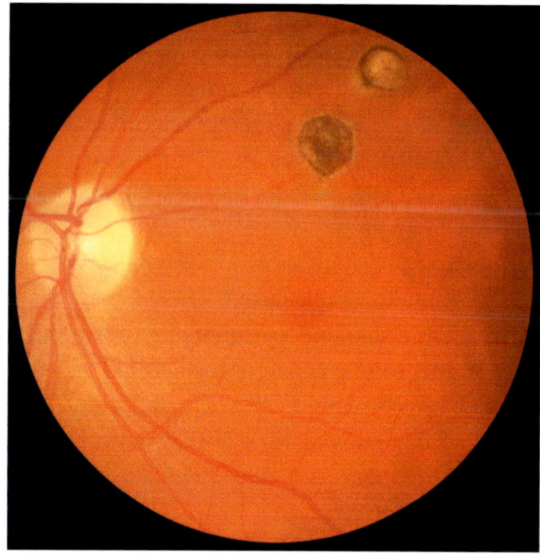

Fig. 10.54 Colour fundus image of a patient with congenital toxoplasmosis with multiple hyperpigmented scars

10.23.2 Investigations

- VDRL—rule out syphilis
- ACE, CXR—rule out sarcoidosis
- HIV serology—rule out HIV
- Pregnancy test
- Anti-toxoplasma IgM & IgG antibodies:
- Negative IgG and negative IgM antibodies implies infection has not occurred
- Positive IgG and negative IgM antibodies implies an infection that was in the distant past
- Positive IgM antibodies may suggest a recently acquired infection.
- PCR: detection of T gondii DNA by PCR in both aqueous humour and vitreous humour fluid is both sensitive and specific

10.23.3 Treatment

- Inflammation
  - (a) In immunocompetent patients, the disease is self-limiting and does not require treatment unless sight threatening

(b) Indications for treatment:
  - Lesions involving the disc, macula, or papillomacular bundle
  - Lesions threatening a major vessel
  - Marked vitritis
  - Any lesion in an immunocompromised patient

(c) No corticosteroids if patient is immunocompromised

(d) Triple therapy: pyrimethamine, sulfadiazine, folinic acid, corticosteroids

(e) Co-trimoxazole (trimethoprim + sulfamethoxazole) + corticosteroids

(f) Intravitreal dexamethasone + clindamycin

(g) Oral clindamycin

(h) Spiramycin or atovaquone if maternal infection acquired during pregnancy (15% in the first trimester and 60% in the third trimester risk of fetal transmission if acquired during pregnancy)

- Cataract extraction once uveitis is inactive for ≥3 months

10.23.4 Other Diagnoses to Consider

- Infectious—TB, syphilis, rubella, CMV retinitis, herpes simplex, toxocariasis
- Non-infectious—sarcoidosis

10.24 Multifocal Choroiditis and Panuveitis (MFC) (Table 10.22)

Table 10.22 Key facts about MFC

Typically affects myopic caucasian women between the second and sixth decades of life (most affected patients are in their 30 s)

10.24.1 Examination

- Acute phase—yellow round or oval lesions in the posterior pole, peripapillary region and midperiphery +/− subretinal fluid, vitritis +/− anterior uveitis, periphlebitis
- Chronic phase—punched out atrophic scars with variable hyperpigmentation (see Fig. 10.55), peripapillary subretinal fibrosis, bridging subretinal fibrosis between atrophic scars, peripheral linear streak chorioretinal scars parallel to the ora, optic disc atrophy, CNV membrane (25–30%), CMO

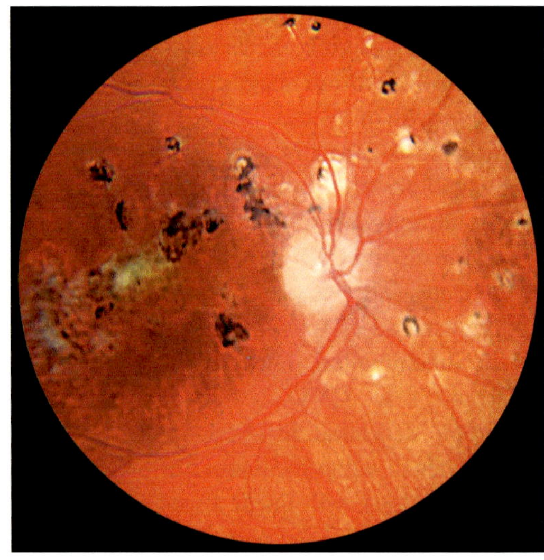

Fig. 10.55 Colour fundus image of a patient with MFC showing multiple hyperpigmented punched out atrophic scars in the posterior pole and peripapillary region

10.24.2 Investigations

- OCT—CMO
- OCT-A—detect CNV membrane
- FFA—early hypofluorescence and late staining of lesions, leakage for CNV membrane
- ICG—hypofluorescent round spots with staining of edges

10.24.3 Treatment

- CMO—topical, periocular, intraocular, and systemic corticosteroids
- CNV—anti-VEGF therapy

10.24.4 Other Diagnoses to Consider

- Inflammatory—POHS (no vitritis), PIC (posterior pole, no vitritis), Sarcoidosis, VKH syndrome/Sympathetic ophthalmia, Serpiginous choroidopathy, Birdshot chorioretinopathy

- Infectious—TB, syphilis
- Degenerative—Myopic degeneration maculopathy
- Neoplastic masquerading diseases—intraocular lymphoma

10.25 Retinal Arterial Macroaneurysm

10.25.1 Risk Factors

- HTN
- Diabetes

10.25.2 Examination

- Fusiform or round dilatations of the retinal arterioles that occur in the posterior fundus within the first 3 orders of arteriolar bifurcation (see Figs. 10.56 and 10.57)
- Hourglass retinal haemorrhage (subretinal, intraretinal, sub-ILM, vitreous) +/− retinal oedema +/− retinal exudation

10.25.3 Investigations

- FFA—hyperfluorescence of macroaneurysm in the early arterial phase with leakage in the late stage

10.25.4 Treatment

- Conservative: most spontaneously thrombose and undergo involution with clearing of exudates
- Laser photocoagulation (if lipid exudation involves or threatens the fovea): treat around the macroaneurysm with a single confluent laser barrier—if leakage persists, repeat procedure with direct laser of the lesion
- Vitrectomy: non-clearing vitreous haemorrhage

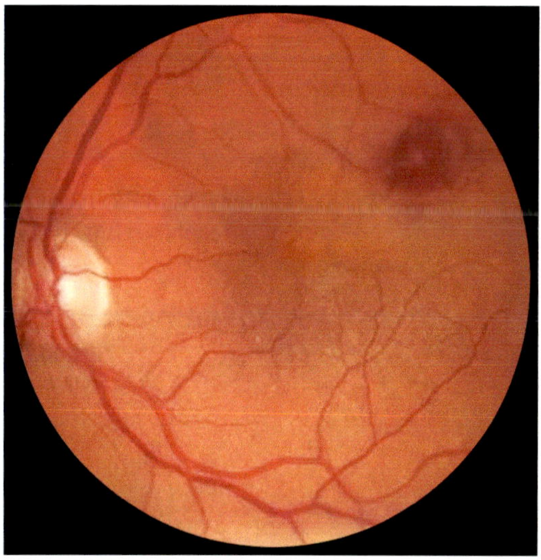

Fig. 10.56 Colour fundus image of a patient with a retinal arterial macroaneurysm

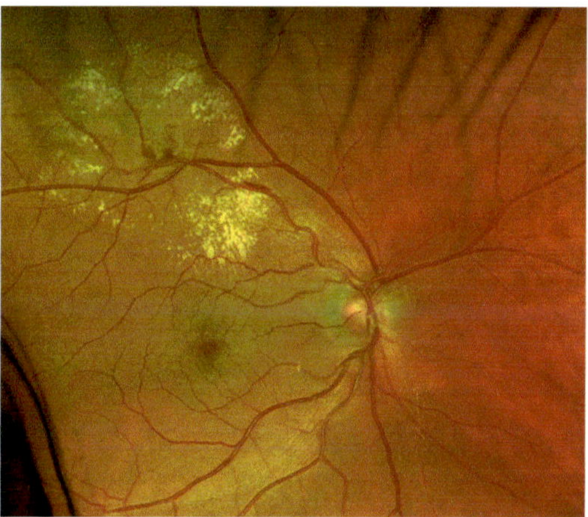

Fig. 10.57 Pseudocolour fundus image of a patient with a retinal arterial macroaneurysm with surrounding exudates

10.25.5 Other Diagnoses to Consider

- Diabetic retinopathy
- Retinal telangiectasia
- Retinal capillary angioma
- Cavernous haemangioma
- Haemorrhagic PED of AMD

10.26 Choroidal Naevus

10.26.1 Examination

- Flat or minimally elevated slate-grey lesion with irregularly defined margins (see Fig. 10.58) +/− surface drusen (see Fig. 10.59)

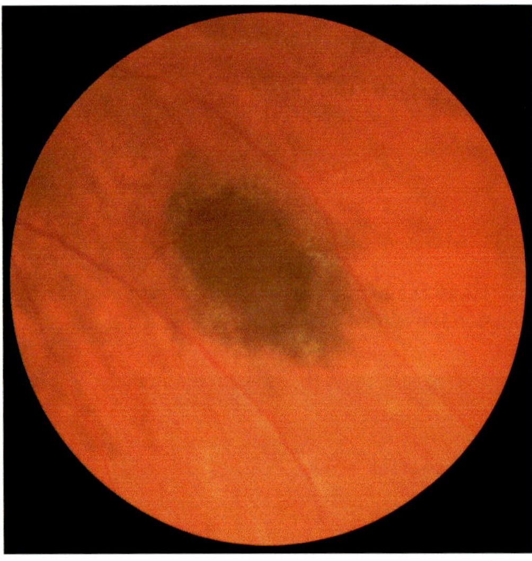

Fig. 10.58 Colour fundus image of a patient with a flat choroidal naevus

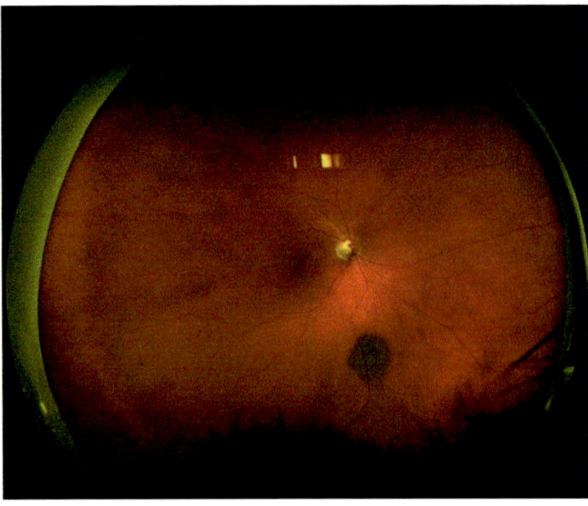

Fig. 10.59 Pseudocolour ultra-widefield image of a patient with a flat choroidal naevus with surface drusen

10.26.2 Investigations

- Colour fundus photography—documentation
- B-scan US—determine tumour thickness
- OCT—subretinal fluid

10.26.3 Treatment

- If no suspicious features are present, these lesions do not require regular ophthalmic review. Naevus photographed and a copy is given to the patient to permit their own optometrist to monitor the lesion (e.g. annually) as part of their routine optometric review
- Refer patients in accordance with the RCOphth guidelines (see Table 10.23) [72]

10.26.4 Other Diagnoses to Consider for a Pigmented Choroidal Lesion

- Choroidal melanoma (see Table 10.24 and Figs. 10.60, 10.61, 10.62,and 10.63)—more elevation, medium- low internal reflectivity on A-scan US, irregular elevated acoustically hollow choroidal mass on B-scan US
- Congenital hypertrophy of the RPE (CHRPE—see Fig. 10.64)—typically unilateral, solitary or grouped ("bear-track"), darkly pigmented, round, well circumscribed, flat lesions at the level of the RPE, intralesional lacunae, CHRPE-like lesions associated with FAP (Gardner syndrome—AD) are similar in appearance but are bilateral multiple and pisciform in shape
- Choroidal metastasis—indistinct or irregular margins, creamy-yellow colour (see Fig. 10.65), often associated with a serous RD out of proportion to size of tumour, B-scan US for an area of mild choroidal elevation with medium-high internal reflectivity on A-scan, +ve hx of prior malignancy, if no prior hx of malignancy—CT chest (lung Ca) and breast imaging (breast Ca)

Table 10.23 When to refer a patient with a choroidal lesion to the ocular oncology service [72]

Risk factor	Severity	Score
Refer patients with the following choroidal tumours:		
Melanocytic choroidal tumour having a MOLES score of 3 or more		
Choroidal haemangioma with subretinal fluid and/or symptoms		
Choroidal osteoma		
Lymphoma		
Do not refer patients with the following choroidal tumours:		
Probable choroidal naevus (i.e., MOLES score < 3)		
Melanocytoma of disc if less than 2 mm in thickness		
Choroidal haemangioma if no serous retinal detachment		
The MOLES acronym and scoring system for categorising melanocytic choroidal tumours according to likelihood of malignancy		
Risk factor	**Severity**	**Score**
Mushroom shape	Absent	0
	Unsure/Early growth through RPE	1
	Present, with overhang	2
Orange pigment	Absent	0
	Unsure/Trace (i.e., dusting)	1
	Confluent clumps	2
Large size		
(ignore thickness if this cannot be measured)	Thickness < 1.0 mm (flat/ minimal thickening) and diameter < 3DD	0
	Thickness 1.0–2.0 mm ('subtle dome') and/or diameter 3-4DD	1
	Thickness > 2 mm ('significant thickening') and/or diameter > 4DD	2
Enlargement	None (or no previous ophthalmoscopy)	0
	Unsure (poor image quality or 'new' lesion but no previous photo)	1
	Definite (confirmed with sequential photography) or assumed, if thickness > 3 mm or diameter > 5DD	2
Subretinal fluid	Absent	0
	Trace (if minimal and detected only with OCT)	1
	Definite (if seen without OCT or extending beyond tumour margins	2
Score of 0—'Common naevus'—mnitoring by optometrist in community		
Score of 1—'Low-risk naevus'—monitoring by optometrist or ophthalmologist		
Score of 2—'High-risk naevus'—monitoring by ophthalmologist		
Score of 3—'Probable melanoma'—urgent referral to ocular oncologist		

Table 10.24 Features suggestive of a choroidal melanoma [58]

"To find small ocular melanomas using helpful hints daily"
Thickness: more than 2 mm
Fluid: presence of SRF (serous RD)
Symptoms: photopsias
Orange pigment: lipofuscin
Margin: tumour margin within 3 mm of the optic disc
Ultrasonography **H**ollowness
Halo absence (in halo choroidal naevus the lesion is surrounded by a depigmented yellow ring)
Drusen absence
Tumours that display a single factor have a 38% chance for transformation
Tumours with 2 or more factors show transformation in over 50% of cases at 5 years

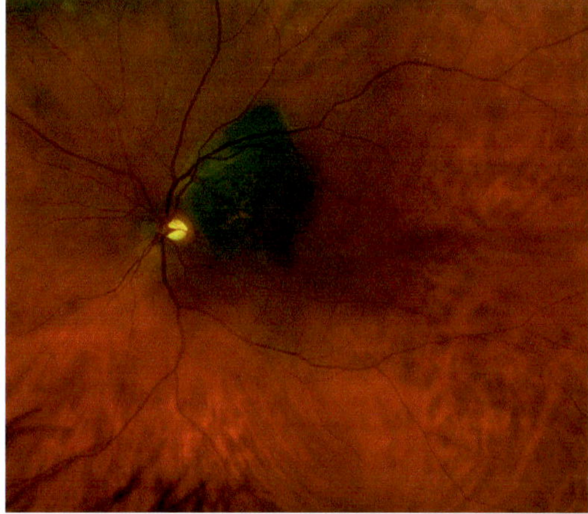

Fig. 10.60 Pseudocolour fundus image of a patient with a peripapillary choroidal melanoma

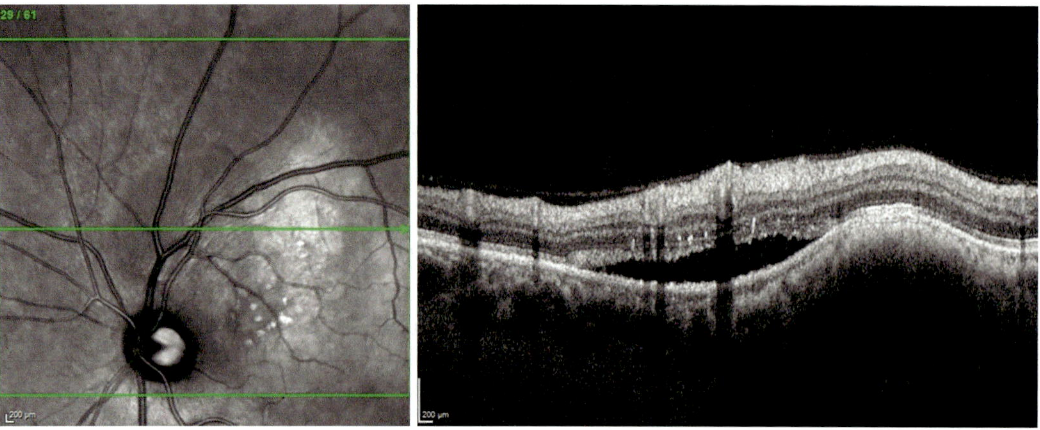

Fig. 10.61 OCT image from the same patient in Fig. 10.60 showing the presence of SRF

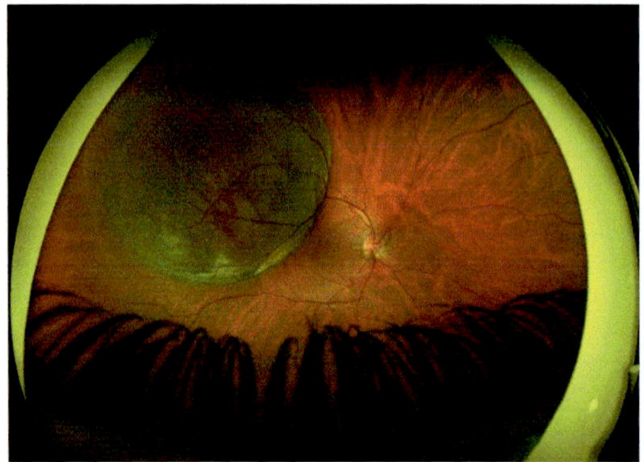

Fig. 10.62 Pseudocolour fundus image of a patient with a large choroidal melanoma with SRF extending to the macula

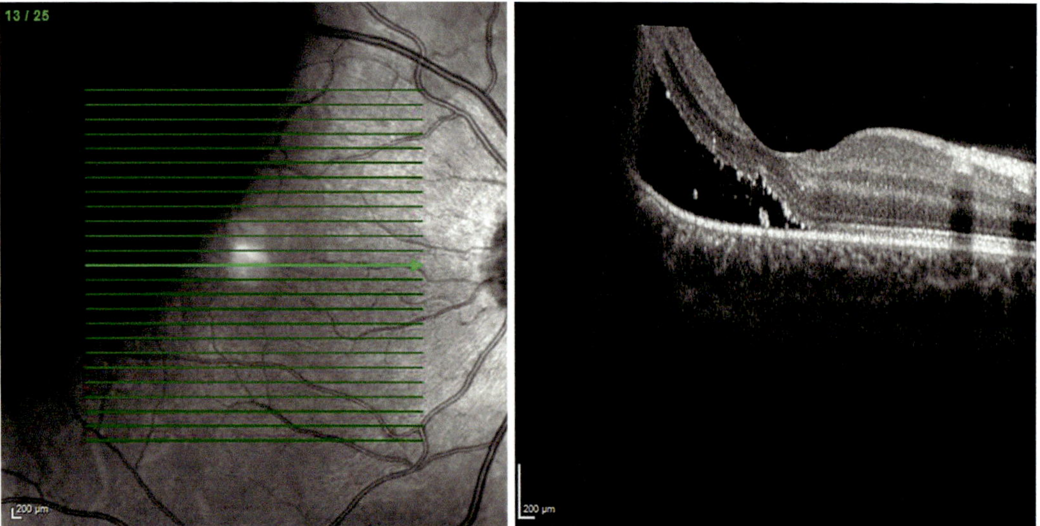

Fig. 10.63 OCT image of the same patient in Fig. 10.62 showing the presence of SRF extending to the macula

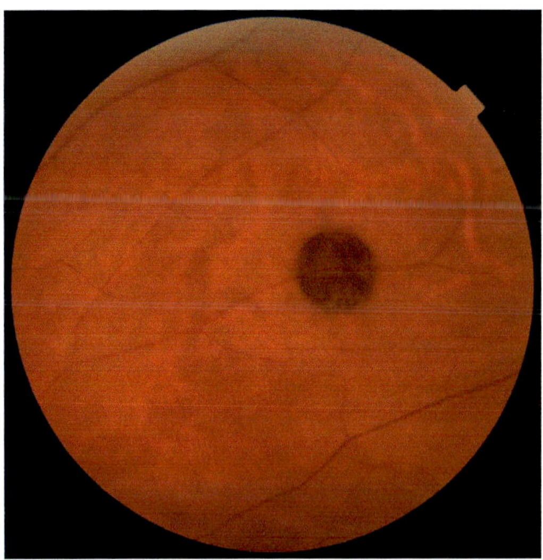

Fig. 10.64 Colour fundus image of a patient with a solitary CHRPE with intralesional lacunae (or loss of RPE hyperpigmentation)

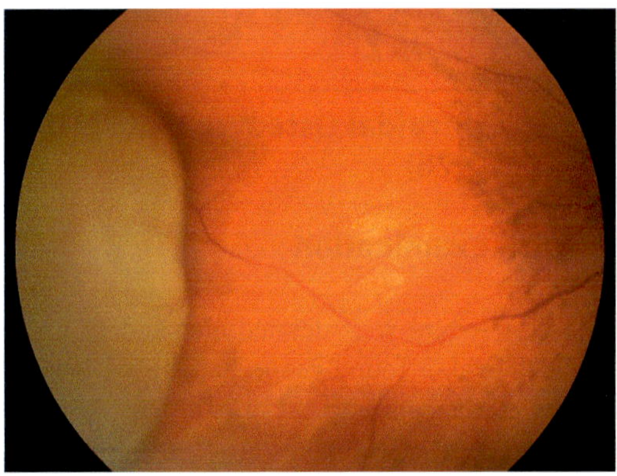

Fig. 10.65 Colour fundus image of a patient with a choroidal metastasis

10.27 Coats Disease (Table 10.25)

10.27.1 Examination

- Localised, yellow, intraretinal and subretinal exudation +/− exudative RD associated with adjacent vascular anomalies, including venous sheathing and beading, telangiectasia (irregular dilation of the capillary bed), tortuosity, arteriolar aneurysmal dilatation ("light bulb" aneurysms) +/− NVD +/− NVE (see Figs. 10.66, 10.67, and 10.68)

Table 10.25 Key facts about Coat's disease

Idiopathic condition characterised by telangiectatic and aneurysmal retinal vessels with intraretinal and subretinal exudation and fluid
Disease affects males 3× as often as females
Unilateral in 80–95% of cases

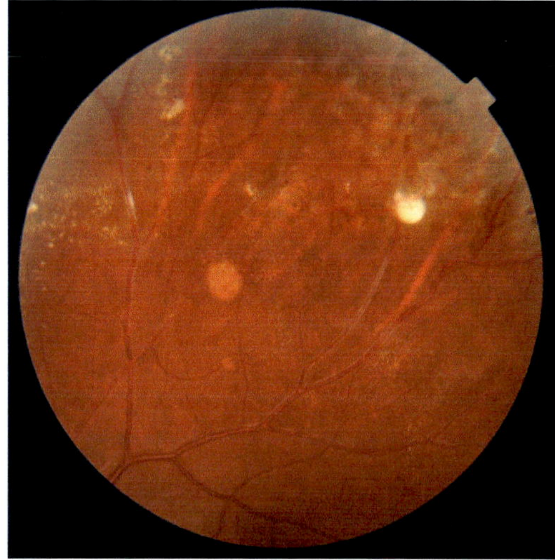

Fig. 10.66 Colour fundus image of a patient with Coats disease showing intraretinal and subretinal exudates, venous sheathing and arteriolar aneurysmal dilations

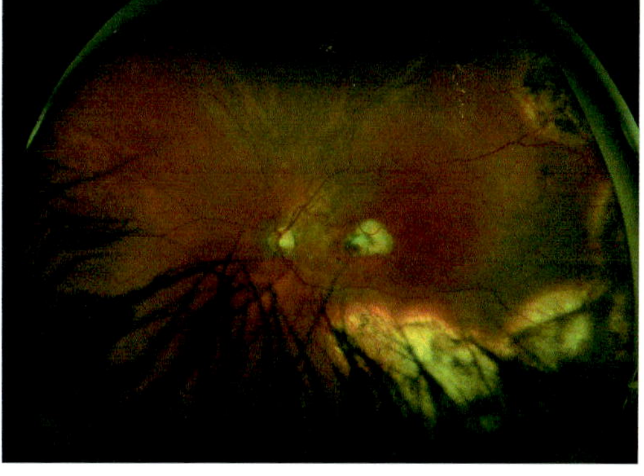

Fig. 10.67 Ultra-widefield pseudocolour fundus image of a patient with Coats disease showing peripheral arteriolar aneurysmal dilations, intraretinal and subretinal exudates, and cryotherapy scars. There is also the presence of a macular scar

- Check IOP (neovascular glaucoma)
- Perform an anterior segment examination to look for NVI and cataract

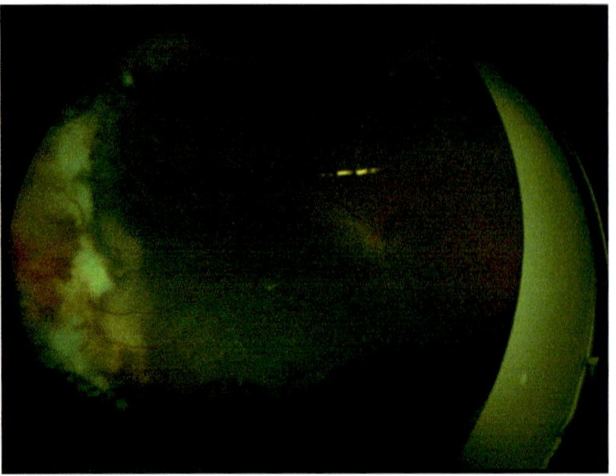

Fig. 10.68 Ultra-widefield pseudocolour fundus image of another patient with Coats disease showing peripheral intraretinal and subretinal exudates, haemorrhage and laser scars

10.27.2 Investigations

- OCT-A—capillary non-perfusion
- FFA—capillary non-perfusion between dilated telangiectatic vessels, leakage of dye from telangiectatic vessels and disc neovascularisation

10.27.3 Treatment

- Retinal telangiectasia present only: follow conservatively
- Subretinal exudation or fluid present: focal laser photocoagulation (first line treatment), or cryotherapy (if extensive subretinal exudation or RD) to areas of leaking telangiectatic vasculature and capillary non-perfusion +/− adjuvant anti-VEGF injection (helps reduce subretinal fluid and macular exudation)
- Surgery for eyes with advanced exudative RD abutting the crystalline lens or those with a rhegmatogenous component to the detachment

10.27.4 Other Diagnoses to Consider

- BRVO
- Peripheral vasculitis (pars planitis)
- Eales disease

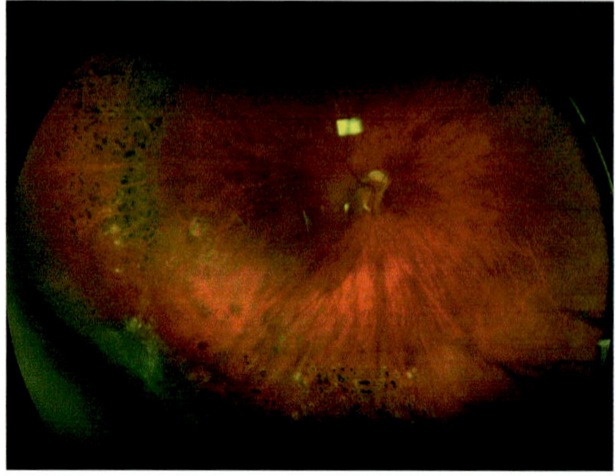

Fig. 10.69 Ultra-widefield pseudocolour fundus image of a patient with FEVR showing the presence of retinal dragging, an inferotemporal tractional RD and old laser scars

- Ocular toxocariasis
- FEVR—retinal dragging (see Fig. 10.69), +ve FHx, bilateral
- Persistent fetal vasculature

10.28 Choroidal Osteoma (Table 10.26)

10.28.1 Examination

- Yellow-white well defined elevated or excavated oval or round geographic lesion located in the juxtapapillary or peripapillary area (see Fig. 10.70) +/− extension into the macula (rarely tumour is confined to the macular region only without involvement of the juxtapapillary area)
- Subretinal haemorrhages—suggestive of CNV
- Overlying retinal vasculature and optic disc is characteristically unaffected by the osseous tumour and there are no associated vitreous or anterior segment abnormalities

10.28.2 Investigations

- OCT—serous SRF +/− retinal thinning over macular portion of the osteoma

Table 10.26 Key facts about a choroidal osteoma

• Benign tumour of the choroid composed of mature bone (mature bone replaces choroid with damage to overlying RPE and retina)
• Typically found in healthy young females in the 2nd or 3rd decade of life
• Tumour usually occurs as a sporadic trait and is usually unilateral

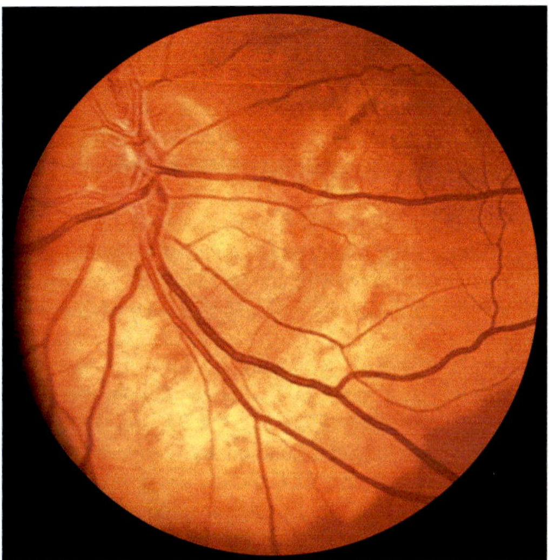

Fig. 10.70 Colour fundus image of a patient with a choroidal osteoma

- FFA (if SRF or haemorrhage present)—look for leakage suggestive of CNV membrane, osteoma produces a mild patchy hyperfluorescence of the tumour that evolves to a diffuse intense late staining
- A-scan US—high intensity echo spike from the inner surface of the tumour
- B-scan US—slightly elevated highly reflective choroidal mass with acoustic shadowing just posterior to the choroidal mass (gives appearance of a pseudo-optic nerve)

10.28.3 Treatment

- Treatment of CNV—extrafoveal (laser photocoagulation or PDT), subfoveal (anti-VEGF therapy)
- Induction of decalcification of tumour—if osteoma in extrafoveal region, argon laser photocoagulation or PDT to prevent growth of osteoma towards foveola (decalcified osteoma does not grow in the direction of the decalcification)

10.28.4 Other Diagnoses to Consider

- Amelanotic choroidal melanoma: less well-defined margin, more elevation, medium- low internal reflectivity on A-scan US, irregular elevated acoustically hollow choroidal mass on B-scan US
- Metastatic carcinoma to the choroid—indistinct or irregular margins, creamy-yellow colour, often associated with a serous RD out of proportion to size of tumour, B-scan US for an area of mild choroidal elevation with medium-high internal reflectivity on A-scan, +ve hx of prior malignancy, if no prior hx of malignancy—CT chest (lung Ca) and breast imaging (breast Ca)
- Disciform macular degeneration—older pt's with AMD, usually centered in the macula with AMD
- Circumscribed choroidal haemangioma—characteristically dome shaped with smooth regular margins with overlying serous SRF with cystoid degeneration of retina, orange-red in colour, high internal reflectivity on A-scan, acoustically full dome-shaped elevated mass
- Posterior scleritis—indistinct margins, US evidence of thickened sclera and choroid with retrobulbar oedema (T-sign)

References

1. Abraham P, Yue H, Wilson L. Randomised, double-masked, sham-controlled trial of ranibizumab for neovascular age-related macular degeneration: PIER study year 2. Am J Ophthalmol. 2010;150:315–24.
2. Age-Related Eye Disease Study Research Group. A randomised, placebo-controlled, clinical trial of high-dose supplementation with vitamins C and E, beta carotene, and zinc for age-related macular degeneration and vision loss. AREDS report no.8., vol. 119. Arch Ophthalmol; 2001. p. 1417–36.

3. Age-Related Eye Disease Study Research Group. The age-related eye disease study severity scale for age-related macular degeneration: AREDS report no.17. Arch Ophthalmol. 2005;123:1484–98.
4. Boyer DS, Yoon YH, Belfort R, Bandello F, Maturi RK, Augustin AJ, Li XY, Cui H, Hashad Y, Whitcup SM. Three-year, randomised, sham-controlled trial of dexamethasone intravitreal implant in patients with diabetic macular edema. Ophthalmology. 2014;121:1904–14.
5. Brown DM, Campochiaro PA, Singh RP, Li Z, Gray S, Saroj N, Rundle AC, Rubio RG, Murahashi WY. Ranibizumab for macular edema following central retinal vein occlusion. Six-month primary end point results of a phase III study. Ophthalmology. 2010;117:1124–33.
6. Brown DM, Emanuelli A, Bandello F, Barranco JJE, Figueira J, Souied E, Wolf S, Gupta V, Ngah NF, Liew G, Tuli R, Tadayoni R, Dhoot D, Wang L, Bouillaud E, Wang Y, Kovacic L, Guerard N, Garweg JG. KESTREL and KITE: 52-week results from two phase III pivotal trials of brolucizumab for diabetic macular edema. Am J Ophthal 2022;238:157–172.
7. Brown DM, Nguyen QD, Marcus DM, Boyer DS, Patal S, Feiner L, Schlottmann PG, Rundle AC, Zhang J, Rubio RG, Adamis AP, Ehrlich JS, Hopkins J. Long-term outcomes of ranibizumab therapy for diabetic macular edema: the 36-month results from two phase III trials: RISE and RIDE. Ophthalmology. 2013;120:2013–22.
8. Brown DM, Schmidt-Erfurth I, Do DV, Holz FG, Boyer DS, Midena E, Heier JS, Terasaki H, Kaiser PK, Marcus DM, Nguyen QD, Jaffe GJ, Slakter JS, Simader C, Soo Y, Schmelter T, Yancopoulos GD, Stahl N, Vitti R, Berliner AJ, Zeitz O, Metzig C, Korobelnik JF. Intravitreal aflibercept for diabetic macular edema: 100-week results from the VISTA and VIVID studies. Ophthalmology. 2015;122:2044–52.
9. Boyer DS, Heier MD, Brown DM, Clark WL, Vitti R, Berliner AJ, Groetzbach G, Zeitz O, Sandbrink R, Zhu X, Beckmann K, Haller JA. Vascular endothelial growth factor trap-eye for macular edema secondary to central retinal vein occlusion. Six-month results of the phase 3 COPERNICUS study. Ophthalmology. 2012;119:1024–32.
10. Brown DM, Kaiser PK, Michels M, Soubrane G, Heier JS, Kim RY, Sy JP, Schneider S. Ranibizumab versus verteportin for neovascular age-related macular degeneration. N Engl J Med. 2006;355:1432–44.
11. Callanan DG, Gupta S, Boyer DS, Ciulla TA, Singer MA, Kuppermann BD, Liu CC, Li XY, Hollander DA, Schiffman RM, Whitcup SM. Dexamethasone intravitreal implant in combination with laser photocoagulation for the treatment of diffuse diabetic macular edema. Ophthalmology. 2013;120:1843–51.
12. Campochiaro PA, Heier JS, Feiner L, Gray S, Saroj N, Rundle AC, Murahashi WY, Rubio RG. Ranibizumab for macular edema following branch retinal vein occlusion. Six-month primary end point results of a phase III study. Ophthalmology. 2010;117:1102–12.
13. Campochiaro PA, Clark WL, Boyer DS, Heier JS, Brown DM, Vitti R, Kazmi H, Berliner AJ, Erickson K, Chu KW, Soo Y, Cheng Y, Haller JA. Intravitral aflibercept for macular edema following branch retinal vein occlusion: the 24-week results of the VIBRANT study. Ophthalmology. 2015;122:538–44.
14. Chakravarthy U, Harding SP, Rogers CA, Downes SM, Lotery AJ, Culliford LA, Reeves BC. Alternative treatments to inhibit VEGF in age-related choroidal neovascularisation: 2-year findings of the IVAN randomised controlled trial. Lancet. 2013;382:1258–67.
15. Cunha-Vaz J, Ashton P, Iezzi R, Campochiaro P, Dugel PU, Holz FG, Weber M, Danis RP, Kuppermann BD, Bailey C, Billman K, Kapik B, Kane F, Green K. Sustained delivery fluocinolone acetonide vitreous implants. Long term benefits in patients with chronic diabetic macular oedema. Ophthalmology. 2014;121:1892–903.
16. Diabetes Control and Complications Trial Research Group. Progression of retinopathy with intensive versus conventional treatment in the diabetes control and complications trial. Ophthalmology. 1995;102:647–61.
17. Dugel PU, Koh A, Ogura Y, Jaffe GJ, Schmidt-Erfurth U, Brown DM, Gomes AV, Warburton J, Weichselberger A, Holz FG. HAWK and HARRIER: phase 3, multicenter, randomized, double-masked trials of brolucizumab for neovascular age-related macular degeneration. Ophthalmology 1995;102:647–661.
18. Early Treatment Diabetic Retinopathy Study Research Group. Early photocoagulation for diabetic retinopathy. ETDRS report number 9. Early Treatment Diabetic Retinopathy Study Research Group. Ophthalmology. 1991a;98:766–85.
19. Early Treatment Diabetic Retinopathy Study Research Group. Fundus photographic risk factors for progression of diabetic retinopathy. ETDRS report number 12. Ophthalmology. 1991b;98:823–33.
20. Fung AE, Lalwani GA, Rosenfeld PJ, Dubovy SR, Michels S, Feuer WJ, Puliafito CA, Davis JL, Flynn HW, Esquiabro M. An optical coherence tomography-guided, variable dosing regimen with intravitreal ranibizumab (Lucentis) for neovascular age-related macular degeneration. Am J Ophthalmol. 2007;143:566–83.
21. Gillies MC, Lim LL, Campain A, Quin GJ, Salem W, Li J, Goodwin S, Aroney C, McAllister IL, Fraser-Bell S. A randomised clinical trial of intravitreal bevacizumab versus intravitreal dexamethasone for diabetic macular edema: the BEVORDEX study. Ophthalmology. 2014;121:2473–81.
22. Haller JA, Bandello F, Belfort R, Blumenkranz MS, Gillie M, Heier J, Loewenstein A, Yoon YH, Jacques ML, Jiao J, Li XY, Whitcup SM. Randomised, sham-controlled trial of dexamethasone intravitreal implant in patients with macular edema due to retinal vein occlusion. Ophthalmology. 2010;117:1134–46.
23. Heier JS, Brown DM, Chong V, Korobelnik JF, Kaiser PK, Nguyen QD, Kirchhof B, Ho A, Ogura Y, Yancopoulos GD, Stahl N, Vitti R, Berliner AJ, Soo Y,

Anderesi M, Groetzbach G, Sommerauer B, Sandbrink R, Simader C, Schmidt-Erfurth U. Intraviteal aflibercept (VEGF Trap-Eye) in wet age-related macular degeneration. Ophthalmology. 2012;119:2537–48.

24. Heier JS, Khanani AM, Ruiz CQ, Basu K, Ferrone PJ, Brittain C, Figueroa MS, Lin H, Holz FG, Patel V, Lai TYY, Silverman D, Regillo C, Swaminathan B, Viola F, Cheung CMG, Wong TY. Efficacy, durability, and safety of intravitreal faricimab up to every 16 weeks for neovascular age-related macular degeneration (TENAYA and LUCERNE): two randomised, double-masked, phase 3, non-inferiority trials. Lancet 2022;399:729–740.

25. Holz FG, Roider J, Ogura Y, Korobelnik JF, Simader C, Groetzbach G, Vitti R, Berliner AJ, Hiemeyer F, Beckmann K, Zeitz O, Sandbrink R. VEGF trap-eye for macular oedema secondary to central retinal vein occlusion: 6-month results of the phase III GALILEO study. Br J Ophthalmol. 2013;97:278–84.

26. Ikuno Y, Ohno-Matsui K, Wong TY, Korobelnik JF, Vitti R, Li T, Stemper B, Asmus F, Zeitz O, Ishibashi T. Intravitreal aflibercept injection in patients with myopic choroidal neovascularization: the MYRROR study. Ophthalmology. 2015;122:1220–7.

27. Khanani AM, Patel SS, Staurenghi G, Tadayoni R, Danzig CJ, Eichenbaum DA, Hsu J, Wykoff CC, Heier JS, Lally DR, Mones J, Nielson JS, Sheth VS, Kaiser PK, Clark J, Zhu L, Patel H, Tang J, Desai D, Jaffe GJ. Efficacy and safety of Avacincaptad pegol in patients with geographic atrophy (GATHER2): 12-month results from a randomised, double-masked, phase 3 trial. Lancet. 2023;402:1449–58.

28. Lalwani GA, Rosenfeld PJ, Fung AE, Dubovy SR, Michels S, Feuer W, Davis JL, Flynn HW, Esquiabro M. A variable-dosing regimen with intravitreal ranibizumab for neovascular age-related macular degeneration: year 2 of the PrONTO study. Am J Ophthalmol. 2009;148:43–58.

29. Lee WK, Iida T, Ogura Y, Chen SJ, Wong TY, Mitchell P, Cheung GCM, Zhang Z, Leal S, Ishibashi T. Efficacy and safety of intravitreal aflibercept for polypoidal choroidal vasculopathy in the PLANET study: a randomised clinical trial. JAMA Ophthalmol. 2018;136:786–93.

30. Mitchell P, Bandello F, Schmidt-Erfurth U, Lang GE, Massin P, Schlingemann RO, Sutter F, Simader C, Burian G, Gerstner O, Weichselberger A. The RESTORE study. Ranibuzumab monotherapy or combined with laser versus laser monotherapy for diabetic macular edema. Ophthalmology. 2011;118:615–25.

31. National Institute for Health and Care Excellence. Ranibizumab and pegaptanib for the treatment of age-related macular degeneration [TA155]. [Online]. London: NICE; 2008. Available at https://www.nice.org.uk/guidance/ta155. Accessed 11 Dec 2019.

32. National Institute for Health and Care Excellence. Dexamethasone intravitreal implant for the treatment of macular oedema secondary to retinal vein occlusion [TA229]. [Online]. London: NICE; 2011. Available at https://www.nice.org.uk/guidance/ta229. Accessed 11 Dec 2019.

33. National Institute for Health and Care Excellence. Ranibizumab for treating diabetic macular oedema [TA274]. [Online]. London: NICE; 2013a. Available at https://www.nice.org.uk/guidance/ta274. Accessed 11 Dec 2019.

34. National Institute for Health and Care Excellence. Ranibizumab for treating visual impairment caused by macular oedema secondary to retinal vein occlusion [TA283]. [Online]. London: NICE; 2013b. Available at https://www.nice.org.uk/guidance/ta283. Accessed 11 Dec 2019.

35. National Institute for Health and Care Excellence. Fluocinolone acetonide intravitreal implant for treating chronic diabetic macular oedema after an inadequate response to prior therapy [TA301]. [Online]. London: NICE; 2013c. Available at https://www.nice.org.uk/guidance/ta301. Accessed 11 Dec 2019

36. National Institute for Health and Care Excellence. Ranibizumab for treating choroidal neovascularisation associated with pathological myopia [TA298]. [Online]. London: NICE; 2013d. Available at https://www.nice.org.uk/guidance/ta298. Accessed 15 Dec 2019.

37. National Institute for Health and Care Excellence. Aflibercept solution for injection for treating wet age-related macular degeneration [TA294]. [Online]. London: NICE; 2013e. Available at https://www.nice.org.uk/guidance/ta294. Accessed 22 Dec 2024.

38. National Institute for Health and Care Excellence. Aflibercept for treating visual impairment caused by macular oedema secondary to central retinal vein occlusion [TA305]. [Online]. London: NICE; 2014. Available at https://www.nice.org.uk/guidance/ta305. Accessed 11 Dec 2019.

39. National Institute for Health and Care Excellence. Aflibercept for treating diabetic macular oedema [TA346]. [Online]. London: NICE; 2015a. Available at https://www.nice.org.uk/guidance/ta346. Accessed 11 Dec 2019.

40. National Institute for Health and Care Excellence. Dexamethasone intravitreal implant for treating diabetic macular oedema [TA349]. [Online]. London: NICE; 2015b. Available at https://www.nice.org.uk/guidance/ta349. Accessed 11 Dec 2019

41. National Institute for Health and Care Excellence. Aflibercept for treating visual impairment caused by macular oedema after branch retinal vein occlusion [TA409]. [Online]. London: NICE; 2016. Available at https://www.nice.org.uk/guidance/ta409. Accessed 11 Dec 2019.

42. National Institute for Health and Care Excellence. Aflibercept for treating choroidal neovascularisation [TA486]. [Online]. London: NICE; 2017. Available at https://www.nice.org.uk/guidance/ta486. Accessed 15 Dec 2019.

43. National Institute for Health and Care Excellence. Age-related macular degeneration [NG82]. [Online].

London: NICE; 2018. Available at https://www.nice.org.uk/guidance/ng82. Accessed 13 Dec 2019.
44. National Institute for Health and Care Excellence. Voretigene neparvovec for treating inherited retinal dystrophies caused by RPE65 gene mutations [HST11]. [Online]. London: NICE; 2019a. Available at https://www.nice.org.uk/guidance/hst11. Accessed 15 Dec 2019.
45. National Institute for Health and Care Excellence. Brolucizumab for treating wet age-related macular degeneration [TA672]. [Online]. London: NICE; 2021. Available at https://www.nice.org.uk/guidance/ta672. Accessed 22 Dec 2024.
46. National Institute for Health and Care Excellence. Faricimab for treating diabetic macular oedema [TA799]. [Online]. London: NICE; 2022. Available at https://www.nice.org.uk/guidance/ta799. Accessed 6 Nov 2024.
47. National Institute for Health and Care Excellence. Faricimab for treating wet age-related macular degeneration [TA800]. [Online]. London: NICE; 2022. Available at https://www.nice.org.uk/guidance/ta800. Accessed 22 Dec 2024.
48. National Institute for Health and Care Excellence. Brolucizumab for treating diabetic macular oedema [TA820].[Online]. London: NICE; 2022. Available at https://www.nice.org.uk/guidance/ta820. Accessed 6 Nov 2024.
49. National Institute for Health and Care Excellence. Faricimab for treating visual impairment caused by macular oedema after retinal vein occlusion [TA1004]. [Online]. London: NICE; 2024. Available at http://www.nice.org.uk/guidance/TA1004. Accessed 7 Nov 2024.
50. National Institute for Health and Care Excellence. Bevacizumab gamma for treating wet age-related macular degeneration [TA1022]. [Online]. London: NICE; 2024a. Available at https://www.nice.org.uk/guidance/ta1022. Accessed 22 Dec 2024.
51. National Institute for Health and Care Excellence. Diabetic retinopathy: management and monitoring [NG242]. [Online]. London: NICE; 2024b. Available at http://www.nice.org.uk/guidance/ta242. Accessed 6 Nov 2024.
52. National Institute for Health and Care Excellence. Type 2 diabetes in adults: management [NG28]. [Online]. London: NICE; 2015c. Available at http://www.nice.org.uk/guidance/ng28. Accessed 7 Nov 2024.
53. National Institute for Health and Care Excellence. Hypertension in adults diagnosis and management [NG136]. [Online]. London: NICE; 2019b. Available at http://www.nice.org.uk/guidance/ta136. Accessed 6 Nov 2024
54. Nguyen QD, Brown DM, Marcus DM, Boyer DS, Patel S, Feiner L, Gibson A, Sy J, Rundle AC, Hopkins J, Rubio RG, Ehrlich JS. Ranibizumab for diabetic macular edema. Results from 2 phase III randomised trials: RISE and RIDE. Ophthalmology. 2012;119:789–801.
55. Oishi A, Miyamoto N, Mandai M, Honda S, Matsuoka T, Oh H, Kita M, Nagai T, Bessho N, Uenishi M, Kurimoto Y, Negi A. LAPTOP study: a 24-month trial of verteporfin versus ranibizumab for polypoidal choroidal vasculopathy. Ophthalmology. 2014;121:1151–2.
56. Regillo CD, Brown DM, Abraham P, Yue H, Ianchulev T, Schneider S, Shams N. Randomised, double-masked, sham-controlled trial of ranibizumab for neovascular age-related macular degeneration: PIER study year 1. Am J Ophthalmol. 2008;145:239–48.
57. Rosenfeld PJ, Brown DM, Heier JS, Boyer DS, Kaiser PK, Chung CY, Kim RY. Ranibizumab for neovascular age-related macular degeneration. N Engl J Med. 2006;355:1419–31.
58. Shield CL, Furata M, Berman EL, Zahler JD, Hoberman DM, Dinh DH, Mashayekhi A, Shields JA. Choroidal nevus transformation into melanoma. Arch Ophthalmol. 2009;127:981–7.
59. Tadayoni R, Paris LP, Danzig CJ, Abreu F, Khanani AM, Brittain C, Lai TYY, Haskova Z, Sakamoto T, Kotecha A, Schlottmann PG, Liu Y, Seres A, Retiere A, Willis JR, Yoon YH. Efficacy and safety of faricimab for macular edema due to retinal vein occlusion: 24-week results from the BALATON and COMINO trials. Ophthalmology 2024;131:950–950.
60. Tan CS, Ngo WK, Chen JP, Tan NW, Lim TH. EVEREST study report 2: imaging and grading protocol, and baseline characteristics of a randomised controlled trial of polypoidal choroidal vasculopathy. Br J Ophthalmol. 2015;99:624–8.
61. The ACCORD Study Group and ACCORD Eye Study Group. Effects of medical therapies on retinopathy progression in type 2 diabetes. N Engl J Med. 2010;363:233–44.
62. The Age-Related Eye Disease Study Research Group. A simplified severity scale for age-related macular degeneration: AREDS no. 18. Arch Ophthalmol. 2005;123:1570–4.
63. The Age-Related Eye Disease Study 2 (AREDS2) Research Group. Secondary analyses of the effects of lutein/zeaxanthin on age-related macular degeneration progression. AREDS2 report no.3. JAMA Ophthalmol. 2014;132:142–9.
64. The Branch Vein Occlusion Study Group. Argon laser photocoagulation for macular edema in branch vein occlusion. Am J Ophthalmol. 1984;98:271–82.
65. The Branch Vein Occlusion Study Group. Prevention of neovascularisation and vitreous hemorrhage in branch vein occlusion. Arch Ophthalmol. 1986;104:34–41.
66. The CATT Research Group. Ranibizumab and bevacizumab for neovascular age-related macular degeneration. N Engl J Med. 2011;364:1897–908.
67. The Central Vein Occlusion Study Group. Natural history and clinical management of central retinal vein occlusion. Arch Ophthalmol. 1997;115:486–91.
68. The Diabetic Retinopathy Study Research Group. Photocoagulation treatment of proliferative diabetic retinopathy. Clinical application of diabetic retinop-

athy study (DRS) findings, DRS report number 8. Ophthalmology. 1981;88:583–600.
69. The Diabetic Retinopathy Vitrectomy Study Research Group. Early vitrectomy for severe proliferative diabetic retinopathy in eyes with useful vision. Results of a randomised trial—diabetic retinopathy vitrectomy study report 3. Ophthalmology. 1988;95:1307–20.
70. The Royal College of Ophthalmologists. Diabetic Retinopathy Guidelines 2012. [Online]. London: The Royal College of Ophthalmologists. Available at https://www.rcophth.ac.uk/wp-content/uploads/2014/12/2013-SCI-301-FINAL-DR-GUIDELINES-DEC-2012-updated-July-2013.pdf. Accessed 11 Dec 2019.
71. The Royal College of Ophthalmologists. Retinal Vein Occlusion (RVO) Guidelines 2022. [Online]. London: The Royal College of Ophthalmologists. Available at https://www.rcophth.ac.uk/wp-content/uploads/2015/07/Retinal-Vein-Occlusion-Guidelines-2022.pdf. Accessed 6 Nov 2024
72. The Royal College of Ophthalmologists Ophthalmic Services Guidance. Referral pathways for ocular tumours 2022. [Online]. London: The Royal College of Ophthalmologists. Available at https://www.rcophth.ac.uk/resources-listing/referral-pathways-for-adult-ocular-tumours/. Accessed 07 Jan 2025.
73. UK Prospective Diabetes Study (UKPDS) Group. Intensive blood-glucose control with sulphonylureas or insulin compared with conventional treatment and risk of complications in patients with type 2 diabetes (UKPDS 33). Lancet. 1998;352:837–53.
74. Vingerling JR, Dielemans I, Hofman A, Grobbee DE, Hijmering M, Kramer CF, de Jong PT. The prevalence of age-related maculopathy in the Rotterdam Study. Ophthalmology. 1995;102:205–10.
75. Wilkinson CP, Ferris FL 3rd, Klein RE, Lee PP, Agardh CD, Davis M, Dills D, Kampik A, Pararajasegaram R, Verdaguer JT, Global Diabetic Retinopathy Project Group. Proposed international clinical diabetic retinopathy and diabetic macular edema disease severity scales. Ophthalmology. 2003;110:1677–82.
76. Wolf S, Balciuniene VJ, Laganovska G, Menchini U, Ohno-Matsui K, Sharma T, Wong TY, Silva R, Pilz S, Gekkieva M. RADIANCE: a randomized controlled study of ranibizumab in patients with choroidal neovascularization secondary to pathologic myopia. Ophthalmology. 2014;121:682–92.
77. Wycoff CC, Abreu F, Adamis AP, Basu K, Eichenbaum DA, Haskova Z, Lin H, Loewenstein A, Mohan S, Pearce IA, Sakamoto T, Schlottmann PG, Silverman D, Sun JK, Wells JA, Willis JR, Tadayoni R. Efficacy, durability, and safety of intravitreal faricimab with extended dosing up to every 16 weeks in patients with diabetic macular oedema (YOSEMITE and RHINE): two randomised, double-masked, phase 3 trials. Lancet 2022;399:741–755.

Strabismus & Orbit

11

Timothy H. M. Fung and Winfried M. K. Amoaku

Abstract

This chapter offers a comprehensive overview of ocular motility disorders and orbital pathologies that are commonly encountered in an OSCE exam for ophthalmologists

11.1 Strabismus Examination Sequence

- Introduce yourself
- Ask the examiner for the patient's visual acuity: ensure that the patient can fixate on the distant target
- Ask the examiner if they would like you to perform the cover test (cover-uncover test and alternate cover test): move straight to ocular movements if not required
- Look for any obvious abnormal head postures
- Ask the patient to remove their glasses (if worn): quickly check the glasses to see if the patient is myopic or hyperopic and whether prisms are present in the glasses
- Perform the Hirschberg's test: ask the patient to fixate on light from a pentorch and ask the patient if they can see one or two images
- Ask the patient to look at a distant target (e.g. letter on a snellen chart or logMAR chart) and position yourself slightly to the side of the midline, facing the patient and at arm's length from the patient (do not obstruct patient's view of distance target):
  - Cover each eye in turn with an occluder to ensure the patient can visualise the distant target with each eye: if the patient has NPL vision then cover-uncover test and alternate cover test is not applicable
  - Perform a cover-uncover test to look for tropias:
    - Swiftly cover the fixating eye with an occluder and observe the other eye for any movement. Carefully note its direction
    - Uncover the eye and allow about 3 seconds for both eyes to be uncovered
    - Swiftly cover the other eye and observe its fellow eye for any movement

Supplementary Information The online version contains supplementary material available at https://doi.org/10.1007/978-3-031-97401-4_11.

T. H. M. Fung (✉)
University Hospitals of Derby & Burton NHS Foundation Trust, Royal Derby Hospital, Derby, UK
e-mail: timothy.fung@nhs.net

W. M. K. Amoaku
Eye, Ear, Nose and Throat Centre, Queens Medical Centre, Nottingham University Hospitals NHS Trust, Nottingham, UK

T. H. M. Fung, W. M. K. Amoaku (eds.), *Viva and OSCE Exams in Ophthalmology*,
https://doi.org/10.1007/978-3-031-97401-4_11

  - Perform the alternate cover test to look for phorias:
    - Rapidly shift the occluder from one eye to the other several times, not allowing any interval of binocularity
    - Ensure that each eye fixes on the target after each movement of the cover
    - Observe for any movement of the eyes
- Ask the patient to look at a near accommodative target and position yourself directly opposite the patient within arm's reach:
  - Cover each eye in turn with an occluder to ensure patient can visualise near accommodative target with each eye
  - Perform a cover-uncover test to look for tropias:
  - Perform an alternate cover test to look for phorias:
- Repeat cover test with the patient wearing glasses (if patient wears glasses): ask the examiner if they would like you to perform this before going ahead
- Examine ocular movements (See Table 11.1):
  - Sit facing the patient. Shine a light from a pentorch at eye level about 10 to 14 inches in front of the patient, with the patient looking in primary position
  - Ask the patient to inform you if they see double vision at any gaze position
  - Ask the patient to follow the light from your pentorch as you move it into the 9 directions of gaze. Elevate the upper eyelid with a finger on your free hand to observe movements in downgaze: note any limitations of movement
  - Examine ductions if you see any limitations on version movements
  - Examine horizontal and vertical saccades: ask patient to look rapidly between targets (e.g. your hands) positioned at 30-degrees on either side of the midline
- Perform a Parks-Bielschowsky 3 step test if hypertropia is present

Table 11.1 Useful information about neurogenic palsies and restrictive/mechanical disorders of ocular motility

Characteristics of Neurogenic Palsies:
The amount of ocular movement elicited is often greater on duction than on version.
Ocular movement ceases gradually in the direction of limitation
Maximal limitation of ocular movement is in the position of main action of the affected muscle
Hess chart: field of affected eye will be smaller, proportional spacing between the inner and outer fields, both fields displaced according to the deviation
Characteristics of mechanical limited ocular movement:
A positive forced duction test (FDT)
Normal saccadic velocity until the point of mechanical restriction is reached—this feature can differentiate a mechanical restriction from a neurogenic palsy
Retraction of the globe, which strongly suggests mechanical limitation—occurs when gaze is directed away from the site of the leash and is best seen by viewing the affected eye from the side
Equal limitation of version and duction
Limited development of muscle sequelae, often confined to overaction of the contralateral synergist in the unaffected eye
Hess chart: outer field of chart will be very close to the inner field in the direction of maximum limitation of movement, field of the affected eye will be very narrow either horizontally or vertically
General principles of management of mechanical disorders of ocular motility:
To centralise and if possible enlarge the field of binocular single vision, reducing the need for an abnormal head posture
To reduce or eliminate anomalous ocular movements caused by mechanical restriction (e.g. up-shoot or down-shoot on attempted adduction)
To correct the cosmetic defect (strabismus, enophthalmos, eyelid anomalies)

11.2 Cranial Nerve III Palsy

11.2.1 Examination

- Nuclear lesion: If unilateral CN III palsy is nuclear in origin: bilateral ptosis, bilateral SR paresis (vertical gaze palsy with failure in voluntary upgaze—supranuclear in origin if eyes elevate with Doll's head manoeuvre, nuclear in origin if eyes do not elevate on Doll's head manoeuvre), unilateral MR, IR and IO paresis
- Fascicular lesion (associated damage to brainstem structures):
  (a) Webers syndrome (damage to cerebral peduncle + fascicular CN III): Ipsilateral CN III palsy + contralateral hemiparesis
  (b) Benedikt's syndrome (damage to red nucleus + fascicular CN III): Ipsilateral CN III palsy + contralateral ataxia with intention tremor
- Ptosis: partial (see Fig. 11.1) or complete (see Fig. 11.2)
- Pupil: involvement (dilated pupil) or non-involvement
- Ocular movements: all muscles affected (exotropia, hypotropia, intorsion), superior division (hypotropia), inferior division (exotropia, hypertropia, intorsion), single muscle palsy (IR, IO, SR, MR—most commonly IR followed by SR)
- Abnormal head posture: all muscles affected (face turn to unaffected side), superior division (head tilt, face turn to affected side and chin elevation), inferior division (head tilt to unaffected side, face turn to unaffected side)
- Aberrant regeneration (feature of compressive and traumatic CN III palsy, does not occur in microvascular lesions): its development without a history of trauma demands a CT/MRI to rule out SOL
- Examine the SO muscle (CN IV): instruct patient to abduct eye (patient unable to adduct eye in CN III palsy) and then look down—look for intorsion (look at iris landmark or conjunctival vessel) to determine CN IV not involved.
- Examine the LR muscle (CN VI): even when eye is exotropic, it is possible to demonstrate LR function by observing the saccadic velocity or performing a force generation test

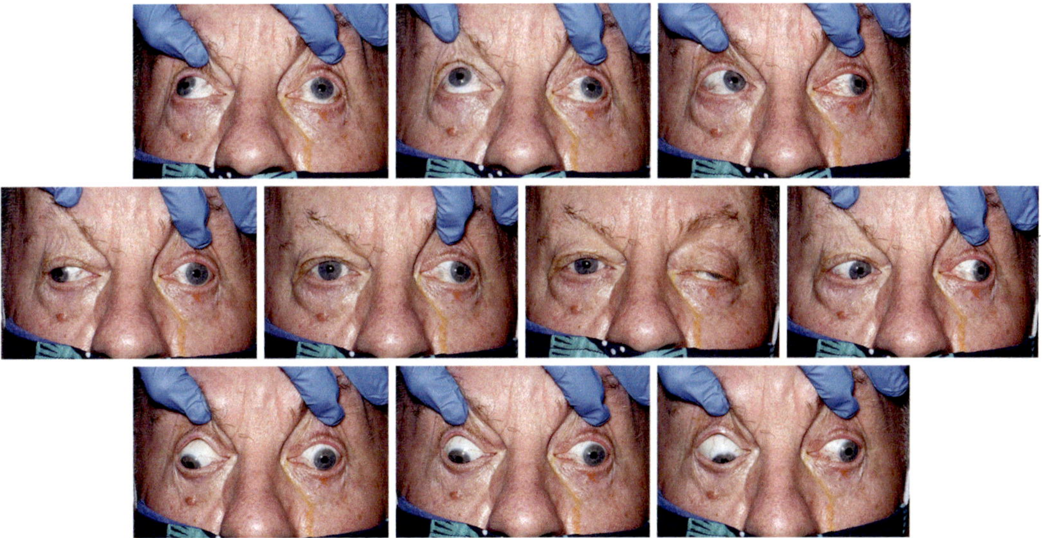

Fig. 11.1 Patient with a left CN III palsy

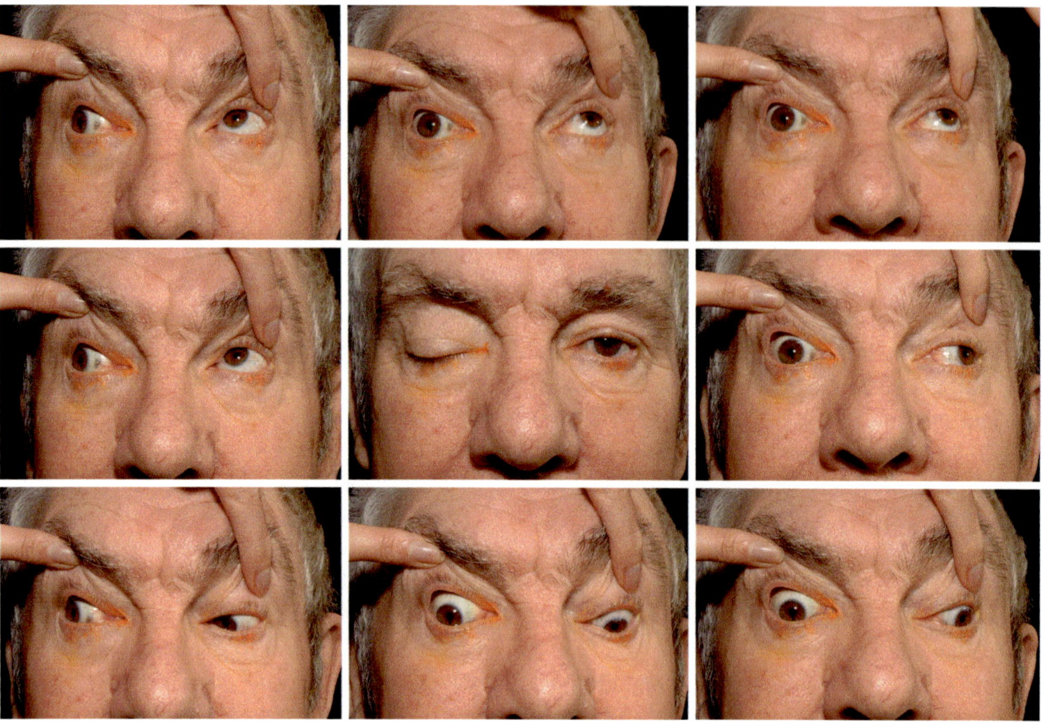

Fig. 11.2 Patient with a right CN III palsy

11.2.2 Discussion Points (Tables 11.2 and 11.3)

11.2.2.1 Anatomy

- CN III nucleus lies in the midbrain, anterior to the periaqueductal grey matter, at the level of the superior colliculus
- CN III nucleus consists of a single central nucleus, innervating both LPS muscles, and separate subnuclei for each SR (contralateral innervation), MR, IR, and IO (all ipsilateral innervation)
- CN III fasciculus travels anteriorly through the MLF, the red nucleus, and the cerebral

Table 11.2 Differentiating SR palsy and contralateral SO palsy

Compare the amount of vertical deviation in extreme positions of gaze by use of the alternate cover test
Deviation increasing on dextrodepression: indicates a left SO palsy
Deviation increasing on dextroelevation: indicates a right SR palsy
Excyclotorsion of globe seen objectively with a fundus photograph: more suggestive of SO palsy
Comparison of the near and distance vertical deviation: hypertropia that increases for near fixation suggests a SO palsy
Compensatory head posture: chin up in SR palsy, chin down in SO palsy
Bielschowsky head tilt test

Table 11.3 Differentiating IO palsy and Brown's syndrome

FDT: restricted in Brown's syndrome, passive movement in IO palsy
A pattern occurs in IO palsy whereas Brown's syndrome shows a V pattern
Incyclotropia usually present in IO palsy but not in Brown's syndrome
Muscle sequelae (can be seen clearly on Hess chart) should develop as expected in IO palsy whereas development is confined to overaction of the contralateral SR in Brown's syndrome, field of the affected eye in IO palsy will be displaced down in IO palsy but that of a pt with Brown's syndrome will show little or no abnormality in the primary position or in the lower field

peduncle. On leaving the midbrain, CN III peripheral nerve emerges within the interpeduncular fossa and passes anteriorly beneath the PCA, above the superior cerebellar artery, and lateral to the posterior communicating artery (PCoA)

- CN III peripheral nerve travels within the lateral wall of the cavernous sinus, dividing into superior (innervates the LPS, SR) and inferior (MR, IR, IO) branches that enter the orbit via the superior orbital fissure and annulus of Zinn.
- Parasympathetic fibers from the Edinger-Westphal nucleus travel in the IO branch as far as the ciliary ganglion and then in the short ciliary nerves to the globe where they innervate the ciliary muscle and pupillary sphincter

11.2.2.2 Causes

- Acquired
  - (a) Compression by a PCoA aneurysm (pupil involvement)
  - (b) Microvascular disease: HTN, DM (usually pupil sparing)
  - (c) Tumours: direct damage from adjacent tumours such as meningioma's, affecting areas of the base of the skull or adjacent to the pituitary fossa and cavernous sinus
  - (d) Closed head trauma (pupillary involvement in most cases) or birth trauma
  - (e) GCA
- Congenital

11.2.2.3 Muscle Sequelae

- All muscles affected: overaction contralateral LR, SO, SR, and IO
- Superior division: overaction contralateral IO, contracture of ipsilateral IR, secondary inhibitional palsy of contralateral SO
- Inferior division: overaction contralateral LR, SR and SO
- MR: overaction contralateral LR, contracture ipsilateral LR, secondary inhibitional palsy of contralateral MR
- SR: overaction contralateral IO, contracture of ipsilateral IR, secondary inhibitional palsy of contralateral SO
- IR: overaction contralateral SO, contracture of ipsilateral SR, secondary inhibitional palsy of contralateral IO
- IO: overaction contralateral SR, contracture of ipsilateral SO, secondary inhibitional palsy of contralateral IR

11.2.2.4 Investigations

- Non-traumatic partial CN III palsy +/− pupil involvement: CTA/MRA to exclude a posterior communicating artery aneurysm
- Non-traumatic complete CN III palsy with pupil sparing (usually ischaemic—likelihood increased if age > 40, known vasculopathy, acute-onset, non-progressive, no other neurological abnormality): bloods (FBC/ESR/CRP to rule out GCA if age ≥ 50 glucose to rule out DM), MRI head if no recovery of function at 3/12. Initial review every 2–3/7 for the first week after presentation to ensure no pupil involvement occurs.
- Aberrant regeneration of CN III palsy without hx of trauma: MRI to rule out SOL
- Hess chart (see Fig. 2.52)

11.2.2.5 Treatment

- Urgent referral to neurosurgeons if posterior communicating artery aneurysm is found on imaging
- Conservative
  - (a) Symptomatic diplopia only present if the ptosis does not cover the visual axis): prisms (limited use though as diplopia

reverses in different positions of gaze), occlusion of an eye with a patch or CL
(b) Mydriasis causing photophobia: tinted glasses, painted CL, constriction of pupil with pilocarpine drops
(c) Ptosis: ptosis crutches fitted to spectacle frames

- Surgical
  (a) Symptomatic diplopia or cosmetic appearance: Botox, muscle surgery
  (b) Ptosis

11.3 Cranial Nerve IV Palsy

11.3.1 Examination

- Congenital—unilateral: head tilt to unaffected side, facial asymmetry (reduction of distance between the lateral canthus and the corner of the mouth on the side of the head posture), large hyperphoria (sometimes exceeding 20PD), manifest vertical deviation with the head straight, vertical deviation increases on near fixation, excyclotorsion in primary position (seen on fundus examination), +ve Bielschowsky head tilt test, large vertical fusion amplitude of ≥10PD
- Congenital—bilateral: alternating hypertropia of non-fixing eye with a constant large V-pattern esotropia (≥25PD), chin down head posture, +ve Bielschowsky head tilt test to either side with reversal of hypertropia on right and left tilt (helps differentiate from primary ET with IOOA), excyclotorsion in primary position, large vertical fusion amplitude of ≥10PD
- Acquired (see Fig. 11.3)—unilateral: hypertropia on affected side that is worse on adduction, head tilt/face turn to unaffected side (to overcome vertical diplopia), +ve Bielschowsky head tilt test (fixation at 3 m target), vertical fusion amplitude of 2–3PD
- Acquired—bilateral (see Table 11.4): chin depression, reversal of hypertropia on right and left gaze and on dextro- and laevo-depres-

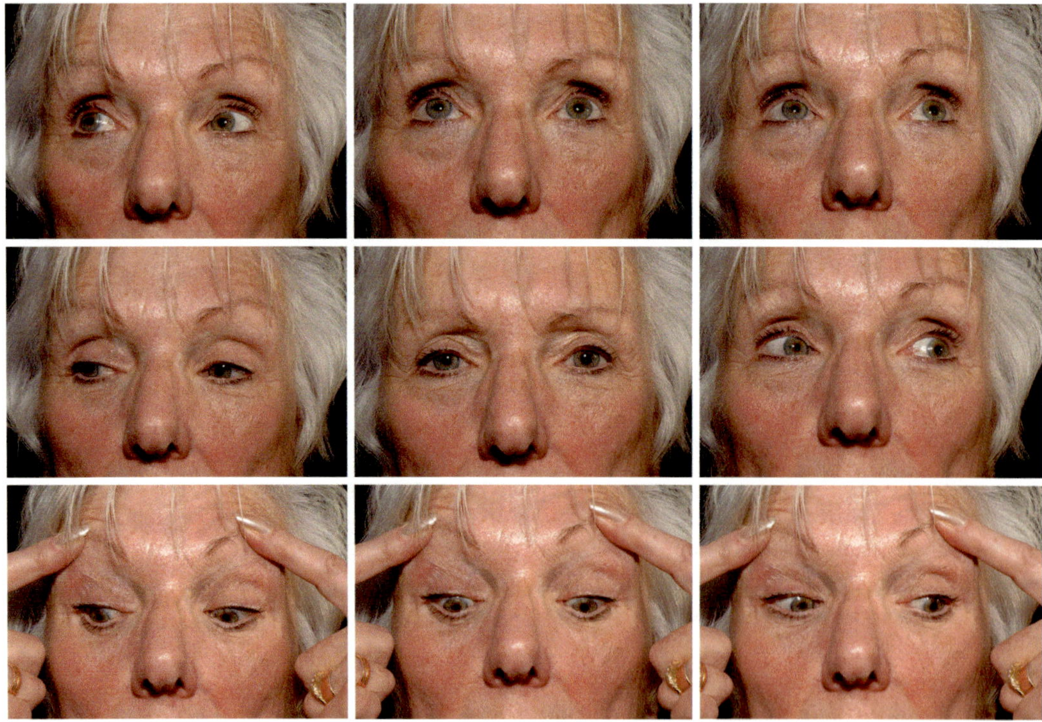

Fig. 11.3 Patient with a right CN IV palsy

Table 11.4 Features suggestive of a congenital CN IV palsy

Facial asymmetry
Old photographs demonstrating head posture
Vertical fusion amplitude well in excess of normal 2–4PD, which is the usual finding in acquired palsies

sion, positive Bielschowsky head tilt test to either side, V-pattern esotropia, symptomatic excyclotorsion >10 degrees in primary position, vertical fusion amplitude of 2–3PD

- Perform a dilated fundus examination to look for excyclotorsion of the fundus (normally an imaginary line drawn horizontally from inferior 1/3 of the disc intersects the fovea. A line drawn in the same manner crosses superior to the fovea in an eye that is excyclotorted)

11.3.2 Discussion Points

11.3.2.1 Anatomy

- CN IV nucleus lies just below CN III nucleus in the lower midbrain at the level of the inferior colliculus
- Fasciculus decussates within the anterior medullary venum and exits the midbrain posteriorly.
- CN IV peripheral nerve curves around the midbrain, passes anteriorly between the posterior cerebral and superior cerebellar arteries, travels within the lateral wall of the cavernous sinus (inferolateral to CN III, superior to V1), enters the orbit through the SOF (but superior to the annulus of Zinn) and terminates in the SO muscle.

11.3.2.2 Causes

- Congenital (1/3 of cases - see Table 11.5)
- Acquired
  (a) Closed head trauma
  (b) Microvascular disease: age > 40, acute onset, non-progressive, no other neurological abnormality, known vasculopath
  (c) Tumours
  (d) GCA

Table 11.5 Features suggestive a bilateral CN IV palsy

Chin down head posture
Alternating hypertropia: confirmed with a bilaterally positive Bielschowsky head tilt test with right hypertropia on right head tilt and left hypertropia on left head tilt
Prominent V pattern esotropia (≥25PD)
Excyclotorsion >10 degrees in the primary position
Bilateral failure of adduction on depression

11.3.2.3 Muscle Sequelae

- Overaction of ipsilateral IO
- Overaction of contralateral IR
- Secondary inhibitional palsy of contralateral SR

11.3.2.4 Investigations

- Double Maddox rod to measure cyclotorsion
- Bloods to rule out GCA (FBC/ESR/CRP if age ≥ 50), DM (glucose)
- MRI head if: age < 40, progressive, no recovery of function at 3/12, associated neurological abnormality
- Hess chart (see Figs. 2.53 and 2.54)

11.3.2.5 Treatment

- Conservative
  (a) Symptomatic diplopia: prisms, occlusion of eye with patch or CL
- Surgical
  (a) Symptomatic diplopia or cosmetic appearance: Botox, muscle surgery (Harada-Ito for excyclotortion)

11.4 Cranial Nerve VI Palsy

11.4.1 Examination

- Esodeviation which increases in the distance (see Fig. 11.4)
- Face turn towards affected side
- Abduction deficit (see Figs. 11.5 and 11.6)
- Examine the fundus to look for optic disc swelling

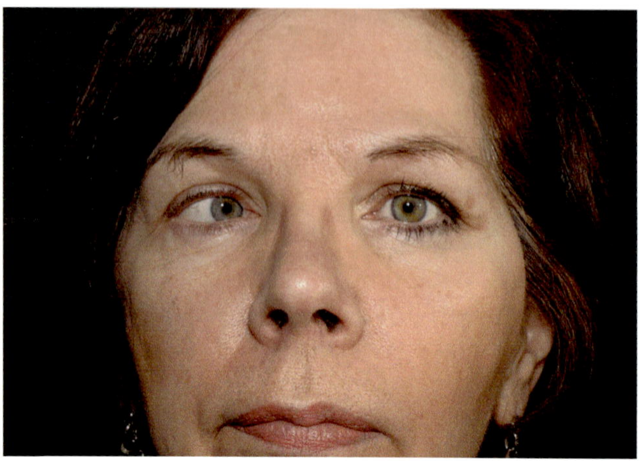

Fig. 11.4 Patient with a right CN VI palsy with an esodeviation in primary gaze

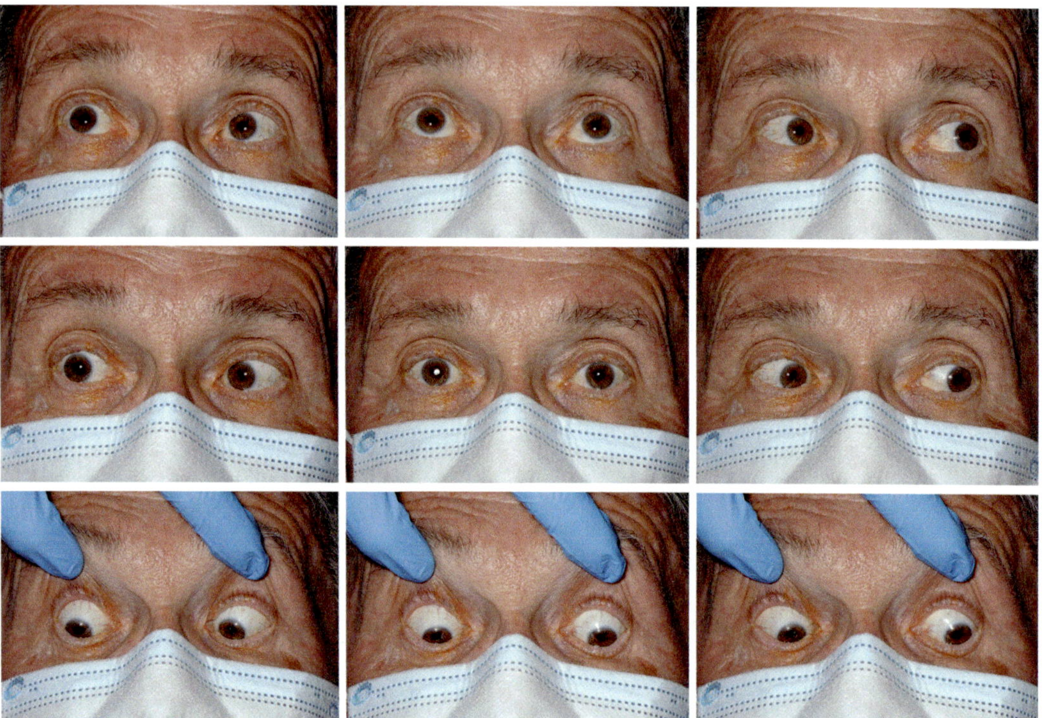

Fig. 11.5 Patient with a right CN VI palsy

11.4.2 Discussion Points

11.4.2.1 Differential Diagnosis of Abduction Deficit

- Neurological
  (a) CN VI palsy (see Table 11.6)
- Mechanical
  (a) Orbital trauma (blow out fracture of medial orbital wall): Hx + CT scan
  (b) TED: proptosis, eyelid signs
  (c) Duane's syndrome: retraction of globe on adduction
- Myopathic:
  (a) Myasthenia gravis

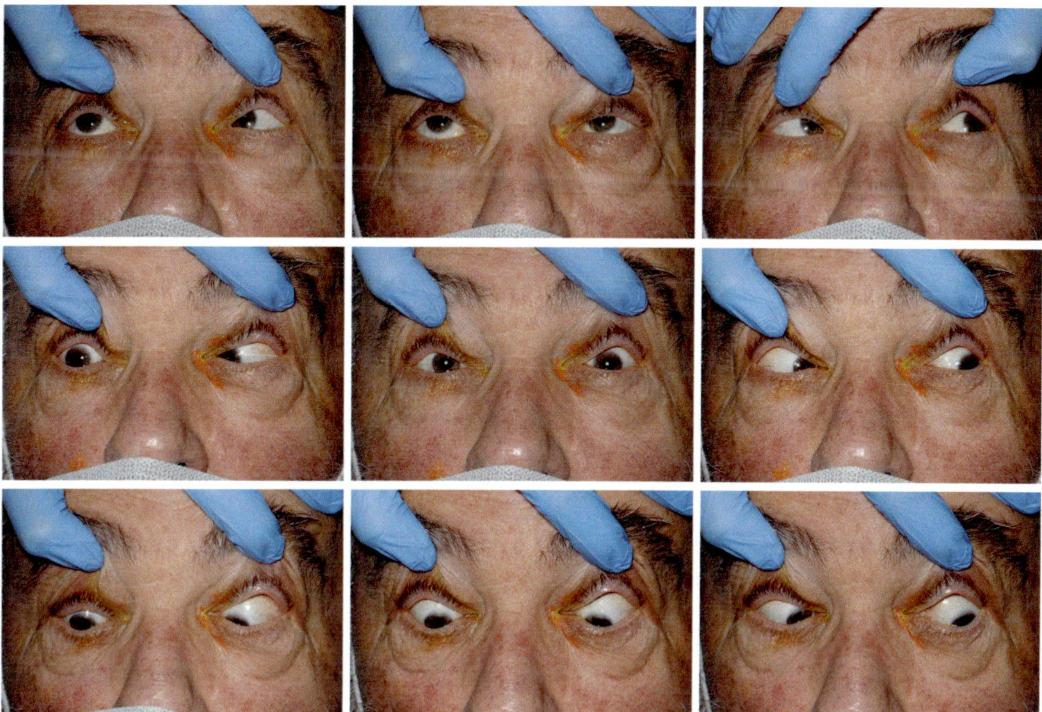

Fig. 11.6 Another patient with a right CN VI palsy

Table 11.6 Factors suggesting a bilateral CN VI palsy

Incomitant ET on both right and left gaze
Bilateral contracture of the MR muscles in long standing total bilateral palsies
Slow peak saccadic velocity on abduction
V-pattern esotropia: more likely in the presence of a bilateral palsy

- Other
  - (a) Distance ET of high myopia: can lead to progressive loss of abduction

11.4.2.2 Anatomy

- CN VI nucleus lies in the lower pons anterior to the fourth ventricle, at the level of the facial colliculus
- CN VI fasciculus travels anteriorly through the medial lemniscus and corticospinal tract, just medial to the trigeminal nuclear complex and vestibular nuclei
- CN VI basilar nerve emerges from the pontomedullary junction, ascends in the subarachnoid space between the pons and clivus, before turning anterior over the petrous apex of the temporal bone and under the petroclinoid ligament to enter the cavernous sinus, where it runs within the sinus itself and then enters the orbit via the SOF and annulus of Zinn to terminate in the LR muscle

11.4.2.3 Causes

- Acquired
  - (a) False localising sign: raised ICP from SOL—CN VI subjected to traction as rise in ICP causes a downward displacement of the brainstem,
  - (b) Fascicular CN VI palsy: demyelination, CVA, metastatic tumours
  - (c) Peripheral CN VI palsy:
    - (1) Microvascular disease
    - (2) Closed head injury
    - (3) Localised compression of the nerve by a primary pituitary tumour, craniopharyngioma or meningioma in the base of the skull or close to the pituitary fossa or cavernous sinus

(4) Basilar artery aneurysm
(5) Metastatic tumours
(6) Bacterial infection of the middle ear: spread to petrous temporal bone, involving the sixth and fifth nerves, presenting as a CN VI palsy with ipsilateral facial pain (Gradenigo's syndrome)

- Congenital

11.4.2.4 Muscle Sequelae

- Contracture of ipsilateral MR
- Contralateral MR overaction
- Secondary inhibitional palsy of contralateral LR

11.4.2.5 Investigations

- Bloods to rule out GCA (FBC/ESR/CRP if age $\geq$ 50), DM (glucose)
- MRI head if no recovery of function at 3/12
- Hess chart (see Figs. 2.55 and 2.56)

11.4.2.6 Treatment

- Conservative
  (a) Symptomatic diplopia: prisms, occlusion of eye with patch or CL
- Surgical:
  (a) Symptomatic diplopia or cosmetic appearance: Botox, Muscle surgery (if total palsy with no recovery of CN VI function—vertical muscle transposition using the Hummelsheim and Jensen operations/if partial palsy with residual CN VI function—LR resect/MR recess)

11.5 Brown's Syndrome

11.5.1 Examination

- Limitation of elevation in adduction (normal depression in adduction): if the restriction of movement is severe, there may also be some limitation of direct elevation and even of elevation in abduction
- Discomfort on attempting elevation in adduction
- Down drift of the affected eye on contralateral version
- Overaction of the contralateral SR muscle: other muscle sequelae do not develop, therefore there is no overaction of the SO on the affected side
- Abnormal head posture, comprising a head tilt to the affected side, a face turn to the contralateral side and chin elevation
- V pattern
- Absence of cyclotropia

11.5.2 Discussion Points

11.5.2.1 Pathogenesis

- Abnormalities of the superior oblique tendon sheath including shortening (tight SO anterior tendon sheath), inflammation or thickening

11.5.2.2 Other Diagnoses to Consider

- Isolated IO palsy: more frequently seen following orbital trauma or in association with MG—SO overaction, A pattern, negative FDT
- Double elevator palsy: limitation of upgaze on both adduction and abduction, presence of ptosis, Bell's phenomenon may be intact, confirming the absence of any mechanical restriction of elevation
- Orbital blow out fracture: limitation of elevation, enophthalmos, infraorbital nerve anaesthesia
- Congenital ocular muscle fibrosis syndrome: fibrosis of IR muscle will result in limitation of upgaze—limitation will be greatest in abduction with retraction of the globe on attempted up-gaze

11.5.2.3 Causes

- Abnormalities of the superior oblique tendon sheath
- Congenital: affecting SO/trochlear complex
- Acquired (inflammation or trauma affecting the trochlear region): inflammation—RA, orbital inflammation, chronic sinusitis/surgery—SO tuck, buckling, orbital

11.5.2.4 Investigations

- Hess chart (see Fig. 2.57)
- FDT: positive test
- Field of binocular single vision: if diplopia can be elicited
- MRI for acquired Brown's syndrome

11.5.2.5 Treatment

- Majority of patients with Brown's syndrome of early onset maintain symptom free binocular single vision with a relatively slight head posture. Field of binocular single vision is usually adequate and in the optimum position on depression of gaze. These pt's do not require treatment
- Conservative: retrotrochlear steroid injection
- Surgical (SO tenotomy): indications—significant head posture or if strabismus in primary position

11.6 Duane's Retraction Syndrome

11.6.1 Examination

- Limitation of horizontal eye movement: usually comprising a moderate or marked limitation of abduction. In most cases, these is little or no limitation of adduction; in others adduction is restricted but to a lesser extent that abduction. Less commonly, the limitation of adduction exceeds the limitation of abduction
- Compensatory head posture (adopted to centralise the often-narrow field of binocular single vision—determined by deviation in primary position and by the pattern of ocular movement): face turn to affected side if ET, face turn to unaffected side if XT
- Retraction of globe on adduction, with narrowing of palpebral fissure
- Manifest strabismus: usually ET (more marked for distance fixation and reduced for near fixation) when head is straight, XT occurs when adduction is more limited than abduction
- Upshoot and/or downshoot on adduction
- Poor convergence
- Associated ocular abnormality: colobomata, heterochromic iridis, lens opacities, microphthalmos and persistent pupillary membrane
- Skeletal and facial abnormalities: Goldenhars and Klippel-Feil syndrome, abnormal ear formation, deafness, syndactyly, cleft palate and spinal meningocoele

11.6.2 Discussion Points

11.6.2.1 Pathogenesis

- Congenital disorder associated with hypoplasia of CN VI with subsequent aberrant co-innervation of LR and MR by CN III

11.6.2.2 Other Diagnoses to Consider

- Congenital CN VI palsy: large angle esotropia with limited abduction but no evidence of limited adduction nor the associated globe retraction and the upshoot or downshoot
- Infantile esotropia: abduction can usually be demonstrated either by occluding the contralateral eye for a period, or by rotating a young child to induce vestibular nystagmus (thus demonstrating movement past the midline), no other characteristics of Duane's syndrome will be present
- Mobius syndrome: bilateral CN VII weakness and loss of abduction, absence of retraction of the globe and narrowing of the palpebral fissures

11.6.2.3 Classification

- Brown's classification (based on clinical features alone):
  (a) Type A: with limited abduction and less marked limitation of adduction
  (b) Type B: limited abduction but normal adduction
  (c) Type C: limitation of adduction exceeds the limitation of abduction with XT
- Huber's classification (based on EMG findings):
  (a) Type I: marked limitation of abduction
  (b) Type II: limitation of adduction
  (c) Type III: limitation of both abduction and adduction

11.6.2.4 Associations

- Goldenhar syndrome
- Klipper-Feil syndrome: short webbed neck, restricted movement of cervical spine
- Wildervanck syndrome: Klipper-Feil, Duane, deafness

11.6.2.5 Investigations

- Hess chart (see Figs. 2.58, 2.59 and 2.60)

11.6.2.6 Treatment

- The vast majority of patients with Duane's syndrome maintain comfortable binocular single vision and remain compensated, usually with a comparatively slight face turn
- Surgical: indications—decompensation giving rise to a manifest strabismus in the primary position in childhood or symptoms at a later stage, cosmetically poor compensatory head posture, cosmetically poor manifest strabismus, severe globe retraction +/− upshoot and downshoot

11.7 Restrictive Myopathy in TED

11.7.1 Examination

- Ocular motility
  (a) Mechanical restriction of ocular movement +/− pain on looking in the direction of limited movement
  (b) Retraction of the globe occurs when movement away from the site of the restriction is attempted (commonly seen on upgaze)
  (c) In order of decreasing frequency the muscles involved are: IR muscle (restricted up gaze), MR muscle (restricted abduction), SR muscle (restricted downgaze), LR muscle (restricted adduction although LR is usually spared even when enlargement is evident on CT scan)
  (d) Common ocular posture is hypotropia of the more affected eye, sometimes with associated ET
  (e) An abnormal head posture, commonly chin elevation, is often adopted, +/− face turn: purpose is to avoid an uncomfortable position of gaze, to centralise a field of binocular single vision
  (f) Enlarged vertical fusion amplitude

11.7.2 Discussion Points

11.7.2.1 Investigations

- Hess chart (see Fig. 2.63)
- Field of binocular single vision (see Fig. 2.77)
- Forced duction test to confirm presence and extent of mechanical restrictions

11.7.2.2 Treatment

- Conservative
  (a) Treatment of diplopia: prisms, Botox, occlusion (last resort)
- Surgical
  (a) Aims of extraocular muscle surgery are to improve the patient's appearance and to establish a field of binocular single vision in the primary position and on down-gaze, extending the area into other fields of gaze if possible
  (b) Patient should be euthyroid and the ocular muscle imbalance should have remained stable for at least 3 months before considering surgery
  (c) Categorise the ocular motility disturbances into recognisable patterns:
    (1) Unilateral or grossly asymmetrical bilateral restriction of elevation
      – Incomitant (increase in vertical deviation on upgaze and a reduction on downgaze, usually with an intact inferior field of BSV): mechanical restriction of ipsilateral IR—tx with ipsilateral IR recession
      – Concomitant (vertical deviation that is the same on upgaze and which decreases minimally or not at all on downgaze, usually with no field of BSV): mechanical

restriction of ipsilateral IR + contralateral SR—tx with IR recession +/− SR recession

(2) Unilateral or grossly asymmetric bilateral restriction of abduction
   - Incomitant (ET which increases in the direction of mechanical restriction and reduces in the opposite field of gaze + face turn away from the side with the mechanical restriction + intact field of BSV): mechanical restriction of ipsilateral MR—tx with ipsilateral MR recession
   - Concomitant (ET in all positions of gaze): bilateral mechanical restriction of both MR—tx with unilateral or bilateral MR recession

(3) Unilateral or grossly asymmetric bilateral restriction of both elevation and abduction: management is the same as for pattern (1) and (2)

(4) Bilateral symmetric restriction of elevation
   - Neither eye is able to maintain fixation in primary position
   - Asymmetrical mechanical restriction of elevation, with a −2 to −3 restriction in the more mobile eye
   - A pattern ET is present on upgaze, with a convergence retraction movement as the eyes attempt to move into the field of maximum restriction
   - Contraction of the SR, if present, will restrict movement on down-gaze
   - Tx with bilateral IR recession

(5) Bilateral restriction of both elevation and abduction

(6) Mechanical restriction of the superior rectus muscles resulting in limited down-gaze
   - Limitation of depression that is greatest in abduction
   - Treat with SR recession

11.8 Orbit Examination Sequence

- Introduce yourself
- Quick inspection of patient to look for features of a craniosynostosis (e.g. frontal bossing and other anomalous bony changes), lid changes (e.g. lid retraction), goitre, temporal fossa fullness (sphenoid wing meningioma)
- Inspect for an apparent exophthalmos or enophthalmos by the following technique
  - Ask patient to tilt head slightly forwards and to look straight ahead
  - Stand behind the patient and look over the patient's forehead and eyebrows from above, sighting the plane of the face. Elevate both upper eyelids.
  - Note the position of the front of each globe in relationship to each other. A disparity between the 2 globes of more than 2 mm is abnormal
- Palpate the circumference of the orbital rim
- Ask the patient to close their eyes and gently touch the patient's closed eyelid for
  - Any thrills or pulsation movements
  - Any anterior extensions of an anterior or retrobulbar orbital mass
- Compare the ease of globe retropulsion for the 2 orbits by gently pushing the globe posteriorly through the patient's closed eyelids.
- Perform exophthalmometry
  - Position yourself directly in front of the patient. Your right eye measures the patient's left eye, and your left eye measures the patient's right eye
  - Place the instrument so that the foot plates of the exophthalmometer rests on the lateral rims at the level of the lateral canthi: note the intercanthal reading on the exophthalmometer
  - Close your right eye and ask the patient to look at your open left eye to achieve straight ahead alignment. Using your open left eye, align the instruments two vertical markers (usually red) on the millimeter scale and read off where the patient's anterior corneal surface of the cornea appears on the millimeter scale. Obtain a similar

measurement for the patients left eye by using your right eye. A difference of more than 2 mm is considered abnormal

- Measure globe displacement
  - Horizontal displacement:
    - Ask the patient to fixate at a distant target straight ahead. Occlude the fellow eye if strabismus is present
    - Imagine a straight vertical line down the middle of the patients face
    - Hold a ruler horizontally across the bridge of the patient's nose, perpendicular to the imaginary vertical line
    - Measure the distance from the center of the nasal bridge to the medial limbus of the right eye. Repeat measurement for the left eye. The difference between the 2 measurements is the amount of horizontal displacement
  - Vertical displacement:
    - Ask the patient to fixate at a distance target straight ahead.
    - Hold a ruler horizontally along the patient's nasal bridge at the level of the lateral canthi
    - Hold another ruler vertically, perpendicular to the horizontal ruler, to pass through the center of the patient's right pupil and measure the distance from the edge of the horizontal ruler to the pupillary center.
    - Repeat measurements for the left eye. The difference between the 2 measurements is the amount of vertical displacement
- Ask the examiner whether the following is required
  - Ocular motility
  - Examination of the pupils
  - Examination of the eyelids

11.9 TED

11.9.1 Examination

- Check proptosis
  - Measure the degree of proptosis using an exophthalmometer
  - Axial, usually bilateral, but can be quite asymmetric
- Examine the eyelids (see Fig. 11.7)
  - Measure the eyelid position and function (PA, MRD1, LF)
  - Look for lid swelling and erythema
  - Look for upper and lower lid retraction
  - Look for temporal flare of the upper eyelid (lid just keeps getting higher toward the lateral canthus—peak of normal eyelid is just nasal to the pupil)
  - Look for lid lag in downgaze
  - Look for lagophthalmos
- Perform ocular motility to look for the presence of any restrictive myopathy
- Slit lamp examination
  - Check corneal sensation
  - Look for conjunctival and caruncular injection and/or chemosis

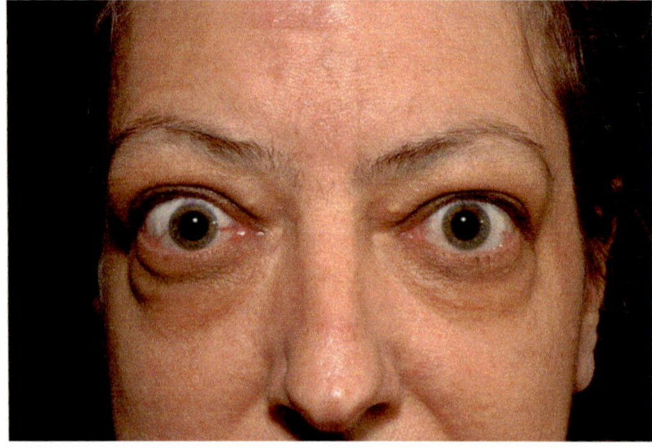

Fig. 11.7 Facial photo of a patient with TED showing bilateral proptosis with upper lid oedema and upper and lower eyelid retraction

  - Look for signs of corneal exposure, superior limbic keratoconjunctivitis
  - Check IOP in primary position and upgaze (more than 5 mmHg difference)
  - Perform a dilated fundus exam to look for optic disc swelling or pallor and choroidal folds
- Systemic examination
  - Examine for goitre, palmar erythema, atrial fibrillation, and pretibial myxedema
  - Look for signs of hyperthyroidism (warm peripheries, tachycardia, atrial fibrillation, hair loss) or hypothyroidism (bradycardia, dry thin hair, dry coarse skin)
- Check optic nerve function for compressive optic neuropathy
  - VA
  - RAPD
  - Colour vision (first sign of early optic nerve compression is reduced colour vision)

11.9.2 Discussion Points

11.9.2.1 Investigations

- Thyroid functions tests (TSH, T4—most patients will have a high T4 and a low TSH level, although in 5–10% of patients, thyroid orbitopathy will be associated with a euthyroid condition) and thyroid autoantibodies (anti-TSH receptor, anti-thyroid peroxidase, anti-thyroglobulin antibodies)
- In some patients, the diagnosis is so obvious that no imaging is necessary
- CT scan with axial and coronal cuts (see Fig. 2.65): enlarged extraocular muscles, proptosis (>1/3 of eye in front of imaginary line from medial to lateral canthus), CT is preferred imaging modality for planning orbital decompression
- MRI (T2 STIR): better soft tissue resolution and used for grading disease activity, enlarged muscle bellies with sparing of the tendons
- Orthoptic review: Hess/Lees chart, field of binocular single vision, field of uniocular fixation
- Serial visual evoked potentials (VEP—provides objective assessment of optic nerve function—important to know that patient is euthyroid before evaluating the result, as hypothyroid patients without optic nerve compression can show a delay in the P100 component of the VEP)
- Forced duction test: confirm presence and extent of mechanical restrictions

11.9.2.2 Treatment

- Achieve a euthyroid state without post-treatment hypothyroidism—seek consultation with an endocrinologist if the patient is not seeing one. Treatment of hyperthyroidism—carbimazole or propylthiouracil, radioactive iodine—short course of prophylactic oral steroid to prevent new onset or progression of TED, thyroidectomy. Treatment of hypothyroidism—levothyroxine
- Promotion of smoking cessation
- Before initiating treatment, determine where the patient's condition falls in the natural history of the disease. Try to determine whether patient is in the "active" stage (swelling or redness of the orbital, lid, and conjunctival tissues—eyelids look "wet" as though you could squeeze oedema fluid out, eyelid swelling and any diplopia are much worse in the mornings) or "chronic" stage (morning eyelid swelling and diplopia are gone, signs of acute inflammation are no longer present, any remaining proptosis and lid retraction probably will not change) of the disease
- Mild TED/CAS < 3—most patients will require only medical management during the active stage—monitor patients for corneal exposure and treat irritation with lubricating drops and ointment, elevate head of the bed to reduce morning swelling or diplopia, sunglasses to decrease photophobia and feelings of dryness, prisms for diplopia
- Moderate-severe TED/CAS ≥ 3—consider immunosuppression (systemic corticosteroids—IV methylprednisolone or oral prednisolone, rituximab, etanercept, AZT) or orbital radiotherapy (2000 rads—for patients

with restrictive myopathy but not for acute optic nerve compression—contraindications include hx of skin cancer, age less than 35 years old)

- Sight threatening TED—admit patient, IV methylprednisolone 1 g every day for 3/7 (maximum total dose of 8 g—if dose exceeds measure LFT's as small risk of acute liver damage). Surgical decompression (fat &/or bony decompression) if the steroid therapy fails and if systemic steroid therapy is contraindicated or has intolerable side effects
- Surgical (decompression then strabismus surgery then lid surgery)—when you have confirmed that there has been no change over 3–6 months, the patient may want to consider procedures to improve the remaining proptosis, lid retraction, and strabismus (to correct diplopia: conservative—prisms, botulinum injection, and Bangerter foils, surgical—indicated when there is diplopia in primary gaze and downgaze and stable inactive TED with stable myopathy for at least 6/12)

11.10 Post Enucleation Socket Syndrome (PESS)

11.10.1 Examination

- Enophthalmos
- Upper eyelid sulcus deformity
- Ptosis or eyelid retraction
- Laxity of the lower eyelid
- A backward tilt of the ocular prosthesis (viewed from side of patient)

11.10.2 Discussion Points

11.10.2.1 Indications for an Enucleation

- Painful blind eye
- Blind unsightly eye
- Intraocular tumour
- Severe irreparable ocular trauma and high risk of sympathetic ophthalmia

11.10.2.2 Treatment

- Correction of orbital volume deficiency
  - Secondary orbital implant surgery:
    - Baseball implant
    - Hydroxyapatite implant
    - Porous polyethylene (Medpor) implant
    - Bioceramic implant
    - Dermis fat graft implant
- Correction of residual orbital volume deficiency (in spite of the insertion of a secondary orbital implant of adequate size):
  - Placement of a subperiosteal implant using pieces of Medpor
  - Structural fat grafting to the orbital apex
  - Intermittent injection of hyaluronic acid filler into the orbital apex
  - Injection of small hydrogel implants into the orbital apex
- Correction of lower eyelid laxity: LTS.

12 Neuro-ophthalmology

Timothy H. M. Fung and Winfried M. K. Amoaku

Abstract

This chapter offers a comprehensive overview of neuroophthalmology pathologies that are commonly encountered in an OSCE exam for ophthalmologists.

12.1 Examination of Patients with Abnormal Pupils

12.1.1 Pupils Examination Sequence

- Introduce yourself
- Quick inspection for the presence of ptosis or heterochromia
- Sit on one side of the seated patient
- In bright lighting
  - Ask patient to look at a distant target (minimise accomodation with its accompanying pupil miosis)
  - Measure and compare pupil size (mm) in each eye with a pupil size gauge on the side of a pen torch
- Ask for room lights to be dimmed
- In dim lighting
  - Ask patient to look at a distant target (minimise accomodation with its accompanying pupil miosis)
  - Measure and compare pupil size (mm) in each eye with a pupil size gauge on the side of a pen torch—use a second pen torch to illuminate both pupils from below the nose if required to discern the pupil sizes
  - Check for direct and consensual light reflex using light source from an indirect ophthalmoscope
  - Check for the presence of a RAPD using light source from an indirect ophthalmoscope
  - Check near reflex: look for any light-near dissociation (significantly better pupillary near reflex than light reflex)

12.1.2 Causes of a RAPD

- Asymmetric optic neuropathies
  - Ischaemic optic neuropathies
  - Advanced glaucoma
  - Optic neuritis
  - Compressive optic neuropathy
- Severe asymmetric retinal diseases
  - Total RD
  - CRAO
  - CRVO

T. H. M. Fung (✉)
University Hospitals of Derby & Burton NHS Foundation Trust, Royal Derby Hospital, Derby, UK
e-mail: timothy.fung@nhs.net

W. M. K. Amoaku
Eye, Ear, Nose and Throat Centre, Queens Medical Centre, Nottingham University Hospitals NHS Trust, Nottingham, UK

T. H. M. Fung, W. M. K. Amoaku (eds.), *Viva and OSCE Exams in Ophthalmology*,
https://doi.org/10.1007/978-3-031-97401-4_12

12.1.3 Causes of Light-Near Dissociation

- Adie (Holmes-Adie) tonic pupil
- Argyll Robertson pupil—syphilis
- Parinaud syndrome
- Myotonic dystrophy

12.1.4 Differential Diagnosis of Anisocoria

- Anisocoria equal in bright and dim illumination
  - Suggests physiologic anisocoria:
    - <1 mm difference in pupillary diameter between the eyes
    - Brisk pupil response to light
    - Brisk pupil response to accommodation
    - No associated ptosis or ocular motility problems
- Anisocoria greater in bright illumination
  - Suggests the bigger pupil is the abnormal one
  - Differential diagnosis:
    - CN III palsy
    - Adie's tonic pupil:
    - Pharmacological dilatation:
      - Fixed large pupil
      - Unreactive to light or accomodation
      - Confirm with 1% pilocarpine: mydriatic pupil will not constrict
    - Traumatic mydriasis
    - Benign episodic unilateral mydriasis
      - More commonly occurs in women
      - Associated with migraines
- Anisocoria greater in dim illumination
  - Suggests the smaller pupil is the abnormal one
  - Differential diagnosis:
    - Horner's syndrome
    - Pharmacological miosis:
      - Fixed small pupil
      - Unreactive to light or accomodation
      - Confirm with 1% tropicamide: miotic pupil will not dilate
    - Posterior synechiae

12.1.5 Clinical Cases for Pupil Examination

12.1.5.1 Horner's Syndrome (Fig. 12.1)

- Causes
  - Congenital:
    - Birth trauma (forceps injury to brachial plexus): ipsilateral arm weakness
    - Idiopathic
  - Acquired:
    - First order neurone lesion:
      - CVA
      - Vertebrobasilar insufficiency causing lateral medullary syndrome:
        - Occlusion of posterior inferior cerebellar artery
        - Ipsilateral loss of pain and temperature sensation in the face
        - Contralateral loss of pain and temperature sensation in the body
        - Ipsilateral Horner's syndrome
        - Ipsilateral cerebellar ataxia
      - Cervical trauma
      - Syringomyelia
      - Neuroblastoma (child: proptosis, ecchymotic eyelid, opsoclonus, Horner's syndrome)
      - Multiple sclerosis (MS): rare
    - Second order neurone (preganglionic) lesion:
      - Tumour: Pancoast, thyroid adenoma, metastasis
      - Thoracic aortic aneurysm
      - Thoracic surgery
      - Brachial plexus injuries (forceps injury at birth)

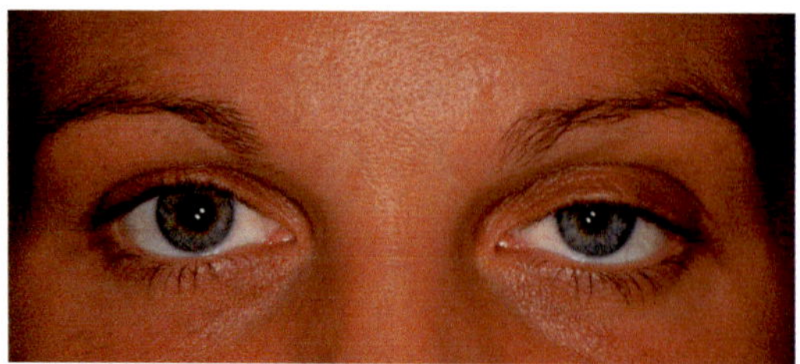

Fig. 12.1 Facial photo of a patient with a left sided Horner's syndrome showing a ptosis and pupil miosis

  - Third order neurone (postganglionic) lesion:
    - Cluster headache
    - Middle ear:
      - Otitis media
      - HZO—ramsay hunt syndrome
    - Neck:
      - ICA dissection
      - Enlarged lymph nodes
    - Cavernous sinus pathology:
      - Inflammation: Tolosa-hunt
      - Vascular: intracavernous carotid aneurysms
      - Tumour
- History
  - First order neurone lesions:
    - Limb weakness, slurred speech: CVA
    - Paraesthesias and weakness of the limbs, urinary incontinence: MS
  - Second order neurone lesions:
    - Haemoptysis, weight loss, SOB, pain in arms or shoulder: lung Ca
  - Third order neurone lesions:
    - Headaches, neck pain, facial or orbital pain, facial numbness and dysesthesia, hx of neck manipulation: internal carotid artery dissection
    - Episodic headaches associated with epiphora and rhinorrhea: cluster headaches
    - Ear pain, discharge, vertigo, tinnitus: Otitis media, Ramsay-Hunt syndrome
    - Diplopia: cavernous sinus pathology
    - Trauma or surgery
- Examination
  - Pupil miosis with a normal light and near dissociation
  - Anisocoria greater in dim conditions
  - 1-2 mm ptosis
  - Apparent enophthalmos due to 1 mm elevation of the lower lid
  - Iris heterochromia: suggests congenital or longstanding lesions
  - Facial anhidrosis: suggests lesion of first- or second-order neurone
  - No involvement of other cranial nerves (II, III, IV, V, VI)
  - Perform a full neurological examination, and perform a systemic examination to look for scars and masses (lung apices, neck, thyroid)
- Investigations
  - Confirm a Horner's syndrome:
    - Apraclonidine 1%:
      - Normally has weak $\alpha1$ agonist activity (greatest effect on $\alpha2$ receptors)
      - Up regulation of $\alpha1$ receptors on iris dilator muscle with sympathetic denervation
      - Test: measure pupil sizes for distance in bright and dark lighting illumination. Instill drops into both eyes. At 60 mins, measure pupil sizes for distance again with the same bright and dark lighting illumination as before
      - Positive test result: miotic pupil will dilate whilst normal pupil will not, resulting in a reversal of anisocoria +/− reversal of ptosis
  - Identify level of lesion:
    - Hydroxyamphetamine 1%:
      - Post-ganglionic lesions will not dilate the miotic pupil whereas the miotic pupil will dilate with first- and second-order neurone lesions
    - Phenylephrine 1%:
      - Dilute 0.1 ml of 10% phenylephrine with 0.9 ml of saline
      - Post-ganglionic lesions will dilate the miotic pupil whereas the miotic pupil will dilate with first- and second-order neurone lesions
  - Further tests based on cause:
    - First order neurone lesion:
      - MRI brain / spinal cord
      - Urinary catecholamines, MRI neck/chest/abdomen: neuroblastoma
    - Second order neurone lesion:
      - CXR: Lung Ca
      - CT thorax: Lung Ca

- Third order neurone lesion:
  - CTA/MRA neck: ICA dissection
  - Lymph node biopsy: tumours
  - ENT assessment: Ramsay Hunt syndrome, Otitis media
- Treatment
  - Treat underlying cause

12.1.5.2 Adie's Tonic Pupil

- Cause
  - Abnormal parasympathetic innervation from ciliary ganglion to the iris and ciliary muscle due to acute viral denervation
- Examination
  - Unilateral and occurs in otherwise healthy women. Mydriatic pupil initially but becomes miotic later on
  - Poor response to light with vermiform eye movements (segmental iris constriction) seen at slit lamp
  - Light-near dissociation
  - Absence of deep tendon reflexes: Adie-Holmes syndrome
- Investigations
  - Confirm diagnosis with 0.125% pilocarpine: constriction of affected pupil (denervation hypersensitivity of sphincter pupillae)
- Treatment
  - Painted CL acting as an artificial pupil for mydriasis
  - Weak strength pilocarpine for mydriatic blurring and accommodative problems

12.2 Examination of Patients with Visual Fields Defects

12.2.1 Confrontation Visual Fields Examination Sequence

- Introduce yourself
- Sit in front of patient at a distance of about 1 meter (3 feet)
- Explain to the patient that you will be moving a white dot in and out of the patient's view and that the patient is to tell you when they first see the white dot
- Begin examining the right eye by asking patient to cover their left eye with the palm of their left hand. Cover your right eye with the palm of your right hand
- Ask the patient to fixate on your nose or on your open eye
- Move a white hatpin held midway between yourself and the patient in one quadrant of the monocular field from the periphery to fixation. Ask the patient to inform you when they first see the white hatpin. Repeat in all four quadrants, testing at least 2 times per quadrant
- Compare the patient's responses to your own visual field
- Repeat process for examining the other eye with the patient asked to cover their right eye with the palm of their right hand and covering your left eye with the palm of your left hand

12.2.2 Differential Diagnosis of Visual Field Defects

- Altitudinal field defects
  - Ischaemic optic neuropathy
  - Hemibranch retinal artery or vein occlusion
  - Glaucoma
  - Optic nerve coloboma
- Arcuate scotoma
  - Glaucoma
  - Ischaemic optic neuropathy
  - Optic disc drusen
- Bitemporal hemianopia
  - Chiasmal lesions
  - Tilted optic discs
  - Sectoral RP
- Binasal hemianopia
  - Glaucoma
  - Bitemporal retinal disease (e.g. RP)
  - Bilateral occipital defect
  - Compressive lesion of both optic nerves or chiasm
  - Functional visual loss
- Blind spot enlargement
  - Papilloedema
  - Glaucoma
  - Optic nerve drusen

- Optic nerve coloboma
- Myelinated nerve fibers
- Myopic discs

- Homonymous hemianopia
  - Optic tract or lateral geniculate nucleus (LGN) lesions
  - Temporal, parietal, or occipital lobe lesions
- Superior quadrantanopia:
  - Temporal lobe lesion
- Inferior quadrantanopia
  - Parietal lobe lesion
- Central scotoma
  - Optic neuritis
  - Optic atrophy
  - Macular lesions
  - Occipital cortex lesions—tip of occipital lobe
- Constriction of peripheral fields
  - Advanced glaucoma
  - Retinal disease e.g. RP
  - Vigabatrin
  - Bilateral extensive PRP

12.3 Examination of Patients with the Direct Ophthalmoscope

12.3.1 Direct Ophthalmoscopy Examination Sequence

- For the exam the patients will likely have non dilated pupils
- Introduce yourself
- Ask for room lights to be dimmed (if not already dimmed)
- Ask patient to look at distant target
- Hold direct ophthalmoscope with dominant hand. Set focusing lens of direct ophthalmoscope at zero (or the user's refractive error) and check the patients red reflex in both eyes from a distance of 2 feet: look for any obvious media opacities (appear as dark shadows)
- Hold direct ophthalmoscope with right hand. Direct light beam of the direct ophthalmoscope into the center of the patient's right pupil and approach as close to the patient's right eye as you can with your left hand on the patient's forehead and your left thumb used to raise the upper eyelid. While holding the patient's eyelid open
  - Dial the ophthalmoscopes focusing lenses into place to clarify the fundus image
  - Angle the ophthalmoscope about 15-degrees temporal to fixation to examine the patient's optic disc (if not visible, find the optic disc by following a retinal blood vessel)
  - From the optic disc, follow the blood vessels outward to examine the superotemporal, inferotemporal, superonasal and inferonasal areas around the posterior pole
  - Examine the macula
- Repeat process with direct ophthalmoscope held in left hand to examine patients left eye

12.3.2 Direct Ophthalmoscopy Clinical Cases

12.3.2.1 Pale Optic Disc (Fig. 12.2)

- Differential diagnosis
  - Congenital:
    - Autosomal dominant optic atrophy
    - Kjer's, Behr's or Wolfram's syndrome
  - Acquired:
    - Ischaemic optic neuropathy: arteritic (GCA), non-arteritic
    - Glaucoma
    - Compressive lesions: optic nerve sheath meningioma, glioma
    - IIH
    - Optic neuritis
    - Trauma
    - Toxic optic neuropathy
    - Severe retinal disease
    - Lebers Hereditary Optic Neuropathy (LHON)

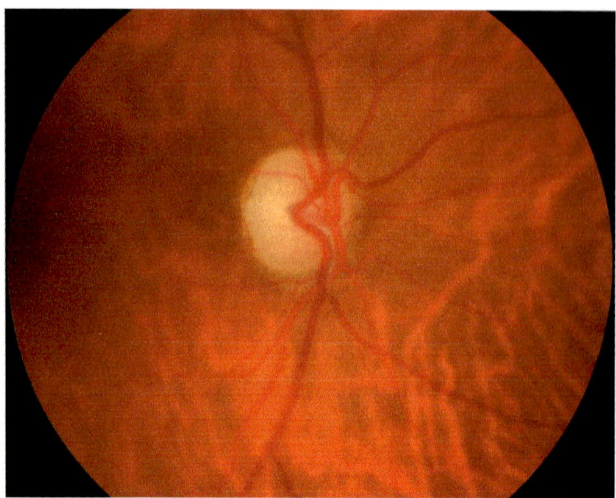

Fig. 12.2 Colour fundus image of a patient with a pale disc

12.4 Examination of Patients with Ocular Motility Disorders

12.4.1 Ocular Motility Examination Sequence

- Introduce yourself
- Ask the examiner for the patient's visual acuity: ensure that the patient can fixate on the distant target
- Ask the examiner if they would like you to perform the cover test (cover-uncover test and alternate cover test): move straight to testing ocular movements if the examiner does not want the cover test performed
- Look for any obvious abnormal head postures
- Ask the patient to remove their glasses (if worn): quickly check the glasses to see if the patient is myopic or hyperopic and whether prisms are present in the glasses
- Perform the Hirschberg's test: ask the patient to fixate on light from a pentorch and ask the patient if they can see one or two images
- Ask the patient to look at a distant target (e.g. letter on a snellen chart or logMAR chart) and position yourself slightly to the side of the midline, facing the patient and at arm's length from the patient (do not obstruct patient's view of distance target)
  - Cover each eye in turn with an occluder to ensure the patient can visualise the distant target with each eye: if the patient has NPL vision then cover-uncover test and alternate cover test is not applicable
  - Perform a cover-uncover test to look for tropias:
    - Swiftly cover the fixating eye with an occluder and observe the other eye for any movement. Carefully note its direction
    - Uncover the eye and allow about 3 seconds for both eyes to be uncovered
    - Swiftly cover the other eye and observe its fellow eye for any movement
  - Perform the alternate cover test to look for phorias:
    - Rapidly shift the occluder from one eye to the other several times, not allowing any interval of binocularity
    - Ensure that each eye fixes on the target after each movement of the cover
    - Observe for any movement of the eyes
- Ask the patient to look at a near accommodative target and position yourself directly opposite the patient within arm's reach
  - Cover each eye in turn with an occluder to ensure patient can visualise near accommodative target with each eye
  - Perform a cover-uncover test to look for tropias:
  - Perform an alternate cover test to look for phorias:
- Repeat cover test with the patient wearing glasses (if patient wears glasses): ask the examiner if they would like you to perform this before going ahead
- Examine ocular movements
  - Sit facing the patient. Shine a light from a pentorch at eye level about 10 to 14 inches in front of the patient, with the patient looking in primary position
  - Ask the patient to inform you if they see double vision at any gaze position
  - Ask the patient to follow the light from your pentorch as you move it into the 9 directions of gaze. Elevate the upper eyelid with a finger on your free hand to observe movements in downgaze: note any limitations of movement
  - Examine ductions if you see any limitations on version movements

- Examine horizontal and vertical saccades: ask patient to look rapidly between targets (e.g your hands) positioned at 30-degrees on either side of the midline

12.4.2 Clinical Cases of Ocular Motility Disorders

12.4.2.1 Internuclear Ophthalmoplegia (INO) (Tables 12.1 and 12.2)

- Causes
  - Multiple sclerosis
  - CVA
  - Tumours (intrinsic or metastatic) of brainstem or fourth ventricle
- Examination
  - Ipsilateral slow adducting saccade (saccadic velocity slowing—saccadic movements are usually impaired to a greater extent than pursuit movements), contralateral abducting nystagmus
  - Ipsilateral adduction deficit overcome with convergence
  - Exophoria or exotropia in the primary position—increase on attempted horizontal gaze in the direction of action of the affected MR muscle in cases of unilateral INO
  - Skew deviation with the hypertropic eye on the side of the lesion
  - Vertical gaze nystagmus
  - Walled eye bilateral INO (WEBINO): bilateral XT on primary gaze, bilateral INO, impaired convergence, +/− vertical gaze palsy, +/− up beat nystagmus, +/− skew deviation
- Investigations
  - MRI brain
  - Hess chart (see Figs. 2.61 and 2.62)

Table 12.1 Key facts about INO

Caused by a lesion of the medial longitudinal fasciculus which is a nerve fiber bundle that connects the CN VI nucleus on one side of the pons to the MR subnucleus of the CN III in the contralateral midbrain
INO should always be suspected whenever there is an acquired limitation of adduction

Table 12.2 Differential diagnosis of an adduction deficit

Neurologic:
INO
Myopathic:
Myasthenia gravis: Variability, Cogan's lid twitch, involvement of vertically acting muscles, positive response to the Tensilon test
Mechanical:
Orbital trauma: History of trauma, evidence of mechanical restriction of abduction
Duane's retraction syndrome: Change in palpebral aperture on horizontal gaze

12.4.2.2 Progressive Supranuclear Palsy (Steele-Richardson Syndrome) (Table 12.3)

- Examination
  - Slowing of the vertical saccadic velocity, usually first affecting downgaze, which is followed in due course by a complete vertical saccadic paralysis
  - Voluntary saccades affected first, convergence, and smooth pursuit later
  - Disorders of horizontal gaze are a late feature; eventually some patients may go on to develop a complete ophthalmoplegia
  - Sparing of the vestibulo-ocular reflex
  - Square wave jerks
  - Apraxia of eyelid opening: difficulty in voluntary opening of the eyelids
  - Axial rigidity with limited neck movement
  - Difficulty with swallowing, speech and balance (postural instability)
- Investigations
  - MRI: midbrain atrophy

Table 12.3 Key facts about progressive supranuclear palsy

Progressive neurodegenerative condition caused by abnormal accumulation of tau proteins
Definitive diagnosis requires histology (tau inclusions on microscopy)

12.5 Approach to Patients with Nystagmus

12.5.1 Description of Nystagmus

- Rhythmical oscillation of the eyes
- One component of the oscillation is a slow phase drift away from the assumed position of gaze; this component differentiates nystagmus from nystagmus-like oscillations which comprise only saccadic (fast) elements
- Description of nystagmus should include:
  - Type of waveform: Jerk nystagmus—a slow phase that drifts away from fixation (abnormal movement), and a fast corrective movement (saccade) in the opposite direction to regain fixation, Pendular nystagmus: equal velocity slow-phase movements in both directions
  - Direction: described by the direction of the fast phase i.e. if the fast phase is to the right then the nystagmus is described as right beating. Both jerk and pendular can be horizontal, vertical or torsional
  - Symmetry: conjugate, disconjugate
  - Intensity
  - Frequency

12.5.2 Classification of Nystagmus

- Early onset
  (a) Horizontal:
    (1) Idiopathic congenital—bilateral jerk (typically) or pendular nystagmus present in the primary position, intensity worse on fixation, better with convergence and in null zone, presence of a face turn, inverted optokinetic response, absent oscillopsia, latent nystagmus
    (2) Latent / manifest latent nystagmus—bilateral jerk nystagmus, fast phase towards the fixing eye, intensity increases on abduction and decreases on adduction, face turn towards fixing eye, associated with infantile ET
  (b) Erratic +/− Roving: sensory deprivation
- Late onset
  (a) Conjugate:
    (1) Horizontal:
      - Peripheral vestibular—bilateral jerk waveform present in the primary position, intensity increases in the direction of the fast phase and decreases in the direction of the slow phase, intensity decreases with fixation, intensity increases with removal of fixation, direction of fast phase opposite to the side of the lesion
      - Central vestibular—bilateral jerk waveform present in the primary position, intensity increases in the direction of the fast phase and decreases in the direction of the slow phase, no change in intensity with removal of fixation
      - Periodic alternating—bilateral jerk waveform present in the primary position in which oscillations change direction every few minutes—seen in patients with albinism
      - Gaze evoked—bilateral jerk waveform that only becomes manifest when gaze is directed away from the primary position, absent in primary position, fast phase always in direction of eccentric gaze
    (2) Vertical:
      - Upbeat
      - Downbeat
  (b) Disconjugate:
    (1) Unilateral:
      - SO myokymia
      - INO
    (3) Bilateral:
      - See-Saw—vertical pendular waveform with synchronous intorsion of the elevating eye and an extorsion of the depressing eye—seen in patients with parasellar tumours

- Acquired pendular: MS if horizontal, ocular palatal myoclonus if vertical

12.5.3 Causes of Nystagmus

- Congenital
- Acquired
  - Sensory deprivation: ocular albinism, oculocutaneous albinism, CSNB, cone-rod dystrophy, LCA, optic nerve hypoplasia
  - Structural abnormalities: Arnold-Chiari malformations, tumours affecting the brainstem or cerebellum
  - Medications: carbamazepine, lithium, phenytoin, amiodarone, morphine, ketamine abuse, fomepizole
  - CVA
  - Demyelination: MS

12.5.4 History

- Age on onset: onset within first 3/12 of life should reliably differentiate congenital nystagmus from other forms
- Visual function: below normal in congenital nystagmus
- Visual symptoms of oscillopsia (illusion of rhythmical movement of stationary objects): suggestive of acquired nystagmus and not congenital nystagmus
- Visual symptoms of diplopia combined with nystagmus: suggest brainstem involvement:
  (a) Horizontal diplopia: INO, Arnold-Chiari malformation
  (b) Vertical diplopia: skew deviation with down-beat nystagmus, and of cavernous sinus spread from a local tumour, which can be associated with see-saw nystagmus
- Systemic symptoms:
  (a) Vertigo, dizziness, nausea, tinnitus: suggests peripheral vestibular dysfunction
  (b) Vertigo, dysarthria, dysphagia, diplopia: suggests a pontomedullary lesion
  (c) Ataxia and coordination difficulty: suggests a cerebellar syndrome
- Medication history: carbamazepine, lithium, phenytoin, amiodarone, morphine, ketamine abuse, fomepizole, nutmeg
- Severe head trauma or brainstem stroke: delayed appearance of an unusual type of nystagmus termed ocular-palatal myoclonus—pendular vertical nystagmus + rhythmical movements of the palate, diaphragm and other structures
- Family history: a number of conditions associated with congenital nystagmus are inherited, including albinism, LCA, idiopathic congenital nystagmus

12.5.5 Examination

- Head posture: feature of congenital nystagmus adopted to improve VA by utilising the null region (e.g. Left head turn implies null zone is in right gaze)
- Nystagmus in the primary position: horizontal—peripheral vestibular, central vestibular, periodic alternating / vertical—upbeat, downbeat
- Nystagmus characteristics on distance and near fixation and on convergence: congenital nystagmus dampens on near fixation and with convergence, subtle forms of see-saw nystagmus may be easier to observe on distance fixation
- Effect of covering one eye (i.e. cover test): latent nystagmus can be identified on cover test—associated with congenital nystagmus, manifest latent nystagmus will show an increase in the intensity of the nystagmus if the non-fixing eye is covered or a dampening or reversal of direction if the fixing eye is covered
- Effect of removing fixation (Spielmann translucent occluder prevents fixation of a non-illuminated target while still observing the eye behind the occluder): peripheral vestibular nystagmus increases when fixation is removed, whereas congenital nystagmus may reduce in intensity, central vestibular nystagmus shows no change

- OKN testing: inverted response with congenital nystagmus (e.g. right beating horizontal nystagmus will continue to show a right beating nystagmus when the drum is rotated to the right)

12.5.6 Investigations

- Refraction: patient's with retinal dystrophies commonly have high levels of refractive error and astigmatism
- Stereoacuity: a near-normal level of Stereoacuity on TNO testing virtually excludes albinism as the cause of congenital nystagmus
- ERG: retinal dystrophies, optic nerve hypoplasia
- VEP: presence of crossed asymmetry in albinism
- MRI of brain, lower brainstem and cerebellum (indications—central vestibular nystagmus, upbeat and downbeat nystagmus, periodic alternating nystagmus, INO, see-saw nystagmus, acquired pendular): exclude the presence of intracranial disease
- In the absence of any evidence of ocular disease and a normal ERG and VEP, the likely diagnosis is congenital idiopathic nystagmus
- Neither latent nystagmus or latent manifest nystagmus require any investigations

12.5.7 Treatment

- Congenital nystagmus
  - Improve VA
    - Refractive error correction
    - Amblyopia treatment
  - Reduction of nystagmus intensity
    - Base out prisms: stimulate convergence can improve VA at distance fixation if pt. has BSV
    - Surgical
  - Reduction in head posture
    - Conservative: prisms with apex pointing towards the null point or base in the direction of the head posture (e.g. right face turn with eyes deviated towards a null region in left gaze, the prism before the right eye is positioned base out and that before the left eye base in)
    - Surgical (for head postures more than 20 degrees):
      - Horizontal head posture: Kestenbaum procedure—surgery on all 4 horizontal rectus muscles with movement of eyes towards head posture (e.g. right head turn—R LR resection, R MR recession, L MR resection, L LR recession)
      - Vertical head posture: Chin down—recession of both SR muscles, Chin up—recession of both IR muscles
- Acquired nystagmus
  - Improve VA by:
    - Correction of any refractive errors
    - Correction of head posture: prisms
    - Correction of oscillopsia: medications (Baclofen for periodic alternating, clonazepam), Botox, surgery
  - Relief of diplopia (involvement of ocular motor nerves from brainstem disease):
    - Prisms
    - Botox
    - Muscle surgery